I have great admiration for the strong writing of this accomplished team of clinicians, researchers, and teachers. This book, their third edition, provides easy-to-use guidance for students, new practitioners, and seasoned mental health clinicians alike. This is truly a desktop essential for all mental health providers aspiring to apply time-efficient and powerful interventions, informed by the current evidence.

—**Patti Robinson, PhD,** coauthor of *Behavioral Consultation and Primary Care: A Guide to Integrating Services, Second Edition*

This book is in my top three recommended books on primary care behavioral health (PCBH). It is a must-have especially for clinicians new to PCBH who are struggling with understanding how behavioral health consultants (BHCs) can achieve substantial results in a 30-minute consult. Chock full of practical tips, forms, and checklists, this resource needs to be on every BHC's bookshelf.

—**Neftali Serrano, PsyD,** Chief Executive Officer, Collaborative Family Healthcare Association, Chapel Hill, NC

I have been waiting for the next edition of this book and here it is! This new edition provides research updates so the busy clinician can be up-to-date with evidence-based approaches for primary care. If you provide clinical services as a behavioral health consultant (BHC) in primary care or supervise BHCs, this book is for you.

—**Stacy Ogbeide, PsyD, ABPP, CSOWM,** Associate Professor of Family & Community Medicine, UT Health San Antonio, San Antonio, TX

T0314924

Integrated
Behavioral Health
in Primary Care

Integrated Behavioral Health in Primary Care

Step-by-Step Guidance for
Assessment and Intervention

Third Edition

Christopher L. Hunter
Jeffrey L. Goodie
Mark S. Oordt
Anne C. Dobmeyer

 AMERICAN PSYCHOLOGICAL ASSOCIATION

The opinions and statements published are the responsibility of the authors, and such opinions and statements do not necessarily represent the policies of the American Psychological Association.

Published by
American Psychological Association
750 First Street, NE
Washington, DC 20002
https://www.apa.org

Order Department
https://www.apa.org/pubs/books
order@apa.org

Typeset in Meridien and Ortodoxa by TiPS Publishing Services, Carrboro, NC

Printer: Lake Book Manufacturing, Melrose Park, IL
Cover Designer: Anthony Paular Design, Newbury Park, CA

Library of Congress Control Number: 2023945494

https://doi.org/10.1037/0000380-000

Printed in the United States of America

10 9 8 7 6 5 4 3 2 1

*To my parents, Norma and Pete, whose love and support
set the foundation for who I am today.*

—Christopher L. Hunter

*To Mary, Alexander, Zachary, and Benjamin, who provide
an endless supply of joy and inspiration every day.*

—Jeffrey L. Goodie

*To my wife, Ruth, and my children, Andrew,
Martha Rose, Carol, Ellen, and Catherine.*

—Mark S. Oordt

To my children, who fill my life with joy.

—Anne C. Dobmeyer

CONTENTS

List of Figures   ix

Introduction   3

I.   FOUNDATIONS OF INTEGRATED BEHAVIORAL
     CONSULTATION SERVICE   15

     1. Population Health and the Patient-Centered Medical Home   17

     2. Core Competencies and Clinical Practice Management Skills   25

     3. Conducting the Initial and Follow-Up Consultation
         Appointments   51

     4. Common Behavioral and Cognitive Interventions in Primary
         Care: Moving Out of the Specialty Mental Health Clinic   65

II. COMMON BEHAVIORAL HEALTH CONCERNS
     IN PRIMARY CARE   103

     5. Depression, Anxiety, Posttraumatic Stress Disorder,
         and Insomnia   105

     6. Health Behaviors: Tobacco Use, Overweight and Obesity,
         and Physical Inactivity   145

     7. Diabetes   177

     8. Chronic Obstructive Pulmonary Disease and Asthma   199

     9. Cardiovascular Disease   227

     10. Pain Disorders   249

11. Unhealthy Substance Use: Alcohol, Illicit Drugs,
    and Prescription Medication   271

12. Sexual Problems   301

13. Special Considerations for Older Adults   327

14. Obstetrics and Gynecology   349

15. Children, Adolescents, and Parenting   373

16. Couple Distress   395

III. SPECIAL ISSUES   417

17. Managing Suicide Risk in the Primary Care Setting   419

18. Developing Clinical Pathways and Implementing Shared
    Medical Appointments   441

References   455
Index   519
About the Authors   553

LIST OF FIGURES

I.1.	The 5As Model of Behavior Change in Primary Care	10
1.1.	Factors Affecting Health Outcomes	18
1.2.	Patient-Centered Medical Home Principles	22
2.1.	BHC Core Competencies	26
2.2.	Marketing Survey	33
2.3.	Consultation Request	35
2.4.	Problem of the Week	37
2.5.	Appointment Template	39
2.6.	Provider Survey	43
2.7.	Note Example	44
2.8.	Additional Training	48
3.1.	Structure for the Initial Consultation Appointment Linked With the 5As	51
3.2.	Behavioral Health Consultation Service	54
3.3.	Functional Assessment of the Problem	57
3.4.	Behavioral Prescription (Rx) Pads	62
4.1.	Deep Breathing	70
4.2.	Cue-Controlled Relaxation	70
4.3.	How to Question Stressful, Angry, Anxious, and Depressed Thinking	79
4.4.	Thinking Mistakes That Increase Stress, Anger, Depression, Anxiety, and Worry	82
4.5.	Disputing/Challenging Thoughts and Beliefs	83
4.6.	Strategies to Improve Motivation to Change	91
4.7.	Problem-Solving Worksheet	92
4.8.	Monitoring Behavioral Triggers	96
4.9.	Stimulus Control Plan	97
4.10.	Assertive Communication	99

4.11.	Recommended Mobile Applications to Support Common Cognitive Behavior Interventions	101
5.1.	Depression Spiral Handout	110
5.2.	Resources for Patients With Depression: Websites, Mobile Applications, and Books	115
5.3.	Mnemonic to Screen for Generalized Anxiety Disorder	118
5.4.	Anxious Worry Handout	120
5.5.	Worry Management Handout	121
5.6.	Anxiety Questions	123
5.7.	Panic Disorder Handout	125
5.8.	Situational Exposure Hierarchy Handout	127
5.9.	Resources for Patients With Anxiety: Websites, Mobile Applications, and Books	129
5.10.	Primary Care PTSD-5 Screen	132
5.11.	Resources for Patients With PTSD: Websites, Mobile Applications, and Books	134
5.12.	Insomnia Severity Index	137
5.13.	Improving Sleep Through Behavior Change Handout	141
5.14.	Sleep Restriction Handout	143
5.15.	Resources for Patients With Insomnia: Websites, Mobile Applications, and Books	144
6.1.	Tobacco Cessation	151
6.2.	Resources for Patients Using Tobacco: Websites, Mobile Applications, and Books	156
6.3.	Personal Food Diary	163
6.4.	The C.A.M.E.S.™ Principle for Improvement	165
6.5.	Modifying Eating Habits	165
6.6.	Resources for Patients Wanting to Lose Weight: Websites, Mobile Applications, and Books/Documents	167
6.7.	Weight Maintenance	168
6.8.	Resources for Patients Who Want to Increase Physical Activity: Websites, Mobile Applications, and Books/Documents	170
6.9.	Examples of Moderate and Vigorous Activities	172
6.10.	Increasing Physical Activity	174
7.1.	Handout for Diabetes Goal Setting	191
7.2.	Handout for Diabetes Self-Monitoring	192
7.3.	Resources for Patients With Diabetes: Websites, Mobile Applications, and Books	193
8.1.	Shortness of Breath Cycle for COPD and Asthma Patient Handout	202
8.2.	COPD Assessment Questions	206
8.3.	Pursed-Lip Breathing Patient Handout	209
8.4.	Resources for Patients With COPD: Websites, Mobile Applications, and Books	211
8.5.	Handout for Asthma Assessment Questions	217
8.6.	Asthma Monitoring Form Patient Handout	221
8.7.	Asthma Allergen and Exposure Checklist Patient Handout	223

8.8. Resources for Patients With Asthma: Websites, Mobile Applications,
        and Books   225
9.1. Classification of Blood Pressure for Adults   228
9.2. Resources for Patients With Cardiovascular Disease: Websites, Mobile
        Applications, and Books   230
9.3. Components of the DASH Eating Plan   231
9.4. Assessment Questions for Patients With Cardiovascular Disease   236
9.5. High Blood Pressure Handout   241
9.6. Diet Change Handout   245
10.1. Understanding Chronic Pain Handout   257
10.2. True or False: Common Pain Beliefs   259
10.3. Pacing Activities Handout   261
10.4. Five Steps for Managing Intense Pain Episodes   262
10.5. Resources for Patients With Chronic Pain: Websites, Mobile Applications,
        and Books   265
10.6. Monitoring Pain Handout   266
10.7. Headache Monitoring Form   268
11.1. Common Mistakes and Assumptions About Alcohol Patient Handout   279
11.2. What Is a "Standard Drink"?   282
11.3. Four As for Managing Alcohol Consumption Patient Handout   284
11.4. Resources for Patients With Unhealthy Substance Use: Websites, Mobile
        Applications, and Books   285
11.5. NIDA Quick Screen V1.01   290
11.6. Questions 1–8 of the NIDA-Modified ASSIST V2.0   291
12.1. Erectile Dysfunction Handout   307
12.2. Resources for Patients With Sexual Problems Handout: Websites and Books   308
12.3. Sexual Problems and Self-Management Interventions Handout   310
12.4. Gaining Control Over Premature Ejaculation Handout   318
12.5. Sample Assessment Questions for Female Orgasmic Disorder   322
12.6. Developing Helpful Beliefs for Enhancing Arousal and Orgasm Handout   324
13.1. Resources for Older Adults: Websites and Mobile Applications   335
13.2. Geriatric Depression Scale 5/15   343
13.3. Bereavement, Grief, and Mourning Handout   347
14.1. Resources for Patients Demonstrating Peripartum Depression: Websites
        and Books   356
14.2. Resources for Patients Demonstrating Chronic Pelvic Pain: Websites, Mobile
        Applications, and Books   362
14.3. Additional Functional Assessment Questions for Women Going
        Through Menopause   366
14.4. Hot Flash Symptom Diary   368
14.5. Managing Menopausal Hot Flashes With Reassuring Thinking   368
14.6. Resources for Patients With Menopause: Websites, Mobile Applications,
        and Books   371
15.1. Resources for Patients With Behavior Management Problems: Websites,
        Mobile Applications, and Books   374

15.2. Age-Appropriate Techniques for Childhood Discipline   379
15.3. Short Screening Instrument for Psychological Problems in Enuresis   385
15.4. Bed-wetting Monitoring Chart   386
15.5. Resources for Patients Who Wet the Bed: Websites and Books   388
15.6. Resources for Patients With Attention-Deficit/Hyperactivity Disorder:
       Websites and Books   392
16.1. Relationship Problems Sample Assessment Questions   402
16.2. Effective Listening Handout   405
16.3. Communication Practice Plan Handout   406
16.4. Problem-Solving Guidelines for Couples Handout   409
16.5. Behavior Exchange Handout   412
16.6. Sample Intimate Partner Violence Safety Plan   413
16.7. Resources for Couples: Websites, Mobile Applications, and Books   415
17.1. Protective and Risk Factors for Suicide   425
17.2. ASQ Suicide Risk Screening Tool   428
17.3. Suicide Risk Assessment Components   429
17.4. Recommended Actions for Primary Care Providers for Levels of Suicide Risk   431
17.5. Crisis Response Planning Worksheet   434
17.6. Sample Crisis Response Plan   434
17.7. Brief Suicide Management Interventions Applicable to Primary Care   436
17.8. Resources for Patients With Suicidal Ideation: Telephone, Websites,
       and Mobile Applications   439
18.1. DIGMA Appointment Introduction   447
18.2. Provider Resources   454

Integrated Behavioral Health in Primary Care

INTRODUCTION

Much has changed since the second edition of this book. In the United States, the shift in primary care service delivery through the patient-centered medical home (PCMH), an increased focus on the Triple Aim (see Chapter 1), and an increasing awareness of the importance of integrated behavioral health service in the PCMH continue to drive change (Dunn et al., 2021; National Committee for Quality Assurance, 2017; Ratzliff et al., 2017). Our goal with this volume is to deliver straightforward information and guidance about what evidence-based/informed screening, assessment, and intervention services a behavioral health provider (e.g., clinical psychologist, clinical social worker) or any provider who has appropriate training to address behavioral health needs can provide to patients in the context of effective integrated primary care service delivery. Every chapter has been updated with the latest research evidence and includes an evidence-informed clinical practice focus. We have added additional information on the primary care Quadruple Aim and a new chapter on behavioral health consultant (BHC) core competencies and clinical practice management skills.

https://doi.org/10.1037/0000380-001

Integrated Behavioral Health in Primary Care: Step-by-Step Guidance for Assessment and Intervention, Third Edition, by C. L. Hunter, J. L. Goodie, M. S. Oordt, and A. C. Dobmeyer

WHAT IS PRIMARY CARE?

The World Health Organization (n.d.) defined primary care as

> a model of care that supports first-contact, accessible, continuous, comprehensive and coordinated person-focused care. It aims to optimize population health and reduce disparities across the population by ensuring that subgroups have equal access to services. There are five core functions of primary care:
>
> - *First contact accessibility* creates a strategic entry point for and improves access to health services.
> - *Continuity* promotes the development of long-term personal relationships between a person and a health professional or a team of providers.
> - *Comprehensiveness* ensures that a diverse range of promotive, protective, preventive, curative, rehabilitative, and palliative services are provided.
> - *Coordination* organizes services and care across levels of the health system and over time.
> - *People-centred* care ensures that people have the education and support needed to make decisions and participate in their own care. (paras. 1–6)

The American Academy of Family Physicians (n.d.) further expanded the definition:

> Primary care is the provision of integrated, accessible health care services by physicians and their health care teams who are accountable for addressing a large majority of personal health care needs, developing a sustained partnership with patients, and practicing in the context of family and community. The care is person-centered, team-based, community-aligned, and designed to achieve better health, better care, and lower costs.
>
> Primary care physicians specifically are trained for and skilled in comprehensive, first contact, and continuing care for persons with any undiagnosed sign, symptom, or health concern (the "undifferentiated" patient) not limited by problem origin (biological, behavioral, or social), organ system, or diagnosis. Additionally, primary care includes health promotion, disease prevention, health maintenance, counseling, patient education, diagnosis and treatment of acute and chronic illnesses in a variety of health care settings (e.g., office, inpatient, critical care, long-term care, home care, schools, telehealth, etc.). Primary care is performed and managed by a personal physician who often collaborates with other health professionals, and utilizes consultation or referral as appropriate. Primary care provides patient advocacy in the health care system to accomplish cost-effective and equitable care by coordination of health care services. Primary care promotes effective communication with patients and families to encourage them to be a partner in health care. (paras. 2–3)

We believe it is important for BHCs to know that the operations and goals of primary care require them to have a skill set for assessing and intervening on the wide range of problems that people bring to this setting.

WHAT IS INTEGRATED CARE?

The terms "collaborative" and "integrated" care are often used interchangeably, which can lead to confusion regarding the type of service that is being delivered or evaluated. Thus, it is important to provide operational definitions of these terms.

Collaborative care is not a fixed model or specific approach. It is a concept that emphasizes opportunities to improve the accessibility and delivery of behavioral health services in primary care through interdisciplinary collaboration (C. L. Hunter & Goodie, 2010; Parkhurst et al., 2022). It can be performed through a range of practice models geared to provide effective patient services across a full spectrum of medical and behavioral health needs.

Models of collaborative care fall on a continuum of integration (Heath et al., 2013; for a review of models, see also C. Collins et al., 2010). On one end, there is collaboration between primary care providers (PCPs) and behavioral health providers who work in separate systems and facilities, delivering separate care. They exchange information regarding patients on an as-needed basis. This type of collaborative care has been referred to as *coordinated care* and involves minimal/basic collaboration at a distance. In the middle of the continuum is *colocated care*. This level of collaborative care can involve closer interactions between behavioral health providers and PCPs who share the same practice space and some shared systems like medical records. The team works together to address specific types of patient presentations. An example of this is the collaborative care model (also referred to as the IMPACT model, care management model, or care facilitation model). This model usually focuses on depression alone, using a specific process of assessing, planning, facilitating, and advocating for options to meet the patient's needs. This model has been shown to improve treatment of depression over standard primary care depression treatment (Katon, 2012).

At the other end of the continuum is *integrated care*. This is care that results from a practiced team of primary care and behavioral health clinicians, working together with patients and families, using a systematic and cost-effective approach to provide patient-centered care for a defined population. This care may address mental health and substance abuse conditions, health behaviors (including their contribution to chronic medical illnesses), life stressors and crises, stress-related physical symptoms, and ineffective patterns of health care utilization (Peek & the National Integration Academy Council, 2013).

An example of an integrated care model is the primary care behavioral health (PCBH) model. Reiter et al. (2018) operationally defined the PCBH model using the "GATHER" acronym detailed in Robinson and Reiter (2016) because it provided a clear initial list of components that were important to operationalize in the definition. In that acronym, "G" is for a "Generalist approach," "A" is for "Accessibility," "T" is for "Team-based," "H" is for "High productivity," "E" is for "Educator," and "R" is for "Routine":

> The PCBH model is a team-based primary care approach to managing behavioral health problems and biopsychosocially influenced health conditions. The model's main goal is to enhance the primary care team's ability to manage and treat such problems/conditions, with resulting improvements in primary care services for the entire clinic population. The model incorporates into the primary care team a behavioral health consultant (BHC), sometimes referred to as a behavioral health clinician, to extend and support the primary care provider (PCP)

and team. The BHC works as a generalist and an educator who provides high volume services that are accessible, team-based, and a routine part of primary care. Specifically, the BHC assists in the care of patients of any age and with any health condition (Generalist); strives to intervene with all patients on the day they are referred (Accessible); shares clinic space and resources and assists the team in various ways (Team-based); engages with a large percentage of the clinic population (High volume); helps improve the team's biopsychosocial assessment and intervention skills and processes (Educator); and is a routine part of biopsychosocial care (Routine). To accomplish these goals, BHCs use focused (15–30 min) visits to assist with specific symptoms or functional improvement. Follow-up is based in a consultant approach in which patients are followed by the BHC and PCP until functioning or symptoms begin improving; at that point, the PCP resumes sole oversight of care but re-engages the BHC at any time, as needed. Patients not improving are referred to a higher intensity of care, though if that is not possible, the BHC may continue to assist until improvements are noted. This consultant approach also aims to improve the PCP's biopsychosocial management of health conditions in general. (Reiter et al., 2018, p. 112)

WHY HAVE A PCBH FOCUS?

The strategies we cover are likely to be useful in any integrated care model, but they are particularly germane to the PCBH model of integrated care. This integrated model has been implemented as the primary model or blended with other types of behavioral health services delivered in primary care in several noteworthy health care system efforts, including the Veterans Health Administration (serving 8.9 million patients), the Department of Defense Medical Health System (3.3 million), Cherokee Health System (66,000+), and Presbyterian Medical Group in New Mexico (190,000+; C. L. Hunter et al., 2018).

In short, the PCBH model is designed to facilitate the delivery of a variety of evidence-based interventions (which we present in this volume) for a range of problems across the lifespan that include prevention as well as treatment of acute and chronic conditions that focus on symptom reduction, functional improvement, and better quality of life. Although care in the PCBH model is typically focused and brief, there is no limit to the number of appointments a patient can have with a BHC. Rather, the number of contacts depends on the patient's progress. Services can occur prior to, within, or after an appointment with a PCP or be provided through psychoeducational groups, shared medical appointments, clinical pathways, or some combination of these, based on the patient population and available clinic and community resources. We discuss the important components of clinical pathways and shared medical appointments and how the BHC might promote these approaches to improve population health impact in more detail in Chapters 1 and 18. We believe the PCBH model can be used effectively in most primary care settings and aligns with the goals of population health care, the Triple Aim, and PCMH goals discussed in Chapter 1.

It has been argued that optimized integrated care models would involve attention to mission, clinical outcomes, physical location, operations, information, and financial and resource integration (Peek, 2008; Strosahl & Robinson, 2008). Integrated behavioral health care brings the skills and expertise for addressing behavioral health needs to a setting in which the patients who can benefit from those services are already receiving care. It normalizes the need for behavioral health support and reduces the stigma associated with it.

Most behavioral health providers have been trained in the traditional specialty mental health care model. In this model, patients either seek help themselves or are referred to a behavioral health provider for problems identified as psychological (e.g., anxiety, depression, interpersonal problems). In specialty mental health care, the practitioner may see the patient in their office for brief psychotherapy (e.g., 8–10 sessions) or for long-term therapy of indefinite duration. In either case, sessions last for 45 to 50 minutes on a regularly scheduled basis (e.g., weekly). This type of behavioral health assessment and intervention can support the lower end of the continuum of integrated care (i.e., collaborative care and colocated care); however, it will not work in an integrated care model. To be an effective primary care team member, the behavioral health provider has to be readily available. Because the integrated approach expects a much wider range of patients to be referred for behavioral health assistance to address not only mental health disorders but also subclinical problems, prevention, adverse health behaviors, and chronic medical conditions, the demand for appointments will quickly exceed the behavioral health provider's ability to meet that need using a specialty mental health model of care. Patients will have extended waiting times for services and, in all likelihood, the behavioral health provider will quickly become an irrelevant team member as a result of not being able to assist the PCP in a timely manner. Thus, behavioral health providers working within an integrated care model must redefine how they think and what they do to provide behavioral health services that will work in the primary care environment. In other words, to be most effective, behavioral health providers must work within the same structures that other PCPs (physicians, physician assistants, and nurse practitioners) use to deliver care.

BECOMING AN INTEGRATED CARE PROVIDER

We have been teaching behavioral health providers to adapt their training and professional practices to the primary care environment for over 20 years. Common questions we have received include "Where do I start?" and "What do I do?" Answers to these questions typically elicit the response "I can't do that in 30 minutes!" We then explain why, in the primary care setting, the typical conventional model of psychological assessment and intervention will not work. The typical 50-minute interview cannot simply be condensed to fit in a 15- to 30-minute appointment. Time demands and practice expectations are structured differently in the primary care setting; behavioral health services must be adapted to this fast pace. The practicalities of adapting one's assessments and interventions to patient problems in the primary care setting are the main focus of this book. We use the abbreviation BHC throughout this volume when referring to a behavioral health provider working in primary care. However, the strategies we describe are applicable to all providers (i.e., behavioral health providers and PCPs) working in this setting.

ETHICAL CONSIDERATIONS

Behavioral health providers engaged in integrated PCBH services quickly learn they face unique circumstances not always addressed by their discipline's ethical guidelines. Ethical guidelines that do address the "content" areas of concern are typically not written to apply to the context of integrated team-based PCBH service delivery, which includes team professionals with different ethical guidelines, expectations, and culture-of-care standards. Common areas of concern for behavioral health providers who are new to primary care include informed consent, confidentiality, complex relationships including whole-family care, multiple relationships, scope of practice, and competence. Ethical guidance for PCBH has received increased attention as BHCs are actively seeking this information. Although a complete review of ethics guidance is beyond the area of focus for this volume, we strongly encourage BHCs to inform this part of their work. Additional information can be found in a special issue devoted to ethics in collaborative care in the journal *Families, Systems, & Health* (Runyan et al., 2013). BHCs might also be interested in reading the journal article "Ethical Challenges Unique to the Primary Care Behavioral Health (PCBH) Model" by Runyan et al. (2018). The authors of this article highlighted conflicting ethical principles and guidelines occurring with PCBH model interprofessional collaboration. They reviewed the extant literature across disciplines, identified gaps, and proposed new ethical guidelines to bridge those gaps. They also discussed common ethical dilemmas unique to the PCBH model of service delivery with case examples and illustrated the application of the proposed guidelines to effectively navigate those dilemmas.

CULTURAL SENSITIVITY AND EVIDENCE-BASED ADAPTATION/TAILORING

Although there is general agreement that cultural sensitivity involves the awareness of cultural influences on patients' behaviors and health beliefs and application of this knowledge to effectively serve culturally diverse patients (one size does not fit all), there is still no uniform definition of cultural sensitivity, and key terms are used interchangeably (Huey et al., 2014; Liu et al., 2021). *Cultural adaptation/tailoring* has been defined as the "systematic modification of an evidence-based treatment (EBT) or intervention protocol to consider language, culture, and context in such a way that it is compatible with the client's cultural patterns, meaning, and values" (Bernal et al., 2009, p. 362). Cultural sensitivity and evidence-based cultural adaptation/tailoring of primary care behavioral health services goes beyond the area of focus for this volume. Nearly all the research in this area has been done in specialty settings, not primary care. In fact, entire books (e.g., Benuto et al., 2020; Bernal & Domenech Rodríguez, 2012; T. B. Smith & Trimble, 2016) have been written on cultural sensitivity and the adaptation/tailoring of EBT for diverse groups. We encourage readers to pursue these resources as a way to improve their awareness of what they might adapt, based on the unique patient populations they serve. A comprehensive review and summary (Huey et al., 2014) of multiple qualitative and meta-analytic reviews on cultural sensitivity and treatment adaptation/tailoring came to the following conclusions:

- Adaptation targeting a specific ethnocultural group is more effective than tailoring targeting a mixed group.

- Some evidence suggests that matching patients with a provider who speaks their preferred (non-English) language might improve treatment outcomes.

- Patient variables like age and acculturation may be particularly important to assess before making cultural adaptations because those adaptations may be most effective for older, less acculturated patients.

- Some evidence suggests that provider–patient agreement on treatment goals and using metaphors/symbols that match the patient's cultural worldview may improve treatment outcomes.

- Myth adaptation that includes the patient's beliefs about symptoms, etiology, course, consequences, and appropriate treatment may improve treatment outcome.

- Addressing cultural factors implicitly rather than explicitly may be a way to get the benefits of cultural adaptation without the risk of iatrogenic effects.

Huey et al. (2014) went on to say,

> These results provide some preliminary guidance to researchers and therapists when deciding what types of cultural tailoring are likely to be most beneficial; however, additional research is necessary to replicate these findings in well-controlled trials before causality can be inferred. (p. 321)

We have included a cultural and diversity considerations section in Chapters 5 to 16 describing information BHCs might want to consider when addressing these clinical content areas.

THE FIVE As

Our format for assessment and intervention is based on the 5As model (Whitlock et al., 2002): assess, advise, agree, assist, and arrange. The 5As format has been strongly recommended for assessment and intervention across a range of problems in primary care (Goldstein et al., 2004). The specific tasks within each of the 5As vary depending on the nature of the problem as well as its severity and complexity (Whitlock et al., 2002). Nevertheless, the 5As model can be applied to any patient in any clinic with any problem. We have found this flexible patient-centered model invaluable in providing behavioral health services in the primary care setting. Figure I.1 provides an overview of how the 5As connect and how they lead to a personal action plan.

The *assess* phase involves gathering information on physical symptoms, emotions, thoughts, behaviors, and important environmental variables, such as family, friends, or work interactions. From a biopsychosocial perspective, the goal is to determine what variables are associated with patients' symptoms and functioning and then, on the basis of patients' values and what they have control over, to determine what they could change or alter that would decrease symptoms and improve functioning.

The *advise* phase involves describing to patients their options for intervention, on the basis of the data gathered in the assessment phase. The goal is to describe the intervention and the expected outcomes.

During the *agree* phase, patients decide on their course of action on the basis of the options discussed. They also might decide that they do not like any of the options, might have other options they would like to pursue, or might take more time to think about their options and discuss them with a significant other. If the patient does not like any of the options initially presented by the BHC or perhaps is ambivalent about moving forward with them, motivational

FIGURE I.1. The 5As Model of Behavior Change in Primary Care

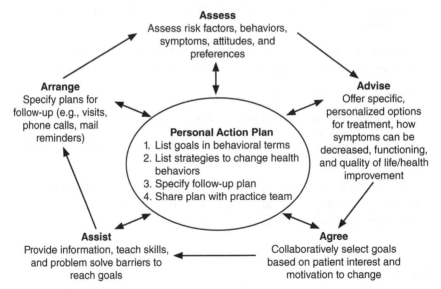

Note. Adapted from "Self-Management Aspects of the Improving Chronic Illness Care Breakthrough Series: Implementation With Diabetes and Heart Failure Teams," by R. E. Glasgow, M. M. Funnell, A. E. Bonomi, C. Davis, V. Beckham, and E. H. Wagner, 2002, *Annals of Behavioral Medicine, 24*(2), p. 83 (https://doi.org/10.1207/S15324796ABM2402_04). Copyright 2002 by Oxford University Press. Adapted with permission.

interviewing strategies (see Chapter 4) may help guide them toward considering other solutions. These strategies may also help to engage them in shared decision making, which is an interactive process in which the BHC and patient work together to come to a decision about care (National Institute for Health and Care Excellence [NICE], n.d.). Shared decision making involves examining care options with a review of the evidence for those options, taking into consideration a patient's values, beliefs, and preferences (NICE, n.d.). It is designed to make sure the patient understands the potential benefits and risk of different options. See the NICE (n.d.) website for additional information and tools to facilitate shared decision making.

If the BHC and patient cannot agree on a course of action to address the presenting problem, they should not move forward to the assist phase. The BHC might let the patient know that they understand the patient's ambivalence about moving forward and that they will talk with the PCP about their appointment and discuss what, if any, additional options might be available.

In the *assist* phase, the BHC's job is to help patients learn new information, develop new skills, solve problems, and overcome environmental or personal barriers to implementing the behavior changes. This is where the formal intervention takes place.

In the *arrange* phase, we specify when or if patients will follow up with the BHC, PCP, or specialty mental health provider. If the patient will be following up with the BHC, we also discuss what will be evaluated or what information or skill will be the focus of the next appointment.

Using the 5As helps produce a meaningful and personalized health care action plan. The plan is specific and focused on health behavior change and is an integrated piece of the patient's overall health care plan. Ideally, the plan is then monitored and managed by the entire health care team.

PURPOSE AND ORGANIZATION OF THIS VOLUME

With the increased need for efficient evidence-based care, this volume provides BHCs working in primary care (e.g., psychologists, social workers, psychiatrists, counselors), PCPs, and other medical care providers (e.g., physician assistants, nurses, health care educators) with practical strategies they can use immediately. Our suggestions are drawn from evidence-based data as well as our experience in translating evidence-based care to our clinical settings. Overall, our book is designed to give practical step-by-step guidance for targeting biopsychosocial factors in primary care. Students may also find this text useful. Undergraduate and graduate courses focused on preparing individuals to work in primary care can use this book as part of a seminar on assessment and intervention in primary care or as part of a larger class focusing on brief treatments for common behavioral health problems.

The book is divided into three parts. Part I consists of four chapters that lay the foundation for an integrated behavioral health care practice. In Chapter 1, we describe foundational concepts of population health service delivery and the PCMH. In Chapter 2, we discuss what we believe are important core competencies and clinical practice management skills necessary to work efficiently and effectively in primary care. In Chapter 3, using the 5As, we outline the steps for an initial consultation appointment. This chapter provides a template for addressing patient problems in the primary care setting and provides the foundation for conducting the initial consultation. In Chapter 4, we describe the basic tools of interventions for behavioral health problems that can be implemented in 15- to 30-minute consultation appointments. These include the following 11 interventions: relaxation training, mindfulness exercises, goal setting, cognitive disputation, acceptance and commitment therapy techniques, motivational enhancement techniques, problem solving, self-monitoring, behavioral self-analysis, stimulus control, and assertive communication. We have found these 11 interventions to be effective for a variety of symptoms and functional impairments. For each intervention, we apply the 5As format and show how to present the intervention to the patient in plain, easily understandable language. In Part II, we apply the foundations presented in Chapters 1 through 4 to the most common patient problems the BHC will encounter in the primary care setting. Each of the 12 chapters in Part II is structured as follows:

- description of the problem area, with emphasis on relevant biopsychosocial factors;

- cultural and diversity considerations;

- review of evidence-based interventions in the problem area;

- adaptation of interventions for the primary care setting;

- use of the 5As format for assessment and intervention;

- websites, mobile applications, and books for patients; and

- assessment and intervention tools, such as BHC scripts, handouts, worksheets, checklists, and monitoring forms (these tools can also be downloaded from the American Psychological Association Books website [https://www.apa.org/pubs/books/integrated-behavioral-health-primary-care-third-edition] and tailored to one's particular needs and setting).

In Part III, we address managing suicide risk, clinical pathways, and shared medical appointments.

For clarity, throughout the volume, the term *specialty mental health* refers to traditional or standard assessment and treatment in an outpatient mental health clinic. The term *behavioral health* refers to activities that are performed within the primary care clinic. Our goal is to provide straightforward, easy-to-use information to assist in addressing particular problems in the primary care setting. We believe readers will find, as we have, that this way of working with patients will result in functional improvement and symptom change over a surprisingly short period.

We include recommended scripts and patient educational handouts throughout the book. These scripts and handouts are meant to serve as starting points; they can and should be altered to meet the needs and values of the patients coming to a given clinic. For ease of adaptation the companion website to this book has the scripts and handouts available to download.

We have had the opportunity to spend thousands of hours in primary care settings, including family medicine, internal medicine, and women's health clinics, as part of successful integrated behavioral health services. We have also taught hundreds of behavioral health providers to deliver effective behavioral health care in integrated settings. We hope that by using these evidence-based assessments and interventions, coupled with our shared experiences, BHCs can become more effective in their primary care work and can continue to improve the health of the population.

FOUNDATIONS OF INTEGRATED BEHAVIORAL CONSULTATION SERVICE

1

Population Health and the Patient-Centered Medical Home

No mass disorder afflicting mankind is ever brought under control or eliminated by attempts at treating the afflicted individual or by attempts at producing large numbers of individual practitioners. (Albee, 1983, p. 24)

POPULATION HEALTH

Data show increasing health outcome gaps between the United States and most developed countries, despite significantly more spending by the United States on medical services (Schneider et al., 2021). To address these gaps, there has been increased focus on improving outcomes through new health care service delivery models. The patient-centered medical home (PCMH; Jabbarpour et al., 2017; Philip et al., 2019) incorporates a population health approach (Caramenico, 2014; John et al., 2020; Saynisch et al., 2021). The PCMH structure meshes well with the primary care behavioral health (PCBH) model of service delivery because both emphasize team-based, population-health-focused services (Reiter et al., 2018). It is important for integrated behavioral health providers to understand basic population health principles as well as the structure and future directions of the PCMH to maximize impact as an effective team member.

The "population" in population health denotes a group of individuals who are organized by categories, such as geographic region, sex, ethnicity, age, health care system or clinic membership, and various risk factors and medical conditions, such as obesity, diabetes or hyperlipidemia, and tobacco use

https://doi.org/10.1037/0000380-002
Integrated Behavioral Health in Primary Care: Step-by-Step Guidance for Assessment and Intervention, Third Edition, by C. L. Hunter, J. L. Goodie, M. S. Oordt, and A. C. Dobmeyer

(Kindig, 2007). Population health management can be broadly defined as a systematic and integrated approach to improving the health of a given population by changing policies and systems that affect health care access, quality, and outcomes (Meiris & Nash, 2008). Using the county health rankings model, Kindig and Isham (2014) illustrated how multiple factors, including health behaviors, physical environments, and social environments, affect health outcomes. As shown in Figure 1.1, clinical care may only account for

FIGURE 1.1. Factors Affecting Health Outcomes

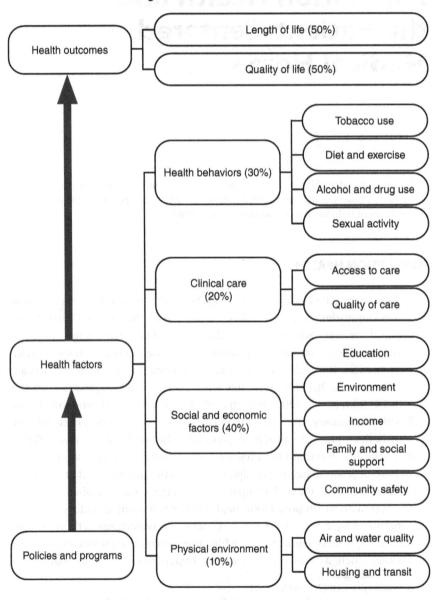

Note. From *County Health Rankings Model*, by University of Wisconsin Population Health Institute, 2014, County Health Rankings & Roadmaps (https://www.countyhealthrankings.org/explore-health-rankings/county-health-rankings-model). Copyright 2014 by UWPHI. Reprinted with permission.

20% of the variance in health outcomes, with another 30% accounted for by modifiable health behaviors, which are potential targets for PCBH intervention. Peterson et al. (2014) made the argument that population health includes interventions and clinical applications focused on the entire patient population, rather than on individual patients. They argued that less intensive (i.e., potentially less effective) interventions, delivered to all beneficiaries who might benefit, have the potential for greater impact on the overall population than more intensive (i.e., potentially more effective) interventions for a smaller number of patients. These interventions can be integrated into clinical pathways that use a set of standard operating procedures, for example, a clinical practice of screening all patients in a certain age group for a specific condition or risk factor. This clinical pathway might involve all personnel, including administrative, nursing, primary care provider (PCP), and behavioral health consultant (BHC) staff. In the population health approach, there is a shift from focusing on only those with an identified problem to identifying everyone in the population at large (e.g., all patients enrolled in a clinical practice) who might benefit from receiving a targeted evidence-based intervention.

As an example of the population health model, a clinic could decide to implement universal screening and intervention for tobacco use. Everyone seen in a primary care appointment, regardless of the problem presentation for that appointment, is screened for tobacco use. Tobacco users are encouraged to quit and offered a brief, low-intensity intervention provided by the PCP or BHC if they want to quit. For this hypothetical example, let us say the successful quit rate is a modest 10%, somewhat lower than the 20% success rate of a more intensive intervention offered by a local wellness center. However, more patients are exposed to the low-intensity intervention because it is offered to all tobacco users in the practice and requires less time and effort by patients. The potential benefits of a population health approach can be seen in this tobacco screening and intervention example (A. Dobmeyer, personal communication, June 23, 2022):

- In 1 year, 1,000 patients received the intervention from a PCP or BHC, and 10% quit (10% = 100 patients).

- During the same year, the wellness center offered high-intensity tobacco cessation counseling (eight 1-hour visits); 100 patients completed the counseling, and 20% quit (20% = 20 patients).

- Thus, although the primary care interventions had a lower success rate (10% vs. 20%), the overall number of patients quitting was greater (100) compared with the wellness center counseling (20).

We expect a lower percentage of tobacco users will quit and stay quit with the lower intensity interventions offered in the primary care setting. However, far more individuals will quit and stay quit because of the number of individuals who are being targeted for tobacco cessation. Consequently, more of the population will quit and stay quit compared with approaches that focus on high-intensity interventions and reach a smaller number of individuals (Fiore et al., 2008). Problem presentations like unhealthy alcohol use, anxiety, chronic pain, depression, diabetes, insomnia, and obesity are also prime targets for a population health approach using evidence-based clinical pathways. We encourage BHCs to work with team leadership to develop clinical pathways for problems in their clinic that might respond well to this approach. To assist with this, we have included on the companion website to this book (https://www. apa.org/pubs/books/integrated-behavioral-health-primary-care-third-edition) materials that can be used to discuss with the BHC's team how they might tailor and launch a standard clinical pathway for unhealthy alcohol use, anxiety, chronic pain, depression, diabetes, insomnia, obesity, and tobacco use. See Chapter 18 for additional information on clinical pathways.

BHCs who bring a population health approach to primary care exponentially increase their value to the team. It puts them in a position to proactively pursue systemic changes in how the clinic engages in screening, assessment, and intervention for a number of problems and highlights how the BHC can participate in the care for everyone in that problem/disease group. For additional information on population health management, see "A Roadmap for Population Health Management" (Cavalieri et al., 2016) and "Population Health Management: Roadmap for Integrated Delivery Networks" (National Committee for Quality Assurance [NCQA] & Jansen, 2019). These documents review population health management definitions; planning for population health care; data collection, storage, and management; population monitoring and stratification; patient engagement; team-based interventions; and outcome measurements.

FROM TRIPLE TO QUADRUPLE AIM

The Triple Aim (Berwick et al., 2008) has served as a leading conceptual population health approach to improving health system outcomes by focusing simultaneously on improving the individual experience of care, reducing the per capita cost of care, and improving the health of populations. Successfully achieving the Triple Aim is influenced by multiple factors, including the redesign and redefinition of primary care services and structures (Berwick et al., 2008). To be effective, primary care redesign needs to include the following (Institute for Healthcare Improvement, 2009):

- basic health care services, including behavioral health, provided by a variety of professionals;

- a team that can deliver at least 70% of the necessary medical and health-related social services to the population they serve;

- health care access that has maximum flexibility for customizing health care to the needs of patients, families, and providers; and

- coordinated and cooperative interactions with hospitals, community services, and other specialty care providers related to the health care management of their patients.

Although the Triple Aim is widely accepted as a path to optimize health system performance and outcomes, there is growing recognition that if the Triple Aim is to meet its full potential, it needs to be expanded to the Quadruple Aim. The additional aim focuses on improving health care team well-being. Bodenheimer and Sinsky (2014) introduced the Quadruple Aim concept, noting that a stressful work environment can lead to increased staff burnout, which can negatively impact Triple Aim goals. The loss of enthusiasm for work, lower sense of accomplishment, and cynicism in staff burnout can lead to increased staff turnover, medical mistakes, decreased medical staff adherence to treatment plans, and lower levels of empathy for patients (Bodenheimer & Sinsky, 2014). They offered practical steps for primary care to improve the work care environment through team documentation (letting other staff enter some or all of the medical documentation in the electronic health record), previsit planning to reduce time wasted during appointments, expanding the roles and responsibilities of team members, synchronizing work flows to save time, having teams work in the same physical spaces, ensuring staff are well trained, and reengineering unnecessary work out of the practice (Bodenheimer & Sinsky, 2014). These recommendations are consistent with the PCBH model of service delivery, and growing evidence shows that integrating BHC services into team-based primary care is helpful in meeting Quadruple Aim goals (American Psychological Association, 2022).

THE PATIENT-CENTERED MEDICAL HOME

Around the time the Triple Aim concept was introduced, the PCMH concept of primary care delivery was being championed as a significant primary care redesign. The PCMH joint principles (see Figure 1.2), consistent with the Triple Aim approach, were published and endorsed by four primary care professional societies in 2007 (American Academy of Family Physicians et al., 2007). A growing body of evidence is showing that primary care practices that fully implement the core principles of the PCMH experience improvements in quality-of-service delivery and reductions of cost, with longer PCMH implementation producing better results (Jabbarpour et al., 2017; John et al., 2020; Philip et al., 2019; Saynisch et al., 2021). Although not expressed in the 2007 joint principles, the PCMH concept presented an opportunity to transform care for patients with behavioral health and medical conditions (R. Kessler et al., 2009; Petterson et al., 2008; Rittenhouse & Shortell, 2009). Six family medicine professional societies formally recognized this opportunity when they published the joint principles for integrated behavioral health services in the PCMH (see Figure 1.2; Baird et al., 2014). These principles detail the integrated behavioral health components believed to be necessary for the PCMH to reach its full potential.

FIGURE 1.2. Patient-Centered Medical Home Principles

2007 joint principles	2014 expanded principles with behavioral health integration
Personal physician	Each patient has a personal physician who knows that patient's situation and biography.
Physician-directed medical practice	The health care team focuses on the physical, mental, emotional, and social aspects of the patient's health care. Behavioral health providers may be part of the primary care practice or may be connected to the primary care practice as part of the medical neighborhood.
Whole-person orientation	To achieve a whole-person orientation, care must focus on both the behavioral and physical aspects of the patient.
Care is coordinated and/or integrated	Behavioral and physical health care must be coordinated and integrated via shared registries, medical records (especially shared problem and medication lists), shared decision making, shared revenue streams, and shared responsibility for patient care plans.
Quality and safety are hallmarks	Care plans are developed in partnership with the patient, family, physician, and behavioral health provider. Electronic health records must incorporate the behavioral health provider's notes, mental health screening, and case finding tools. Behavioral health outcomes must be tracked.
Enhanced access to care	This includes access for patients, families, and physicians to behavioral health care resources through systems of collaboration, shared problem solving, flexible team leadership, and enhanced communication.
Payment recognizes the added value of the PCMH	Payment recognizes the added value of behavioral health care as part of the PCMH and the value of behavioral health clinicians as members of the team. Funding streams should be pooled and applied flexibly such that fragmented care ends.

Note. PCMH = patient-centered medical home. Adapted from *Advancing Behavioral Health Integration Within NCQA Recognized Patient-Centered Medical Homes* (p. 3), by SAMHSA-HRSA Center for Integrated Health Solutions, 2014 (https://brsstacs.center4si.com/Behavioral_Health_Integration.pdf). In the public domain.

When clinics are evolving their primary care services to include PCMH core principles, they often look to outside organizations for an objective evaluation and endorsement of their efforts. Many clinics use the NCQA to evaluate how well they are delivering care in accordance with PCMH principles. NCQA recognition is used by payers (e.g., insurance companies) to determine whether clinics are providing services in a manner likely to produce better outcomes, improved patient satisfaction with care, and cost savings (i.e., meeting the Triple Aim). There is a growing focus on payers requiring a set level of PCMH recognition in order to receive the highest level of reimbursement for services (Philip et al., 2019). The importance of integrated behavioral health services in PCMH recognition standards was further highlighted in 2017 when NCQA launched their PCMH Distinction in Behavioral Health Integration as a way to recognize that

> the practice has resources to support the needs of patients with behavioral health related conditions within the primary care practice. It integrates behavioral health trained staff (e.g., care managers, clinical social workers, psychiatrists) within the practice workflow and creates integrated/coordinated treatment plans that can be shared within and outside the practice. The practice identifies and addresses behavioral health needs using evidence-based guidelines and uses quality measures to monitor the care delivered. The intent is to enhance the care provided in a primary care setting and to improve access, clinical outcomes and patient experience. (NCQA, 2017, p. 5)

See the NCQA website (https://www.ncqa.org/) for additional information and current criteria and standards.

SUMMARY

So what does this all mean? BHCs need to be knowledgeable about the PCMH core principles that are driving service delivery changes. These changes reinforce the need for integrated behavioral health care and the use of BHCs. BHCs should be familiar with the importance of integrated behavioral health services they may be expected to provide as part of a PCMH team and understand that these services are essential parts of establishing and realizing the full impact of PCMH primary care. Understanding the BHC role in implementing and advancing a population health approach to care is also an essential component. Doing so puts BHCs in a position to work with the team in a manner that maximizes their contribution to the care of the population. That impact can be enhanced through the implementation of clinical pathways. Working with the team to set these pathways can enhance a clinic's level of PCMH recognition status and reimbursement and set a process for delivering care that is team-based, proactive, and sustainable and can produce better overall health for the population served by the PCMH team.

2

Core Competencies and Clinical Practice Management Skills

Most mental health providers have not been trained to a set of core competencies that will allow them to effectively work as behavioral health consultants (BHCs) in primary care (Serrano et al., 2018). Fortunately, a number of organizations, including the Agency for Healthcare Research and Quality (Kinman et al., 2015), American Psychological Association (McDaniel et al., 2014), and Substance Abuse and Mental Health Services Administration–Health Resources and Services Administration (Hoge et al., 2014), and subject matter experts (e.g., Dobmeyer et al., 2016; C. L. Hunter & Goodie, 2010; Robinson & Reiter, 2016) have detailed the competencies and clinical practice management skills believed to be important to work as an effective BHC. We have had the opportunity to train and evaluate hundreds of BHCs on core competencies and clinical practice management skills. In this chapter, we review the core competencies and clinical practice management skills we believe are necessary to work effectively in primary care.

SIX COMPETENCY DOMAINS

There are six competency dimensions (Robinson & Reiter, 2016) we believe capture the foundational skill sets that lead to successful integrated behavioral health services in primary care:

I. Clinical practice knowledge and skills

II. Practice management skills

https://doi.org/10.1037/0000380-003
Integrated Behavioral Health in Primary Care: Step-by-Step Guidance for Assessment and Intervention, Third Edition, by C. L. Hunter, J. L. Goodie, M. S. Oordt, and A. C. Dobmeyer

III. Consultation skills

IV. Documentation skills

V. Administrative knowledge and skills

VI. Team performance skills

Figure 2.1 lists the core competency dimensions, elements in those dimensions, and attributes of those elements. The chapters in this book are designed as a launching pad to help a BHC develop these skill sets. To enhance that effort, this chapter focuses specifically on these foundational core competencies and practice management skills.

FIGURE 2.1. BHC Core Competencies (*continues*)

Dimension	Element	Attribute	
I. Clinical practice knowledge and skills	1. Role definition	Says introductory script smoothly, conveys BHC role to all new patients, and answers patient's questions	
	2. Problem identification	Identifies and defines presenting problem with patient within first half of initial 30-minute appointment	
	3. Assessment	Focuses on current problem, functional impact, and environmental factors contributing to/maintaining problem; uses tools appropriate for primary care	
	4. Problem focus	Explores whether additional problems exist, without excessive probing	
	5. Population-based care	a.	Understands difference between population-based and case-focused approach
		b.	Provides care along a continuum from primary prevention to tertiary care; develops/uses pathways to routinely involve BHC in care of chronic conditions
	6. Biopsychosocial approach	Understands relationship of medical and psychological aspects of health	
	7. Use of evidence-based interventions	Utilizes evidence-based recommendations/interventions suitable for primary care for patients and PCPs	
	8. Intervention design	a.	Bases interventions on measurable, functional outcomes and symptom reduction
		b.	Uses self-management, home-based practice
		c.	Uses simple, concrete, practical strategies, based on empirically supported treatments for primary care

FIGURE 2.1. BHC Core Competencies (*continues*)

Dimension	Element	Attribute
I. Clinical practice knowledge and skills (*continued*)	9. Multipatient intervention skills	Works with PCPs to provide classes and/or groups in formats appropriate for primary care (e.g., drop-in stress management class, group medical visit for a chronic condition)
	10. Pharmacotherapy	Can name basic psychotropic medications; can discuss common side effects and common myths; abides by recommended limits for nonprescribers; consults psychopharmacology prescribing expert when needed
II. Practice management skills	1. Visit efficiency	Demonstrates adequate introduction, rapid problem identification and assessment, and development of intervention recommendations and a plan in 30-minute visits
	2. Time management	Stays on time when conducting consecutive appointments
	3. Follow-up planning	Plans follow-up for 2 weeks or 1 month, instead of every week (as appropriate); alternates follow-ups with PCPs for high-utilizing patients
	4. Intervention efficiency	Uses consultant approach to planning follow-up by working with patients only until symptoms or functioning begin to improve and there is a plan in place for continued improvement; structures behavioral change plans consistent with briefer courses of care
	5. Visit flexibility	Appropriately uses flexible strategies for visits: 15 minute, 30 minute, phone contacts, telehealth visits, secure messaging
	6. Triage	Attempts to manage most problems in primary care but does triage to mental health, unhealthy substance use, or other clinics or services when symptoms or functioning are not improving with PCBH services
	7. Case management	a. Uses patient registries (if they exist); takes load off of PCP (e.g., returns patient calls about behavioral issues); advocates for patients
		b. Communicates and coordinates care with care coordinators and case managers
	8. Community resource referrals	Is knowledgeable about and makes use of community resources (e.g., refers to community self-help groups)
III. Consultation skills	1. Referral clarity	Is clear on referral questions; focuses on and responds directly to referral questions in PCP feedback

FIGURE 2.1. BHC Core Competencies (*continued*)

Dimension	Element	Attribute
III. Consultation skills (*continued*)	2. Curbside consultations	Successfully consults with PCPs on demand about a general issue or specific patient; uses clear, direct language in concise manner
	3. Assertive follow-up	Ensures PCPs receive verbal and/or written feedback on patients referred; interrupts PCP, if indicated, for urgent patient needs
	4. PCP education	Delivers brief presentations in primary care staff meetings (e.g., PCP audience; focus on what BHC can do for them, what PCPs can refer, what to expect, how to use BHC optimally)
	5. Recommendation usefulness	Tailors recommendations to the pace of primary care (e.g., interventions suggested for PCPs can be done in 1–3 minutes)
	6. Value-added orientation	Makes recommendations that are intended to reduce PCP visits and workload (e.g., follow-up with BHC instead of PCP)
	7. Clinical pathways	Participates in team efforts to develop, implement, evaluate, and revise pathway programs needed in the clinic
IV. Documentation skills	1. Concise, clear charting	Records clear, concise notes in detail: referral problem specifics, functional analysis, pertinent history, impression, specific recommendations, and follow-up plan
	2. Prompt PCP feedback	Provides written and/or verbal feedback to PCP on the day the patient was seen
	3. Appropriate format	Delivers chart notes that are consistent with expected clinic/system format
V. Administrative knowledge and skills	1. BHC policies and procedures	Understands scheduling, templates, codes for primary care work, criticality of accurate medical coding
	2. Risk-management protocols	Understands limits of existing BHC practices; can describe and discuss, for example, how and why informed consent procedures differ
	3. Coding documentation	Routinely and accurately completes coding documentation
VI. Team performance skills	1. Fit with primary care culture	Understands and operates comfortably in fast-paced, action-oriented, team-based culture
	2. Knows team members	Knows the roles of the various primary care team members; both assists and utilizes them
	3. Responsiveness	Readily provides unscheduled services when needed (e.g., sees patient during lunchtime or at the end of the day, if needed)
	4. Availability	Provides on-demand consultations via wireless communication when not in the clinic; keeps staff aware of whereabouts

Note. BHC = behavioral health consultant; PCP = primary care provider.

Integrating Seamlessly Into Primary Care

For most BHCs, working in primary care is similar to living in a different country for the first time. Upon arriving, one would quickly note that many things are different. The people speak a language that cannot be understood. Customs, mores, and norms are different. Work habits and hours are unfamiliar. People relate to time differently, with some things done more leisurely and some more urgently. Even dealing with money requires some adjustment. If one is not aware of these differences and is not prepared to accept and adjust to them, one will find it impossible to thrive in the new country or be accepted by its inhabitants. If, however, one embraces this different way of life and does one's best to fit in, it is likely that the uniqueness of the culture and background one brings will be viewed as a positive factor that enriches the community rather than challenges it.

Mental health providers and primary care providers (PCPs) are trained differently, think differently, relate to patients and colleagues differently, and practice under different standards and rules. Specialty mental health providers work under different time constraints than their PCP colleagues. Reimbursement systems are typically dissimilar as well. Similar to the ethnocentric visitor, a mental health provider who attempts to integrate into primary care without adapting to the culture of primary care will likely not be accepted by medical peers, making true integration of behavioral health care into the medical practice difficult. Such adaptation is much easier when a BHC has access to a travel guide to explain the culture in sufficient detail.

A Travel Guide

Any worthwhile travel guide tells the reader not only about the sights to see and places of interest but also about how things work at the destination, such as transportation, tipping, laws, and customs. This chapter is intended to provide similar guidance for the mental health provider entering the primary care world. We review step-by-step strategies on what to consider when delivering services within a primary care behavioral health (PCBH) model of service delivery. Key recommendations can serve as a road map for mental health providers to navigate the culture of primary care and build a foundation for PCBH services. We review core competency skills and practice management strategies we have found important to successfully make the transition from specialty behavioral health to PCBH.

The Road Map

Every good travel guide possesses a clear road map. Although there is increasing interest in integrating mental health provider services into primary care settings, many health care organizations and individual physicians are still unfamiliar with the concept and the overall benefits of integrated PCBH services. In our experience, the majority of PCPs, nurse managers, and clinic administrators are enthusiastic about these services once they learn about and experience the benefits. Patients with psychosocial and behavioral health needs are prevalent in primary care (Jetty et al., 2021), and therefore many clinic personnel welcome behavioral health expertise within a specific clinical practice. Integrated behavioral health means better care for patients, targeted referrals to specialty mental health providers outside the primary care practice, and better collaboration between professionals.

Funding

We realize that funding for integrated behavioral health services can be a significant barrier. The funding landscape is continually changing and is not the intended focus of this book. At the same time, we do think it is important that BHCs have knowledge in this area. To that end, we recommend reading Corso et al. (2016). Their book *Integrating Behavioral Health Into the Medical Home: A Rapid Implementation Guide* includes a section on business development, policy, and operations. This section focuses on how to make a business case to payers, develop a basic business plan, and use data reporting and monitoring to show value. The authors reviewed how to engage administrators, calculate a BHC business case and revenue cycles, and generate revenue and maximize reimbursement through fee schedules and provider type. They also discussed the importance of understanding rates and codes for billing and how to deal with those challenges. They walked through examples of how to calculate the return on investment for BHC services as well as a detailed example of how to create a pro forma, which is a method of calculating current or project fiscal results to create financial metrics for program accountability and fiscal sustainability. We also recommend reviewing the D. S. Freeman et al. (2018) article "Financing the Primary Care Behavioral Health Model." Dr. Freeman was the chief executive officer for Cherokee Health Systems at the time of this publication. He and his colleagues reviewed the history of financing the PCBH model of service delivery, how to build a financial infrastructure for the model, opportunities within the funding landscape, increased accountability, and the future of PCBH model funding.

TEAM PERFORMANCE AND CONSULTATION SKILLS DIMENSIONS

Do not underestimate the lack of team understanding or misperception of what a BHC can do and how they can work as a team member. Success begins with effectively communicating to clinic leadership and the team about the breadth and depth of skills one brings to team health care and how that can improve patient outcome and team job satisfaction. It may be particularly important to have clinic leadership communicate the importance of having a BHC and their expectations of care changes and outcomes as a result. Without clinic leadership support, it can be challenging for a BHC to work at peak scope of practice as an integrated team member. Despite what may seem obvious to a BHC as the inherent logic of integrating behavioral health services into primary care, numerous factors can hamper acceptance, including biases about mental health care, reimbursement issues, financial issues related to overhead and support staff costs, workspace concerns, territorial issues, use of support staff, and simple resistance to changing the customary ways in which mental health services have been used in the past (e.g., through referral to an outside source).

Marketing

It will be important to market the BHC skill set, repeatedly. Approach clinic management to ensure that they know what a BHC brings and to assist with marketing BHC services as a new team member. Clinics typically have a set of onboarding activities that are required of all new staff. We recommend that one of the onboarding activities be for new staff to meet with the BHC. During that meeting, a BHC can explain what their role is on the team, answer any questions team members might have, describe how patients can access care with the BHC, and share what they bring to the clinic.

Flexibility

BHCs should be as flexible and accommodating as possible. Although the patient is the BHC's external customer, the primary care team is the BHC's internal customer. BHCs are there to help the rest of the team help patients. Responsiveness and availability show that BHCs are team players, and these qualities are then likely to be reciprocated by others. Flexibility can include actions such as

- seeing unscheduled patients as warm handoffs,

- seeing patients over lunch or prior to or just after regular clinic hours,

- changing offices daily or weekly in the clinic if there is a shortage of clinical office space, and

- briefly pausing an appointment to do a "curbside" consultation with a team member.

It is important to remember BHCs are entering a world and culture that belongs to other professions, and they are the ones who will have to be flexible.

Optimally, in the long term, a BHC will need their own office space and equipment, reception and appointment services, and coding/billing support, just like all the other providers in the clinic. Initially, however, it may be necessary to accept minimal support while the details of what a BHC needs are being implemented and course corrected. With time, PCBH services commonly become viewed as an indispensable component to how health care is delivered, and colleagues may actually advocate on a BHC's behalf with clinic management for improvements to make their work easier and more productive.

Being a Team Member

Functioning well as a team requires each member to know their role and perform well in that role. Flexible collaboration, knowing the target audience, and succinct and timely feedback are keys to being a successful team member.

Collaboration

Collaboration with everyone on the team to help meet the needs of patients is key to a successful PCBH practice. It is essential for BHCs to keep their scope of care as broad as possible within the limits of their training and experience. Accept all referrals and find ways to assist anyone, including but not limited to the following:

- patients with potential mental health diagnoses,

- patients needing help with health-related behavior change (e.g., tobacco cessation, increasing exercise, diet changes, unhealthy substance use),

- patients with stress or coping difficulties,

- grieving or dying patients,

- family members of patients with illnesses or disabilities,

- patients with medical adherence difficulties, and

- patients whom PCPs find challenging to work with or for whom there is no significant benefit derived from repeatedly seeing a PCP.

If it feels like one's scope of practice is limited (i.e., feeling uncomfortable or lacking experience with assessing and treating common problem presentations), then one of a BHC's early goals is to determine what is needed to increase scope and competency. The more of a generalist a BHC is, the more of a team player they will be. A marketing brochure for PCPs that outlines the full range of services a BHC can provide can help establish a BHC in this vein. Figure 2.2 is a sample brochure. When presenting this brochure, consider introducing it like this:

> I was wondering if there was a time today or later this week when I could speak with you for about 2 minutes to go over the types of patients and problems I might be able to help you manage.

Part of a BHC's job is to help the team think about using BHC services for more than the obvious patient presentations such as depression and anxiety. It might be helpful to let them know not to think twice about bringing a BHC in to assist with any patient. Sometimes team members are concerned that they will overwhelm a BHC and do not want to burden them too much. Letting them know that a BHC can do an assessment for every patient of their symptoms, functional problems, and relevant biopsychosocial factors and make a recommendation for a way forward (whether that is in primary care with the BHC or another team member or with a referral to another specialist or a community resource) is a win for everyone.

FIGURE 2.2. Marketing Survey

Providing the Right Care, for the Right People, at the Right Time

Family Medicine Behavioral Health Consultant

Services: Consultation (30 minutes) for assessment and behavioral health treatment planning, recommendations, and interventions.

Referrals: ANYTHING you think might be helped through habit, behavioral, cognitive, or emotional changes.

Goals of Service: To help you and your patients develop practical knowledge and skills to promote and improve physical and emotional health.

The following is a list of common problems for which I may be helpful.

General Mental Health Problems	**Clinical Health Problems**
❏ Stress	❏ Insomnia
❏ Anxiety/fears	❏ Chronic pain
❏ Depression	❏ Headache
❏ Anger	❏ Fibromyalgia
❏ Relationship problems	❏ Temporomandibular disorders
❏ Grief or bereavement	❏ Low back pain
❏ Attention-deficit/hyperactivity disorder	❏ Tobacco use
❏ Posttraumatic stress disorder	❏ Alcohol use
❏ Suicidal thoughts	❏ Diet (weight loss, dietary adherence)
❏ Workplace stress	❏ Exercise
❏ Burnout	❏ Diabetes
❏ Eating disorders	❏ Gastrointestinal problems
❏ Obsessive–compulsive disorder	❏ Chronic obstructive pulmonary disease
❏ Memory concerns	❏ Medication adherence
❏ Parenting concerns	❏ Chronic illness management

PCPs as the BHC's Primary Customer

Another way to establish a BHC as a team player is to view the referring PCPs as the BHC's primary customers. This involves focusing on the PCP's reason for referring the patient before addressing other problems the patient may present. It also involves providing feedback to the PCP in a way that is most helpful to them. BHCs must take care that their services are consistent and supportive of the health care being provided by the PCP; that is, the BHC and the PCP should be working on the same goals in collaboration with the patient. The BHC is working as a consultant to the PCP and is there to assist as a team member with assessment, intervention, and coordination of services, but the BHC does not "own" the patient as they would in a specialty mental health setting. Be diligent both in ensuring one knows what the referring PCP's reason is for referring the patient and in responding back specifically about the referral problem. Other concerns may be identified during a BHC assessment that may need to be addressed in treatment; however, the provider's referral question must not be overshadowed. In an example scenario, a PCP refers a woman to a BHC to learn behavioral strategies for improving sleep. During the evaluation, the BHC learns of significant marital distress, which is the primary concern of the patient and which is believed to be a contributing factor to the sleep difficulties. A treatment plan centered on resolving marital issues is developed and implemented. However, the education on behavioral sleep strategies requested by the PCP is never delivered.

In this example, the BHC and the PCP are working on somewhat different agendas. Although it is appropriate and ethically necessary to offer or facilitate services that address identified problem areas, the primary reason for referral should also be addressed. In this example, the BHC might simply have added an educational component on behavioral strategies to improve sleep as part of the treatment plan so the patient can benefit from both what the PCP determined was needed and what the BHC assessed as an additional problem area. This would represent better collaboration. Of course, there may be times when one believes the intervention requested by the PCP is inappropriate. In those instances, a BHC should discuss their opinions and recommendations with the referring PCP. Never ignore or neglect the referring issue or request. An easy-to-use yet sufficiently detailed referral form can help facilitate communication about what the referring provider is requesting. An example is provided in Figure 2.3.

Assessment/Intervention Feedback for the PCP

Providing feedback to the PCP is a key factor to working as a team. In a busy practice, this can get neglected. However, feedback is the foundation for reaping the benefits of integrating BHCs into primary care. Take time to find out what PCPs find helpful when giving them feedback on a patient.

- How much detail do they want?

- Do they prefer written (clinical notes) or verbal feedback?

- Do they want feedback immediately following the patient visit, or do they prefer feedback about all patients together at the end of the day?

At minimum, BHC feedback should include significant findings, impressions, and recommendations, and effort should be made to provide this feedback on the same day the patient is seen. It is best to keep feedback focused on the PCP's referral question and avoid unnecessary discussion of extraneous issues. Target verbal feedback to be 2 minutes or less. If the PCP wants more information, they will ask. For example,

> I saw Ms. Bennet today. Is now a good time to give you some feedback, or would another time work better? Her sleep problems were kicked off by marital

distress. She is engaging in sleep behaviors that are making her sleep worse, like getting into bed when not sleepy, staying in bed awake for several hours, thinking about the future of her marriage, and taking naps when she comes home from work. We set a plan to change sleep behaviors, to include getting into bed only when sleepy, getting out of bed if not asleep in 15 minutes, thinking about her marriage in her living room and not her bedroom, and stopping naps. I also taught her the basics of assertive communication. She is following up with me in 2 weeks to reassess sleep. When you see her again, I'd encourage you to ask if she is getting into bed only when sleepy and getting out of bed if not asleep in 15 minutes. If not, you might encourage her to do so if she wants her sleep to improve.

FIGURE 2.3. Consultation Request

Consultation Request

Patient Name and ID: _____ **Referring PCP:** _____

Circle Consult Problem: Anxiety, Panic, IBS, Hyperventilation, Depression, Stress, Insomnia, Chronic Pain, GERD, COPD, Diabetes, ETOH Problems, Adherence, Tobacco Cessation, Obesity, Anger, Relational Problems, Bereavement, Memory Problems, Other: _____

*Requesting Provider, please circle requested skills training/patient education:

Anxiety/Panic/IBS/Hyperventilation: 1. Deep Breathing Training; 2. Cue-Controlled Relaxation; 3. Modify Thoughts That ↑Sx; 4. Educate on Physiology of Autonomic Arousal; 5. Decrease Avoidance Behaviors That Maintain Problem; 6. Educate on Medication Side Effect

Depression: 1. Educate on Depression Cycle; 2. ↑Exercise; 3. ↑Social Support; 4. ↑Meaningful/Valued Activities; 5. ↑Medical Tx Adherence; 6. Education on Medication Side Effect

Stress Management: 1. Deep Breathing Training; 2. Cue-Controlled Relaxation; 3. Modify Thoughts That ↑Sx; 4. ↑Exercise; 5. ↑Social Support; 6. ↑Meaningful/Valued Activities; 7. Assertive Communication

Insomnia: 1. Sleep Behavior Change, Stimulus Control, Sleep Restriction; 2. Relaxation Skills Training

Weight Management: 1. Improve Exercise Habits; 2. Eating Behavior Change; 3. Educate on Weight Management; 4. Modify Thoughts That Perpetuate Problem

Chronic Pain (Musculoskeletal/Headache): 1. Pace Activities; 2. Relaxation Training; 3. ↑Exercise; 4. ↑Social Support; 5. ↑Meaningful/Valued Activities; 6. Modify Thoughts; 7. Educate on Pain

Medical Illness Management: 1. Educate on Depression Cycle; 2. Relaxation Skills Training; 3. ↑Social Support; 4. ↑Pleasant Activities; 5. Modify Thoughts That Perpetuate Problem

Other: _____

Note. PCP = primary care provider; IBS = irritable bowel syndrome; GERD = gastroesophageal reflux disease; COPD = chronic obstructive pulmonary disease; ETOH = ethyl alcohol; Sx = symptoms; Tx = treatment.

Build Key Relationships

Few factors contribute to the success of an integrated behavioral health service as much as the relationships BHCs build with the primary care team members. Establishing collegiality with administrative staff, technicians, nurses, and PCPs makes BHC work easier and ensures the best patient care possible. There are several steps BHCs can take to promote a good working relationship with the team.

Get Support From Informal Leaders

Determine who within the clinic are the informal leaders, that is, those to whom others look to shape opinion, those who have a track record of making changes happen, and those whom people come to with organizational issues and problems. These people may or may not be those in formal leadership positions. Talk with them about what a BHC can offer patients and how BHC services can help them to perform their roles better and more easily. Gaining acceptance from these individuals can facilitate others actively seeking a BHC out for assistance.

Get to Know the Whole Team

Take time to get to know all support personnel within the clinic, including medical assistants, reception staff, billing personnel, and housekeepers. Learn their names and their history with the clinic and discuss their role and the challenges they face. These relationships will establish goodwill and may be essential when you need their assistance in the future.

BHCs should ask the PCPs if they can sit in on their appointments for a morning or afternoon clinic. This will ensure the BHC knows each provider and they know the BHC. It will help a BHC understand how they operate a little better and can serve as a crash course in the primary care culture. In addition, a BHC may have an opportunity to point out areas where a referral to a BHC would benefit patients, thus increasing the range of referrals to the BHC practice. Finally, take steps to make oneself part of the clinic by attending formal and informal gatherings along with the other providers, including lunch-and-learn activities, holiday parties, and provider/staff meetings. This will help establish the BHC as part of the clinic team and not just a visiting provider.

Market BHC Services

A new PCBH service will not just happen. It will require persistent marketing to PCPs and frequent reminders that BHC services are available to assist their patients in ways that can both improve care and make PCP jobs easier. A variety of marketing strategies are recommended here to keep one's services in the minds of colleagues.

Problem of the Week

First, consider distributing a "Problem of the Week" flyer to all clinical staff highlighting a specific clinical condition one is seeking referrals for and what services one can offer. Examples would be flyers on obesity, smoking cessation, stress management, medication compliance, depression, worry control, panic control, physical inactivity, or motivational issues. To be useful to busy primary care staff, these marketing materials must be brief; the information must be gleaned by scanning for a few seconds because longer materials are unlikely to be read. Simply state the clinical problem area and what one can do to help in a few bulleted lines. Figure 2.4 shows an example.

FIGURE 2.4. Problem of the Week

Stress

Is STRESS a factor in your patients' well-being?
I can help your patients in the following ways:

- Recognizing the signs and symptoms of stress
- Identifying triggers for stress reactions
- Training in relaxation strategies
- Teaching healthy thinking strategies
- Improving balance between work and leisure
- Enhancing problem-solving skills

Patients can be scheduled for behavioral health consultation appointments at the reception desk or can be seen promptly on the day they have an appointment with you. I can be contacted at XXX-XXX-XXXX.

Daily Check-Ins
Second, consider conducting daily check-ins with each provider. This could be done as part of the morning and/or afternoon clinic group huddle or by asking at the beginning of the day if they have any patients on their schedule who might benefit from seeing a BHC after their appointment. A BHC's schedule should be arranged so that some patients can be seen shortly after their scheduled medical appointment, when needed. A recommended practice is to leave a percentage of clinical time unscheduled or reserved for same-day appointments to maintain availability. This practice allows for what is commonly referred to as a *warm handoff*. A warm handoff begins when the PCP identifies a biopsychosocial concern in their current appointment and requests BHC assistance (Reiter et al., 2018). The BHC immediately responds. They get a brief history and PCP referral concern before the PCP introduces the patient to the BHC in the exam room. The BHC will meet with the patient on the same day, when possible, and immediately start addressing the referral concerns, but there may be times the patient has to wait if the BHC is not immediately available. The goal is to structure the BHC service to always have same-day access for a patient appointment (Reiter et al., 2018). However, there will be times when the patient is unable to stay. The percentage of unscheduled or same-day appointment slots for same-day warm handoffs could range from 20% to 50% of a BHC's template, based on how frequently PCPs initiate same-day warm handoffs to the BHC. Again, this will likely help keep BHC services in the minds of the PCPs as they see their patients throughout the day.

Be Highly Available

PCPs are more likely to use a BHC who is responsive and easily accessible. Therefore, one will benefit from removing as many barriers to care as possible. Potential barriers include the following:

- difficulty reaching a BHC for consultation or warm handoff when needed,

- problems accessing appointments,

- patients having to leave the clinic and return later in the day or week before seeing the BHC, and

- lack of feedback to the provider following a consultation.

BHCs can overcome these barriers by carrying a cell phone and encouraging colleagues to make contact anytime a question arises. Although many outpatient specialty mental health providers use a "do not disturb" sign to avoid interruptions during treatment appointments, this is not the norm within primary care settings. In primary care, knocks on the door and phone calls should be answered promptly even during patient appointments. If a BHC is working in primary care on a part-time basis, arrange a method (e.g., via cell phone) for contacting the BHC when the need arises and the BHC is outside the clinic. It is essential to reinforce PCPs' use of BHC services with quick responsiveness. In addition, be available during times when other providers are likely to be free to consult with a BHC. These times include early morning before the first patient appointment, lunch, and at the end of the business day.

Learn the Primary Care Culture

BHCs should not expect the primary care environment to adapt in response to their presence. The following suggestions are likely to help one fit in.

- Speak the same language. Use practical, no-nonsense language and avoid psychological jargon. Reading medical journals and texts can help one become more familiar with common medical terms to help communicate. Do not try to go beyond one's working knowledge.

- Adopt the primary care pace; 15- to 30-minute appointment slots will help ensure prompt access and will demonstrate the BHC's commitment to working as part of the primary care team. Although many behavioral health providers are unaccustomed to such brief appointments, this schedule is realistic if BHCs are providing focused assessments and brief interventions appropriate to the primary care setting. Figure 2.5 is an example of what a BHC appointment template might look like and how a day in the life of a BHC might look.

- Provide brief, focused interventions to a large number of the patients within the practice (see Chapter 1), rather than provide comprehensive care to a few more severe cases. For instance, avoid providing extended psychother-

FIGURE 2.5. Appointment Template

BHC Schedule Template

• 7:30: Team huddle • 8:00: Book • 8:30: Book • 9:00: Book • 9:30: Open time • 10:00: Book • 10:30: Book • 11:00: Book • 11:30: Book	• 12:00: Lunch • 12:30: Book • 1:00: Book • 1:30: Book • 2:00: Open time • 2:30 Book • 3:00: Class (60 minutes)

A Day in the Life of a BHC

7:30:   Attend huddle(s), touch base with PCP

8:00:   Planned follow-up, diabetes self-management

8:30:   Adult with depressed mood

9:00:   Child with stomach pain who has had a full/clear medical workup

9:30:   Slot not filled; complete remaining notes from earlier

9:45:   Join PCP in exam room to assist patient in identifying support resources

10:00:   (Started at 10:05): Initial appointment for stress related to work

10:30:   Risk assessment for patient in acute distress

11:00:   Initial appointment for pain

11:30:   Adult with relationship concerns

12:00:   Lunch

12:30:   Planned follow-up, second appointment for insomnia

12:45:   Interruption by medical administrative support regarding appointment scheduling for anxiety patient

1:00:   Adult assessment to clarify attention problems in patient requesting ADHD medication

1:30:   Planned follow-up on patient with PTSD

2:00:   Warm handoff for anxiety symptoms

2:30:   Planned follow-up for weight loss

3:00:   Group: Living Well Class, teach and practice stress coping skills

4:00:   PCP feedback, close out notes, and preappointment planning for next day

Note. BHC = behavioral health consultant; PCP = primary care provider; ADHD = attention-deficit/hyperactivity disorder; PTSD = posttraumatic stress disorder.

apy for chronic mental health conditions. This will allow a BHC to integrate into the routine care provided in the clinic and not be relegated to a specialist role. At the same time, it is important to keep in mind that primary care can be episodic. Patients could come in and out of BHC care for the same presenting issues or different treatment presentations, or they might benefit from continuity consultations. A continuity consultation involves seeing a patient consistently over a longer period of time (e.g., 12 months) for the same presenting problem with appointments spread out (e.g., 1 or more months apart), to ensure ongoing improvement or health maintenance. Although many patients can get significant benefit within one to four BHC appointments, there is no rule on capping the number of appointments for a given patient. That decision should be made collaboratively with the patient, looking at the potential benefits of ongoing BHC appointments balanced with the need for the BHC to be available to serve the entire primary care population (see Chapter 1). Some patients would likely benefit from extended psychotherapy or other specialty-level mental health care that goes beyond what would be appropriate for primary care. For these patients, it may be helpful to engage them in a shared-decision-making conversation (see Introduction) to discuss specialty referral options and get their thoughts on pursuing that course of treatment.

- Ensure feedback to providers is succinct and prompt. Comprehensive assessment reports are not the norm within the primary care setting. Verbal feedback should typically be delivered in 2 minutes or less; if more detail is needed, PCPs will ask for clarification.

The primary care culture is also one in which professionals take care of each other. PCPs consult with each other on difficult or complex cases. Personal problems, both medical and social, are discussed and advice is given. Ethical issues are discussed formally and informally. Interpersonal problems between staff members and between patients and staff are addressed. This culture is essential to creating the supportive environment in which people can successfully face the personal and professional challenges of working in health care.

A trained and experienced BHC is a valuable resource for this process, which is generally quickly recognized. In our experience, staff at all levels within the organization from senior executives to the most junior medical assistant will talk with the BHC about personal problems, interpersonal conflicts, difficult patients, and personal or family mental health concerns. It can be helpful to the primary care organization if a BHC embraces this role as caregiver of the staff. Take the time to offer whatever assistance one can. Often, this simply entails listening to, normalizing, and validating people's perceptions and experiences. Sometimes one will be able to give practical advice. To avoid dual relationships, it is important to keep firm boundaries on what one does in this role. Keep the BHC role to one of support, advice, and consultation and avoid formal assessment or treatment with coworkers. If one determines that behavioral health services are indicated, a BHC can encourage or facilitate care with a provider outside the immediate organization. In addition, ensure that coworkers have opportunities to informally access a BHC without drawing excessive attention to themselves. For example, allow them to talk after clinic hours when fewer staff members are present, avoid putting them on the BHC schedule as patients, or talk with them somewhere other than the BHC treatment office so it is not apparent they are coming to the BHC for help. Of course, it is essential that confidentiality be maintained when talking with staff. If a BHC can provide helpful, nonthreatening assistance to a colleague, that colleague will not hesitate to send patients to the BHC as well.

CLINICAL PRACTICE KNOWLEDGE AND PRACTICE MANAGEMENT SKILLS DIMENSION

Global Patient Assessment Measure

Throughout this book we recommend problem-specific measures BHCs can use with their patients. Some BHCs will also screen/assess with multiple specific measures (e.g., Patient Health Questionnaire-9, Generalized Anxiety Disorder-7, Alcohol Use Disorders Identification Test), which could be useful, depending on clinical priorities and time. In addition to those problem-specific measures, when/if indicated, we recommend BHCs use a measure that assesses a range of domains and functioning for all patients at every appointment. The measure should be administered and scored in a short period of time, for example 5 minutes or less, with actionable information that can be incorporated into the appointment as well as be used to track changes over time on functioning and symptoms. Although not originally designed for use in primary care, in our system, the Behavioral Health Measure-20 (Kopta & Lowry, 2002) has been an excellent measure to meet our global assessment measure needs. It assesses well-being (distress, life satisfaction, motivation), symptoms (alcohol/drug abuse, anxiety, bipolar disorder, depression, eating disorder, panic disorder, suicidality, risk of violence), and life functioning (work/school, intimate relationships, social relationships, life enjoyment) over the last 2 weeks. BHCs can incorporate the information from this measure into the first appointment by discussing results with patients, using it to assist with treatment planning and intervention, and monitoring change over time. Other measures that might be viable for the clinic include the Outcome Questionnaire Short Form (Seelert et al., 1999). This 10-item measure assesses psychological well-being and psychological distress over the past week. Some BHCs prefer to use the Duke Health Profile (Parkerson et al., 1990). This 17-item measure contains six health measures (physical, mental, social, general, perceived health, and self-esteem) and four dysfunction measures (anxiety, depression, pain, and disability) over the last week. Even if one chooses to use additional problem-specific measures, global measures like these allow a BHC to assess changes in different areas and can serve as a pre/post measure of BHC intervention effectiveness. In our system we can extract Behavioral Health Measure-20 data from our electronic health record (EHR) to evaluate BHC impact across a range of patient problem presentations. If one does not have the ability to pull data like this, individually, one could still track impact on patients and use that data to demonstrate BHC impact and value.

Identify Clinic Priorities

BHCs should take steps to identify the priorities and needs of the clinic and work to establish initial services that address these needs. Discussions with personnel at all levels within the organization can shed light on what the clinic prioritizes. Perhaps providers are struggling to meet the needs of a few patients with chronic medical conditions who are "overutilizing" medical services; the BHC might offer to see these patients as soon as possible. Ask what personnel find most challenging in providing good care, and then assist with that if desired. For example, PCPs might discuss challenges in getting patients on a diabetes registry to come in for overdue preventive health assessments. BHCs might take the initiative to call these patients, gauge their availability to get those assessments, and engage them in a motivational intervention manner if they are ambivalent about completing the assessments. Perhaps the clinic is establishing a new clinical pathway for obesity. The BHC can offer to contribute by running a weight management group. A brief provider survey may also help identify areas that could benefit from BHC assistance. An example of such a survey can be found in Figure 2.6. When presenting this survey, it may be useful to introduce it in a manner similar to this:

> I was wondering if you had 5 minutes this week to circle the numbers on this sheet so I can get a better idea of the types of patients you see and how you would like me to work with you and your patients to help meet your needs. When would it be a good time for me to pick this up from you?

Letting the PCPs know that what the BHC is asking them to do is geared directly toward helping them is likely to increase the chances they will complete the survey. In addition, knowing the BHC will be coming back when the PCPs say it will be finished may increase the chances they will complete the survey and will give the BHC the opportunity to reengage with them if it is not complete. Responding to the clinic's priorities will likely elicit enthusiasm for the BHC as a new team member and more rapidly get the BHC involved with patients than if one first markets their own specialty areas or interests.

DOCUMENTATION SKILLS DIMENSION

A BHC note will be visible to all providers and the patient. BHC-written documentation should be more abbreviated than what is typical for specialty mental health care. Mimic the writing style of the PCPs with use of similar abbreviations and format. Avoid psychological jargon whenever possible. Each clinic's standards, focus, and unique EHR content and limitations will determine to some extent the uniqueness of a given BHC note. If a BHC is not already doing so, we encourage them to complete the note as they are assessing the patient. We suggest the note be written in a manner that informs anyone on the team about the patient's symptoms and functioning. It should include factors associated with symptoms and functioning getting better or worse, as well as the treatment plan the BHC and the patient have started. The note is also a reminder for the BHC. When and if the BHC sees the patient again, they can go directly to the plan part of the note to inform what they might focus on in that follow-up appointment. Consider using bullet statements and preexisting/loaded EHR text that can be modified as needed to speed up documentation. Being able to check boxes or click buttons in the EHR that produce answers or text to frequently used questions can also be useful. See Figure 2.7 for an example of what an initial and return note might look like. Make recommendations that are brief, specific, and action oriented. Remember PCPs may be spending as little as 5 to 7 minutes

FIGURE 2.6. Provider Survey

A BHC can provide a broad range of services, including assessment, education, and brief intervention for your patients. To help ensure that I provide services that meet the needs of you and your patients, please complete the following survey.

In sections **B** and **C** below, use the following scale to rate your responses:

Never	Rarely	Sometimes	Often
1	2	3	4

	A. Please circle the number of any item below in which you are unclear on how a BHC can help or for which your confidence is low that a BHC can help.	B. How often in your practice do you see patients who present with the following problems?				C. When working with a patient with this problem, how often might you request assistance from a BHC?			
1	Mental health disorders (e.g., depression, anxiety/panic)	1	2	3	4	1	2	3	4
2	Subclinical emotional symptoms (e.g., sadness, worry, guilt)	1	2	3	4	1	2	3	4
3	Difficulties coping with stress	1	2	3	4	1	2	3	4
4	Marital problems	1	2	3	4	1	2	3	4
5	Child behavior problems	1	2	3	4	1	2	3	4
6	Other family problems	1	2	3	4	1	2	3	4
7	Chronic pain	1	2	3	4	1	2	3	4
8	Tension or migraine headache	1	2	3	4	1	2	3	4
9	Chronic insomnia	1	2	3	4	1	2	3	4
10	Grief and bereavement	1	2	3	4	1	2	3	4
11	Noncompliance with medication	1	2	3	4	1	2	3	4
12	Tobacco use (wanting to quit)	1	2	3	4	1	2	3	4
13	Tobacco use (not wanting to quit)	1	2	3	4	1	2	3	4
14	Overweight/obesity	1	2	3	4	1	2	3	4
15	Sedentary lifestyle impacting health	1	2	3	4	1	2	3	4
16	Stress-related medical conditions	1	2	3	4	1	2	3	4
17	Self-esteem issues	1	2	3	4	1	2	3	4
18	Unhealthy alcohol use	1	2	3	4	1	2	3	4
19	Drug abuse	1	2	3	4	1	2	3	4
20	Overutilization of health care	1	2	3	4	1	2	3	4
21	Coping with chronic/terminal illness	1	2	3	4	1	2	3	4
22	White-coat hypertension	1	2	3	4	1	2	3	4
23	Anxiety interfering with medical care	1	2	3	4	1	2	3	4

Please indicate by number the top five items or clinical areas above in which you would like to see services from the behavioral health consultant.

1. _____ 2. _____ 3. _____ 4. _____ 5. _____

Thank you for completing the survey. Please add any comments to the back of this form.

Note. BHC = behavioral health consultant.

FIGURE 2.7. Note Example (*continues*)

S/O

Chief Complaint: Depression

Referring Provider: Dr. Kevin Brown (PCP); feedback was provided to PCP.

History of Present Illness:
- Patient is a 32 y/o female. Source of information was self.
- Pt was given brochure describing PCBH services.
- Discussed with patient the PCBH model of service delivery including limits of confidentiality and the team-based, consultation approach to care. Pt indicated understanding and was seen in a 30-minute BHC appointment.

Health Habits:
OTC/Supplements/Vitamins: None
Medication Relevant to HPI: Prozac 20 mg
Caffeine: 24 ounces of coffee in AM
ETOH: 1 glass of wine 3 days a week
Nicotine: 1 pack of cigarettes a day; no desire to quit at this time
Physical Activity: Walks 30 minutes 2 days/week

Personal History: Social hx reviewed, med tech in hospital

Family History: Married 10 years, one child age 7 years

Description of Depressed Sx: Sad mood, tearfulness, trouble falling asleep, decreased interest, poor concentration, decreased libido

Duration of Depressed Mood: 2 years

Factors Related to Onset: Death of father, increased job stress

Frequency and Severity: Depressive sx daily, rated as a 6 (over last 2 weeks) on 0–10 scale with 0 being no sx and 10 being the most severe imaginable.

Course of Depression: Worse 2 years ago around time of father's illness and death. Sx improved a moderate amount after 6 months. Reported additional mild improvement since starting Prozac 6 months ago.

Hospitalized for Depression: No

Anyone suggested or you noticed mood seems unusually high at times? No

Psychosocial Factors: Death of father 2 years ago, work stress although resolving, supportive husband

Aggravating Factors: Worsened by staying in bed on weekends, withdrawing from friends/ social activities

Alleviating Factors: Improved by doing fun activities with spouse and child

Current Tx: Prozac 20 mg for last 6 months

Past Tx: None

Review of Systems:
Systemic: Feeling tired (fatigued)
Gastrointestinal: Normal appetite
Neurological: No disorientation
Psychological: Sleep disturbance and loss of pleasure. A desire to continue living, not thinking about suicide, no plan or intent. No homicidal thoughts.

Physical Findings:
General Appearance:
Alert, well developed, well nourished, in no acute distress
Neurological:
OX4, no hallucinations, memory did not appear to be impaired, judgment seemed good
Speech: normal rate, appropriate tone and volume

FIGURE 2.7. Note Example (*continued*)

Psychiatric:

    Demonstrated behavior: Good eye contact

    Mood: Depressed

    Affect: Constricted and congruent with mood

    Thought process: linear, logical, and goal directed

BHM-20 Measure Scores:

Global Mental Health	2.80: Mild Distress
Well-Being Scale	1.33: Moderate Distress
Life Functioning Scale	2.00: Mild Distress
Symptoms Scale	3.38: Within Normal Limits
Anxiety Subscale	3.25: Within Normal Limits
Depression Subscale	2.33: Mild Distress
Alcohol/Drug Use Subscale	4.00: Within Normal Limits
Bipolar Subscale	4.00: Within Normal Limits
Eating Disorders Subscale	4.00: Within Normal Limits
Harm to Others Subscale	4.00: Within Normal Limits
Suicide Monitoring Scale	4.00: No Indication of Risk

PHQ-9 Measure Score: 16 Moderate Severity Level

Functional Impact: Accomplishing less at home (housework, yard work). Spending less time with family. Stopped seeing friends. Spending more time in bed on weekend. Denies significant impact on work functioning.

Depression Intervention:

    [X] Provided patient education handout on depression

    [X] Provided education on use of medications to treat depression

    [X] Discussed factors related to development and maintenance of depression

    [X] Discussed and set plan for behavioral activation

A/P

Depression: 32 y/o WF with depressive sx that started 2 years ago around time of father's death and increased work stress. Although grief response has improved and job stress is lower, pt continues to have sig sx of depression. Reports some improvement since starting Prozac 6 mos ago. Pt's sx likely maintained by social withdrawal and decreased rewarding activities. Pt interested in learning self-management skills for improving mood.

Depression recommendations for pt:

1. Continue Prozac as rx by PCP. Pt not interested in change/increase right now.
2. Read handout on increasing rewarding activities for mood management. Plan and do one enjoyable and one mastery activity per day; keep record on monitoring form.
3. Plan one social activity with friends each weekend.
4. On weekends get out of bed at 8 a.m. Eliminate naps.
5. F/u with BHC in 2 weeks.

Depression recommendations to PCP and team:

1. Encourage pt to follow plan above.
2. If sx do not improve in 6–8 wks discuss with pt whether modification in psychotropic meds is indicated.

Note. S/O = subjective and objective; PCP = primary care provider; Pt = patient; PCBH = primary care behavioral health; BHC = behavioral health care; OTC = over the counter; HPI = history of present illness; ETOH = ethyl alcohol; Hx = history; Sx = symptoms; Tx = treatment; OX4 = alert and oriented; BHM-20 = Behavioral Health Measure; PHQ-9 = Patient Health Questionnaire; A/P = assessment and plan; WF = White female; Rx = prescription; F/u = follow-up.

with the patient and recommendations the BHC would like them to incorporate into their care will need to be practical within that context.

ASSESSING PERFORMANCE ACROSS ALL SIX CORE COMPETENCY DIMENSIONS

Sometimes it can be challenging to assess the efficiency and effectiveness of BHC service delivery. In addition, over time, BHCs can start to slip back into a specialty mental health service delivery model. Using the Primary Care Behavioral Health Provider Adherence Questionnaire (PPAQ-2) is one way to assess BHC performance and how consistent it is with a PCBH model of service delivery. This measure can be used if BHCs are working in a PCBH model or a collaborative care management (CCM) model of service delivery (Beehler et al., 2020). The PPAQ-2 is a psychometrically sound measure with factor analyses demonstrating adequate fit with the data and acceptable to excellent composite reliabilities across five PCBH domains and five CCM domains. Validity was demonstrated by correlations between adherence scores and measures of clinic integration and barriers to fidelity (Beehler et al., 2020).

Primary Care Behavioral Health Domains (Items 1–42)

- *Clinical Scope and Interventions*: This domain refers to integrated care provider behaviors related to providing clinical services to patients, including the type and nature of interventions utilized.

- *Practice and Session Management*: This domain refers to integrated care provider behaviors that characterize their overall approach to integrated health care using a population-based model.

- *Referral Management and Care Continuity*: This domain refers to integrated care provider behaviors related to the types of referrals they accept from PCPs, as well as advice given to PCPs about referring to specialty mental health.

- *Consultation, Collaboration, and Interprofessional Communication*: This domain refers to integrated care provider behaviors related to communicating and collaborating with other members of the primary care team.

- *Prohibited*: This domain refers to integrated care provider behaviors that are inconsistent with the PCBH population-based model and more indicative of engagement in specialty mental health care. *These behaviors should be avoided.*

Collaborative Care Management Domains (Items 43–93)

- *Patient Identification*: This domain refers to integrated care provider behaviors related to proactively identifying patients for intervention and being receptive to referrals from the primary care team.

- *Patient Education, Self-Management Support, and Psychological Intervention*: This domain refers to integrated care provider behaviors related to providing care management clinical services to patients, including education, motivational enhancement, and related behavioral or psychological intervention.

- *Supervision and Care Coordination*: This domain refers to integrated care provider behaviors related to facilitating communication, care coordination, and treatment decision making between the primary care provider and supervising mental health prescriber.

- *Measurement-Based Care and Protocol Adherence*: This domain refers to integrated care provider behaviors related to using protocolized care procedures to engage in measurement-based care, including the use of standardized measures from baseline through follow-up.

- *Panel Management*: This domain refers to integrated care provider behaviors related to population-level monitoring and evaluation of patients who have received care management services.

This self-report instrument is completed by the BHC and/or care manager to assess adherence to key features of the service delivery models using a 5-point scale ranging from *never* to *always*. For those interested in using this measure or learning more about it, we recommend going to the Center for Integrated Healthcare (2022) website, where BHCs will find a self-report form, user guide, and toolkit that will further inform and assist in using the measure.

Additional Training

BHCs can pursue a variety of options to attain additional training. There are university and society certificates and continuing education programs that focus on helping providers improve the breadth and depth of their PCBH skills. Figure 2.8 details programs and professional societies that offer asynchronous and in-person training BHCs might find useful. We encourage BHCs to examine these offerings and determine if any are a good fit for improving their clinical acumen in integrated primary care.

SUMMARY

Working in a primary care medical setting can be a highly rewarding and positively challenging experience for a behavioral health provider. It is a setting that provides opportunities to contribute to the well-being of patients who might otherwise never use behavioral health care and to assist PCPs in delivering more effective behavioral health services.

Not all behavioral health providers are well suited for the primary care environment. This setting does not allow for time-intensive, long-term psychotherapy modalities or comprehensive psychological testing batteries. Behavioral health providers in primary care must accept working in a hierarchical system in which physicians have a higher position than nonphysicians. They must be willing and able to work as independent practitioners but also be part of a team. For those who are willing to work with these issues, however, the primary care environment can be a fulfilling work environment. Primary behavioral health care is a journey, and building a solid foundation to one's practice will help the BHC thrive and enjoy this unique application of behavioral health care knowledge and skills.

FIGURE 2.8. Additional Training (*continues*)

University of Massachusetts Certificate Course in Primary Care Behavioral Health (https://www.umassmed.edu/cipc/continuing-education/pcbh-certificate-course/)	"This course acknowledges the skills of specialty mental health clinicians and helps to translate prior knowledge and experience to the fast-paced, evidence-based, generalist culture of primary care. PCBH includes a range of topics from orientation to integrated behavioral health models, to specific health care issues like substance use and depression to cultural influences on health care. . . . The program consists of 22 pre-recorded e-learning modules that can be watched at any time and at your own pace; each takes about 1.5–2 hours to view and engage. PCBH is given four times each academic year, we collect completion data for CE/CME at the end of each session; you must finish the requirements of the course during the session you have registered for in order to receive CE/CME credit, you have access to all materials for one month after the semester deadline date." (paras. 1, 5–6)
University of Michigan Certificate in Integrated Behavioral Health and Primary Care (https://interprofessional.umich.edu/faculty/integrated-health-certificate-program/)	"This web-based interdisciplinary certificate is designed for clinicians—social workers, nurses, care managers, psychologists, and physicians—who deliver or plan to deliver integrated health services. Participants will gain assessment, intervention, and consultation skills; will learn how to apply these skills in the workplace; and will engage with a peer distance-learning community to practice new skills and share ideas." (para. 1) They offer a pediatric track, adult track, and combined pediatric adult track.
National Register of Health Service Psychologists (https://www.nationalregister.org/education-training/ihts/)	"The National Register created a training series to help position Health Service Psychologists as essential team members in integrated healthcare. There are 42 videos (more than 11 total hours) available on the National Register's continuing education site, CE.NationalRegister.org. These videos cover theory, models, and implementation as well as discussion of the medical, pharmacological, and psychosocial management of conditions that commonly present in integrated settings. Continuing education is awarded as the videos are completed. This training series includes a comprehensive review of clinical and administrative facets of integrated care: • **Key concepts** such as the behavioral healthcare consultation, the Triple Aim, reverse integration, and collaborating with medical personnel. • **Medical conditions** including hypertension, diabetes, cardiovascular disease, respiratory disease, arthritis, and obesity. • **Psychosocial conditions** including depression, ADHD, insomnia, chronic pain, trauma, and substance abuse. • **Healthcare overview** such as establishing and financing integrated care, EHRs and privacy, billing and coding." (paras. 1–6)

FIGURE 2.8. Additional Training (*continued*)

Society for Health Psychology (https://societyforhealthpsychology.org/training/integrated-primary-care-psychology-curriculum/)	"The course modules can be used/reviewed as a collection or separately depending on program needs or self-study participant interest. There are four foundation modules that set the stage for working in primary care. Eighteen topic modules related to specific patient behavioral health challenges and physical health conditions and the varied roles of integrated primary care psychologists along the prevention to intervention continuum, complete the curriculum. Each module includes PowerPoint lectures, notes, exercises, illustrative videos, resources, and references. Supplementary training manuals that elucidate key concepts and offer additional readings and resources accompany the modules. The curriculum was developed by a core group of nine primary care psychologists with vast experience working and training in integrated primary care. Some of the topic modules, such as working with older adults and managing chronic pain, were written by experts in particular subject areas in collaboration with the core team to ensure that they retained a foundation in primary care." (para. 2)
Collaborative Family Healthcare Association (https://www.cfha.net/about-us/)	"The Collaborative Family Healthcare Association (CFHA) is a multi-guild member association whose goal is to make integrated care the standard of care across the United States and beyond. For us, collaboration is not just a word in our name; it defines who we are, how we interact with each other and other organizations. We believe deeply that collaboration across professions is an essential element necessary for revisioning healthcare." (para. 1) Their annual conference offers a number of workshops and presentations focused on improving integrated behavioral health care skills. In addition, there is a Primary Care Behavioral Health Special Interest Group that offers year-round webinars.
Society of Behavioral Medicine (https://www.sbm.org/about)	"SBM is a nonprofit organization composed of researchers, clinicians, educators, industry professionals, and policy-makers from more than 20 healthcare disciplines. They focus on behavioral, psychosocial, environmental, and biomedical theory, knowledge, and interventions relevant to health and disease. SBM members conduct research on conditions such as cardiovascular diseases, respiratory diseases, obesity, diabetes, chronic pain, and cancer. They conduct research on specialty populations like children, women, veterans, aging adults, and minority groups. And they conduct research on clinical care and healthcare delivery, from in-person appointments to telemedicine and health apps. SBM members then use research findings to improve their own clinical practice and the lives of their patients. They also use research findings to improve public health policies and to make healthcare cheaper and fairer. They do this through individual work and in strategic partnerships with community groups, corporations, government entities, legislators, and other professional organizations." (paras. 3–5) There is an Integrated Primary Care Special Interest Group, which sponsors preconference and conference training on integrated behavioral health services.

Note. PCBH = primary care behavioral health; CE/CME = continuing education/continuing medical education; ADHD = attention-deficit/hyperactivity disorder; EHRs = electronic health records; SBM = Society of Behavioral Medicine.

3

Conducting the Initial and Follow-Up Consultation Appointments

In this chapter, we detail the steps to follow in an initial and follow-up consultation appointment. These include reviewing the electronic health record (EHR), using screening and assessment measures, introducing the behavioral health consultant (BHC) service to the patient, identifying and clarifying the problem for which the patient was referred, conducting a functional assessment of that problem, sharing a problem summary and formulation with the patient, suggesting change options, and starting the change plan. We presented the basic 5As structure in Figure I.1 in the introduction. Figure 3.1 illustrates how these steps fit into a 30-minute time frame. In this chapter, we focus on a general format for any initial and follow-up consultation. The chapters in Part II suggest additional material to cover in the initial consultation specific to a particular problem area.

FIGURE 3.1. Structure for the Initial Consultation Appointment Linked With the 5As

1. Introduction of behavioral health consultation service (1–2 minutes)	**Assess**
2. Identifying/clarifying consultation problem (10–60 seconds)	
3. Conducting a functional assessment of the problem (12–15 minutes)	
4. Summarizing your understanding of the problem (1–2 minutes)	
5. Listing possible change plan options (selling it; 1–2 minutes)	**Advise/Agree**
6. Starting a change plan (5–10 minutes)	**Assist**
7. Determine if a follow-up appointment is needed (30–60 seconds)	**Arrange**

https://doi.org/10.1037/0000380-004

Integrated Behavioral Health in Primary Care: Step-by-Step Guidance for Assessment and Intervention, Third Edition, by C. L. Hunter, J. L. Goodie, M. S. Oordt, and A. C. Dobmeyer

Throughout the book, we weave in the recurring thread of patient self-management. The majority of patient change, health care improvement, and health maintenance may be dependent on what the patient does outside of their medical appointments. Self-management broadly includes management or change in physical, social, emotional, cognitive, and environmental domains (Taylor et al., 2014). There is no universally accepted definition of self-management, but it generally includes a focus on providing education and information to patients on their problem presentation, collaboratively working with them on an individualized treatment plan, improving symptom self-monitoring skills, and developing strategies to support adherence to the plan (Lean et al., 2019). Self-management strategies have been found to effectively improve outcomes on a range of patient presentations from severe mental illness (Lean et al., 2019) to chronic medical conditions such as diabetes and asthma (Taylor et al., 2014). Self-management focus is consistent with shared decision making (see Introduction) and fits well with the primary care behavioral health model of service delivery.

REVIEWING CLINICAL DATA FROM THE EHR

Whenever possible the BHC should review the patient's EHR prior to seeing them. Most EHRs contain a wealth of information that will assist the BHC in understanding medical history, current treatments, and concerns. This can reduce the time needed for information collection during the assessment phase of an initial consultation; it also communicates to the patient that the BHC already knows something about their health status and is proactive and engaged. Helpful information in the EHR includes current and past medical and behavioral health conditions, treatment, and outcome; medication use; social and family history; preventive services; pain; weight; physical activity level; alcohol and tobacco use; over-the-counter medications; and depression, anxiety, and alcohol screening measure scores.

BHC SCREENING AND ASSESSMENT MEASURES

In addition to the population health screening measure approach discussed in Chapter 1, the BHC can also have patients complete appropriate primary care screening or assessment measures prior to the initial consultation appointment as well as at follow-up appointments. We discuss the use of global measures in Chapter 2. Global or problem-specific measures can be used at follow-up appointments as one source of objective information on change in patient symptoms, functioning, or quality of life. We have included screening and assessment measures for consideration in Chapters 4 through 16.

INTRODUCING THE BEHAVIORAL HEALTH CONSULTATION SERVICE

Patients are often unclear about what to expect when they see a BHC. Therefore, it is essential to provide the patient with information about what the BHC does early in the first encounter. In our experience, patients who do not have this information often have more difficulty answering questions, are more likely to believe the BHC is going to provide a service they cannot provide (e.g., specialty mental health services), and are more likely to feel uncertain about how the BHC is going to help them. Start the appointment by making the following clear to the patient:

- BHC profession and training,

- BHC role in the clinic,

- the amount of time the BHC will be spending with them during the appointment,

- who will have access to the information they discuss, and

- what the BHC is going to do to try to help them.

To assist with this process, we suggest providing an information sheet to patients that summarizes the information they are being told. Figure 3.2 is an example of an information sheet. The BHC might say the following:

> I'd like to begin by explaining who I am and what I do in the clinic. I'm a [psychologist, social worker, licensed professional counselor, etc.], and I work with primary care providers in situations where good health care involves paying attention to physical health, habits, behaviors, emotional health, and how these might interact with each other. This pamphlet describes my services in more detail, and you may want to read it over after our appointment today. Your provider has asked me to consult with you today. My job is to help you and your provider better address the problems you're having right now. To help the two of you do this, I'm going to spend about 30 minutes with you in a consultation appointment. During this time, I'd like to get a snapshot of your life and determine what's working well and what's not working so well. I'll take the information that you give me, and together you and I will come up with a plan to help you better manage what's going on. The plan might include things you try on your own, such as reading some self-help material or practicing various skills. Or we may decide to have you come back for follow-up appointments to help monitor your progress or to help you learn additional skills. We might also decide that you would benefit from seeing a more intensive specialty service. If that were the case, I would help your provider arrange that referral. I'm going to write a note that will go into your medical record, and I'm going to give your provider some feedback on the plan we come up with today. Do you have any questions about any of this before we begin?

If patients have questions, spend the time needed to make sure they understand the purposes of this service. It is important to allow at least a brief time for patients to ask any questions they have about the BHC role before starting, as this will help prevent misunderstanding and confusion later.

FIGURE 3.2. Behavioral Health Consultation Service

What Is the Behavioral Health Consultation Service?

The Behavioral Health Consultation Service offers assistance when habits, behaviors, stress, worry, or emotional concerns about physical or other life problems are interfering with a person's daily life and/or overall health. The behavioral health consultant (BHC) works with your primary care provider (PCP) to evaluate the mind–body–behavior connection and provide brief, solution-focused interventions.

The BHC has specialty training in the behavioral and cognitive management of health problems. Together, the BHC and your PCP can consider the physical, behavioral, and emotional aspects of your health concern and help determine a course of action that will work best for you.

What Kind of Health Concerns Do You See?

The BHC can help you reduce symptoms associated with various chronic medical conditions or help you cope better with these conditions. A few of these are *Headaches, Sleep, High Blood Pressure, Asthma, Diabetes, Obesity, Chronic Pain*, and *Irritable Bowel Syndrome*.

The BHC can help you and your PCP develop behavioral change plans for smoking cessation, weight loss, alcohol use, exercise, or other lifestyle modifications. The BHC can also help you and your PCP develop skills to effectively manage emotional or behavioral difficulties such as *Anger, Anxiety, Bereavement, Depression*, and *Stress*.

Who Is Eligible to Receive These Services?

The service is available to all patients within the Family Health Center as a part of good overall health care.

What Should I Expect When I See the BHC?

You can expect the BHC to ask you specific questions about your physical symptoms, the emotional concerns you are experiencing, your behaviors, and how all of these might be related. You can expect your appointments to last approximately 30 minutes and for the BHC to provide brief solution-focused assessment and intervention. You can also expect to be seen in this clinic and for the BHC to have a close working relationship with your PCP. Remember, you and your PCP remain in charge of your health care; the BHC's primary job is to help you and your PCP develop and implement the best integrated health care plan for you!

How Is This Service Different From Mental Health Services?

The services provided by the BHC are simply another part of your overall health care and are not specialty mental health care. Documentation of your appointment and recommendations from the BHC will be written in your medical record and shared with your medical provider(s). A separate mental health record will not be kept when you see the BHC.

Communications with your BHC may not be entirely confidential. Your BHC will make every effort to protect your privacy. However, like all providers, they may have to report information regarding child or spouse abuse or share information regarding those at risk of harming themselves or others.

The BHC does not provide traditional psychotherapy. If you request, or the BHC believes that you would benefit from specialty mental health services, the BHC will recommend that you and your PCP consider those services.

How Do I Schedule a Behavioral Health Consultant Appointment?

Discuss with your PCP the desire to access this service. If you and your provider agree this service would be helpful, call the Family Health Center at XXX-XXX-XXXX to schedule a BHC appointment.

We include recommended scripts and patient educational handouts throughout the book. These scripts and handouts are meant to serve as starting points. They can and should be altered so they best meet the needs and values of the patients coming to a given clinic. For ease of adaptation, the companion website to this book has the scripts and handouts available to download.

IDENTIFYING AND CLARIFYING THE CONSULTATION PROBLEM

After one has verbally introduced the BHC service, one should aim to rapidly reach agreement with the patient on the reason for the appointment. The BHC might say something such as the following: "[Medical provider's name] would like me to assist the two of you in better managing or targeting [referral reason]. Is that what you see as the main problem, or is it something different?" If they say yes and agree with the main problem focus for the appointment, then begin the functional assessment by saying something such as, "Okay, then I'd like to ask you several questions about [referral reason] to get a better understanding of what's involved." Then begin the functional assessment. If the answer is no, then ask the patient what they see as the main problem. This is important because primary care providers (PCPs) sometimes misunderstand what the patient considers the main problem, and sometimes the PCP and the patient disagree about the main problem. However, if one spends time assessing a problem the patient is not concerned about, they are likely to have an unproductive appointment.

Sometimes the BHC may encounter a patient that identifies multiple problems they would like to address. It is common for primary care patients to have more than one significant symptom or problem (Ee et al., 2020; Funderburk et al., 2013; Wallace et al., 2015). We suggest asking the patient which of their problems is most important to target at that appointment and focus the assessment on that problem first. Let the patient know there may be time to discuss the additional problem(s) if time allows, but if not, the patient and BHC would target the other problem(s) at a follow-up appointment. If the problem area assessed in the initial appointment differs from the referral problem, discuss with the PCP the rationale for focusing on a different area at that point in time and the plan to follow up on their referral concern.

CONDUCTING A FUNCTIONAL ASSESSMENT OF THE PROBLEM

After the introduction, the primary focus is information gathering. A common mistake made by behavioral health and medical providers when initially gathering information is overuse of ambiguous and open-ended questions. Although open-ended questions are certainly useful in specialty mental health care settings, time limitations make this strategy impractical as a primary way to gather information in primary care. Open-ended or ambiguous questions may elicit lengthy or ambiguous answers that may not provide much useful information. As such, BHCs may find themselves at the end of a 30-minute appointment without having obtained sufficient information from which to make recommendations or start an intervention.

Focused questions that are closed-ended or menu driven (e.g., providing patients with several choices to pick from when answering) allow the BHC to gather information needed to identify the primary problem, determine contributing factors, and make a diagnosis, if necessary, in a limited time frame. However, we recommend the use of open-ended questions once one thinks they have collected all the information they need to understand the patient's problem. For instance, one might say,

- Is there anything I haven't asked about that you think is important for me to know?

As time allows, one may also choose to ask the following:

- Take me through what a typical day (workday, if they work) looks like for you.

- What does your nonworkday look like?

Questions such as these can yield information one might not get by asking closed-ended or menu-driven questions, and sometimes that information can be valuable for understanding the factors related to that problem and for intervention planning.

Another common mistake involves the frequent use of empathic or reflective statements and restatement of what the patient has just said in a manner consistent with what is done in a traditional specialty mental health service. This is typically not necessary and can be an inefficient use of time. This manner of assessment and interaction can feel awkward to behavioral health providers first starting in primary care. That makes sense, as it is a different type of clinical behavior than they are used to doing. We are not saying one must be robotic in their assessment; one can still joke, laugh, and actively engage the patient and at the same time be very precise in their functional assessment of their current situation. Patients will know the BHC is listening by eye contact, head nods, and brief verbalizations (e.g., "uh huh"). Patients will also know the BHC has understood them when they hear the summary and conceptualization statement given after one has finished the functional assessment of the problem.

General areas to assess that can elicit more information on the primary referral problem include the nature of the referral problem; triggering events; duration, frequency, and intensity of the problem; factors that make the problem better or worse; functional impairment at home, work, or school; and their social environments, as well as changes in symptoms relevant to the presenting problem (e.g., sleep, energy, mood). Screening for suicidal or homicidal risk should be done at each encounter. Examples of closed-ended or menu-driven questions one might ask for each category, using depression as the example, are presented in Figure 3.3. Keep in mind that answers to some of the questions in Figure 3.3 might be obtained from reviewing the EHR prior to seeing the patient, thus eliminating the need to ask about them in the consultation, unless the information in the EHR is unclear or out of date. These examples demonstrate questions that are likely to get clinically rich information in a relatively short period of time; however, we are not suggesting that all of these questions should be or need to be asked of every patient. To demonstrate follow-up questions that might be asked, we have also included individual responses to some

FIGURE 3.3. Functional Assessment of the Problem (*continues*)

Examples of closed-ended or menu-type questions the behavioral health consultant (BHC) might ask in each category, using depression as the example.

1. **Nature of the referral problem** (the first question to ask after the introduction)
    BHC Question:
    - Dr. Smith would like me to assist the two of you to better manage your depressed mood. Is depressed mood what you see as the main problem, or is it something different?
    Patient Response: Yes, it's depression.
2. **Duration of the presenting problem**
    BHC Questions:
    - Is feeling depressed something that has been going on for the past 2 or 3 weeks, or has it been longer or shorter than that?
    - About how long ago was it that you first noticed you were feeling depressed?
    - How many months or weeks ago did you start to notice you were getting more depressed?
3. **Triggering events of the presenting problem**
    BHC Question:
    - Was there anything different going on in your life or anything that happened to trigger your depressed mood, or did it just seem to come out of the blue?
4. **Frequency and intensity of the presenting problem**
    BHC Questions:
    - How many times a day, week, or month would you say you feel depressed?
    - On a scale of 0 to 10, with 0 being not depressed at all and 10 being the most depressed you've ever felt in your life, what was your average level of depression over the past 2 weeks?
5. **Factors associated with the presenting problem getting better or worse**
    Physical (what is going on in the person's body): sleep, pain, blood pressure, blood glucose, etc.
    Emotional (how they feel): sad, happy, angry, worried, anxious, depressed, frustrated, stressed, etc.
    Behavioral (what do they do or not do): too much or too little activity, saying or not saying things, etc.
    Environmental/social (place, time of day, friends, family, coworkers): afternoon, when boss is there, etc.
    Cognitive (thoughts): what are they thinking in association with symptoms and/or poor functioning?
    BHC Questions:
    - Is there anything that you do or anything that happens that helps you feel less depressed?
    - Is there anything that you do or anything that happens that leads you to feel more depressed?
6. **Patient functional impairment**
    Changes in work performance
    BHC Question:
    - Have you noticed any changes in your ability to do your job as your depressed mood has gotten worse?

    Changes in work, friend, or social relationships
    BHC Questions:
    - Have you noticed changes in your work relationships as your depression has gotten worse?
    - Were there any changes in friend or social relationships just before or around the time your difficulties started?

    Changes in significant familial relationships (e.g., spouse, children)
    BHC Questions:
    - Were there any changes in family relationships just prior to or around the time your difficulties started?
    - Since you started getting depressed, has there been an impact on your relationships with your (spouse, children, friends)?

FIGURE 3.3. Functional Assessment of the Problem (*continues*)

Patient Response: Yes, with my wife.
BHC Question Based on Patient Response:
- What seems to be the biggest problem with your wife since you've been more depressed?

Changes in social activities (e.g., going out with friends, church)
BHC Question:
- Often people will decrease or stop their social activities when depressed. Has that happened to you?
Patient Response: Yes.
BHC Question Based on Patient Response:
- What have you cut back on or stopped?
Patient Response: Going to church and going to dinner with my wife.
BHC Question Based on Patient Response:
- Before your depression symptoms worsened, how often did you go to church and go out to dinner with your wife?

Changes in fun/recreational/relaxing/meaningful activities
BHC Question:
- Sometimes when people get depressed, they cut back or stop meaningful or enjoyable activities. Have you cut back or stopped enjoyable or meaningful activities?
Patient Response: Yes.
BHC Question Based on Patient Response:
- What have you cut back on or stopped?
Patient Response: Playing with the kids.
BHC Question Based on Patient Response:
- How often did you used to play with the kids?

Change in exercise
BHC Question:
- Do you exercise now?
Patient Response: No.
BHC Question Based on Patient Response:
- Have you exercised in the past?
Patient Response: Yes.
BHC Question Based on Patient Response:
- Have you stopped since you started feeling depressed?
Patient Response: Yes.
BHC Questions Based on Patient Response:
- What did you used to do and how many days a week did you do it?
- When you were exercising before, what benefits did you get from it?

7. **Changes in sleep, energy, concentration, appetite**
   BHC Question:
   - Are you sleeping about the same, more, or less than before you started getting depressed?
   Patient Response: Less.
   BHC Question Based on Patient Response:
   - Are you having trouble falling asleep, staying asleep, or both?
   Patient Response: Both.
   BHC Question Based on Patient Response:
   - Over the past 2 weeks, on average, how long does it take you to fall asleep?
   Patient Response: 2 hours.
   BHC Question Based on Patient Response:
   - Over the past 2 weeks, on average, how many times do you wake up at night?
   Patient Response: Three.
   BHC Question Based on Patient Response:
   - About how long does it take you to fall back to sleep?
   Patient Response: 45 minutes.
   BHC Questions Based on Patient Response:
   - Have you noticed a decrease in energy?
   - Has your ability to concentrate decreased?

FIGURE 3.3. Functional Assessment of the Problem (*continued*)

- Have you seen any increase or decrease in your appetite, or is it about the same as usual?
- Have you lost or gained any weight since you started getting depressed?

8. **Caffeine use**
   BHC Question:
   - Do you drink caffeinated drinks?
   Patient Response: Yes.
   BHC Question Based on Patient Response:
   - What kind: tea, coffee, soda?
   Patient Response: Coffee.
   BHC Question Based on Patient Response:
   - How many in a typical day?
   Patient Response: Two.
   BHC Question Based on Patient Response:
   - How many ounces in each drink?
   Patient: Twelve.

9. **Alcohol use**
   BHC Question:
   - Do you drink alcoholic drinks?
   Patient Response: Yes.
   BHC Question Based on Patient Response:
   - What kind: beer, wine, mixed drinks?
   Patient Response: Beer.
   BHC Question Based on Patient Response:
   - How many in a typical day, week, or month?
   Patient Response: Three a day.
   BHC Question Based on Patient Response:
   - How many ounces in each drink?
   Patient Response: 24.

10. **Medications or supplements**
    BHC Question:
    - Are you taking any prescribed or over-the-counter medications or supplements?
    Patient Response: Yes.
    BHC Question Based on Patient Response:
    - What are you taking, how much are you taking, and what are you taking it for?

11. **Mood over past 2 weeks**
    BHC Question:
    - Over the past 2 weeks would you describe your mood as down, sad, depressed, anxious, angry, frustrated, something different, or is it a combination of things?
    Patient Response: Sad and anxious.
    BHC Question Based on Patient Response:
    - How many days a week would you say you feel sad and anxious?
    Patient Response: Six.

12. **Suicide or homicide risk**
    BHC Questions:
    - In the past month have you had thoughts of killing yourself?
    - Have you ever tried to kill yourself?
    - In the past month have you had thoughts of harming or killing anyone else?
    - Have you ever tried to harm or kill anyone?

13. **Open-ended questions**
    BHC Questions:
    - Is there anything I haven't asked you about that you think is important for me to know?
    - [If time allows.] Take me through what a typical weekday is like for you from the time you get up to the time you go to bed.
    - Take me through what you typically do on the days you're not working or on the weekend.

questions as examples of what a patient might say. Answers to the questions under these content areas will allow one to get a reasonable understanding of the frequency, duration, and severity of the patient's symptoms and functional impairments. Responses will also shed light on what the patient is doing or not doing that might be related to their symptoms and poor functioning.

Another approach BHCs might find useful in assessing a patient's functioning and symptoms is the contextual interview detailed by Robinson et al. (2011) and Robinson (2019). This assessment strategy includes focused questions on life context (love, work, play, and health) and problem context (time, trigger, trajectory, and workability of current way of living). We encourage BHCs to review these works for additional information on the contextual interview.

SUMMARIZING AND CONCEPTUALIZING ONE'S UNDERSTANDING OF THE PROBLEM

Once the BHC has a working understanding of the patient's symptoms and functional impairments as well as the factors adding to, perpetuating, or driving the problem, provide a summary and formulation of the problem as one has understood it. In the brief formulation of the problem, one should discuss at least one biopsychosocial factor that appears to be causing or maintaining the problem. Ideally, the factors one highlights in the formulation should be factors over which the patient has some control. Describing these links in a formulation helps to build the rationale for suggested interventions. This vital step provides patients with an opportunity to clarify any key information one has missed or misunderstood. A summary and conceptual statement does not have to be 100% accurate to be effective; minor clarification by a patient is likely to help increase rapport and increase their confidence that the BHC has an accurate understanding of their problems. In addition, a summary and conceptualization provides a cue to patients that the BHC is moving on to the next stage of the appointment. This type of cue is important for effective time management. Skipping the summary and conceptualization can be problematic. First, patients may not be sure the BHC completely understands the problem. Second, they may think the BHC is still in the interview and information-gathering stage and continue to try to give the BHC information. It is helpful to communicate directly to patients that one is preparing to switch away from the information-gathering mode. For example, one might state the following:

> Let me stop here. I'd like to summarize my understanding of what you've told me to make sure I have it right. If I don't have it right or I've missed something important, I want you to tell me what I've missed. I have some specific suggestions I'd like to review with you in a moment that are based on my understanding of what you've told me. So it is important that I have it right, or my recommendation may be off target.
> Your experience of depression might be best understood as an interaction between physical factors, behaviors, emotions, thoughts, and your social envi-

ronment. This is what we call taking a biopsychosocial perspective, and doing this puts us in a better position to identify specific factors that contribute to your symptoms, functioning, and quality of life. In your case, it sounds like you've been depressed for the last 3 months associated with the death of your father and having your work time cut in half. You've noticed you're having more thoughts about what you missed out on with your father and if you are going to be able to support your family. Those thoughts lead you to feel depressed and worried; leave you not feeling motivated to engage in fun and valuable activities like going to church, going out to eat with your wife, and playing with your kids; and keep you from being able to fall asleep or back to sleep after waking. You feel exhausted every morning with low energy, and you're not sure what to change to get back to the old you. Does that sound right, or did I miss some things?

Once the BHC has finished their summary and formulation, ask the patient whether it was right or whether there is something that one missed. This invites the patient to correct misperceptions and add additional information that one may have missed.

LISTING POSSIBLE CHANGE PLAN OPTIONS

Once one is confident they have a good understanding of the problem, shift to discussing possible goals or areas of change. One might say something such as the following:

> I have some ideas about what you might focus on and things you might do differently that could decrease your symptoms and improve your functioning. I would like to tell you what those things are and how I think they might be helpful. Then you can tell me if you think you want to try one, some, or maybe none of the things I suggest. Or maybe you have some different ideas of what might be helpful to focus on. You might also want to discuss these options with friends, family members, or someone else before making a decision.

Once the BHC presents the options, ask whether any of those options sound like they might be helpful. Typically, patients will think one or several of the options will be useful. Asking which option(s) they see as the easiest can be a good place to start. If none of the options for change are of interest to the patient, it is important to address this ambivalence toward change before moving on. Chapter 4 of this book offers additional details on motivational enhancement strategies, including motivational interviewing (W. R. Miller & Rollnick, 2013; Rollnick et al., 2022), to use when patients are ambivalent about change.

Sometimes one might find at the end of the summary that patients are functioning well, given their limitations. In this case, the BHC's primary recommendations may involve letting them know they are doing a good job of managing their difficulties, encouraging them to continue what they are doing, discussing their prognosis or the course of symptoms to expect, and identifying red flags or symptoms that should trigger them to return to the BHC in the future.

STARTING A CHANGE PLAN

Once the BHC and the patient have mutually agreed on a change plan, briefly write the plan out. A *behavior prescription pad* can be a helpful tool for writing these recommendations (see Figure 3.4). Patients can use the written prescription as a reminder of the recommendations. In the following chapters, we present various forms and educational handouts the BHC can use for education and treatment interventions. During this phase, a BHC may also teach the patient a specific skill to practice and use as part of their plan. It can be helpful to ask if the patient sees any barriers in following the change plan (e.g., money, time, friends, family members) and to deal with those barriers before starting the plan. Before concluding the first appointment, one will need to determine whether a follow-up consultation appointment with the BHC would be useful to help assess the success of the plan or to teach additional skills. We recommend that this decision be made collaboratively with the patient. If one thinks it would be helpful to have a follow-up appointment to reinforce the intervention, to monitor progress, or to get a significant other (e.g., family member, friend) involved with the plan, one should make that recommendation. In addition, if one did not have time to start or complete

FIGURE 3.4. Behavioral Prescription (Rx) Pads

Behavioral Rx
Your Name Here

_____
_____
_____

Behavioral Health Consultation at the Family Health Center
XXX-XXX-XXXX

— —

Behavioral Rx
Your Name Here

Deep breathing: two times a day for 5 minutes at 10:00 a.m. and 5:00 p.m.

Cue-controlled relaxation:
   a) *External cue.* Take two to three slow breaths; let your shoulders drop when you look at your watch.
   b) *Internal cue.* Take two to three slow breaths; let your shoulders drop when you think, "I can't stand this."

Increasing valuable enjoyable activities:
   a) Read on Monday, Wednesday, and Friday at 7:00 p.m. for 30 minutes in the living room.
   b) Question distressing thinking.

Behavioral Health Consultation at the Family Health Center
XXX-XXX-XXXX

the intervention, a follow-up appointment will be needed. The BHC might say the following:

> We can go one of two ways here. Either way is fine with me, and I'd like to know what you think is best for you. We can set a follow-up appointment to help monitor how you're doing and discuss any problems you may be having, or you can try this on your own and follow up with me or Dr. Sullivan as needed.

Alternatively, the BHC might say the following:

> I'm glad you're willing to try out the plan we've developed. I think you'll begin to see improvements in how you're doing. But given how much this problem has been affecting you, I'd like to see you back in about 2 to 3 weeks to see how you're doing and whether we should change or add to the plan. Does that sound okay to you?

FOLLOW-UP APPOINTMENTS

The follow-up visit structure looks like this and also loosely follows the 5As, with some differences:

- Assess patient's adherence to the plan, reinforce successes, and address barriers.

- Assess changes in symptoms and functioning: Use standardized measures when feasible, assess changes in symptom intensity/severity/frequency, and assess changes in functioning in major life areas.

- Select and provide intervention (advise/agree/assist): Consider modifying/ improving the existing plan, teach new skills when appropriate (limit to one or two interventions), and end appointment when content has been covered (may be 15 or 20 minutes).

- Arrange follow-up:
  - When patient begins showing improvements in symptoms and/or functioning and a plan for continued improvement is in place, further BHC follow-up is not planned and care continues with the PCP, who may refer again if needed.
  - When patient is not benefiting from services or needs a higher level of care, recommend referral to a specialty behavioral health clinic.

- If patient has shown improvements on the focal problem but has an identified second problem, discuss whether to start a new episode of care focused on the second area.

In particular, the assess phase is more targeted, with a focus on assessment of progress and any changes in symptoms and functioning. Rather than 10 to 15 minutes, the assess phase of a follow-up appointment may just take a few minutes. From there, the BHC moves into shared decision making about the focus of the follow-up visit, such as what intervention/skill will be worked on. The BHC may want to again briefly share a biopsychosocial formulation to help the patient understand the rationale for the proposed intervention (advise/agree). The majority of the follow-up visit is usually spent providing the intervention (assist).

SUMMARY

Each stage of the first appointment is designed to accomplish a specific purpose. Shifting between stages within the 30-minute consult is like shifting gears on a car as one drives down the road. Each gear is distinct and allows one to travel a certain distance at a certain speed; one shifts when they want to go another speed. The amount of time one spends in each gear may vary depending on the terrain and how fast one wants to go. The same concept applies to the phases of the BHC consultation appointment and to the unique problems and interaction styles of each patient.

We have made multiple recommendations in this chapter for conducting the 30-minute initial consultation. We expect that one will adapt the steps of this plan to their unique setting and style. In Chapter 4, we describe the interventions that we have found to be most helpful to BHCs working in the fast-paced world of primary care. The following chapters conceptually flow from the model we have presented, with an emphasis on additional assessment questions, practice strategies, and specific interventions developed on the basis of evidence-based care and our own field experience.

4

Common Behavioral and Cognitive Interventions in Primary Care

Moving Out of the Specialty Mental Health Clinic

The American Psychological Association's competencies for psychological practice in primary care (McDaniel et al., 2014) highlight the importance of using current evidence-based interventions that are appropriate for primary care to treat health- and mental-health-related issues. Behavioral health consultants (BHCs) should "focus on patient self-care, symptom reduction, and functional improvement with interventions such as deep breathing, cue-controlled relaxation, cognitive disputation, sleep hygiene, stimulus control, increased exercise, problem solving, assertive communication, and disease management" (McDaniel et al., 2014, p. 421). To be successful in primary care, behavioral health providers must be skilled at providing interventions that can be implemented in appointments that are 30 minutes or less, that help patients begin to experience improvements in symptoms or functioning in a relatively brief course of care, and that can be supported by the primary care provider (PCP) once the BHC is no longer involved with direct care of the patient. Furthermore, providers must be able to deliver these interventions while maintaining empathy; respecting patient autonomy; and tailoring them to the clinical, personal, and cultural needs of each individual.

We have found that 11 interventions have been effective for addressing a wide variety of symptoms and functional impairments seen in primary care. The first group of interventions includes common behavioral interventions: (a) relaxation training, (b) mindfulness exercises, (c) goal setting, (d) cognitive disputation, and (e) acceptance and commitment techniques. The second group

https://doi.org/10.1037/0000380-005

Integrated Behavioral Health in Primary Care: Step-by-Step Guidance for Assessment and Intervention, Third Edition, by C. L. Hunter, J. L. Goodie, M. S. Oordt, and A. C. Dobmeyer

includes interventions that enhance motivation to change and adhere to treatment regimens: (f) motivation enhancement techniques, (g) problem solving, (h) self-monitoring, and (i) behavioral self-analysis. The last two interventions, (j) stimulus control and (k) assertive communication, are holistic interventions that can be important parts of the BHC's practice. These interventions were selected based on empirical evidence and their compatibility with a self-management model of care. Regarding empirical support, we looked for interventions that have been tested in multiple well-designed studies, have been found to be effective, and are of low risk to patients. Although research specific to integrated behavioral health care in the primary care setting is growing, it is still limited in many areas, which has required us to generalize and adapt these interventions to the fast-paced setting of primary care.

Consistent with the self-management model of care, we have selected those skill-based interventions that patients can apply and practice outside of the office setting. The time the patient spends with the BHC is viewed as a coaching appointment in which skills are first taught and then refined and monitored as needed. Patients are expected to practice the interventions on their own, and BHCs may use strategies to decrease barriers and increase motivation for home-based practice.

The intervention strategies we describe are not the only interventions that can or should be used in primary care settings. However, we believe that these interventions provide a foundation for the BHC practice in primary care. Experience in the primary care setting will allow BHCs to adapt their clinical training and experience to fit within this setting.

THE BHC TOOLKIT

We have found that the 11 interventions discussed in this chapter have been effective for addressing a wide variety of symptoms and functional impairments seen in primary care. We first describe the intervention and how it fits into the 5As model (i.e., assess, advise, agree, assist, arrange). Within the structure of the 5As, we describe how to present the intervention to a patient in plain, understandable language. For several of the interventions, handouts and worksheets are included and can also be downloaded from the American Psychological Association website (https://www.apa.org/pubs/books/integrated-behavioral-health-primary-care-third-edition). Part II of this volume focuses on how to apply these interventions to specific patient problems.

Relaxation Training

For decades, relaxation training has been one of the most used behavioral interventions because it can be quickly taught, is easily learned by many patients, and can have immediate effects on physiological arousal and symptoms (Kim & Kim, 2018; Park & Han, 2017; Perciavalle et al., 2017; F. Zhang et al., 2021). As such, it is applicable and versatile for use in primary care (Cully et al., 2010; Kaplun et al., 2021; Minen et al., 2020; Perciavalle et al., 2017; Posadzki & Ernst, 2011; Pourdowlat et al., 2019; Roy-Byrne et al., 2009). We believe relaxation skills are most effective when tailored to the individual.

Assess

A functional assessment of each patient's problem (see Chapter 3) is essential to determine contributing factors and to decide whether relaxation training is an appropriate intervention. Once its appropriateness has been established, further assessment of several factors will provide a basis for tailoring the intervention for optimal benefit. The following are suggested assessment questions:

- What do you do to relax (e.g., napping, television, reading, conversation, hobbies)?

- How often do you engage in these activities?

- How effective are these strategies for you?

- Have you ever been trained in relaxation techniques? If so, what have you been trained to do and when? How well did the relaxation techniques work for you?

- Do you currently practice any relaxation techniques? If so, how often? When?

- What are the primary barriers for you in using relaxation strategies?

- What are the common triggers that increase your stress?

- How do you think your stress response and your current problem are connected?

Advise

The findings from the assessment phase will shape what needs to be done in the advise phase. If the patient has relaxation strategies that have been effective in the past but are currently being neglected, it may be sufficient to establish a connection between relaxation and the patient's concerns and advise the patient to dedicate more time to these activities. Patients who are currently engaging only in recreational relaxation activities, such as reading, watching television, or participating in hobbies, might be advised to use more focused relaxation techniques that specifically target physiological arousal.

Some patients perceive themselves as being unable to relax despite efforts with numerous techniques and approaches. It is important that these concerns are heard in a nonjudgmental manner and advice on relaxation is presented in such a way that instills hope that change can occur. Relaxation should be presented as a skill that can be learned with sufficient training and practice. The following metaphor may be helpful:

> It sounds like your difficulties relaxing are similar to someone with no musical training trying to play the piano. They may sit down at a piano and try to pound out tunes, but it may never sound very good. And why would it? They have

never had lessons or practiced proper techniques to develop good skills. They may even feel frustrated that others have more natural musical talent and are self-taught. It's true that some people are natural musicians, but that doesn't mean the rest of us can't try to learn to play the old-fashioned way: with training and practice. I have worked with a lot of people who, like you, don't feel very skilled at relaxation. My experience is that most people can learn to improve their ability to relax if they work at it and consistently practice the right skills. Do you think you may be expecting relaxation to come more naturally than it does and, therefore, feel you can't do it? Are you interested in developing a plan to practice and improve your relaxation skills?

Agree

If the patient expresses interest, the BHC can move toward agreeing on relaxation-oriented goals. It is essential that the BHC and the patient reach mutually agreeable goals before moving on with the intervention. It may be tempting to rush into this step; however, a lack of acceptance from the patient will ultimately sabotage the treatment effectiveness in almost every case. If the patient does not express willingness to learn and use relaxation, go back to the assessment phase and further explore the barriers. If the patient cannot move past these obstacles, relaxation may not be the right treatment at this time and other options should be explored.

Assist

In this phase, the patient is ready to learn the behavioral skills of relaxation. Relaxation exercises fall into three primary categories: (a) breathing exercises, (b) muscle relaxation exercises, and (c) guided imagery. Patients can be taught either a single technique or multiple techniques that they can use in different situations. We recommend that the assist phase include instruction in the relaxation technique followed by practice of that technique during the appointment with the BHC coaching the patient through the exercise.

The use of a simple self-rating scale before and after the exercise can help a patient recognize acute changes that occur with relaxation and build confidence in their ability to effectively use relaxation techniques. This can be presented in the following way: "Before we start, I'd like you to rate your level of stress, anxiety, or tension on a 0-to-10-point scale. Let 10 represent high stress, anxiety, or tension; 0 means you are thoroughly and completely relaxed." At the completion of the relaxation exercise, the BHC can say, "Now rate your stress, anxiety, or tension level again using that 0-to-10 scale."

Verbally praise changes and highlight that the patient was able to bring about that change. Small reductions of one to two points in self-ratings can be framed as a good start, and the patient should be reminded that skills such as relaxation improve with regular and frequent practice. If the self-rating does not decrease or if it increases, the BHC can emphasize that this is normal for individuals at the beginning and that sometimes when they try too hard, their symptoms can get a little worse at first; practice is required to begin seeing benefits.

BHCs should develop their own style for instructing and coaching; however, the following scripts for each technique can provide a basic structure.

Deep (diaphragmatic) breathing. Breathing exercises focus on controlled respiration to induce the relaxation response (for the patient education handout, see Figure 4.1). Deep breathing is an easy-to-learn technique that can be a good first step for people who have never used relaxation exercises previously. The following script can be used to teach the technique:

> Let me explain to you what deep breathing is and how it might be useful. Deep breathing is using the muscles below your lungs to take in more oxygen than you normally would. This helps relax your nervous system and can lead to lower heart rate, lower blood pressure, and increased muscle relaxation. Let me show you what deep breathing looks like. [Demonstrate by putting one hand on your chest and one hand on your stomach and take two deep breaths by pushing your stomach out as you breathe in and letting it fall as you breathe out.] Did you notice how my bottom hand went up and down and my top hand was still? This is what it might look like if you are doing it correctly. For some people, both hands will go up at the same time, and this can work as well. You can breathe through your mouth or nose, whatever is most comfortable for you. Many people find this difficult when they first try, but it usually starts to feel more natural with practice. As you start to relax, you might notice a sense of heaviness, warmth, or floating. As we're going through this exercise, you may notice sounds inside and outside of the room you haven't noticed before or thoughts popping into your mind that distract you from the relaxation. This is normal. As a way to help you focus, you can repeat the words "calm" or "relax" to yourself silently each time you breathe out. You might also notice your heart beating or muscles twitching, which is nothing to be concerned about. Some people get dizzy when they first try this because their body has gotten used to running on a higher level of carbon dioxide, and suddenly providing more oxygen can temporarily disrupt the body and cause dizziness. Don't be alarmed if that happens; usually that dizziness goes away. If you're getting dizzy and feel like you are going to fall out of your chair, I want you to stop and practice at another time. When that happens, it is best to start with only a few deep breaths and work your way up to more as your body adapts. Do you have questions about what deep breathing is or how it might help?
>
> I'd like to walk you through about a 3-minute deep-breathing exercise. I'm going to look away from you as we do this so you don't feel like you're under a big magnifying glass. This usually makes it a little easier for people to do.
>
> So go ahead and place one hand on your chest and one hand on your stomach, and I will just walk you through this exercise. If you would like, you can lightly close your eyes as we go through the deep breathing. First, just notice your breathing. Don't try to change it just yet but notice the sound and feel of the air as you breathe in and the sound and the feel of the air as you breathe out. You might notice that the air is dry and cool as you inhale and a little warmer as you exhale. Remember to repeat silently to yourself the word you chose ("calm" or "relax") each time you breathe out as a way to help you focus. Continue to breathe slowly and easily at your own pace. You can start to shift the focus of your breathing so that, as you breathe in, it feels as if the air is going past your chest and filling your stomach. As your stomach moves out, hold it there for just a moment then let all the air leave your body at once. As you let the air out, you can allow yourself to feel more comfortable and more at ease. It might be helpful to imagine, as the air is leaving your body, that you're sinking deeper into the chair, getting more comfortable, and feeling more at ease. As you continue to breathe at your own pace, you can take three more comfortable, easy breaths, and as you exhale on the last breath, you can open your eyes and get adjusted to the light in the room.

FIGURE 4.1. Deep Breathing

What Is Deep Breathing?

Deep breathing involves using your diaphragm muscle to help bring about a state of physiological relaxation. The diaphragm is a large muscle that rests across the bottom of your rib cage. When you inhale, the diaphragm muscle drops, opening up space so air can come in. When watching someone do this, it looks like their stomach is filling with air. This type of breathing helps activate the part of your nervous system that controls relaxation. It can lead to decreased heart rate, blood pressure, decreased muscle tension, and overall feelings of relaxation.

Why Be Concerned With How I'm Breathing?

- To increase your awareness of the role that breathing plays in stress
- To lower your level of stress
- To give you a method of taking calm, relaxing breaths in order to break the cycle of stress

What Is the Best Way to Use Deep Breathing Exercises?

- Use deep breathing frequently.
- Take deep breaths at the first signs of stress, anxiety, physical tension, or symptoms.
- Schedule time for relaxation. My scheduled time for deep breathing will be: _____

Cue-controlled relaxation. Cue-controlled relaxation is a technique for associating a specific environmental cue or cues with the relaxation response (for a patient education handout, see Figure 4.2). The cue helps the individual remember to engage in relaxation exercises, developing a daily environment that promotes relaxation and stress relief. This strategy involves selecting a cue that patients will encounter frequently throughout their day. Each time the patient encounters this cue, they should engage in a brief relaxation-inducing behavior such as taking two deep relaxed breaths. Examples of cues include visual stimuli (e.g., looking at their watch, seeing small reminder notes that they have placed around the house or office), auditory stimuli (e.g., the phone ringing, a watch alarm at the top of each hour), and situational stimuli (e.g., getting into the car, sitting down at a desk). With repetition, the cue will become

FIGURE 4.2. Cue-Controlled Relaxation

Cue-controlled relaxation is a quick and easy relaxation technique.

- There are two different types of cues:
  - **External cues:** Things you hear, see, or do. Examples might include looking at your watch, ending a phone call, going to the bathroom, checking your email, hearing a tone or alarm from your cell phone or fitness device, or seeing something in your home or office.
  - **Internal cues:** Thoughts, emotions, or physical sensations. Examples might include feeling stressed, frustrated, anxious, or panicky or having thoughts about negative events.
- It is important that once you set your cue, you do the relaxed breathing every time the cue occurs so that being relaxed becomes more of an automatic habit.
- When the cue occurs, relax by
  - Taking a slow deep breath
  - Exhaling comfortably and easily
  - Saying a word to yourself as you exhale (e.g., "relax" or "calm")
- External cue: _____
- Internal cue: _____

associated with the relaxation response and will begin to automatically induce relaxation.

The following script can be a foundation for providing training in this technique:

> We can take the deep breathing you just learned and start to make it a habit so that you are relaxing throughout the day. We can do that with something called cue-controlled relaxation. A cue is a kind of reminder. Cue-controlled relaxation involves using that reminder to help you remember to take two to three slow deep breaths.
>
> There are two kinds of cues, external and internal. External cues are things you hear, see, or do. Examples of external cues might be looking at your watch, ending a phone call, going to the bathroom, checking your email, hearing a tone or alarm on your cell phone or fitness device, or seeing something in your home or office. A good external cue is something that occurs at least once or twice an hour. Internal cues are thoughts, emotions, or physical sensations. These don't necessarily happen once or twice an hour. In fact, they may not happen with regularity at all; however, they should occur in situations in which you would benefit from relaxation. Examples might include feeling angry, feeling your heart beating rapidly, or having thoughts about a specific problem. You might pick the first thing you're aware of when you are more distressed than you would like to be.
>
> The idea is to take something that is already occurring frequently in your daily life and use it as a reminder to take two to three slow deep breaths. By doing this, you help turn down the "volume" on any stress response that might have been building up and of which you were not aware. If you use external cues throughout the day, you will help keep yourself as physically relaxed as possible. Likewise, if you regularly relax as soon as you are aware of specific internal cues, you will be actively working to manage some of your high-risk situations. People commonly report that doing this can help them to feel less stressed or anxious, have better concentration, have more energy, and sleep better at night. I recommend that you identify and use both external and internal cues. What can you think of that you hear, see, or do once or twice an hour? You could also set an alarm on your phone to prompt you. Additionally, what would be good internal cues for you: a thought, an emotion, or a physical sensation?

Progressive muscle relaxation. Progressive muscle relaxation (PMR) is another relaxation technique that is easily adapted to the primary care setting. It involves the patient progressively tensing and relaxing muscles throughout the body. It generally takes more time to use this exercise compared with diaphragmatic breathing; therefore, it may be less convenient for a patient with a busy lifestyle. However, many patients report that it produces deeper relaxation. We recommend it be used as one of several techniques so that the patient has a variety of relaxation strategies to use in different settings.

PMR is typically conducted by isolating muscle groups (e.g., feet, calves, thighs, abdomen) for tensing and relaxing. The number of muscle groups used can vary. Given the time constraints of a primary care visit, we find it useful to train patients in using only four muscle groups: legs, arms, shoulder and abdomen, and face and neck. This shortens the time needed for training and for conducting the exercise. If a patient has difficulty getting relaxed using only four muscle groups, the BHC might expand this to eight or 16 groups. The following script can be used as a foundation for coaching this exercise:

> The technique I am going to help you learn is called progressive muscle relaxation. It involves tensing and relaxing muscle groups throughout your body to bring about a state of relaxation. As I ask you to tense your muscles, only tighten them enough to feel some tension—maybe a third to a half of their fully tense state. Make sure you don't strain yourself or hold your breath when you tense your muscles. The goal is to notice what the muscles feel like when they are tense so you can more fully relax them. I'll have you hold the tension for about 4 to 5 seconds and then ask you to relax. Focus on the sensations of letting go of the tension and study the feelings of the muscle being completely relaxed. We'll have you do that for about a minute before moving on to the next muscle group.
>
> Before we begin, get into a comfortable relaxation posture: feet on the floor, legs apart, neck straight, back against your chair, teeth slightly apart, eyes gently closed, and head upright. Take a few slow, deep, comfortable breaths. Breathe in deeply, hold for a moment, and exhale. As you breathe in, concentrate on the sound and feel of the air. As you exhale completely, notice the warmth of the air and silently say the word "calm" to yourself with each breath you let out. Take a few more slow, deep breaths. Be sure to exhale slowly and completely each time. Imagine your body becoming more relaxed and feeling heavier in your chair each time you exhale. [Pause.]
>
> Now we'll begin the progressive muscle relaxation. First, we'll start with your legs. Lift your legs slightly off the ground, tense your thighs, and flex your toes toward your head. Hold that position and feel the tension. Now let your legs drop to the ground and release all the tension at once. Notice the difference between the way your legs feel now when relaxed and how they felt when they were tense.
>
> Now we will move to your arms. With your palms facing the ceiling, make fists and raise your forearms, bringing your fists as close to your shoulders as you can while at the same time pressing your arms to your sides. Feel the tension in your fingers, hands, and arms. And now relax. As you relax you may notice your arms feel warm and heavy. Notice the difference between the relaxation and tension in your arms. Continue to breathe slowly and deeply.
>
> While your legs and arms remain relaxed, we will now move to your shoulders and stomach. Lift both shoulders as if you were trying to touch your ears with them and at the same time suck your stomach in as if someone were pushing on it. Feel the tightness and tension across both shoulders and in your stomach muscles and hold it. And now relax. Let your shoulders fall back down and enjoy the heaviness, warmth, and relaxation in your shoulders.
>
> Continue to breathe slowly and deeply, and scan your legs, arms, and shoulders, releasing any excess tension you notice. Focus on the sensation of relaxation in these areas. We'll now move to your face and neck. To tense your neck, press your chin to your chest or the back of your head to the back of your chair. While doing this, squint your eyes and slightly bring your back teeth together, tensing just enough to feel the muscles in your jaw. Notice the tension in your face and neck: Hold it. And now relax. Let all the tension go from your face and neck.
>
> Continue to breathe slowly and enjoy the relaxed feelings throughout your entire body. Scan your body from your head to your toes and notice what your muscles feel like. As you are doing this, take five more slow deep breaths at your own pace. After you exhale on the last breath, open your eyes.

Once patients have learned the techniques of PMR and have practiced them, introduce the use of the body scan component as a separate relaxation technique that can be used independently of a full PMR exercise. Once they have become more aware through PMR of how tense muscles feel, they can do a body scan by drawing their attention to each muscle group and letting go of any tension there without tensing the muscle first. This is useful in stressful situations in which the patient wants to relax their muscles without others noticing that they are doing so.

Guided imagery. Guided imagery exercises use mental pictures to induce relaxation. By bringing to mind images that already are associated with relaxation, the patient can reduce autonomic arousal when needed or desired. Using all five senses in the imagery will often enhance the relaxation experience. The following script can be used:

> Close your eyes and begin to relax. Breathe deeply and slowly and let your entire body feel relaxed and at ease. Now, imagine yourself at the back of a movie theatre. Picture a scene or a place that you associate with feeling relaxed and calm and imagine it on the screen at the front of the theatre. It can be a real place that you have been to or an imaginary place. Do you have a scene in your mind? Now imagine yourself moving closer and closer to the screen, and as you get closer, the picture becomes clearer and more vivid, almost as if you're in the image. Imagine that there are three steps right in front of the screen. Walk up the first, then the second, and now the third step. You are right in front of the screen and can see the image with perfect clarity. Now walk through the screen and put yourself in that image, not as if you were outside looking in, but actually in that place. [Pause.] Now look around you. Be aware of all the details of what you see. Notice the colors of everything around you, notice how vivid those colors are and areas of light and darkness. You might notice the various shades or textures and the intensity, softness, or brightness of the light. [Pause.] Be aware of the sounds you hear or don't hear in this place. Are the sounds close or far, loud or soft? [Pause.] Become aware of the smells. [Pause.] Notice the things that you can feel and the temperature of the air. [Pause.] Enjoy the sensation of being in this place where you can feel very, very relaxed. You can use any distracting, stressful, or anxious thoughts as reminders to easily travel back to this image and relax yourself. This can be your relaxation place, and you can come here whenever you wish.

Encourage the patient to practice imagery exercises daily to build the skills for relaxation and to manage daily stress. Advise the patient to use the same image every time so that it becomes a familiar, comfortable place that is associated with relaxation.

Following the practice of these relaxation techniques during the appointment, it is important to explore the patient's experience while doing the exercise and attempt to identify barriers or problems. Assist the patient in problem solving around these issues. For example, if they did not really try the exercise, explore that hesitancy and provide further education on the rationale for using relaxation. If they do not understand the technique, provide further training. Some patients will experience anxiety related to letting go or fearing they will be out of control if they release tension. Further exploration and questioning of thoughts contributing to this anxiety may be necessary before the patient is ready to use a relaxation technique. These patients may also benefit from progressive exposure to relaxation to allow them to get used to the sensations of a more relaxed state. This can be accomplished with various relaxation strategies that produce progressively deeper relaxation states. Start with coaching them in a relaxed posture. Once the patient is comfortable with that posture, teach them to take a few deep breaths. When the patient can tolerate that state, progress to deeper relaxation using muscle relaxation techniques or guided imagery. Some people will also not allow themselves to relax because they perceive the techniques to be a form of hypnosis or to be inconsistent with their religious or moral beliefs. Although relaxation is similar in some ways to meditation that is practiced by followers of most of the major religions, individuals may have concerns. These concerns can be explored, and misinformation (e.g., that relaxation will put them in a hypnotic trance) can be corrected. Religious and cultural beliefs should be respected and understood. It may be necessary to find alternative strategies for treatment if the patient has concerns based on their faith or culture.

Arrange

Once individuals have learned relaxation techniques, discuss potential times during their daily routine when relaxation can be scheduled. Encourage the patients to dedicate themselves to relaxing during this scheduled time. Many BHCs advise patients to use relaxation-based mobile applications to assist with relaxation practice. Applications such as Breathe2Relax (available from various app stores) allow users to record their stress level before and after relaxation practice and also use graphics and narration to assist with relaxation. We also advise arranging a follow-up appointment after 1 to 2 weeks. The purpose of this follow-up is to assess the effectiveness of relaxation on symptoms, identify problems associated with incorporating relaxation practice into the patient's lifestyle and schedule, and reinforce changes made. We highly recommend repeated coaching of the techniques in subsequent appointments to enhance their skills.

Mindfulness Exercises

Similar to relaxation exercises, mindfulness is a means of reducing arousal and emotional distress. Often patients present in the clinic hoping the BHC can help them eliminate symptoms or problems over which they can have little direct control. Mindfulness exercises allow the patient to focus on the present moment in an open way without judgment, thereby decreasing suffering and distress associated with overfocus on the past or worry about the future. With mindfulness, the individual observes thoughts and emotions rather than reacting to them. Mindfulness is associated with self-regulated behavior and positive emotional states, and an increase in mindfulness over time is related to declines in mood disturbance and stress (D. M. Davis & Hayes, 2011; Li & Bressington, 2019; Seshadri et al., 2021; Sundquist et al., 2015) and has been successfully applied to management of pain and reduction of opioid use (Cherkin et al., 2016; Garland et al., 2020, 2022; Hilton et al., 2017).

Assess

As with relaxation exercises, a functional analysis can be helpful to determine whether mindfulness exercises may be useful. Because mindfulness is directed toward the here and now, it can be particularly helpful when patients are experiencing anxiety about the future or distress about the past. Briefly exploring the nature of these anxieties can be an avenue for introducing the concept of mindfulness and its potential benefits:

- What types of issues do you get most concerned or worried about?

- How often does this anxiety occur?

- What triggers for worry or anxiety have you identified?

- What methods do you use to calm yourself?

- How effective are these strategies for you?

- How effective do you feel you are at pulling yourself back from worrying about what might happen to focus on the present moment?

The Five Facet Mindfulness Scale–Short Form (Bohlmeijer et al., 2011) can also be beneficial for assessing skills in mindfulness. This short assessment instrument has 24 items, which can be completed in about 5 minutes to help the BHC and patient identify where mindfulness can be focused to obtain the most benefit.

Advise

Individuals can often feel powerless to control worry and distress. Distressing emotions can spiral out of control as a person feels distress about the negative emotions they are experiencing, which in turn compounds the negativity. By advising them that skills can be learned to help them respond to emotional events in a way that is consistent with their personal/life goals and values, the BHC will be offering hope for breaking this cycle. A simple introduction such as the following is one approach:

> Would you be interested in learning a technique for responding in a more effective way to your distressing emotions? Rather than worrying about the future or dwelling on the past, you can learn to focus on the here and now and just observe, without reacting, to what you are experiencing. Some people find this unusual at first because they are so used to making judgments about things. However, you can learn to change that with a little practice. I think this could improve your confidence and skills in responding to your emotions in a way that is consistent with how you want to live your life. Would you be interested in trying this?

Agree

If the patient expresses interest, the BHC might suggest teaching a mindfulness exercise if they are willing to practice it at home daily. Suggest a 2-week trial of daily practice to allow time for them to develop the skill.

Assist

There are many approaches to mindfulness, and no single method is necessarily better than another. Some people are comfortable with the concept of meditation and will be open to trying a variety of mental exercises that fall under the umbrella of mindfulness. Other people are quite uncomfortable with these exercises and will easily dismiss them if they fall too far outside their comfort zone. Therefore, a simple set of instructions using straightforward language may be most acceptable to a broad range of people.

The following script is one such approach that helps the patient focus on their experiences of thoughts, feelings, and sensations in the present:

> Close your eyes and let whatever comes into your mind be there. Pay attention to whatever is in your awareness and observe it with curiosity and without judgment. Let things come and go as they happen. In your mind, label what you are experiencing: Are they thoughts? Are they feelings? Are they physical sensations? Are they smells? Maintain this observation of your experience for a couple of minutes.

Another approach is to guide the patient in focusing on their sensations in the here and now:

> Close your eyes and focus on your breathing. Take slow, deep breaths and feel the sensation of air coming into your lungs and back out. Notice the feeling of your lungs being full and then the feeling of them being empty. Take a few deep breaths and focus on those sensations. Now shift your attention to the sensations within your body as you sit in your chair. Notice your legs and your back against your chair. Feel the sensation of your arms resting in your lap. Feel the weight of your arms and your legs. Focus on those sensations for a few moments. Now shift your focus to the sounds you hear in the room. Pay attention to noises in the background that you might not ordinarily hear. Carefully study the details of those sounds as you focus on them for a few moments. Now return your attention to your breathing.

Arrange

Collaborate with the patient to identify times when one of these exercises can be used each day. If needed, arrange for a follow-up visit in 2 weeks to discuss how the mindfulness exercises are working and to address any problems experienced in practicing them.

Goal Setting

Patients often come to primary care with a complaint or concern; however, they often do not have a clear idea of how to address that problem. Others can articulate what changes they want but do not have appropriate and achievable goals relevant to those changes. In both of these situations, patients can benefit from focused assistance with goal setting to help attain improved health and well-being, especially if goals are difficult, set publicly, or group goals (Epton et al., 2017). Goal setting has been found to have a unique positive effect across a range of behaviors (Epton et al., 2017), including physical activity behavior (McEwan et al., 2016), weight management (Samdal et al., 2017), diabetes self-management (Fredrix et al., 2018), physical rehabilitation (Levack et al., 2016), and substance use disorders (Magill et al., 2022).

Assess

The assessment phase of goal setting involves identifying what the patient would like to change in their life. Questions for the assessment phase might include the following:

- What will it take for you to look back 1 month from now and say, "I'm glad I went to see that BHC?" In other words, what will have to change for you to feel this visit or series of visits was a success?

- If you were to change one thing in your life, and one thing only, what would it be?

- List five things you would like to see changed in your life. Rank order them from most important to least important.

Advise

Once general goals are identified, the BHC can advise the patient on their goals. The SMART acronym (specific, measurable, achievable, relevant, and time-bound) is a commonly used mnemonic device to highlight areas of importance when setting goals. Consider the following when discussing goals with patients:

- Are the goals well defined? Nonspecific goals are difficult to achieve. Patients can be encouraged to make general goals more specific to increase their chance of success. For example, if a patient's goal is "to be a better husband," advise him to specify behaviors he wants to engage in and make those his goals (e.g., criticize less, help bathe the children every evening, ask his wife about her day and spend time listening). A well-defined goal also allows progress to be measured. A goal to "eat better" can be defined as "eat five servings of fruits and vegetables daily" or "eat dessert only 1 day per week."

- Are the goals realistic and achievable? Those with unrealistic goals are setting themselves up for failure. Advise them to reframe the goals in realistic and achievable terms. For example, a goal to eliminate a 10-year chronic pain problem may be unrealistic, whereas a goal to reduce the number of pain-related sick days away from work might be more achievable. A goal to eliminate lifelong public-speaking anxiety may be unrealistic, whereas managing anxiety enough to give a sufficient and successful presentation may be reasonable.

- Are the goals within the patient's realm of control or influence? Goals that require someone or something besides the patient to change may be unrealistic. Examples of goals outside the patient's control may be presented as follows: "I want my boss to stop yelling at me" or "My mother is always telling me what to do; I'm a grown woman and she needs to let me live my own life." Advising the patient to refocus on goals that are within their control can help. In the first example, the patient might set a goal to be less upset when the boss yells or to find another job. In the second example, the patient might set a goal to be more assertive with her mother.

- Can the goals be broken down into subgoals that are more easily accomplished? Patients are most likely to succeed with small goals that have a high chance of success. If large goals can be broken down into small, achievable subgoals, the individual will likely be rewarded by short-term success and continue making progress toward the larger goal. For example, a goal to lose 50 pounds might best be broken down into subgoals of losing 5 pounds per month.

- Are the goals personally important to the patient or are there other factors driving the goal? Patients who do not have sufficient intrinsic motivation to make a change are not likely to succeed. Examples of this include individuals who try to stop smoking to please a spouse or who try to exercise more to satisfy a physician. These motives are not bad; however, they are likely to be insufficient to bring about success if the change is not also personally meaningful. Advice might include having the patient examine their own priorities and values related to the change.

- Are there more important goals that need to be addressed first? A patient may seek help from a behavioral health provider for a worthwhile goal; however, there may be other issues that should take priority. Safety issues such as domestic violence, suicide risk, or adherence to lifesaving medical treatment regimens may need to take precedence over other goals.

Agree, Assist, and Arrange

Once these issues are addressed, the BHC and patient should agree on a goal or set of goals. We recommend these be written down in specific behavioral terms with target dates and strategies for reaching them. This will ensure that both parties are in clear agreement about what they are working toward. The BHC can assist the patient in defining these goals, establishing subgoals, and determining realistic time frames. It is important, however, that the patient has a sense of ownership of the goals. At this point, you are ready to arrange the treatment plan for working on these goals.

Cognitive Disputation

Cognitive therapy can be a lengthy and complex endeavor unsuited to the primary care setting. At the same time, we believe there are cognitive disputation skills that are relatively easy for BHCs to apply in primary care. Cognitive disputation is adaptable to the brief interventions conducted in this environment, and empirical evidence shows the effectiveness of cognitive therapy for problems commonly presenting in primary care (J. K. Carpenter et al., 2018; Roy-Byrne et al., 2010). This section, therefore, is intended to help those who have cognitive therapy skills adapt those skills to primary care (for patient education handout, see Figure 4.3).

Assess

An assessment of a presenting problem should include exploration of contributing factors from a variety of sources. These include physiological, emotional, cognitive, behavioral, spiritual, social, and environmental components as well as the interaction between these elements. The cognitive component includes the thoughts and beliefs the patient holds that contribute to their physiological stress reaction, emotional distress, maladaptive or unhealthy behaviors, interpersonal conflict, problematic choices, and so forth. BHCs should attempt to identify these thoughts or beliefs as part of the assessment process.

A simple structure for assessing relevant cognitions in a brief primary care assessment is to listen for and explore three cognitive areas: (a) predictions, (b) expectations, and (c) evaluations.

FIGURE 4.3. How to Question Stressful, Angry, Anxious, and Depressed Thinking

1. Am I upsetting myself unnecessarily? How can I see this another way?
2. Is my thinking working for or against me? How could I view this in a less upsetting way?
3. What am I demanding must happen? What do I want or prefer, rather than need?
4. Am I making something too terrible? Is that awful? What would be so terrible about that?
5. Am I labeling a person? What is the action that I don't like?
6. What's untrue about my thoughts? How can I stick to the facts?
7. Am I using extreme language? What words might be more accurate?
8. Am I fortune telling or mind reading in a way that gets me upset or unhappy? What are the odds or chance that it will really turn out the way I'm thinking or imagining?
9. What are my options in this situation? How would I like to respond?
10. What are more moderate, helpful, or realistic statements to replace the upsetting ones?
11. Have I had any experiences that show that this thought might not be completely true?
12. If my best friend or someone I loved had this thought, what would I tell them?
13. If someone I cared about knew I was thinking this thought, what would they say to me?
14. Are there strengths in me or positives in the situation that I am ignoring?
15. When I am not feeling this way, do I think about this situation any differently? How?
16. Have I been in this type of situation before? What happened? What have I learned from prior experiences that could help me now?
17. Five years from now, if I look back on this situation, will I look at it any differently? Will I focus on any different part of my experience?
18. Am I blaming myself for something over which I do not have complete control?

Predictions.

- What negative events or circumstances does the patient anticipate or worry about?

- How convinced is the patient that their prediction will occur?

- Are there facts to support the prediction?

- What is the patient's belief about their ability to tolerate or cope with the predicted event?

Expectations.

- How does the current situation conflict with what the patient believes should be happening?

- How rigid or flexible are the patient's expectations about others' behavior or their own behavior?

Evaluations.

- Is the patient using emotionally loaded or exaggerated language in evaluations of situations or people that may be contributing to the distress (e.g., disaster, terrible, horrible, awful, unbelievable, unbearable, miserable, intolerable)?

Advise

Once the cognitive distortions or unhelpful thinking patterns that are contributing to the patient's problem are identified, the patient may benefit from evaluating the role these thoughts may play in their problem. Recommend that they focus on these thoughts and beliefs as part of the treatment plan.

Agree

The patient's receptivity in the advise phase can help the BHC determine where to go with this next phase. Those who are receptive to the potential role of their thought processes in their problems and who express a willingness to engage in this aspect of treatment are most likely to benefit from a primary care level of intervention. We recommend that those with little understanding of or receptivity for the role their thoughts play in their current problems may be better suited for traditional psychotherapy, where more time can be dedicated to establishing rapport, overcoming barriers to change, and addressing issues more pressing for the patient. However, those who express eagerness or openness to learn more might be appropriate for a brief cognitive disputation intervention in primary care, and an agreement can be established for this plan. Alternatively, focusing on concrete behavioral interventions may be the best option.

Assist

We suggest a stepped approach when helping people learn to question their thoughts. In our experience, Step 1 is a basic way to help people learn to notice and question their thinking, and, frequently, we will start here. Step 2 is often used when Step 1 fails to achieve the objective for which it is being used. It is also used when the patient might benefit from a more specific, directed way of questioning their thinking.

Step 1: Basic. The goal of this step is to help patients learn to respond to situations in ways consistent with their values instead of reacting to their initial thoughts. Patients can identify these thoughts that are not helpful and change them or use their value system to help them think and respond in a useful manner even if they are unable to change or alter the initial way of thinking.

The following script is one example of how to teach patients to examine and question unhelpful thinking in the primary care setting. The idea is to let them know they can manage distress differently by questioning how their thoughts are working or not working for them.

> Often when people get stressed, anxious, or depressed, their minds will tell them all kinds of things that can make them more distressed than they would like to be. You can't stop your mind from talking to you, that's its job; however, you can improve your skills for recognizing what your mind is telling you and step back from those thoughts to ask yourself how useful they are. The idea here is to increase your ability to choose how you want to respond to situations instead of just reacting automatically. Questioning your thoughts gives you the opportunity to respond in a manner consistent with your values and with how you want to represent yourself to others. This can allow you to turn the volume down on any distressing responses you might be having. This does not mean you will think happy or positive thoughts that will make everything better. It is beneficial, however, to be able to look at your initial thinking and determine if it is helpful, useful, and/or accurate and ask yourself how you would need to think differently to change how you feel.
>
> Questioning your thoughts is a skill that you can learn and get better at with practice. Look at this list of 18 groups of questions [see Figure 4.3] and when you come to one that really jumps off the page as something that would be good to ask or tell yourself, tell me what it is.

Once the patient finds a question or statement they think might work, say,

> If you were to ask or tell yourself that, how do you think it would be helpful? What would it allow you to do?

Typically, patients say it would allow them to look at the situation in a different, less extreme way.

> So, by asking or telling yourself that, it can interrupt how you typically think and react to situations, help you look at the big picture, and decide how you want to respond instead of reacting, and you can start to change your thinking so it works for you instead of against you.

Step 2: Advanced. This component, which is more like traditional cognitive therapy, is geared toward helping the patient identify faulty ways of thinking. It can help patients learn how their thoughts affect them physically, emotionally, and behaviorally and how they can develop more accurate, evidence-based ways of thinking that can change physical, emotional, and behavioral responses.

Several patient handouts are provided for Step 2 to introduce cognitive therapy concepts to patients in an educational format and get them started recognizing and disputing dysfunctional thoughts. These include suggested questions for identifying cognitive distortions (Figure 4.3), descriptions of common patterns of unhealthy thinking (Figure 4.4), and a cognition monitoring form (Figure 4.5). In our experience, cognitive disputation, including identifying thinking mistakes and evaluating evidence for and against beliefs, can be effectively delivered in 30-minute appointments. Cognitive disputation helps patients distance themselves from their thinking and develop skills to respond instead of react to their initial thoughts.

Arrange

Following the presentation and discussion of these questions or statements, a follow-up appointment should be arranged to determine whether additional help with questioning unhelpful thoughts is needed, and if so, whether further learning and practice is sufficient or a referral for traditional cognitive therapy is indicated.

FIGURE 4.4. Thinking Mistakes That Increase Stress, Anger, Depression, Anxiety, and Worry

All-or-Nothing Thinking: You see things as either all one thing or all another, with no room for anything in between. *"I'm 100% healthy or I must have a fatal disease."*

Jumping to Conclusions: You make a negative interpretation even though there are no definite facts that convincingly support your conclusion. *"My husband is late because he is in a car accident injured on the side of the road."*

Fortune Telling: You anticipate things will turn out badly and are convinced the prediction is a fact. *"Not getting this job will cause us to lose the house."*

Should Statements: "Musts" and "oughts" are also offenders. Emotional consequences can include anxiety and anger. *"I should be able to handle this."*

Overgeneralization: Assuming one event is actually a pattern. *"My hand is a little shaky today; I must have Parkinson's disease."*

Disqualifying the Positive: Filtering out or rejecting positive experiences to maintain negative beliefs. Upon hearing that your spouse has checked all the doors and windows and they are all locked, you think, *"But someone could cut out a piece of glass and open the window."*

Catastrophizing: Predicting the worst possible outcome imaginable. "Terrible," "awful," "horrible," and "worst ever" might be key words. *"If I can't get my heart to stop pounding, I'm going to die."*

Superstitious Thinking: The thought that something you do prevents something awful from happening. *"Telling my spouse to be careful before going to work will prevent her from getting in a wreck. I do it every morning and she hasn't gotten in a wreck yet."*

Emotional Reasoning: The belief that because you feel a certain way means that the assumptions and associations you have with that feeling are true. *"The fear, doom, and constant anxiety must mean something is seriously wrong with me."*

FIGURE 4.5. Disputing/Challenging Thoughts and Beliefs

Activating event (What happened?)	Consequences (How did I get myself to respond?)	Thoughts/beliefs (What am I telling myself? What thinking mistake am I making?)	Evidence for thoughts/beliefs/self-talk	Evidence against thoughts/beliefs/self-talk	What different thoughts can I have based on the evidence for and against my original way of thinking?	How did or might my responses change with my new way of thinking?
	Physically (What are my body responses?)					Physically (What are my new body responses?)
	Emotionally (How do I feel?)					Emotionally (How do I feel?)
	Behaviorally (What did I do?)					Behaviorally (What did I do?)

Acceptance and Commitment Therapy Techniques

Acceptance and commitment therapy (ACT) and the brief form of this treatment approach, called focused ACT, emphasizes the use of acceptance, mindfulness, commitment, and behavior change strategies to enhance psychological flexibility and promote living life in a manner that is consistent with one's values (Hayes, 2016; Strosahl et al., 2012). Patients learn skills for accepting the experiences and circumstances that they cannot control. They also learn to see their emotions as appropriate reactions to situations and come to understand that these experiences and internal responses do not need to impede them from moving forward in their lives and achieving goals. Acceptance-based interventions may also include components to increase planned actions that are aligned with a patient's core values. These approaches help patients move in valued directions despite the presence of continued unwanted symptoms, which sometimes cannot be eliminated from life experience. ACT is clinically effective for a range of psychological and somatic outcomes, including depression, anxiety, addictions, chronic pain, tinnitus, and stress (A-Tjak et al., 2015; Bai et al., 2020; Hughes et al., 2017; Öst, 2014; Thompson et al., 2021). For the primary care context, focused ACT interventions (often administered in group formats) have been found to have efficacy for improving psychological and physical functioning as well as health-related quality of life (Glover et al., 2016; Kanzler et al., 2022; Majumdar & Morris, 2019; Vasiliou et al., 2021; Wynne et al., 2019). Practitioners of ACT should have training in the theory and techniques of this approach, which are beyond the scope of this book. Numerous resources are available (see Luoma et al., 2007, and https://www.contextualscience.org/). This section is intended to help clinicians already trained in ACT to apply it in the primary care setting. Readers may also find Strosahl et al.'s (2012) book, *Brief Interventions for Radical Change*, helpful as the authors describe multiple ACT-based interventions that are brief and appropriate for primary care settings.

Assess

A brief acceptance-focused intervention may be useful for many issues that present in primary care. The Acceptance and Avoidance Questionnaire, Version 2 (Bond et al., 2011), is a commonly used tool that assesses a person's experiential avoidance and immobility as well as acceptance and action. The items are rated on a 7-point Likert-type scale, and high scores indicate greater experiential avoidance and immobility, whereas low scores reflect greater acceptance and action. The Acceptance and Avoidance Questionnaire can be used as a pre/post measure to help assess the impact of acceptance-based interventions.

Advise

Individuals often believe they must resolve a situation, symptom, or struggle before they can move forward in their life. They can feel stuck when life circumstances are outside their control. This is sometimes why they seek professional therapy or counseling. Optimism for change can be increased by advising them that there are effective strategies for taking action toward what they value most in life even though they may be experiencing distress. An introduction such as the following is suggested:

> It sounds like you are struggling with how these challenges are interfering with how you want to live your life, and at the same time, you feel they are part of your life now and can't be changed. Often people believe they need to eliminate certain difficulties before they can take concrete steps to move forward toward doing what they value most, but that is not always the best approach. Would you be interested in working on moving toward some of the goals you have despite the difficulties you are having?

If the patient answers yes, continue with the following:

> The thoughts, emotions, memories, and discomfort you have are often appropriate reactions. When you learn to be less judgmental about these reactions, you won't dwell on them so much and you can allow yourself to do the things you value, even though those internal experiences are still there. Essentially, you can come to accept them so they don't have so much control over you. Some people find this approach to be very helpful, especially when life has given them some challenges that they cannot control. This doesn't mean being passive about every bad circumstance, but it can help you to deal with some of your challenges and focus on living your life consistent with your values. Would you be interested in learning more about this approach?

Agree

If the patient expresses interest, collaborate to identify one specific behavior goal that would move them toward living the life they want to live. The BHC and the patient can agree to work together over a couple of follow-up visits.

Assist

Tell them that you would like to start by teaching them a mindfulness exercise (see the previous section) for them to practice at home daily. Suggest a 2-week trial of daily practice to allow time for them to develop the skill. During the follow-up visit, ask how the mindfulness exercise practice has been going and address any difficulties. Next, talk through the steps the patient may take toward their goal. Talk through barriers to achieving the goals using ACT principles and approaches (Luoma et al., 2007). Examples might include helping them to stay in the here and now; recognizing judgments about internal experiences and encouraging nonjudgmental acceptance of thoughts, feelings, memories, and experiences; and reinforcing committed action toward valued goals.

Arrange

Set another follow-up appointment in 2 weeks to assess progress toward the goal the patient has set for themselves. Review the ACT principles already discussed. Encourage continued use of the mindfulness exercises.

Enhancing Motivation to Change and Adhere to Treatment Regimens: Motivation Enhancement Techniques, Problem Solving, Self-Monitoring, and Behavioral Self-Analysis

Poor adherence to medical treatments or lifestyle-change recommendations is often attributed to negative characteristics of the individual; they are seen as lazy, stubborn, unmotivated, unconcerned for their own health, and so forth. Many times, however, there are contingencies operating independently of personality characteristics and, fortunately, many of these are modifiable. Thus, BHCs can play an important role in identifying factors contributing to inadequate follow-through on recommended changes and work with individuals to improve confidence in making behavioral changes, stressing the importance of those changes and related medical outcomes (DiMatteo et al., 2002).

We have found that four interventions are particularly useful in this situation: (a) motivational enhancement techniques, (b) problem solving, (c) self-monitoring, and (d) behavioral self-analysis. In this section, we apply the 5As model to motivation and adherence in general by discussing factors that often contribute to medical adherence, and we suggest questions to ask to help determine which factors are relevant to a particular patient. Following this, we describe how each of the four interventions can assist the patient to follow through with treatment recommendations.

Assess
The reasons for nonadherence can be numerous. Examples include overly complex treatment, insufficient communication by the health care provider, poor understanding by the patient, lack of treatment coordination, patient beliefs, a range of psychosocial factors, and medication side effects. In addition, patients are sometimes not motivated to adhere to their treatment regimens because they do not believe the treatment will help, they are not confident they can successfully follow the medical advice, or they feel that the health problem is not a high priority for them. The readiness-to-change ruler, discussed later and in Figure 4.6, can be a useful tool for assessing both the patient's confidence level for making changes and the level of importance the patient assigns to making the change. When a patient feels the behavior change is important but their confidence is low, a skills training approach may be most helpful, whereas when the importance is low and confidence is high, it may be necessary to use motivational enhancement strategies before starting on any behavior change. The following questions also can help to assess factors that may be affecting individual follow-through on change or adherence to treatment recommendations.

Complexity of the patient's treatment regimen.

- Is the treatment easy, medium, or hard for you to carry out?

- What are some of the challenges it poses for you?

- Do you ever get confused or mixed up about what you are supposed to do?

- What do you do to help keep it straight?

Communication between PCPs and patients.

- How is your relationship with your doctor?

- Are there things your doctor says that you don't understand?

- Are there cultural, ethnic, or gender issues that your provider does not understand or consider in your health care?

- Do you feel like they listen to your concerns?

- Are you getting answers to your questions?

- Do you feel you have input into the medical decisions that are being made?

Patient's understanding of the treatment and its relationship to the medical problem.

- Tell me what your doctor wants you to do, and be specific.

- How often are you supposed to take your medication? How much? At what time of day?

- What is your medication supposed to do for you?

- Why does your doctor want you to change your habits (e.g., eating, exercise, smoking, drinking, sleeping)?

- Why do you think your doctor wants you to see a BHC?

Coordination of how and when treatment is administered.

- Are you able to get medical appointments at times that are convenient for you?

- Do work or family responsibilities get in the way of following your treatment regimen?

Inaccurate beliefs and unrealistic expectations about treatment.

- What do you anticipate will be the worst part of following your treatment?

- What do you worry about regarding the treatment?

- Do you know anyone who has used this treatment before? What did they say?

- What do you think the result of this treatment will be?

Social/cultural factors that serve as barriers to effective disease management.

- Are there any cultural or religious issues that are relevant to what your doctor has recommended?

- Does the medication or treatment cause a financial strain?

- Do you have transportation problems that get in the way of receiving health care you need?

- How does your family feel about your health problems and the recommended treatment?

- How do your family members and friends help you make changes (e.g., eat better, exercise, drink less, avoid tobacco use)? What do they do that is not helpful?

- Does your living environment/community support a healthy lifestyle (e.g., safety in exercising outdoors, access to healthy foods)? What are your concerns?

- Do you experience discrimination in ways that affect your health or health care?

- Are there any ways in which your medical treatment interferes with your work? Are there ways that people at work support you? What do they do that is not helpful?

- How do you think this treatment or lifestyle change will affect your social life or intimate relationships?

Medication side effects.

- What side effects do you experience from your medications or treatments?

- On a scale from 0 to 10, how bad are the side effects, with 0 being *no side effects* and 10 being *severe side effects*?

- Do the side effects make it hard for you to take the medicines?

Motivational factors.

- How satisfied are you with your health right now?

- How important is it to you to manage your health problem better?

- How confident are you that you will do something that will improve your health?

- How confident are you that what your doctor recommended will help bring about the change you desire?

- Is there something going on in your life right now that is more important to you than your health, something you are more focused on?

Advise

Once factors have been identified that may be interfering with treatment adherence or lifestyle change, summarize these with the patient. Taking time to truly understand the patient's experience and express empathy is highly important for building trust and rapport necessary for successful intervention. Discuss how difficult it would be for anyone to adhere to a doctor's recommendation when there are significant barriers. Communicate to the patient that you recognize them as the expert on their own life experience and you will need them to help you understand these issues. Advise the patient that treatment will involve working collaboratively on managing or overcoming these difficulties.

Agree

Attempt to reach an agreement about which factors will be worked on together. In discussing this, you might consider which factors are most important to the patient, which are within the patient's control, and which will most likely result in improved adherence.

Assist

Four strategies are reviewed here for assisting patients with treatment adherence within a primary care visit. Again, these are (a) motivation enhancement techniques, (b) problem solving, (c) self-monitoring, and (d) behavioral self-analysis.

Motivation enhancement techniques. Change is difficult for all of us. Obstacles to changing health-related behavior can be internal (e.g., cognitions, emotions, learned habits) and external (e.g., environmental cues, reinforcement and punishment, social conditions). Behavioral health providers typically encounter some level of resistance to change when helping patients, regardless of whether the individual has never contemplated making the change, is ambivalent about change, or is expressing high motivation but has yet to alter their behavior. Motivation enhancement techniques have been developed and used effectively by clinicians for many years to bolster patients' readiness to change and to address obstacles along the way. By maintaining empathy and understanding for where patients are in their readiness to make changes, respecting their decision-making autonomy, and assuming a collaborative role alongside the patient, clinicians can play a meaningful role in a patient's journey toward better health and well-being.

One of the most used and well-researched approaches to motivational enhancement is motivational interviewing (MI). MI strategies help people recognize problems and resolve ambivalence toward health behavior change (Rollnick et al., 2022). Through MI, the BHC or PCP attempts to elicit self-motivational statements that reflect an underlying desire of the patient to change. MI strategies are neither coercive nor confrontational; rather, strategies involve open-ended questions, reflective listening, affirmation, and summarizing to help the patient evaluate the pros and cons of change. When signs of resistance to change are observed, the skilled motivational interviewer attempts to accept the resistance rather than confronting it head on. The scope of this volume does not permit a thorough overview of MI strategies; interested readers should consult Rollnick et al. (2022) for further information and evidence supporting this approach. Various strategies from MI can be useful for helping patients address intrapersonal obstacles to medical adherence and lifestyle change (D'Amico et al., 2018; Lindson-Hawley et al., 2015; Rollnick et al., 2022). Three useful strategies to enhance motivation based on MI techniques are examining readiness to change: importance of change, self-efficacy of change (the confidence a patient has that they can change), and the pros and cons of change.

Patients must be ready to change before they will put the time and effort into altering how they think or what they do. Assessing readiness can provide information that can help improve readiness or motivation to change. One way to assess readiness is with the use of a simple readiness-to-change ruler (see Figure 4.6), followed up with questions such as, "A rating of 0 would indicate you are not at all ready to change. A rating of 10 would suggest you are completely ready to change. You rated yourself as a 5. Why are you at a 5 and not a lower number?" "Right now, you are at a 5. What would have to happen or change for the number to be one or two points higher?"

In their responses, patients may articulate strengths of which they had been previously unaware or identify barriers they had not discussed before. You can then build on those strengths and help eliminate the barriers to increase motivation to change. In addition to being ready to change, patients also need to see the change as important and have confidence that they can do what is necessary to attain the objectives. Assessing importance and confidence (see Figure 4.6) and engaging in additional assessment of these areas when rated as low can help decrease ambivalence about changing. Follow-up questions such as the following might be asked: "What would have to happen or change for this to be more important? What keeps you from moving up to a higher number on the importance scale?"

It can be helpful for some patients to discuss or view the specific pros and cons of making a change. Do this verbally or use the cost–benefit analysis table in Figure 4.6. It has frequently been our experience that patients who are ambivalent about making changes experience decreases in ambivalence after expressly listing the benefits and costs of change. The patients, rather than the BHC, make the argument for why it would be in their best interest to change. However, if the costs outnumber the benefits of change, it could be that change is not in the best interest of the patient at the time. This exercise can also provide the opportunity to review possible benefits of change that the patient was not aware existed. BHCs should also be mindful that not all individuals have a strong internal locus of control and may have difficulty engaging in this task.

Problem solving. Often, patients understand the factors that interfere with medical adherence but have poor problem-solving skills. Therefore, they are unable to address these factors in a productive way. Teaching a simple problem-solving strategy and working together can help patients address target problems as well as equip them with a skill that can help them in other aspects of their lives. Studies have found problem-solving training to be effective for

FIGURE 4.6. Strategies to Improve Motivation to Change

Readiness-to-Change Ruler

At this moment what number best reflects how ready you are to _____?

0	1	2	3	4	5	6	7	8	9	10

Not Ready   *Unsure*   *Ready*

Importance and Confidence in Change

How important is it that you _____?

0	1	2	3	4	5	6	7	8	9	10

Not at all   *Most important*

How confident are you that you can _____?

0	1	2	3	4	5	6	7	8	9	10

Not at all   *Most confident*

Decisional Balance

Benefits of Changing	Costs of Changing

improving common mental health problems (Bell & D'Zurilla, 2009) and for aiding management of health issues such as diabetes (F. L. Wu et al., 2021). A seven-step problem-solving model is recommended for the primary care setting: (a) Specifically define the problem; (b) brainstorm possible solutions without being critical; (c) critically evaluate each possible solution, discarding those that are clearly unreasonable or impossible using a listing of pros and cons to help evaluate them; (d) select the best option; (e) implement the chosen solution; (f) assess the outcome, likely in a follow-up visit; and (g) if the outcome is favorable, fine-tune the solution as needed and continue to monitor the patient. If the outcome is unfavorable, return to step (d). The patient handout in Figure 4.7 can be used to guide the progression through these steps either during an appointment (or multiple appointments, if necessary) or as a homework assignment.

FIGURE 4.7. Problem-Solving Worksheet

1. Write out the problem: _____
2. Brainstorm all possible solutions. Write down anything you can think of. The goal is to get your mind flowing with ideas: _____
   _____
3. Evaluate your ideas:
   a) Cross out any that are clearly unrealistic, outside your control, or impossible.
   b) Of those that remain, circle the top three. Write the top three below in any order:

   _____   _____   _____

   c) For each one, list all the possible pros and cons:
   Pros: _____   Pros: _____   Pros: _____
   _____   _____   _____
   Cons: _____   Cons: _____   Cons: _____
   _____   _____   _____

4. Based on your pros and cons, select one that you feel has the best chances of working.
5. Implement the chosen solution. Define how you will know if the solution is working:
   _____
6. Assess the outcome on the following scale:

   _____   _____   _____   _____   _____

   No   Little   Some   A lot of   Total
   Improvement   Improvement   Improvement   Improvement   Improvement

7. If the outcome is positive, fine-tune the solution as needed and continue to monitor; if the outcome is not positive, return to Step 4.

Self-monitoring. Self-monitoring can help patients track their progress toward a goal, stay focused on the target of change, and facilitate naturally occurring rewards as they see tangible evidence of positive change. Methods for self-monitoring will vary depending on what is being monitored; however, it is generally helpful to keep monitoring simple and brief. The following are useful strategies:

- Mark on a calendar each day that the target behavior is accomplished. This is useful for behaviors that are to occur daily (e.g., exercises, physical therapy, taking medicines).

- Keep a tally. Tallies can be successfully used both for increasing behaviors that occur several times per day (e.g., servings of fruits and vegetables, glasses of water) and for decreasing behaviors that occur several times per day (e.g., cigarettes smoked).

- Chart the behavior on a graph. Graphing can be particularly useful when working with behaviors you want to change in a slowly progressing manner (e.g., minutes of walking for chronic back pain patients).

Behavioral self-analysis. Behavioral self-analysis is a model for teaching patients to analyze events or activities that immediately precede a behavior (antecedents) and immediately follow a behavior (consequences) to optimize success at managing their health and disease. The following script, which uses diabetes management as an example, can easily be applied within a primary care visit:

I would like to introduce you to a helpful strategy that can assist you in changing health-related behavior. We call it the ABC model. The A stands for antecedents. These are events or activities that come before the behavior. B stands for the behavior itself. C stands for consequences, which include things that can happen after the behavior and either increase or decrease the likelihood that you will engage in that behavior again.

The concept is one I'm sure you are familiar with, as we use it in a lot of everyday events.

For example, if you wanted to learn a new skill, such as driving a car for the first time, we could apply the ABC model. First let's consider A, which again are antecedents, or things you would want to do before getting behind the wheel. What are some things you would want to do before you just start driving on your own for the first time?

- *Instruction.* Learn how to turn the car on, how to work the controls, what the rules of the road are, what strategies help others to be successful, and what pitfalls to be cautious of.
- *Practice.* Drive around an empty parking lot, then move to residential streets, then busier streets. Have an advanced driver or instructor in the car with you to coach you. Repeatedly practice the more difficult aspects, such as parallel parking, until you develop the skill.
- *Define the goal and determine the best route.* Decide where you are going and map out the route.
- *Identify potential problems.* What are some of the hazards that could interfere with success? How is the weather? What are the road conditions? Is the car well maintained?

Okay, good. Now let's think about B, which is the actual behaviors while you are driving. What are some important behaviors while driving (e.g., staying focused; avoiding distractions, such as eating, listening to music, or talking; not getting discouraged if you make a mistake; applying the skills you have learned and practiced; assessing how you are doing and making adjustments when necessary; taking safety precautions, such as wearing a seatbelt)?

Finally, let's identify the Cs in our driving examples, which are the consequences. What are some of the consequences that will make it likely that you will drive again (e.g., arriving safely at your destination, gaining pride in learning a new skill, enjoying the freedom of getting around more easily)?

By analyzing the ABCs of any new skill, you can increase your chances of success.

Now that you have the idea, let's apply this ABC model to learning to manage your diabetes. What are some of the antecedents (events or activities) you may want to pay attention to when developing the skill of managing diabetes?

- *Instruction.* What is diabetes? How can medical science help control the disease and optimize quality of life? What skills do you need to learn? What lifestyle behaviors do you need to change? How can your family help? What equipment is available? What books or education programs are available? How often do you need to visit the doctor?
- *Practice.* Practice testing blood sugars, giving insulin injections, checking feet, and investigating new diets and exercise plans. Use a diabetes educator to help coach you. Keep working on those aspects that are difficult for you until you become good at it.
- *Define the goal and determine the best route.* Set behavioral goals for diet, exercise, weight loss, medication use, and doctor visits. Establish reasonable subgoals and target dates, taking small, achievable steps.

- *Identify potential problems.* What are some of the hazards that could interfere with success? Is there anyone in your life who will work against you achieving success, even unintentionally? How is your motivation and attitude; are they working for you or against you? Do you believe you can make healthy changes in your life? Are you getting depressed?

Next is the Bs or behaviors. What are some of the important factors in making lifestyle changes? Many are the same as when talking about driving: (a) Stay mentally focused; (b) avoid distractions; (c) don't get discouraged if you make a mistake; (d) apply the skills you have learned; (e) assess how you are doing and make adjustments when necessary; and (f) take safety precautions, such as not keeping sugary desserts readily available at home.

Finally, let's talk about the Cs or consequences. When you do well, what are some of the consequences that will increase the likelihood that you will continue to make those changes? Again, there are parallels to our driving example: (a) Arriving safely at your destination is the same as achieving better health and quality of life, (b) feeling pride in learning a new skill is similar to gaining a sense that you are in control of your diabetes, and (c) enjoying the freedom of getting around more easily is like maintaining high levels of functioning and not letting diabetes limit your potential.

Now that we have identified some of the ABCs related to managing your diabetes, would you be willing to come back to work on some of these things together with me with the goal of helping you to be more successful?

Arrange

Once the barriers to adherence have been addressed, it is often helpful to arrange follow-up care to monitor progress. One helpful strategy is to schedule the patient to see the BHC as part of medical follow-up visits.

Stimulus Control

Another useful strategy for helping patients change health-related behavior involves the behavioral principle of stimulus control (Dunkel & Glaros, 1978; Jacobson, 1978). Similar to the ABC model just discussed, stimulus control involves collaborating with the patient to identify stimuli that naturally precede a target behavior and then taking steps to alter these stimuli to bring about a desired result. Stimuli can be environmental, interpersonal, emotional, behavioral, or cognitive. Stimulus control strategies can help to increase desirable behaviors, such as increasing exercise, and to decrease undesirable behaviors, such as eating too many unhealthy snacks (L. H. Epstein et al., 2004; Wilfley et al., 2011).

Assess

The following script is a suggested way of using stimulus control in a primary care visit. The example uses eating unhealthy snack foods as a target behavior.

When you eat an unhealthy snack, a variety of things happen before you actually start eating it. Over time, these factors become associated with eating. In other words, they start to become triggers for eating. Triggers can be things you see, hear, smell, feel, or do. What triggers for eating junk food have you recognized in yourself?

Have the patient list factors. Categorize them as follows: (a) behaviors (e.g., watching television), (b) emotions (e.g., anger), (c) thoughts (e.g., "I'm hungry"), (d) other people (e.g., family not home), and (e) environmental (e.g., sitting at my desk at work).

This is a good start. It's good that you are aware of many of the factors that are triggering your eating. As you can see, I've organized the triggers you listed into different categories.

There may also be some of which you are not aware. The more triggers of which you are aware, the greater are the chances of being successful at managing your eating.

I would like to suggest that, over the next week, you monitor your eating outside of meals. For this week, don't try to make any changes, just monitor your eating. This form [see Figure 4.8] can be used to help you recognize additional triggers. Every time you eat something or get the urge to eat something, apart from mealtime, log it on the form. Let's meet in 1 week and we'll review what you've observed.

At the next appointment, you could say,

Let's look at your eating log. What did you observe were the most important or most frequently occurring triggers for you? Were there any that you hadn't recognized before?

Advise and Agree

It looks like you have done a good job recognizing some of the triggers related to your consumption of snack foods. I suggest we work together on trying to control these. Is that something you would be willing to do? Let's list the factors you identified on this worksheet [see Figure 4.8]. Now, which of these triggers are within your ability to control, and which do you feel are outside your control?

Check off in the corresponding column those that the patient has direct control over, those they can learn to control better, and those outside their control.

Assist and Arrange

Now let's come up with a plan for avoiding some of these triggers so that we can help you control your eating.

Discuss each of the triggers and steps that can be taken to control them. List each idea that the patient is willing to start under the plan column. Examples are provided in Figure 4.9. After using the worksheet to develop a stimulus control plan, arrange follow-up care to monitor and assist efforts to change the target behaviors.

Assertive Communication

Assertive communication training is often used as an important component of comprehensive treatment packages for problems such as eating disorders (Shiina et al., 2005), anxiety (Kubany et al., 2004), chronic pain (Merlijn et al., 2005), depression (Ball et al., 2000; Ghazavi et al., 2016; Kubany et al., 2004),

FIGURE 4.8. Monitoring Behavioral Triggers

Date	Behavior	What was I doing?	How was I feeling?	What was I thinking?	What were others around me doing?	Time of day, location, and other environmental factors

Controlling Trigger Worksheet

Trigger	Level of control			Plan
	Lots	Some	None	

FIGURE 4.9. Stimulus Control Plan

Trigger	Level of control			Plan
	Lots	Some	None	

Stimulus Control Plan (Sample)

Trigger	Level of control			Plan
	Lots	Some	None	
Watching TV	X			Not willing to give up watching TV. Make a commitment to only eat while sitting at the kitchen table.
Anger		X		Avoid the kitchen when feeling angry. Take an anger management class or read a book on the topic.
Thinking "I'm hungry"		X		Rethink with realistic thinking: "I'm not hungry. I just ate dinner an hour ago. I have an urge to eat but it is not physiological hunger."
Family not home			X	Can't avoid being home alone; however, access to snack foods can be controlled. Avoid going in the kitchen when family is not home. Don't buy unhealthy food.
Sitting at my desk at work			X	Avoid access to snack foods at work. Don't carry small change so vending machines and snack cupboards are not convenient.

and partner-relationship difficulties (Alipour et al., 2020; Benson et al., 2012). Poor communication with others is not frequently identified as the presenting problem. However, in our experience, passive and aggressive communication problems can exacerbate symptoms and impede functioning and goal attainment. Thus, being able to teach the patient assertive communication skills can be an important part of the BHC's practice.

Assess

As part of a standard first assessment, asking the following questions can help you determine whether communication is a problem that deserves further inquiry: "Do you find that you sometimes have difficulty communicating what you think or how you feel? Do you feel that others do not respond to you in a manner that you would like them to?" If the answer to these questions is no, then you might move on to other functional assessment questions. If the answer is yes, follow up with questions such as these, to further clarify and determine whether assertive communications skills training might be helpful:

- With what people, or in what situations, do you have these communication difficulties?

- Is this communication difficulty something new, or has it happened with other people or in other situations during your life?

- What thoughts do you have when you are in these situations?

- What makes the communication better? What makes it worse?

- Do you notice any physical changes when you are in these situations?

Advise and Agree

> It sounds like there are times when you do not communicate as effectively as you would like to. You find that you get nervous in these situations and your words do not come out the way you would like them to. You feel humiliated, which leads you to not want to say things in future situations, but you feel angry and frustrated by not saying anything because people take advantage of your generosity. One of the things we can do is to help you learn to communicate more effectively so that you can improve the chances that situations such as this can turn out differently. Is learning how to communicate more effectively something you are interested in doing?
>
> This is a handout [see Figure 4.10] I would like you to review between now and our follow-up appointment. When you come back, I'll teach you some assertiveness skills and we'll review this handout to make sure you understand it, and then we'll set a specific plan for you to improve.

Assist

The primary goal is to help the patient learn the differences between passive, assertive, and aggressive communication and how to speak assertively when needed. Use the handout in Figure 4.10 to assist with this teaching. We use the HARD acronym (honest, appropriate, respectful, direct) to help the individual

FIGURE 4.10. Assertive Communication

Assertiveness Is Simple but HARD

Nonassertive	Assertive	Aggressive
(Passive)	(Tactful)	(Rude)
☹ **H** onest	✓ **H** onest	✓ **H** onest
✓ **A** ppropriate	✓ **A** ppropriate	☹ **A** ppropriate
✓ **R** espectful	✓ **R** espectful	☹ **R** espectful
☹ **D** irect	✓ **D** irect	✓ **D** irect

Assertiveness involves respecting your rights and the rights of others.

Important Facts About Assertiveness

- "I statements" such as "When _____ happens, I feel _____" are more effective than blaming or accusing statement such as "You make me so angry when you _____."
- Your voice tone, eye contact, and body posture are important parts of assertiveness.
- Use a steady calm voice, stand or sit up straight, look the other person in the eyes.
- Feelings are usually only one word (e.g., angry, anxious, happy, sad, hurt, frustrated, joyful).
- Remember, assertiveness doesn't guarantee that you will get what you want or that the other person will understand your concerns or be happy with what you said. It does improve the chances that the other person will understand what you want or how you feel and thus improve your chances of communicating effectively.

Four Essential Steps to Assertive Communication

1. Tell the other person how you feel.
2. Tell them the specific situations in which you feel that way (again, don't blame or accuse the person; just describe the situation).
3. Tell them how their behavior affects you and your relationship with them.
4. Tell them what you would prefer them to do instead.

XYZ* Formula for Effective Communication

Goal: To express the way you feel (internal world) in response to others' behavior (external world) in specific situations.

You are the only person who has access to your feelings. Others have no access to your internal world. The only way they will know what you are feeling is if you tell them.

Similarly, you only have access to other people's external world. It is very easy to make a mistake when trying to guess what others are feeling or intending.

Examples of the XYZ* model:

I feel X	when Y occurs	because of Z,	and I would like *
I feel angry	when socks and underwear are on the bedroom floor	because we just talked about keeping your room neater,	and I would like you to put them in the hamper.
I felt annoyed	when I saw an empty gas tank this morning	because I had to stop on my way to work and I was late,	and I would like you to leave the car with at least a quarter tank of gas.
I feel scared	when I don't hear from you if you are staying late at work	because I don't know if something happened to you,	and I would like you to call as soon as you know you will be late.
I feel loved	when you kiss me when you get home	because it says to me you are glad to see me,	and I would like you to do that every day.

assess their communication style in any situation. We also teach the XYZ* formula in Figure 4.10 as a format for practicing direct communication that may be healthier and more effective in meeting their needs. The XYZ* formula is a way for the patient to assertively express thoughts by putting the appropriate words in the XYZ* positions, with X being the patient's emotional reaction, Y being the action of the other person that is eliciting the patient's emotional response, Z being the specific situation, and * being desired change the patient would like to see from the other person. We recommend the following to help the patient learn effective assertive communication:

- Review the HARD acronym handout, explaining differences in communication styles.

- Demonstrate the differences between speaking passively, assertively, and aggressively. Change voice tone, affect, body posture, and eye contact appropriately.

- After demonstrating each of these, ask the patient which was the easiest to listen to.

- Highlight the point that if the words do not match what the listener sees (nonverbal communication), the listener may pay more attention to what they see than to what they hear.

- Develop appropriate statements for situations and demonstrate how those might be verbalized using the XYZ* formula.

- Ask the patient to role play assertive communication with you during the appointment. Provide constructive feedback.

- Set a plan for the patient to practice the statements at home in front of a mirror.

- You might also recommend that the patient obtain a self-help book on assertive communication (e.g., Murphy, 2011) for further information and skill development.

Arrange

We recommend having patients return for a follow-up consult to demonstrate their practiced skill through role play. This allows the opportunity to provide additional feedback and modeling, as necessary. At this point, the patient may be ready to set a specific plan to use the skill. The BHC may decide not to schedule any follow-up consults at this point or may recommend additional follow-ups as necessary if the patient's communications skills plans are not as effective as predicted.

SUMMARY

The cognitive and behavioral skills discussed in this chapter are applicable to a broad range of medical and behavioral health concerns. We reviewed strategies and suggested methods of application that we have found to be suitable for the demands and limitations of the primary care environment. Figure 4.11 lists several mobile applications that are applicable to the strategies discussed.

Even within the brief/focused context, however, it is important the BHC deliver interventions in a person-centered, empathetic manner that is tailored to the clinical needs, personal characteristics, culture, and limitations of each individual. In other words, these interventions should be skillfully applied using the full scope of the BHC's clinical training. The chapters in Part II that address specific patient problems will often refer to these interventions, and many of the scripts in this chapter can be easily modified to address these problems.

FIGURE 4.11. Recommended Mobile Applications to Support Common Cognitive Behavior Interventions

Intervention	Mobile application
Relaxation skills	Breathe2Relax
Mindfulness exercises	Mindfulness Coach
Cognitive disputation	CPT Legacy, Self CBT
Acceptance and commitment techniques	ACT Coach
Self-monitoring	Mood Tracker
Assertive communication	Self CBT

Note. CPT = cognitive processing therapy; CBT = cognitive behavior therapy; ACT = acceptance and commitment therapy.

II

COMMON BEHAVIORAL HEALTH CONCERNS IN PRIMARY CARE

5

Depression, Anxiety, Posttraumatic Stress Disorder, and Insomnia

Behavioral health concerns such as depression, anxiety, posttraumatic stress disorder (PTSD), and insomnia are prevalent in primary care. One of the greatest advantages of integrating behavioral health professionals into primary care systems is the potential to identify and use evidence-based behavioral and cognitive interventions with individuals who demonstrate subclinical or mild to moderate depression, anxiety, PTSD, and insomnia. Consultation and treatment for these behavioral health problems in primary care is efficacious, although it is unclear how long the impact of these interventions lasts (D. Gillies et al., 2015). Each topic covered could constitute its own chapter or even its own book. Our intent in this chapter is to provide an overview of the main areas we often target when confronting these problems in primary care.

DEPRESSION

National surveys suggest that the lifetime prevalence rate of major depressive disorder is 20.6% (Hasin et al., 2018). The number of adults in the United States experiencing major depressive disorder increased 12.9% between 2010 and 2018, which is estimated to be associated with an economic burden of $326.2 billion (Greenberg et al., 2021). A meta-analysis suggests that the prevalence of depressive symptoms for those being seen in U.S. primary care settings

https://doi.org/10.1037/0000380-006

Integrated Behavioral Health in Primary Care: Step-by-Step Guidance for Assessment and Intervention, Third Edition, by C. L. Hunter, J. L. Goodie, M. S. Oordt, and A. C. Dobmeyer

is 12.5% (Mitchell et al., 2011). The U.S. Preventive Services Task Force recommends screening adults, pregnant and postpartum persons, older adults, and adolescents 12 to 18 years old for depressive symptoms (Mangione et al., 2022; Siu et al., 2016). A major depressive episode is defined in the fifth edition of the *Diagnostic and Statistical Manual of Mental Disorders, Text Revision* (*DSM-5-TR*; American Psychiatric Association, 2022) as a depressed mood or loss of interest or pleasure for at least 2 weeks in addition to at least four other symptoms, including significant weight changes, insomnia or hypersomnia, psychomotor agitation or retardation, fatigue or loss of energy, feelings of worthlessness or inappropriate guilt, difficulty concentrating or indecisiveness, or recurrent thoughts of death or suicide (pp. 183–192). Individuals diagnosed with major depressive disorder must have had a major depressive episode, whereas individuals with fewer symptoms or those who have experienced the symptoms for shorter periods of time may be diagnosed with other specified or unspecified depressive disorder. Major depressive symptoms may occur in the context of a bipolar I disorder (i.e., the individual has had a manic episode) and bipolar II disorder (i.e., no manic episodes but a history of a hypomanic episode), and depressive symptoms may also occur in the context of other disorders (e.g., cyclothymic disorder, persistent depressive disorder, adjustment disorders). It is beyond the scope of this chapter to discuss each of these conditions; however, we broadly discuss methods for targeting depressive symptoms.

Cultural and Diversity Considerations

Those identifying as Black (15.2%), Hispanic (16.2%), or Asian/Pacific Islander demonstrate lower lifetime prevalence of major depression compared with Native American (28.2%) or White (23.1%) adults (Hasin et al., 2018). Women are twice as likely to demonstrate major depressive symptoms in their lifetime compared with men (Hasin et al., 2018). Depression is 2 times more prevalent among lesbian, gay, and bisexual (LGB) populations (King et al., 2008); therefore, it is particularly important to screen for depression in these populations. These statistics only touch on the surface of the complexity of how diversity and cultural factors may influence the risks associated with depression. It is beyond the scope of this chapter to fully describe this complexity. Behavioral health consultants (BHCs) should continually educate themselves on how depressive symptoms can present differently across cultural backgrounds and remain aware of how biases and self-identities may influence assessments and intervention guidance. Such education and awareness can facilitate the adaptability of the BHC for helping to manage not just depressive symptoms but all behavioral health concerns.

Specialty Mental Health

Although a wide variety of therapies are offered for the treatment of depressive symptoms, evidence-based guidelines suggest that the strongest evidence exists for psychological therapies, including behavioral, cognitive behavioral, interpersonal, psychodynamic, and supportive therapies, as well as second generation antidepressants (i.e., selective serotonin reuptake inhibitors [SSRIs], serotonin and norepinephrine reuptake inhibitors [SNRIs]; American Psychological Association [APA], 2019). Cognitive behavioral treatments involve techniques such as behavioral activation, cognitive restructuring, problem solving, and relaxation. Interventions drawn from acceptance and commitment therapy (ACT) are also effective (Bai et al., 2020).

Behavioral Health in Primary Care

BHCs play particularly important roles as collaborative partners on the primary care team for individuals demonstrating mild to severe depression. Collaborative care models (i.e., using a care manager to assist with monitoring medication adherence and specialty mental health care appointments) for depression have been widely studied and found to be effective in treating depression (Archer et al., 2012; McNaughton, 2009). Although there are fewer well-controlled studies, time-limited, depression-targeted psychotherapies (i.e., cognitive behavioral, interpersonal, problem-solving) have also been found to be effective in primary care settings (Linde et al., 2015). Studies examining large populations of individuals have found that care provided by BHCs results in clinically reliable functional improvements (Wilfong et al., 2022). BHC-delivered care has been found to reduce depressive symptoms among diverse populations (Robinson et al., 2020; Wolff et al., 2021). Given the breadth of data in specialty mental health settings and the developing evidence in primary care settings, our recommendations for assessments and interventions for depressive symptoms rely heavily on cognitive and behavioral techniques.

Primary Care Adaptation

Assessing and targeting depressive symptoms in primary care requires the BHC to use focused questions and interventions. The 5As provides a useful guide.

Assess

Several self-report measures are available that are both short and easily scored and therefore can be useful for screening or assessing depressive symptoms in primary care. Given the prevalence of depression, it may be helpful to implement population-screening approaches for depressive symptoms, as we discuss in Chapters 1 and 3. El-Den et al. (2018) provided a broad review of depression-screening measures for use in primary care. Several popular measures used to screen for depression in primary care include the Patient Health Questionnaire-9 (PHQ-9: 10 items; Kroenke et al., 2001) and the Center for Epidemiologic Studies Depression Scale-Revised (20 items; Eaton et al., 2004). These two measures, and their derivatives (e.g., the PHQ-2), were the most studied measures for screening for depression in primary care (El-Den et al., 2018).

The Patient Health Questionnaire-2. The PHQ-2 (Kroenke et al., 2003) was adapted from the PHQ-9, using the first two questions to screen for depression:

> Over the last 2 weeks, how often have you been bothered by any of the following problems:
>
> 1. Little interest or pleasure in doing things?
> 2. Feeling down, depressed, or hopeless?

Given its brevity, the PHQ-2 is a good measure to use for population screening. Across studies, sensitivity ranged from 42% to 95% and specificity ranged from 61% to 95% (El-Den et al., 2018). The PHQ-9 and other versions of the PHQ can be retrieved from https://www.phqscreeners.com/.

Sleep, interest, guilt, energy, concentration, appetite, psychomotor retardation or agitation, suicidal ideation mnemonic. Even relatively brief measures can be difficult to administer in fast-paced primary care environments. In addition to or instead of the PHQ-2, we suggest that BHCs ask about mood and then incorporate the commonly used SIGECAPS mnemonic (sleep, interest, guilt, energy, concentration, appetite, psychomotor agitation or retardation, suicidal ideation):

- Mood: How would you describe your mood? Happy? Mad? Sad? Irritable? On a scale of negative 5 to positive 5, where negative 5 is the *most depressed or worst you can imagine yourself feeling* and positive 5 is the *happiest or best you could imagine yourself feeling,* with 0 right in between where you feel neither sad nor happy, how would you rate your mood on average? Right now? At its worst? At its best?

- Sleep: Are you sleeping more? Less? Do you wake before your alarm?

- Interest: Do you have less interest in activities that you used to enjoy?

- Guilt: Do you have increased feelings of guilt? Worthlessness?

- Energy: Do you have less energy to do things that you want to do?

- Concentration: Do you have difficulty concentrating?

- Appetite: Has your appetite increased? Decreased? Has your weight changed?

- Psychomotor retardation or agitation: Do you feel slowed down or keyed up?

- Suicidal ideation: Do you think about hurting or killing yourself?

Functional assessment. As with any functional assessment, it is important to determine the onset, duration, intensity, and frequency of the symptoms. A review of the medical record prior to meeting with the patient can help guide these questions. We use targeted and more closed-ended questions than would likely be used in specialty mental health clinics. In Figure 3.3 of Chapter 3, we present specific questions BHCs can ask during a functional assessment of depression. As in any situation, when BHCs are screening for depressive symptoms it is important to be mindful of medical causes of depression, such as endocrine disorders (e.g., hyper- and hypothyroidism, hyper- and hypopara-thyroidism), infectious diseases (e.g., HIV, hepatitis, mononucleosis), nutritional deficits (e.g., vitamin B_{12} deficiencies), diseases of the central nervous system (e.g., stroke, traumatic brain injuries), and substance use (e.g., excessive caffeine use interfering with sleep, excessive alcohol or hypnotic use).

Positive responses to any question related to depressive symptoms may result in further follow-up questions, but this is particularly the case if there are positive responses to questions about suicidal ideation. We discuss how to manage suicidal behaviors in Chapter 17. Clinic leaders and providers should establish policies and guidelines to help them determine whether someone should be managed in primary care, referred to specialty mental health care, or hospitalized. Similarly, if the BHC suspects that the patient may meet criteria for bipolar disorder I or II, they may want to consider arranging further assessment and care in a specialty mental health setting.

Advise

Following the functional assessment, and depending on the data gathered by the BHC, they might use the analogy of a spiral to describe to patients how removing activities from their lives and doing less can affect their mood and increase negative thinking. In turn, their negative mood and thoughts can contribute to doing still less, and hence they spiral in a downward direction. We show how this process works on the first page of the depression handout (see Figure 5.1). To begin to move upward on this spiral, patients might consider a variety of options, including (a) developing a plan for change, (b) pursuing specialty mental health care, (c) taking medications (i.e., antidepressants), and (d) doing nothing (i.e., keep doing what they are doing and evaluate whether their depressive symptoms improve).

We typically suggest that the interventions we offer would be a useful place to start as part of a stepped-care approach. If a patient has been started on an antidepressant, BHCs can help the primary care provider (PCP) by assessing adherence to the prescribed regimen and asking whether the patient has any concerns or questions about the use of the medication. For this reason, it is important to be familiar with the most commonly prescribed antidepressants.

We recommend and refer patients to specialty mental health care providers when patients demonstrate complex depressive symptoms that are beyond the scope of management in a primary care setting (e.g., psychotic features, prolonged and severe symptoms, multiple failed treatments with antidepressants) or when they exhibit significant suicidal risk (e.g., evidence of a plan or intent) that is difficult to adequately monitor and address in a primary care environment (e.g., weekly return appointments would be required over time).

When advising on a plan for change, describe what the option involves and how it will help target their specific problems. For instance,

> One of the things we might do is set a plan to increase the potentially enjoyable and valued activities in your life. You've noticed that as you've cut back or cut

out these activities, your mood has gotten worse. The idea is, if you're not doing fun, enjoyable, and valued activities in your life, your life will not feel very fun, enjoyable, or valuable. So this plan would be like the old Nike commercials where you "just do it." We could set a specific day, time, and plan for what you might add back into your life.

BHCs could also say,

Another thing we might do is to help you work on your ability to challenge the depressive thoughts you have. Your mind will tell you things that are not true, not helpful, and inconsistent with your values. You can't stop your mind from telling you things, but you can work on questioning those thoughts and developing new ways of thinking that can decrease depressed mood and make it easier for you to live your life in a way that is consistent with your values.

FIGURE 5.1. Depression Spiral Handout (*continues*)

Depression Spiral

Depression often involves feelings of sadness, irritability, or ambivalence (e.g., "I don't care"), doing fewer enjoyable activities (e.g., withdrawing from others), and thinking more negatively (e.g., "I'm worthless," "Why bother?"). As the spiral downward on the left represents, negative thoughts and withdrawal can lead to feeling "depressed." As shown on the right, focusing on valued thoughts and engaging in valued activities can reverse that spiral, leading to living the life that you choose. Use the blocks on the left spiral to write the thoughts that are leading to a downward spiral and feeling depressed. Use the blocks on the right spiral to write the thoughts and activities that could lead you to live a more valued life.

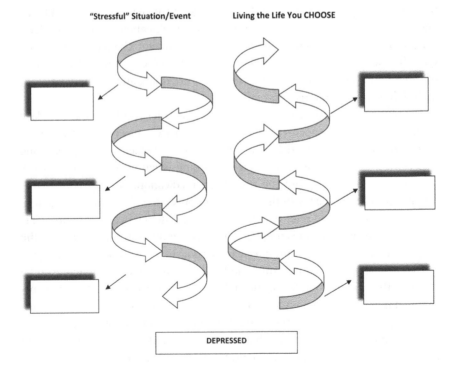

FIGURE 5.1. Depression Spiral Handout (*continues*)

Recognizing Depression

How do you know when you or someone else is depressed? What are the signs? Some signs include the following:

Physical	Behavioral	Cognitive	Emotional
Tired/fatigued	Doing less	Difficulty concentrating	Sadness
Appetite change (increase or decrease)	Sleeping more/less	Expecting the worst	Anger/irritability
More aches and pains	Withdrawing from others	Thoughts of suicide	Guilty feelings

What are the physical, behavioral, cognitive, and emotional signs of depression that you have noticed in yourself?

Physical	Behavioral	Cognitive	Emotional

Improving Your Mood

To identify the situations that affect your mood, it can be helpful to monitor how your mood changes. Consider using this diary to track how your mood changes from day to day and try to identify patterns that occur.

Daily Mood Record

–5	–4	–3	–2	–1	0	+1	+2	+3	+4	+5

Very Sad   Neutral   Very Happy

1.   Using the scale above, rate your general level of sadness/happiness at the end of each day.
2.   This rating is based on how you felt on average over the course of each day.
3.   If you felt great, mark "+5."
4.   If you felt really bad (e.g., the worst you have ever felt or can imagine feeling), mark "–5."
5.   If you felt "so-so" or neither sad nor happy, mark "0."

FIGURE 5.1. Depression Spiral Handout (*continued*)

	Mon	Tues	Wed	Thurs	Fri	Sat	Sun	Average
Week 1								
Week 2								
Week 3								
Week 4								
Week 5								
Week 6								
Week 7								
Week 8								

Increasing Activities

When we perceive ourselves as overwhelmed or not feeling well, we often choose to avoid activities that we once enjoyed, but by not spending time on those activities, we have fewer opportunities for enjoyment. One of the most important steps to help reduce depressive symptoms is to engage in potentially enjoyable/meaningful activities

Setting Enjoyable/Meaningful or Physical Activity Goals

1. Is the goal realistic?
2. Is a target date set for completion?
3. Is the goal measurable?
4. Is the goal broken down into small, realistic parts?
5. Once accomplished, what rewards will you use?
6. Is the goal personally meaningful?
7. Is a relapse plan clearly established?
8. Example of goal setting:

Week 1: Walk 8 mins/day, 3 days/week.   Week 6: Walk 16 mins/day, 4 days/week.
Week 2: Walk 10 mins/day, 3 days/week.   Week 7: Walk 16 mins/day, 5 days/week.
Week 3: Walk 12 mins/day, 3 days/week.   Week 8: Walk 18 mins/day, 5 days/week.
Week 4: Walk 12 mins/day, 4 days/week.   Week 9: Walk 20 mins/day, 5 days/week.
Week 5: Walk 14 mins/day, 4 days/week.   Week 10: Walk 20 mins/day, 5 days/week.

Agree

It is important for patients to agree to do something before BHCs try to start an intervention, even if that something is just doing a little more than what they are currently doing. If they seem unwilling to try any of the options, then a BHC might ask them whether they have additional ideas on how a BHC might assist them. Another option is to have a follow-up appointment to discuss the options further. The follow-up appointment itself may start to help decrease depressed mood because it provides increased social activities with BHCs and others in the clinic and thus may make it easier for the patient to choose a viable evidence-based plan.

Assist

We use a handout such as the one in Figure 5.1 to introduce evidence-based components of cognitive and behavioral interventions, including behavioral activation, cognitive disputation, and problem solving for intervening with depressed mood.

Behavioral activation. Our experiences suggest that one of the simplest and most effective initial interventions is behavioral activation (Stein et al., 2021; Uphoff et al., 2020). The functional assessment usually identifies activities patients have decreased or stopped. We use the depression handout (see Figure 5.1) to help patients recognize the symptoms of depression, get them started with monitoring their mood, and start them on a behavioral activation plan with realistic goals. We suggest starting with a plan to add these activities back into their daily or weekly schedule and to set specific goals, including time, place, duration, and frequency (for specifics on goal setting, see Chapter 4). The activities might involve little effort and represent doing just a little more than they do currently. For example, a BHC might say,

> You mentioned that you used to go out with your friends once a week. Would it be realistic for you to plan an outing with your friends at least once between now and the next time we meet?

An even simpler change plan might be to say,

> You indicated that you used to walk your dog in the neighborhood for 20 minutes a day. Would it be realistic for you to start to do that again?

We use the goal-setting sheets in the handout in Figure 5.1 to develop a plan for how patients will begin their behavioral activation plan. As part of behavioral activation, we encourage individuals to increase physical activity or exercise because evidence suggests increasing physical activity prevents and treats depressive symptoms (Gianfredi et al., 2020; Nyström et al., 2015). The available evidence suggests that at least 30 minutes of aerobic or anerobic activity at least three times per week is helpful for treating depressive symptoms (Nyström et al., 2015). Current physical activity guidelines for improving overall health recommend 30 minutes of moderate activity at least 5 days per week or 30 minutes of vigorous activity three times per week (Physical Activity Guidelines Advisory Committee, 2018). It is important for the goal to be specific and realistic for the patient. For individuals who have not exercised in the past, we often start with a simple walking program, whereas for those individuals who have exercised regularly in the past, we build on what they used to do.

Changing thinking. In addition to behavioral activation, we discuss methods for changing the way patients think. We may use cognitive restructuring techniques or ACT techniques (Bai et al., 2020) that are effective for improving functioning. Rather than focusing on trying to change or control negative or depressive thinking, ACT interventions use the premise that people cannot control or stop their negative thinking. Instead, ACT encourages patients to allow thoughts and emotions to happen and to focus on making changes in areas of their life that they can control (Hayes, 2016; Hayes et al., 2011). In Chapter 4 (see Figures 4.3–4.5), we discuss how we use two levels of cognitive disputation, which can target the negative and alarming thinking associated with depressive symptoms. Identifying thoughts that are inconsistent with how individuals want to live their life and either changing those thoughts or living with them can be an important component of improving functioning in individuals demonstrating depressive symptoms. We often encourage patients to write down the three or four questions that seem most applicable to them on a note card to help them remember the questions. We focus on the demands that patients place on themselves and discuss issues related to what they can and cannot control (for additional information, see Chapter 4).

Problem solving. Problem solving is another skill we discuss with patients to help them to effectively manage their depressive symptoms. Using the outline found in Chapter 4, we take time with the patient to identify a problem they are struggling with, then we brainstorm on solutions, evaluate those solutions, help them choose the best ones to try, and discuss how to evaluate the outcome and decide whether they will need to try another possible solution. Often, problem solving involves engaging in an activity and can become a part of the behavioral activation plan.

The BHC can also provide the patient with a variety of additional resources that might be used in conjunction with BHC appointments or might be used by patients who will be following up with their PCP only. Patients might be interested in websites, mobile device applications, or self-help books to assist in managing depressive symptoms. Some of these resources are summarized in Figure 5.2.

Arrange

Follow-up appointments can vary greatly between individuals. Some return after the initial appointment having successfully increased their participation in activities, exceeding their goals and appearing to demonstrate significantly improved functioning and mood. However, some individuals may return for two or three appointments and will not have changed their thinking or behaviors; BHCs might consider recommending these individuals for specialty mental health treatment if obvious barriers cannot be overcome. For individuals demonstrating suicidal thoughts, the BHC should consider frequent appointments or even multiple appointments in the same week to monitor whether the intensity and frequency of the thoughts change over time. This may need to continue until the patient can be successfully linked with specialty behavioral health care. Feedback should always be provided to the PCP about the plan for managing the depressive symptoms and existing suicidal thoughts. Additional guidance for managing suicide risk in primary care is found in Chapter 17.

ANXIETY DISORDERS

Among U.S. adults, 33.7% experience an anxiety disorder during their lifetime (R. C. Kessler et al., 2012) and an estimated 20% of the patients seen in primary care clinics meet the criteria for an anxiety disorder (Kroenke et al., 2007). One study found that patients who were eventually diagnosed with

FIGURE 5.2. Resources for Patients With Depression: Websites, Mobile Applications, and Books

Depression Resources

Type	Location	Descriptions
Websites	Anxiety and Depression Association of America (http://www.adaa.org/)	Provides information and resources for patients about anxiety and depressive disorders; professional organization for researchers and therapists who specialize in these areas
	National Institute of Mental Health (https://www.nimh.nih.gov/health/topics/depression/index.shtml)	Provides information for patients about depression
Mobile application	ACT Coach (https://mobile.va.gov/app/act-coach)	Supplements interventions using acceptance and commitment therapy
Books	*Mind Over Mood: Change How You Feel by Changing the Way You Think*, 2nd edition (Greenberger & Padesky, 2015)	Uses principles of behavior and cognitive therapies to help patients improve their mood
	The Mindfulness and Acceptance Workbook for Depression: Using Acceptance and Commitment Therapy to Move Through Depression and Create a Life Worth Living, 2nd edition (Strosahl & Robinson, 2017)	Uses principles of acceptance and commitment therapy to help patients target depressive symptoms
	Overcoming Depression and Low Mood: A Five Areas Approach, 4th edition (C. Williams, 2017)	Uses cognitive and behavioral methods to target negative mood and depressive symptoms

these disorders had been seen in primary and specialty care clinics an average of six times before being identified as having an anxiety disorder (Deacon et al., 2008). Often patients will present with somatic complaints rather than with anxiety symptoms as the presenting problem (Combs & Markman, 2014). In addition, anxiety disorders have been associated with the occurrence of multiple medical problems, including irritable bowel syndrome, asthma, cardiovascular disease, and chronic pain (Roy-Byrne et al., 2008). In this section, we discuss methods for managing generalized anxiety disorder (GAD) and panic disorder, as these are two of the most common anxiety disorders presenting in primary care (Combs & Markman, 2014; DeGeorge et al., 2022).

In a U.S. national survey between January and June 2022 (National Center for Health Statistics, n.d.), 12.6% of adults reported having feelings of worry, nervousness, or anxiety. In that same survey, 13.6% of White non-Hispanic adults, 10.8% of Black non-Hispanic adults, and 10.8% of Hispanic adults reported those feelings. Previous data have shown that Black adults (23.8%)

have a lower lifetime prevalence of any anxiety disorder compared with White adults (29.4%); Black adults also have lower lifetime prevalence of GAD (5.1% vs. 8.6%) and panic disorder (3.1% vs. 4.9%) compared with their adult White counterparts (Breslau et al., 2006). Hispanic and White adults demonstrate statistically similar lifetime rates of anxiety disorders (24.9% vs. 29.4%) and of panic disorder (5.4% vs. 4.9%); but Hispanic adults (4.8%) demonstrate lower lifetime prevalence of GAD compared with White adults (8.6%; Breslau et al., 2006). When examining both sexes among LGB populations, there is a 2.3 times higher lifetime risk of any anxiety disorder. This finding seems to be true of men, but when women are examined separately, the data are less consistent about whether there is a difference between LGB and heterosexual women (King et al., 2008). These statistics highlight the need for increased awareness of anxiety symptoms among White adults and particularly among men who identify as gay or bisexual.

GENERALIZED ANXIETY DISORDER

According to *DSM-5-TR* criteria (American Psychiatric Association, 2022, pp. 250–254), GAD is associated with difficult-to-control excessive anxiety and worry, with symptoms of restlessness, fatigue, difficulty concentrating or mind going blank, irritability, muscle tension, and/or disturbances of sleep. The source of the worry cannot involve features of other disorders (e.g., embarrassment in public [social phobia], fear of contamination [obsessive-compulsive disorder], the patient's belief that they have multiple health problems [hypochondriasis]). The 12-month prevalence rate of GAD was found to be 2.9% among a U.S. population (American Psychiatric Association, 2022).

Specialty Mental Health

In systematic reviews of the literature, cognitive behavioral therapy has been shown to be effective for treating GAD (J. K. Carpenter et al., 2018). Cognitive behavioral treatments for GAD focus on reducing physiological symptoms using relaxation training (e.g., progressive muscle relaxation), managing anxious and worried thinking, behaviorally reducing avoidance of feared situations, and improving problem-solving and time-management skills (Shapiro, 2022).

Behavioral Health in Primary Care

Meta-analyses have found that brief cognitive and behavioral interventions are effective for anxiety in primary care settings (Cape et al., 2010). Multiple individual studies have found that CBT interventions for GAD are effective, but these studies often use eight to 12 appointments (e.g., Bogucki et al., 2021; Roy-Byrne et al., 2010; Stanley et al., 2003). These models of care are more similar to a colocated model of treatment than to an integrated model using time-limited interventions. Some data have suggested that GAD symptoms have improved using self-help or physician-guided, evidence-based interventions (van Boeijen et al., 2005).

Primary Care Adaptation

Combining what is known from specialty mental health and behavioral health in primary care informs BHCs how to implement the 5As, as described next.

Assess

To begin screening for GAD, BHCs can simply ask individuals,

- Do you worry most days?

- Is it difficult to control your worry?

- How does worry affect your life?

Generalized Anxiety Disorder-7. A systematic review of the Generalized Anxiety Disorder-7 (GAD-7) found that with a cutoff score of 8, the GAD-7 has good sensitivity (83%) and good specificity (84%) for screening for GAD (Plummer et al., 2016). Cutoff scores between 7 and 10 had similar sensitivity and specificity findings. The even shorter GAD-2, with a cutoff score of 3, may be a useful screening measure for identifying individuals who would benefit from additional assessments for GAD (sensitivity, 76%; specificity, 81%) and other anxiety disorders (sensitivity, 65%–72%; specificity, 88%–92%; one study found specificity to be low, at 39%; Plummer et al., 2016).

Functional assessment. We suggest using a screening mnemonic such as AND I C REST, proposed by Seitz (2005), which we present in Figure 5.3, to help guide the functional assessment of worry symptoms. It is also important to assess whether the patient demonstrates other anxiety disorders or other conditions (e.g., depressive symptoms, substance abuse, pain). Reviewing the electronic health record can assist with this process. In addition, whenever BHCs are assessing anxiety symptoms, it is important to work with the PCP to rule out medical conditions (e.g., hyperthyroidism) that may cause anxiety like symptoms.

Advise

GAD is generally treatable by cognitive and behavioral interventions, although in the primary care setting it is common to see individuals who have been prescribed anxiolytics to help manage symptoms. When physicians know that they can easily help their patients access nonpharmacological evidence-based strategies, they may be more likely to try those interventions before starting medication. Nonetheless, it is important to be familiar with the medications often prescribed for anxiety disorders. First-line medications that are effective for GAD include SSRIs (e.g., escitalopram) and SNRIs (e.g., venlafaxine); these

FIGURE 5.3. Mnemonic to Screen for Generalized Anxiety Disorder

Letter	*DSM-IV-TR* symptoms[a]	Screening questions
A	**A**nxious, nervous, or worried	Do you feel anxious, nervous, or worried most of the time? Do you worry about several things?
N	**N**o control over worry	Do you find it difficult to control the worry?
D	**D**uration of 6 months	How long has worrying been a problem for you?
I	**I**rritability	Do you find that you are more irritable than usual? Do you find that you are more easily frustrated by others than usual?
C	**C**oncentration impairment	Are you having any troubles with concentration? Do you find your mind going blank at times?
R	**R**estlessness	Are you feeling restless, fidgety, or that you can't sit still?
E	**E**nergy decreased	Are you feeling more tired than usual? Do you find that you are tiring more easily?
S	**S**leep impairment	Are you having any difficulties with falling asleep or staying asleep?
T	**T**ension in muscles	Do your muscles feel tense? Do you feel wound up like a spring?

Note. Adapted from "Screening Mnemonic for Generalized Anxiety Disorder," by D. P. Seitz, 2005, *Canadian Family Physician, 51*, p. 1342. Copyright 2005 by College of Family Physicians of Canada. Adapted with permission.
[a]The mnemonic designed to screen for generalized anxiety disorder (GAD) based on diagnostic criteria in the *Diagnostic and Statistical Manual of Mental Disorders*, fourth edition, text revision (*DSM-IV-TR*) remains relevant for diagnostic criteria in the *DSM-5-TR*. The diagnostic criteria for GAD have not substantially changed between these diagnostic manuals.

may be supplemented by benzodiazepines for short-term use (e.g., alprazolam; DeGeorge et al., 2022). Based on a meta-analysis, duloxetine (e.g., Cymbalta); venlafaxine (Effexor); escitalopram (Lexapro); and pregabalin (Lyrica), which is an antiepileptic medication, had the largest evidence base, were the most effective, and were the best tolerated (DeGeorge et al., 2022; Slee et al., 2019).

When introducing cognitive and behavioral interventions, it is important to discuss what changes patients will be asked to make and how those changes will help them manage symptoms and function more effectively. For example, a BHC might say the following:

> The interventions that I can discuss with you are skill based, that is, they require practice to be effective. The interventions are intended to help you change the way that you think and what you do to help you become distressed less often. Research has demonstrated that these interventions help most individuals who have difficulty managing their worry.

If the individual is taking an anxiolytic, a BHC could say,

> Changing your thoughts and what you do may help you reduce your need for taking medications, if that is something you and your medical provider are interested in accomplishing.

Agree

To effectively target worrying, patients must be willing to consider methods of accepting and managing their thinking. Relaxation exercises may help to reduce the physiological effects of worried thinking; however, without thinking differently about their worries, relaxation will likely not be sufficient to have an impact on the frequency, duration, and intensity of those worries. We suggest BHCs carefully explain that the goal is not to eliminate anxiety or worry; instead, the goal is to reduce anxiety and worry to a level that does not interfere with functioning. Therefore, a key aspect of targeting worried thinking is to discuss with patients possible methods of managing their worries and eliciting a willingness from patients to pursue those changes. For example, a BHC might say the following:

> It sounds as if you spend a significant amount of your time worrying about things that you have very little control over. To reduce your worrying, we can discuss several methods, such as writing your worries down, which can help reduce the frequency, duration, and intensity of your worrying. However, these techniques won't eliminate all of your worries. Worrying is a normal part of human existence, and it would be unrealistic to totally eliminate worries. Nevertheless, the techniques that we'll discuss require practice for them to work. Are you willing to use and practice these techniques with the goal of reducing your worrying?

As part of the agree phase, BHCs are beginning to educate patients and lead them into the assist phase.

Assist

Once a patient demonstrates a willingness to engage in an intervention for worrying, we always spend some time normalizing the behavior and educating them about the factors involved in worrying. We use handouts, such as the one provided in Figure 5.4, to guide patients through understanding worry, overcoming barriers associated with changing worry behavior, and practicing interventions that can help reduce worry. We take time to discuss the effects of worry, how to distinguish between helpful worry and unhelpful worry, and how the intensity of worry symptoms may interfere with their functioning. We also highlight how thinking can interfere with attempts to change their responses to anxiety.

We also suggest the use of a worry log, such as the one in Figure 5.5, as an effective way to manage worry. The goal of a worry log is to decrease overall daily worry by creating a specific place and time the individual can engage in worry. The changes can be tracked as the patient implements worry management strategies.

As a primary worry management strategy, patients are encouraged to have a 30-minute worry period that occurs at the same place and time each day. They are asked to write out their worries during this time, identifying data to support or not support the worries. Worry outside of this period is delayed, and the individual is asked to instead focus on the present moment: what they are doing, what others are doing, the environment, what they see, and what they hear.

FIGURE 5.4. Anxious Worry Handout

Common Symptoms of Anxious Worry

Anxiety is a normal human emotion that is experienced by everyone at one point or another. Anxiety is an adaptive function that motivates us to correct or flee situations that may be stressful or hazardous. Because of its protective function, the body is designed to experience anxiety. The body is also designed to counteract this response in time, once the danger is over.

Here are some signs that worrying may be a problem for you:

Worrying more often than not for at least 6 months

Difficulty falling or staying asleep

Worrying interfering with some aspect of your life

Chronic muscle tension

Feeling restless, on edge, or "keyed up"

Feeling irritated

Getting fatigued easily

Difficulty controlling your worries

Difficulty concentrating, mind going blank

Is Worrying Bad?

The anxiety associated with worry can be helpful. We can be motivated by worry. If we have deadlines or goals that we want to meet, anxiety can be useful. But, once anxiety gets too high, our performance can begin to decline, so the goal is to keep worrying and anxiety in a healthy range.

Barriers to Treatment

Sometimes the way we think can affect whether we can change our worry. Here are some examples of worried thoughts:

My worries are perfectly justified because of all the stress in my life. Since the stress will never go away, I will never stop worrying.

No one could realistically guarantee you that all of the stress in your life could possibly be removed. You can change the way that you interpret and deal with the events in your life. A fact of life is that some worry is justified. However, individuals experiencing difficulties with anxious worry often overestimate the amount of justifiable worry in their lives and stand to gain from skills aimed at improving this judgment.

Worrying about things is how I prepare. If I don't worry about how I will handle different situations beforehand, I won't be prepared when situations arise and I'll be overwhelmed.

For those with anxiety, worrying does serve a purpose. It can serve as a form of avoidance for the worrier because of the distraction it provides. For others, worrying is a coping strategy, a form of busywork that provides the worrier a small degree of control over the situation. You've probably had some experience with successfully handling one or two of these unexpected crises, even though you had no time to worry about it beforehand. Treatment for anxiety replaces worry with more adaptive ways of coping.

My life is so stressful. I don't have time to relax.

When crises arise, we often sacrifice personal time to meet deadlines. For individuals with chronic anxiety who spend most of their time worrying, even small "time-outs" for relaxation can be beneficial. Most people can find just 15 minutes a day to devote to relaxation.

I'm afraid to focus on my anxiety because I think it might be a sign that I'm going crazy.

People experiencing difficulty with anxious worry often report that it is difficult to stop worrying once they get started. This perceived loss of control is very disturbing. Difficulty controlling anxious thoughts or feelings is different from an inability to control one's behavior or perceptions of reality. There is very little evidence to suggest that anxiety disorders can develop into the various thought disorders that people often think of when they describe "going crazy."

FIGURE 5.5. Worry Management Handout

Worry Management

1. **Worry Place and Time:** Set a 30-minute worry period that will take place at the same time and same place each day. Your worry place and time will be:

   _____

2. **Worry Log:** Record all your worries during your worry time on the Worry Log, then take time to categorize these worries. You can choose categories that are helpful for you. You might organize them by "Big Concerns," "Medium Concerns," and "Small Concerns." Another option would be to categorize them by content area, such as "Work Concerns," "Family Concerns," "Financial Concerns," and "Relationship Concerns." Any means of categorizing can be used; however, it is important not to use too many categories. Usually between three and seven works best. In the next column of your worry log, you can write how you will manage the problem. If the problem is something you have absolutely no control over, you might write down, *"I'm not going to worry about this problem because there is nothing I can do about it right now."*

3. **Delay Worry:** If you notice you are worrying outside of your scheduled worry time, tell yourself, *"I have plenty of time to focus on this later. Right now I'm just going to be in the moment and notice what I'm doing, what others are doing, the environment, and other things I see, hear, or smell."*

Worry Log

Worrisome Thought	Category	Management Strategy

In addition to methods for addressing cognitive changes, we may also teach relaxation methods (e.g., relaxed breathing) and ways to reduce alarming thinking (see Chapter 4) to help lower sympathetic arousal and alarming thinking associated with worrying.

Arrange

Often patients who adopt new patterns of thinking will quickly notice decreases in their worrying. Follow-up appointments may focus on teaching new skills or overcoming barriers associated with modifying thinking habits. For those individuals who demonstrate difficulty in making changes in their thinking or behaviors, specialty mental health may be useful for providing a more intensive treatment for worrying.

PANIC DISORDER

DSM-5-TR (American Psychiatric Association, 2022, pp. 235–245) criteria for panic disorder include recurrent panic attacks (i.e., an abrupt surge of intense fear or discomfort that peaks within a few minutes and is associated with at least four physical or cognitive symptoms, such as heart racing, sweating, nausea, fear of death, fear of losing control). In addition, there is concern about having attacks in the future, worry about the implications or consequences of the attack (e.g., having a heart attack, going crazy), and/or significant behavior changes caused by the attacks. Panic disorder may be associated with agoraphobia (i.e., anxiety about places or situations that may be difficult or embarrassing to escape; those situations are avoided or are associated with marked distress or anxiety). Lifetime prevalence data suggest that panic disorder affects approximately 4.8% of the population; 23.5% experience isolated panic, without panic disorder (R. C. Kessler et al., 2006). Patients demonstrating panic disorder have higher rates of utilization of medical services compared with individuals with other anxiety disorders (Deacon et al., 2008).

Specialty Mental Health

Behavioral therapies and cognitive behavioral therapies have been found to be effective treatments for panic disorder either alone or combined with pharmacotherapy (e.g., escitalopram [Lexapro], sertraline [Zoloft], citalopram [Celexa], paroxetine [Paxil], venlafaxine [Effexor]; DeGeorge et al., 2022; Rabasco et al., 2022). Ultrabrief interventions (e.g., five sessions) for panic disorder have also been found to be effective (Otto et al., 2012). Interventions for panic disorder typically incorporate education, cognitive restructuring, in vivo and imaginal exposure, breathing retraining, and relaxation (Otto et al., 2012). Similar to those of GAD, panic symptoms have been improved through the use of self-help or physician-guided, evidence-based interventions (van Boeijen et al., 2005).

Behavioral Health in Primary Care

Some data have shown that cognitive and behavioral interventions delivered by BHCs in primary care, as well as SSRIs, can be effective for the treatment of panic disorder (DeGeorge et al., 2022; Roy-Byrne et al., 2009; Shepardson et al., 2018).

Primary Care Adaptation

The 5As help to guide BHCs through the process of assessing and treating panic disorder in primary care.

Assess

To screen for panic disorder, a BHC can ask targeted questions about experiences with panic-related symptoms, as follows:

- Have you ever had an episode when you suddenly felt your heart racing; had difficulty breathing; started feeling shaky or dizzy; and/or were worried that you might die, suffocate, or have something bad happen?

- How long did that episode last? How many experiences have you had like that?

- Are you worried that it will happen again? Did you change what you do because you were concerned about the attacks?

- Have you avoided places that might be difficult to get out of or might be embarrassing if you had one of these attacks?

- What do you do to avoid having an attack? Have you avoided driving? Going to the store? Going to social gatherings?

The goal of the questioning is to determine whether the individual experienced a panic attack and how they changed their behavior in response to concerns about the attacks. The GAD-7 and GAD-2 may be helpful as screening tools for panic disorder. Using five questions from the panic module in the PHQ has resulted in the best sensitivity (81%) and specificity (99%) for detecting panic disorder (Herr et al., 2014; Spitzer et al., 1999); these questions are provided in Figure 5.6.

Advise

Once our functional assessment has identified a patient with panic disorder, we discuss the various treatment options. Patients diagnosed with panic disorder commonly use medications to manage their symptoms. Medication recommendations for panic disorder include SSRIs or possibly imipramine or clomipramine; however, benzodiazepines are not recommended (National Institute

FIGURE 5.6. Anxiety Questions

Questions About Anxiety From the PHQ

	No	Yes
In the last 4 weeks, have you had an anxiety attack—suddenly feeling fear or panic?	❏	❏
Has this ever happened before?	❏	❏
Do some of these attacks come suddenly out of the blue—that is, in situations where you don't expect to be nervous or uncomfortable?	❏	❏
Do these attacks bother you a lot or are you worried about having another attack?	❏	❏
During your last bad anxiety attack, did you have symptoms like shortness of breath, sweating, your heart racing or pounding, dizziness or faintness, tingling or numbness, or nausea or upset stomach?	❏	❏

Panic disorder may be indicated if all questions are endorsed with "Yes."
Note. PHQ = Patient Health Questionnaire. Data from Spitzer et al. (2016).

for Health and Care Excellence [NICE], 2011). We discuss with patients the importance of education and the possibility of using cognitive and behavioral techniques to manage their anxiety symptoms. We tell them that these techniques have been shown to be superior for long-term treatment of panic symptoms. This is often a good time to use some of the motivational enhancement techniques that we review in Chapter 4. Thus, a BHC could say the following:

> It sounds as if you have used medications to manage the uncomfortable symptoms of your anxiety. I'm wondering whether it would be beneficial for you to learn other ways to manage this anxiety so that you don't need to use the medication as often. We know that, over the long term, these techniques can be as or more effective interventions for panic symptoms. What would be the benefits of changing? What would be the risks?

Agree

As with depressive symptoms, it is necessary to assess what the patient is willing to attempt regarding change. Cognitive and behavioral interventions often involve a willingness to tolerate the uncomfortable physiological symptoms that occur with anxious thinking. Relaxation techniques can reduce the intensity of these symptoms, but the patient must be willing to think about their exaggerated physiological symptoms in a different way and be willing to implement and practice a new set of skills for managing these symptoms. Review the options for treatment (e.g., continue taking medication, learn cognitive and behavioral techniques, do nothing) and ask patients what they want to pursue.

Assist

We have included a patient handout in Figure 5.7 that guides the patient through the interventions for panic disorder. In general, we educate the patient about panic, teach ways to manage their alarming thoughts, and may teach relaxation and ways to decrease behavioral avoidance.

Education. To decrease symptoms associated with panic disorder, we start by educating patients about panic attacks and discussing how these attacks are due to exaggerated sympathetic responses, which are usually helpful for managing stressful situations. It is often important to draw on the fact that the medical provider has ruled out any serious medical problems. Thus, we might say the following:

> Your doctor has ruled out any significant medical problems at this point, so we think the physical symptoms you are experiencing are related to what we call the fight-or-flight response, a reflex that helps all of us to react to potentially dangerous situations. This response does everything possible to allow us to respond as quickly as possible to these situations, including increasing our heart rate, tightening our muscles, and slowing down our digestive system, so we can fight or flee from something that is potentially dangerous. In individuals who have panic attacks, this system seems to activate for no reason, and people notice an intense unexpected physiological response. The symptoms can feel as if they are life threatening, and all you want is for those symptoms to stop.

FIGURE 5.7. Panic Disorder Handout (*continues*)

Panic Disorder

What Is a Panic Attack?

Sometimes we experience a sudden and severe onset of symptoms that can be scary. These symptoms can include some or all of the following:

Pounding heart or increased heart rate	Feeling dizzy, unsteady, lightheaded, or faint
Sweating, nausea	Feelings of unreality or being detached from yourself
Trembling or shaking	Fear of losing control or going crazy
Shortness of breath	Fear of dying
Feeling of choking	Numbness or tingling
Chest pain	Chills or hot flashes

Although we don't fully understand why some people experience panic attacks and other people don't, we do know that these symptoms are related to a very normal response called the fight-or-flight response. This response allows our body to react quickly when we think that something is dangerous, like being attacked or someone cutting us off when we are driving.

How Do Panic Attacks Affect Our Lives?

Because these symptoms come out of the blue, we can become worried about the symptoms and we may begin to avoid situations that we think will result in these panic symptoms, like crowded stores, public transportation, or driving. What situations have you avoided because of panic attacks?

_____
_____
_____

Changing Thinking Patterns

One of the most important changes associated with panic attacks is changing how we think. The fear associated with having a panic attack may increase the likelihood of having an attack. Therefore, a willingness to experience a panic attack, knowing that the symptoms, while uncomfortable, will not harm you, is an important aspect of managing the symptoms of panic.

Thinking that increases panic	Thinking that decreases panic
I'm having a heart attack!	This is not an emergency.
I'm going to die.	This doesn't feel good, but it won't hurt me.
I can't stand this.	I can feel uncomfortable and still be okay.
I have to get out of here.	This will go away with time.
Oh no, here it comes!	I can handle this.

What are the things that you say to yourself that may increase panic symptoms?

_____
_____
_____

What could you say to decrease panic symptoms?

_____
_____
_____

FIGURE 5.7. Panic Disorder Handout (*continued*)

Breathing Retraining

People who have panic attacks show some signs of hyperventilation or overbreathing. When people hyperventilate, certain blood vessels in the body become narrower, which can contribute to numbness or tingling in the hands or feet or the sensation of cold, clammy hands and increased heart rate. You can help overcome overbreathing by learning breathing control.

Instructions for Breathing Retraining

1. Find a comfortable, quiet location.
2. Count "1" on breath in and think "relax" on breath out.
3. Focus attention on breathing and counting.
4. Maintain a normal rate and depth of breathing.
5. Expand abdomen on breath in and keep chest still.
6. Count up to 10 and back to 1.
7. Practice twice per day, 10 minutes each time.

Decreasing Avoidance

Regardless of whether you can identify why you began having panic attacks or whether they seemed to come out of the blue, the places where you began having panic attacks often can become triggers themselves.

To break the cycle of avoidance, it is important to first identify the places or situations that are being avoided and then to do some relearning. Just as the negative experience of a panic attack can result in learning to avoid certain locations, having positive, successful experiences can result in learning that the location is nothing to be afraid of.

Which item on your list of avoided locations or situations would you like to target first? Please list this situation here: _____

Now, you can develop a hierarchy for this situation or location. This hierarchy will help guide you as you gradually begin to expose yourself to this situation or location that you have been avoiding.

Changing thinking. We then focus on discussing how thoughts and fears associated with these responses, as well as attempts to avoid panic-related symptoms, can increase the intensity and frequency of these symptoms. This component, which is more like traditional cognitive therapy, is geared toward helping the patient identify ways of thinking that exacerbate their symptoms (for further details, see the discussion of cognitive disputation in Chapter 4). We also incorporate simple analogies used with ACT, such as the Chinese finger trap (Hayes et al., 1999, pp. 104–105), to help illustrate this point. Therefore, we might say the following:

> When we experience these physical symptoms, often our first instinct is to want them to go away. Sometimes we may leave the situation, we may try to gain control of our breathing, we may try to distract ourselves, but if the symptoms don't go away, we get more worried. Sometimes our attempts to control these symptoms may make the symptoms worse. For example, have you ever played with Chinese finger cuffs? [Explain that you put one finger of each hand into each end of a woven tubelike device; when you try to quickly pull your fingers out of it, the tube holds your fingers in place.] If you try to quickly pull your fingers out of the finger cuff, the cuff gets tighter. Panic symptoms can be very similar to that finger cuff; the harder we try to control the symptoms, the tighter or the more intense the symptoms can become. So instead of trying to make the symptoms go away, maybe it would be possible to let the symptoms occur, and relax our fingers in the cuff, knowing that, in time, the symptoms will go away.

Relaxation training. We may teach relaxation methods, such as controlled breathing, to help manage hyperventilation or overbreathing, which is experienced by some patients with panic disorder. Such breathing strategies provide a way for the patient to cope with a panic attack when it occurs.

Situational exposure. Situational exposure involves having the patient come in contact with the object, person, or place that results in fear. It is used to desensitize the patient to people, places, and objects the patient avoids because of fear. Detailed explanations for behavioral exposure treatments are explained in many publications (e.g., Richard & Lauterbach, 2007; Rosqvist, 2005). The goals of exposure are to decrease general fear, avoidance, and safety behaviors. Have the patient complete the Situational Exposure Hierarchy in Figure 5.8 on their own. At a follow-up consult, discuss specifics and devise a plan to go through the hierarchy and set times for exposure.

Interoceptive exposure. Interoceptive exposure involves exercises that produce a physical symptom (e.g., breathing through a straw for 2 minutes to produce a rapid heartbeat and short shallow breaths). Interoceptive exposure can be done in a 30-minute appointment in much the same way as in a specialty mental health appointment. This exercise should be geared toward the feared body sensations. The goal is to help patients learn that their feared prediction about

FIGURE 5.8. Situational Exposure Hierarchy Handout (*continues*)

Situational Exposure Hierarchy

Example: Fear of driving List situations from least to most anxiety provoking. 1. Visualizing driving to the store 2. Sitting in car in the driveway, with car off 3. Sitting in car in the driveway, with car idling 4. Driving to end of driveway and back 5. Driving to end of street and back 6. Driving from driveway to main street and back 7. Driving car from house to store	Your fear: _____ List situations from least to most anxiety provoking. 1. 2. 3. 4. 5. 6. 7.

Situational Exposure Rating Form

Date	Number of times practiced	Exposure situation	Maximum anxiety (0–10)

FIGURE 5.8. Situational Exposure Hierarchy Handout (*continued*)

Interoceptive Exposure
Activities That Can Produce Feared Body Sensations

Activity	Physical sensation
Hold breath as long as you can	Tight chest, out of breath
Overbreathe, take short and shallow breaths with chest going out for 60 seconds	Numb, racing heart, tingling fingers
Spin in a chair for 90 seconds	Dizzy, nauseous
Breathe through a straw for 2 minutes	Increased heart rate, breathless
Shake head from side to side for 30 seconds	Blurred vision, dizzy
Tense all muscles in body while sitting in a chair for 60 seconds	Trembling, shaky
Swallow six times quickly	Sore, uncomfortable throat
Clear throat six times quickly	Sore, uncomfortable throat
Jog in one place for 3 minutes	Racing heart, tight chest

Feared Physical Sensation Exercise

Physical activity	Feared prediction/ belief about the physical sensations of the activity	Alternative/ rational prediction/ belief about the sensations of the activity	Physical sensations produced by the activity	How similar were the sensations to what you experience naturally 0–10	Anxiety in response to the sensations 0–10

what might happen is not true and to desensitize them to these sensations (for patient handouts, see Figure 5.8).

Arrange

Many individuals treated with brief interventions for panic disorder improve quickly. If significant improvement is not seen in a short period or if there are comorbid disorders (e.g., substance abuse) that significantly complicate the treatment of the anxiety disorder, then consider a referral to specialty mental health care. If possible, the specialty mental health provider should be trained in cognitive and behavioral interventions for panic disorder, which evidence-based guidelines suggest are the most effective interventions (NICE, 2011).

For both GAD and panic disorder, a variety of additional resources, including websites, mobile device applications, and self-help books, are available that might be used in conjunction with BHC appointments or might be used by patients who will be following up with their PCP only. Some of these resources are summarized in Figure 5.9.

POSTTRAUMATIC STRESS DISORDER

The *DSM-5-TR* (American Psychiatric Association, 2022, pp. 301–313) diagnosis of PTSD is dependent on (a) exposure to a traumatic event, involving actual or threatened death, serious injury, or sexual violence; (b) intrusion symptoms associated with the traumatic event (e.g., recurrent memories, distressing

FIGURE 5.9. Resources for Patients With Anxiety: Websites, Mobile Applications, and Books

Type	Location	Descriptions
Websites	Anxiety and Depression Association of America (http://www.adaa.org/)	Provides information and resources for patients about anxiety and depressive disorders; professional organization for researchers and therapists who specialize in these areas
	National Institute of Mental Health (https://www.nimh.nih.gov/health/topics/anxiety-disorders?rf=32471)	Provides information for patients about anxiety
Mobile applications	Breathe2Relax (Apple iOS and Android)	Guides patients through deep breathing exercises
	Self-Help for Anxiety Management (Apple iOS and Android)	Provides self-help information for patients to manage anxiety
Books	*The Mindfulness and Acceptance Workbook for Anxiety: A Guide to Breaking Free From Anxiety, Phobias, and Worry Using Acceptance and Commitment Therapy*, 2nd ed. (Forsyth & Eifert, 2016)	Uses acceptance and commitment therapy techniques to help patients target a broad range of anxiety symptoms
	The Anxiety and Phobia Workbook, 7th ed. (Bourne, 2020)	Provides practical guidance for patients to target anxiety and phobia symptoms
	Face Your Fears: A Proven Plan to Beat Anxiety, Panic, Phobias, and Obsessions (Tolin, 2012)	Provides step-by-step guidance for targeting a range of anxiety symptoms

dreams, dissociative reactions, distress or physiological reactions with exposure to cues related to the event); (c) avoidance of stimuli associated with the traumatic event; (d) negative alteration in thoughts or mood associated with the event (e.g., inability to remember important aspects of the event, persistent negative emotional state, detachment from others, inability to experience positive emotions); and (e) alterations in arousal and reactivity (e.g., irritable behavior and angry outbursts, reckless or self-destructive behavior, hypervigilance, concentration problems, sleep disturbance). The symptoms (b), (c), (d), and (e) must last longer than 1 month and cause significant distress or impairment.

Cultural and Diversity Considerations

The lifetime prevalence of PTSD is statistically similar across Hispanic (5.9%), Black (7.1%), and White (6.8%) adults. Studies have found significantly higher lifetime prevalence of PTSD among American Indian/Alaska Native populations (22.9%). LGB individuals are more likely to be exposed to childhood abuse and traumatic events and have a 1.6 to 3.9 times greater risk of PTSD compared with their heterosexual peers (Sayed et al., 2015). Among the best studies, the lifetime prevalence of PTSD is higher for military populations (7.7%–13.4%) compared with civilian populations (3.4%–8.0%; Schein et al., 2021). Lifetime prevalence of PTSD is also higher for women (i.e., 6%–26.9%) compared with men (2.6%–17.1%), with American Indian/Alaska Native women demonstrating the highest lifetime prevalence rate (26.9%; Emerson et al., 2017; Schein et al., 2021).

Specialty Mental Health

Clinical practice guidelines for the assessment and treatment of PTSD have been developed by the APA (2017) and the U.S. Department of Veterans Affairs and Department of Defense (VA/DoD; 2017). Both of these sets of guidelines concluded that trauma-focused psychotherapy involving exposure and/or cognitive restructuring (e.g., prolonged exposure, cognitive processing therapy, cognitive therapy, eye movement desensitization and reprocessing) were effective treatments. Regarding medications, SSRIs (e.g., fluoxetine, paroxetine, sertraline) and SNRIs (e.g., venlafaxine) have the strongest support as first-line medication treatment or for augmenting psychotherapy for PTSD (APA, 2017; VA/DoD, 2017)

Behavioral Health in Primary Care

Providers are encouraged to offer education and evidence-based treatment in primary care or through a referral to specialty mental health. Several studies have demonstrated benefits of brief PTSD interventions adapted for primary care environments (Cigrang et al., 2011, 2015; Corso et al., 2009; Harmon et al., 2014, Ogbeide et al., 2021; Possemato, 2011). However, more robust studies are needed to determine whether these brief interventions result in lasting functional improvements.

Primary Care Adaptation

Using what is known about treating PTSD in specialty mental health and primary care environments, in conjunction with the 5As approach, can help BHCs efficiently integrate evidence-based care in an effective manner.

Assess

The need for improved identification of PTSD in primary care has been discussed repeatedly (e.g., NICE, 2018; VA/DoD, 2017; Wilson, 2007). Particularly with individuals who demonstrate affective distress, it is important to ask about exposure to traumatic events and to provide possible examples, such as assault, rape, motor vehicle accidents, and childhood abuse (NICE, 2018). Individuals demonstrating PTSD symptoms often demonstrate other behavioral health conditions, including depression, anxiety, and/or substance use disorders (Galatzer-Levy et al., 2013); therefore, it is important to assess whether the patient is struggling with these concerns as well. Most individuals demonstrate PTSD symptoms within the 1st month of the traumatic event; however, some individuals (15%) may not demonstrate symptoms of PTSD for years after the event (McNally, 2003). The Primary Care PTSD Screen for the *DSM-5* (PC-PTSD-5), which was adapted from the PC-PTSD (Prins et al., 2003), is a useful screening measure for PTSD. In one study (Prins et al., 2016) using a sample of veterans, a cutoff score of 3 optimized sensitivity (94.8%), while providing acceptable specificity ($\geq 80\%$). Bovin et al. (2021) found that a cutoff score of 4 maximized sensitivity and specificity for male veterans, whereas a cutoff score of 3 worked better for female veterans. Williamson et al. (2022), using a sample of civilians, found that a cutoff score of 4 maximized sensitivity (100%), while providing acceptable specificity (85.2%). BHCs using the PC-PTSD-5 will need to consider the populations that they serve when selecting the most appropriate cutoff score (i.e., 3 vs. 4). The PC-PTSD is available in Figure 5.10.

Advise

In primary care settings, SSRIs or SNRIs will likely be a first line of treatment for the symptoms of PTSD, given the systematic review evidence supporting their use (APA, 2017; VA/DoD, 2017). As with depression, it is important to advise patients to use the medication as prescribed. In addition to medications, it is often necessary to recommend psychotherapy in a specialty behavioral health setting. A BHC can play a vital role in discussing what psychotherapy might involve and in advising the patient about the importance of pursuing treatment and the likelihood of improvement.

FIGURE 5.10. Primary Care PTSD-5 Screen (*continues*)

PC-PTSD-5

Description

The Primary Care Posttraumatic Stress Disorder Screen for *DSM-5* (PC-PTSD-5) is a five-item screen designed to identify individuals with probable PTSD. Those who screen positive require further assessment, preferably with a structured interview.

Scoring

The measure begins with an item designed to assess whether the respondent has had any exposure to traumatic events. If a respondent denies exposure, the PC-PTSD-5 is complete with a score of 0. If a respondent indicates a trauma history—experiencing a traumatic event over the course of their life—the respondent is instructed to answer five additional yes/no questions (see below) about how that trauma has affected them over the past month. Respondents can score a 0–5, which is a count of "yes" responses to the five questions below. Research in a large sample of VA primary care patients found that a cut point of 4 ideally balanced false negatives and false positives for the overall sample of men. However, for women, a cut point of 4 resulted in high numbers of false negatives. Practitioners may consider a lower cut point for women in some settings if evaluation resources are available. In contrast, a higher cut point may be preferable if resources are such that false positives will substantially decrease clinician availability. Because performance parameters will change according to the sample, clinicians should consider sample characteristics and screening purposes when selecting a cut point.

Example

In the past month, have you . . .

had nightmares about the event(s) or thought about the event(s) when you did not want to?	YES	NO
tried hard not to think about the event(s) or went out of your way to avoid situations that reminded you of the event(s)?	YES	NO
been constantly on guard, watchful, or easily startled?	YES	NO
felt numb or detached from people, activities, or your surroundings?	YES	NO
felt guilty or unable to stop blaming yourself or others for the event(s) or any problems the events may have caused?	YES	NO
Total score is sum of "YES" responses in items 1–5.	TOTAL SCORE	

PC-PTSD-5

Sometimes things happen to people that are unusually or especially frightening, horrible, or traumatic. For example,

- a serious accident or fire,
- a physical or sexual assault or abuse,
- an earthquake or flood,
- a war,
- seeing someone be killed or seriously injured, or
- having a loved one die through homicide or suicide.

Have you ever experienced this kind of event?

                    YES   NO

If no, screen total = 0. Please stop here.

FIGURE 5.10. Primary Care PTSD-5 Screen (*continued*)

If yes, please answer the questions below.

In the past month, have you . . .

had nightmares about the event(s) or thought about the event(s) when you did not want to?	YES	NO
tried hard not to think about the event(s) or went out of your way to avoid situations that reminded you of the event(s)?	YES	NO
been constantly on guard, watchful, or easily startled?	YES	NO
felt numb or detached from people, activities, or your surroundings?	YES	NO
felt guilty or unable to stop blaming yourself or others for the event(s) or any problems the events may have caused?	YES	NO
Total score is sum of "YES" responses in Items 1–5.	TOTAL SCORE	

Note. Adapted from *The Primary Care PTSD Screen for* DSM-5 *(PC-PTSD-5)*, by A. Prins, M. J. Bovin, R. Kimerling, D. G. Kaloupek, B. P. Marx, A. Pless Kaiser, and P. P. Schnurr, 2015, U.S. Department of Veterans Affairs (https://www.ptsd.va.gov/professional/assessment/screens/pc-ptsd.asp). In the public domain.

Agree

The BHC can help the medical team by establishing a plan of treatment, even if it is a wait-and-see approach, as well as by maintaining appropriate medication use and/or pursuing psychotherapy. The BHC may also contribute by developing a treatment plan that the patient agrees to and by helping the patient to identify situations that may indicate the treatment is not working. The BHC might say the following:

> So you are going to continue with the medication and consider pursuing psychotherapy. If your symptoms worsen, such as if the nightmares become more intense or more frequent, or if you notice your irritability negatively affecting your relationships at work or at home, we want you to come back to see what other services might be helpful. Does that seem reasonable to you?

Assist

Prolonged exposure techniques, as well as other treatments requiring extended and repeated appointments, are not appropriate for a primary care environment given the extended time necessary for such interventions. However, modified versions of these techniques (e.g., using at-home writing and reading of events) used in studies exploring PTSD treatment in primary care may be useful for PTSD treatment (e.g., Cigrang et al., 2011, 2015). Although the VA/DoD (2017) guidelines suggest that brief interventions (i.e., 4–5 sessions) in specialty behavioral health care may be effective, it remains unclear whether brief interventions provided in primary care are effective. However, there may be opportunities for BHCs to intervene with subclinical symptoms of PTSD and assist with monitoring symptoms that may indicate acute stress disorder. Once responses have been normalized for these individuals, the interventions, including relaxation exercises, cognitive disputation, and problem solving (as discussed in Chapter 4) may be particularly helpful for reducing symptoms associated with increased physiological arousal. In addition, writing down negative or worried thoughts, in a manner similar to strategies used with GAD, and using acceptance-based techniques may help in the management of the distressing symptoms (e.g., Walser & Westrup, 2007).

Arrange

When making a referral to specialty mental health providers for PTSD, it is important to ensure that they have experience treating PTSD. Specialty mental health providers should be offering prolonged exposure, cognitive processing therapy, eye movement desensitization and reprocessing, specific cognitive behavioral therapies for PTSD, brief eclectic psychotherapy, narrative exposure therapy, and/or written narrative exposure, which have strong evidence for their effectiveness (VA/DoD, 2017). Websites, mobile device applications, or self-help books may also be helpful as an adjunct to treatment for PTSD. Some of these resources are summarized in Figure 5.11.

FIGURE 5.11. Resources for Patients With PTSD: Websites, Mobile Applications, and Books

Type	Location	Descriptions
Websites	National Center for PTSD (https://www.ptsd.va.gov/)	Provides information and resources about PTSD for individuals and family members
	National Institute of Mental Health (https://www.nimh.nih.gov/health/topics/post-traumatic-stress-disorder-ptsd)	Provides information about PTSD for patients
Mobile applications	PTSD Coach (https://mobile.va.gov/app/ptsd-coach; Apple iOS and Android)	Helps patients manage symptoms associated with PTSD
	CPT Coach (https://mobile.va.gov/app/cpt-coach; Apple iOS and Android)	Intended as a supplement for those involved in CPT treatment with a provider
	PE Coach (https://mobile.va.gov/app/pe-coach; Apple iOS and Android)	Intended as a supplement for those involved in PE treatment with a provider
Books	*Overcoming Trauma and PTSD: A Workbook Integrating Skills From ACT, DBT, and CBT* (Raja, 2012)	Incorporates trauma-related interventions from ACT, DBT, and CBT
	The PTSD Workbook: Simple, Effective Techniques for Overcoming Traumatic Stress Symptoms, 3rd ed. (M. B. Williams & Poijula, 2016)	Provides self-help tools to assist those exposed to trauma

Note. PTSD = posttraumatic stress disorder; CPT = cognitive processing therapy; PE = prolonged exposure; ACT = acceptance and commitment therapy; DBT = dialectical behavior therapy; CBT = cognitive behavior therapy.

INSOMNIA

The prevalence of sleep complaints in primary care has been estimated to be as high as 69%, with 49% of patients reporting occasional insomnia and 10% to 15% reporting chronic insomnia (Ram et al., 2010). Insomnia tends to be persistent over time if not treated (Morin et al., 2020). However, the percentage of outpatient office visits in which insomnia is listed as a reason for the visit is only 0.7% (Ford et al., 2014). Primary care providers often focus on prescribing medicine, adjusting medications that may affect sleep, and discussing healthy sleep habits (Ulmer et al., 2017) but not on the treatments (e.g., stimulus control, sleep restriction) that have been shown to be most effective and longer lasting (Trauer et al., 2015). According to the *DSM-5-TR* (American Psychiatric Association, 2022, pp. 409–417), primary insomnia occurs when an individual has difficulty initiating or maintaining sleep or experiences early-morning awakening with an inability to return to sleep 3 nights per week for at least 3 months. The sleep disturbance must result in clinically significant distress or impairment. The sleep disturbances cannot be due to other sleep or mental health disorders or to the physiological effects of an illicit drug, medication, or medical condition.

Cultural and Diversity Considerations

Studies have found that those with a lower socioeconomic status experience more sleep-related problems and that Black adults tend to demonstrate shorter, less efficient sleep but fewer symptoms of insomnia compared with their White counterparts (T. J. Cunningham et al., 2015). As White adults rise in their socioeconomic status, sleep tends to improve; however, this same pattern is not seen among Black, Hispanic, and Asian adults (T. J. Cunningham et al., 2015). Additional risk factors for insomnia include female sex, a family history of insomnia, and severe and chronic life stressors (Morin et al., 2015).

Specialty Mental Health

Evidence from meta-analyses and systematic reviews highlight that cognitive behavior therapies for insomnia are effective (Trauer et al., 2015) and superior to pharmacotherapy over the long term (van der Zweerde et al., 2019; Y. Zhang et al., 2022). Cognitive and behavioral interventions usually involve a combination of sleep hygiene, stimulus control, sleep restriction, and relaxation. Sleep hygiene involves lifestyle (e.g., caffeine, nicotine, alcohol, diet, exercise) and environmental factors (e.g., noise, room temperature, body temperature, air quality, light, bed comfort) that patients can potentially control (Morin & Espie, 2003).

Increasing the degree to which the bed and bedroom are associated with sleep rather than other activities (e.g., watching television, eating, using the computer) is called *stimulus control* (Bootzin & Epstein, 2000). To maximize stimulus control, patients are encouraged to avoid all activities in the bedroom except sleep and sex, and they are encouraged to get out of bed in 15 minutes if they are not asleep. Sleep restriction requires that individuals reduce the amount of time that they are in bed to the amount of time that they are actually asleep. Therefore, if someone only sleeps 5.5 hours but typically stays in bed for 7 hours, the time between getting in and out of bed would be reduced so that the total time in bed would only be 5.5 hours. Developing a wind-down routine and engaging in relaxation training help reduce sympathetic arousal before bedtime, increasing the likelihood that the patient can fall asleep. An excellent review of insomnia and treatments is provided by Morin and colleagues (2015).

Behavioral Health in Primary Care

Evidence has shown that brief interventions, including self-help programs, can successfully reduce insomnia (Morin et al., 2006). These interventions can be successfully delivered in primary care (e.g., Buysse et al., 2011; Falloon et al., 2015; Fernando et al., 2013; Goodie et al., 2009; Jernelöv et al., 2012). Brief behavioral treatment for insomnia (Troxel et al., 2012) uses four appointments, two of which could be conducted by phone, to deliver the core components of cognitive behavioral therapy for insomnia. Brief behavioral treatment for insomnia has been found to be effective for improving insomnia and is well suited for use in primary care (Gunn et al., 2019; Troxel et al., 2012).

Primary Care Adaptation

As demonstrated with brief behavioral treatment for insomnia, the assessments and interventions developed and evaluated in specialty mental health settings can be adapted and implemented by BHCs using the 5As in primary care.

Assess

Typically, in outpatient specialty mental health settings, sleep diaries are used as part of a sleep assessment; however, in primary care environments we rely more heavily on patient self-reports. We suggest that a BHC's primary assessment involves asking targeted questions to assess sleep behaviors, factors that may prompt and maintain insomnia (stimulus control), and sleep hygiene. Brief standardized self-report measures exist that can be appropriate for the primary care environment. The Insomnia Severity Index (Bastien et al., 2001) uses seven items to assess sleep impairment. Using a cutoff score of 14, this measure correctly identified 82.2% of the individuals in primary care settings diagnosed with insomnia and is considered a valid index of insomnia severity (Gagnon et al., 2013). The Insomnia Severity Index is presented in Figure 5.12.

Supplementing a review of the electronic health record, a focused functional assessment of a sleep problem might focus on the following areas:

FIGURE 5.12. Insomnia Severity Index

The Insomnia Severity Index

1.   Please rate the current (i.e., last 2 weeks) severity of your insomnia problem(s).

		None	Mild	Moderate	Severe	Very
a.	Difficulty falling asleep	0	1	2	3	4
b.	Difficulty staying asleep	0	1	2	3	4
c.	Problem waking up too early	0	1	2	3	4

2.   How satisfied/dissatisfied are you with your current sleep pattern?

Very satisfied	Satisfied	Neutral	Dissatisfied	Very dissatisfied
0	1	2	3	4

3.   To what extent do you consider your sleep problem to interfere with your daily functioning (e.g., daytime fatigue, ability to function at work/daily chores, concentration, memory, mood)?

Not at all interfering	A little	Somewhat	Much	Very much interfering
0	1	2	3	4

4.   How noticeable to others do you think your sleeping problem is in terms of impairing the quality of your life?

Not at all noticeable	A little	Somewhat	Much	Very much noticeable
0	1	2	3	4

5.   How worried/distressed are you about your current sleep problem?

Not at all worried	A little	Somewhat	Much	Very much worried
0	1	2	3	4

Guidelines for Scoring/Interpretation
Add scores for all seven items (1a + 1b + 1c + 2 + 3 + 4 + 5) =
Total score ranges from 0–28; if total score falls between:

> 0–7 = No clinically significant insomnia
> 8–14 = Subthreshold insomnia
> 15–21 = Clinical insomnia (moderate severity)
> 22–28 = Clinical insomnia (severe)

Note. From *Insomnia: A Clinical Guide to Assessment and Treatment* (p. 137), by C. M. Morin and C. A. Espie, 2003, Springer Nature. Copyright 2003 by Springer Nature. Reprinted with permission.

History.

- When did you first start having difficulty with your sleep?

- Did anything happen that started your sleep problem?

- How many nights of the week do you have difficulty with your sleep?

Sleep environment.

- Is your bedroom generally quiet and comfortable?

- Are there any sources of light in your bedroom after you lay down to go to sleep?

- Is there anything that wakes you up throughout the night, such as noises, pets, or children?

- Do you have a bed partner? Does your partner affect your sleep?

Presleep behaviors.

- Do you take or use anything to help you fall asleep, including alcohol or sleeping medication?

- What time of day do you exercise?

- Do you use any tobacco? (Information may be obtained from medical record.) If so, what is the latest time you use tobacco before you go to bed?

- How much caffeine, including coffee, tea, and soda, do you consume? What is the latest time you have any caffeinated beverages before getting into bed?

In-bed behaviors.

- What time do you go to bed? How long does it take you to fall asleep once you are in bed?

- How many times do you wake up throughout the night? How long are you awake? What do you do when you wake up? Do you worry about not sleeping?

- What time do you wake up? Is that before or after the time you set on your alarm?

- How many naps do you take during the day? For how long? When you are awake in bed, do you watch TV, read, or eat?

- How long do you stay in bed when you are awake?

Consequences.

- Do you feel rested or tired when you wake up?

- Does that change during the day?

- Do you feel sleepy throughout the day?

- Have you fallen asleep in inappropriate places (e.g., in your car, in a waiting room)?

- Do you have difficulty concentrating?

- What are some ways that your sleep affects your functioning?

- Do you nap? If so, how long are your naps?

Exclusions.

- Sleep apnea: Do you snore at night? Do you wake up with a headache or a tight chest? Has anyone told you that you gasp for air when you are sleeping?

- Periodic limb movements: Has a bed partner ever told you that you kick them at night? Do your legs suddenly move and wake you up?

- Restless leg syndrome: Do you experience uncomfortable feelings in your legs, such as burning, itching, or crawling sensations that might go away for a little bit when you move your legs but make it difficult to fall asleep?

- Narcolepsy: Do you have unwanted/unplanned periods of sleep that help you feel refreshed? If you become frightened or have another intense emotional response, do you suddenly lose your balance or fall? Do you find that you are unable to move or speak when waking after you have fallen asleep? Do you see or hear things when you are falling asleep?

- Bruxism: Do you grind your teeth at night? Do you wake with a headache?

Advise

Similar to dealing with individuals with depressive and anxious symptoms, BHCs need to be prepared to discuss the role of medication in managing sleep. In primary care settings, we see a wide range of individuals with sleeping problems, from those who have recently developed insomnia to those who have had insomnia for decades. We discuss the value of trying to minimize the use of medications to manage sleep over the long term but acknowledge the possible short-term benefits of medications. We encourage patients to consider behavioral changes as alternatives to medications and explain that these behavioral changes have been shown to work for 70% to 80% of patients struggling with insomnia. In a discussion about sleep medication, the BHC might say the following:

> In the short term, sleep medications can be very useful for helping people to get sleep when they really need to sleep. However, we know for most people with sleep problems, there are things they can do differently that can significantly improve their sleep if they stick with those changes for about a month. By making these changes, most individuals don't need sleep medications.

We believe it is important to make clear the types of behaviors the individual can change and why those changes are important to improve sleep. We might say the following:

> There are several things you might consider doing to improve your sleep. I'd like to tell you what those are and how they might work, and then you can tell me whether you think you want to do them. Going to bed when you are not sleepy and lying in bed awake is a sure way to make your sleep problem worse. The longer you stay in bed awake, the more you associate your bed with a place to be awake; the bed becomes a signal to be awake instead of asleep. I'd suggest you stop watching TV in bed as well. Watching TV is not compatible with sleep, so your bed becomes your couch or easy chair and is a reminder to watch TV, not sleep. I would also recommend stopping your 2-hour nap in the afternoon. That nap interrupts your sleep–wake cycle so you are not sleepy at night or, if you do fall asleep, your sleep is light and you wake frequently. Increased stress and worry are also a target for change. Stress and worry are not compatible with sleep, and, in fact, you have experienced this so much that often when you are sleepy and get into bed, you immediately become alert and start worrying about the next day. Your bed has become your worry place. Learning relaxation strategies and getting out of bed when worry starts can help improve sleep and allow the bed to become a place to sleep and not be awake.

If there are indications that other medical factors (e.g., obstructive sleep apnea, restless leg syndrome, narcolepsy) are contributing to sleep difficulties, it is important to coordinate with the patient and their PCP about the next steps for care (e.g., referral to a sleep study).

Agree

Typically, patients will agree to start the recommended changes; then a BHC can begin to help them learn what they need to do, set a specific plan, and teach them the skills required. Behavioral interventions for sleep require commitment, and sometimes the prospect of getting out of bed if the patient does not fall asleep or fall back to sleep after waking can be concerning. It is important to answer all questions and discuss the reasons why it is important to change. If the patient continues to hesitate over the recommended change(s), a BHC can ask,

> Is what you are currently doing to manage your sleep working?

When they say no, then say the following:

> The one thing we know for sure is that if you keep doing what you are doing it will continue to not work. In fact, you've really proven this by doing it for the last 6 months. To get a different outcome, you are going to have to do something different. Are you willing to try these recommendations for the next 3 weeks to see what happens?

Assist

We suggest using the handout in Figure 5.13 to help patients learn about sleep and interventions for improving sleep. When reviewing the handout, target those areas that appear to be of particular concern based on the functional assessment.

FIGURE 5.13. Improving Sleep Through Behavior Change Handout

Improving Sleep Through Behavior Change

Stimulus Control Procedures

Go to Bed Only When You Are Sleepy
The longer you are in bed, the more the bed is associated with a place to be awake instead of asleep. Delay bedtime until sleepy.

Get Out of Bed When You Can't Fall Asleep or Go Back to Sleep in About 15 Minutes
Get out of bed if you don't fall asleep fairly soon. Return to bed only when you are sleepy. When you feel sleepy return to bed. The goal is to reconnect your bed with being asleep.

Use the Bed for Sleep and Sex Only
Do not watch TV, listen to the radio, eat, or read in your bed or bedroom.

Sleep Hygiene Guidelines

Caffeine: Avoid Caffeine 6 to 8 Hours Before Bedtime
Caffeine disturbs sleep. Thus, drinking caffeinated beverages should be avoided near bedtime.

Nicotine: Avoid Nicotine Before Bedtime
Nicotine can keep you awake. Avoid tobacco near bedtime and during the night.

Alcohol: Avoid Alcohol After Dinner
Alcohol often promotes the onset of sleep but interrupts your natural sleep pattern. Do not consume it any closer than 4 hours before going to bed.

Sleeping Pills: Sleep Medications Are Effective Only Temporarily
Sleep medications lose their effectiveness in about 2 to 4 weeks when taken regularly. Over time, sleeping pills can make sleep problems worse and withdrawal from the medication can lead to an insomnia rebound. Keep use of sleep pills infrequent, but don't worry if you need to use them on an occasional basis.

Regular Exercise
Do not exercise within 2 hours of bedtime, as it may elevate nervous system activity and interfere with your ability to fall asleep.

Bedroom Environment: Moderate Temperature, Quiet, and Dark
Noises can be masked with background white noise (such as the noise of a fan) or with ear-plugs. Bedrooms may be darkened with blackout shades, or sleep masks can be worn.

Eating
A light bedtime snack, such a glass of warm milk, cheese, or a bowl of cereal, can promote sleep. Avoid snacks in the middle of the night since awakening may become associated with hunger.

Avoid Naps
Avoid naps. The sleep you obtain during the day takes away from your sleep need that night. If you must nap, schedule it before 3:00 p.m. and do not sleep more than 15 to 30 minutes.

Allow Yourself at Least an Hour Before Bedtime to Unwind
Find what works for you in winding down. Give yourself perhaps an hour to do so.

Regular Sleep Schedule
Keep a regular time each day, 7 days a week, to get out of bed. Keeping a regular awaking time helps set your circadian rhythm so that your body learns to sleep at the desired time.

Set a Reasonable Bedtime and Arising Time and Stick to Them
Set the alarm clock and get out of bed at the same time each morning, weekdays and week-ends, regardless of your bedtime or the amount of sleep you obtained on the previous night. This guideline is designed to regulate your internal biological clock and reset your sleep-wake rhythm.

Sleep hygiene. Focus on prebedtime rituals that may be influencing sleep as well as possible influences of the substances that the patient is using. For example, if we were discussing alcohol, we might say the following:

> Although alcohol can help you fall asleep, it can disrupt the quality of your sleep and contributes to less restful sleep. Having one to two drinks with dinner is probably okay, if you're not getting into bed for 4 hours. Is it reasonable for you to avoid alcohol before bedtime?

We suggest going through each lifestyle and environmental factor that may be contributing to the sleep problem and briefly discussing which of and how these factors can be changed.

Stimulus control. When discussing stimulus control, we emphasize using the bed only for sleep and sex and avoiding all other activities in bed. We focus on the activities that patients indicated that they do in bed and discuss alternatives for those activities. For example, we might say the following:

> You mentioned that you sometimes watch TV in bed before trying to fall asleep. Sleep is an automatic process, and our bodies can learn to stay awake in bed, rather than associate the bed with sleep. It is important to reteach your body that the bed is a place where you sleep. Would you be willing to watch TV in another room before getting into bed?

If patients tend to stay in bed when they are not asleep, we discuss possible alternatives, as follows:

> You mentioned that when you cannot fall asleep, you tend to lie awake in bed. Because we want you to associate your bed with sleep and sex, and nothing else, it is important to get out of bed and do something boring when you cannot sleep. We recommend that if you've been awake for longer than 15 minutes, that you get out of bed and go into another room where you can sit quietly until you feel sleepy, that is, when your eyes feel heavy and you think that you'll fall asleep.

Sleep restriction. Most often, we do not have a sleep diary to estimate total sleep time. Based on self-reports of how long it takes to fall asleep, whether the patient is waking before their alarm clock, and their estimated total sleep time, we develop a plan for when the patient should get into bed and plan to wake. Figure 5.14 is an interactive handout. We suggest having the patient read it and then explaining it to them verbally, as follows:

> The idea of sleep restriction is to take the amount of time you are asleep in bed—for you it is 5 hours—and limit the time you can be in bed to that—5 hours. Because you get up at 8:00 a.m. every morning, the earliest you would be able to get into bed would be 3:00 a.m. By staying up so late you will get very sleepy and are more likely to fall asleep quickly and limit the time you are awake in bed, both of which will help improve your sleep. Once you are regularly falling asleep within 15 minutes, we can move back your bedtime by about 20 minutes and continue to do that until we get the best time range determined.

Relaxation. If patients report sympathetic arousal before bedtime, we may teach them the brief relaxation techniques presented in Chapter 4; however,

FIGURE 5.14. Sleep Restriction Handout

Sleep Restriction

One of the Keys to Changing Your Sleep Behavior

What Is It?
Sleep restriction involves restricting the amount of time you spend in bed and the amount of time that you currently spend asleep.

Why Would This Be Helpful?
Research has shown sleep restriction to be an effective technique for improving sleep. In general, most people notice their sleep improves within just a few weeks. Sleep restriction initially produces a mild state of sleep deprivation, which helps people fall asleep faster, stay asleep longer, and improve their overall quality of sleep.

How Do I Do It?
Example: Your usual bedtime is 10:00 p.m., and you get out of bed in the morning at 6:00 a.m. (8 hours in bed). However, if it takes you 1 hour to fall asleep and you wake up for 30 minutes during the middle of the night and spend 30 minutes awake before you get out of bed, you are spending 6 hours sleeping and 2 hours awake. Your sleep efficiency (the percent of time you are actually asleep during the time period you are trying to sleep) is 75%. Sleep restriction in this case would mean decreasing time in bed (8 hours) to the estimated time actually spent sleeping (6 hours).

In this example you would adjust either your bedtime or the time you get up in the morning so that the maximum amount of time you spend in bed is 6 hours. You could go to bed at 12:00 a.m. (midnight) and get up at 6:00 a.m. or continue to go to bed at 10:00 p.m. and get up at 4:00 a.m. After sleep efficiency reaches 85% or greater, time in bed can be increased in 15- to 20-minute blocks. Time in bed each week is increased if sleep efficiency is 85% or greater until sleep efficiency starts to fall below 80%, then time in bed is decreased in 15- to 20-minute blocks. This process of increasing or decreasing time in bed is done until sleep efficiency falls between 80% and 85% on a regular basis.

this often requires a separate follow-up appointment. Similarly, if patients report that they worry in bed, we may discuss using a worry log in which to write their worries before getting into bed. You should inform patients that it may take 2 to 4 weeks for their sleep to improve and that their sleep may get worse before it improves. Identify patients' barriers to implementing the recommendations and set appropriate follow-up appointments to assess change and solve difficulties. A typical follow-up might occur about 2 weeks after the previous appointment.

Together, sleep hygiene, stimulus control, sleep restriction, and relaxation can significantly improve insomnia. Websites, mobile device applications, and self-help books may assist in managing insomnia symptoms. Some of these resources are summarized in Figure 5.15.

Arrange

Most cases of insomnia likely can be treated in primary care. One or two return appointments after the interventions for sleep have been taught can help assess whether the interventions are working for the patient. If interventions in primary care are not effective and the patient is being referred to a specialty mental health care setting, consider making the referral to a provider who has experience treating sleep disorders, such as a clinical health psychologist.

FIGURE 5.15. Resources for Patients With Insomnia: Websites, Mobile Applications, and Books

Type	Location	Descriptions
Website	National Sleep Foundation (https:// sleepfoundation.org/sleep-disorders-problems)	Provides information and resources about insomnia and other sleep disorders for patients and professionals
Mobile application	CBT-i Coach (https://mobile.va.gov/ app/cbt-i-coach; Apple iOS and Android)	Designed to supplement care for those receiving cognitive behavior therapy for insomnia
Books	*Overcoming Insomnia: A Cognitive-Behavioral Therapy Approach, Workbook (Treatments That Work)*, 2nd ed. (Edinger & Carney, 2014)	Provides guidance to patients for targeting insomnia and has a complementary therapist book
	The Insomnia Workbook: A Comprehensive Guide to Getting the Sleep You Need (Silberman, 2008)	Provides guidance to patients about sleep and how to improve sleep using cognitive behavior therapy for insomnia techniques

SUMMARY

Subclinical and clinical depression, anxiety, PTSD, and sleep problems will be the mainstays for most BHCs in primary care settings. Evidence suggests that brief interventions can help many of the symptoms associated with these presentations and improve function. The recommendations and handouts in this chapter provide a place to start; building on these ideas to develop time-limited effective interventions for these problems will be essential for any BHC.

6

Health Behaviors

Tobacco Use, Overweight and Obesity, and Physical Inactivity

As described in the National Academy of Medicine's Vital Directions for Health and Health Care series, tobacco use, obesity and dietary habits, and physical inactivity are among the top contributors to chronic disease in the United States (Dietz et al., 2016; Salinas et al., 2011). It is remarkable, therefore, that health care professionals often do not address these health risks with individuals who display them. Medical providers must assess and overcome multiple barriers with these health behaviors, including lack of time, perceived ineffectiveness of behavior change strategies, and low confidence in their abilities and knowledge to effect behavior change (Rojewski et al., 2019; Salinas et al., 2011). Despite these barriers, the primary care setting is an opportune place, if not the most important place, to target health behavior change. In this chapter, we provide systematic methods for addressing these health behavior problems in a busy primary care setting.

TOBACCO USE

Fifty-six years after the first Surgeon General's report on smoking, and despite decreases in cigarette use, the 2020 Surgeon General's report on smoking cessation stated that smoking remains the leading cause of premature disease and death in the United States (U.S. Department of Health and Human Services [DHHS], 2020). Among U.S. adults in 2020, 19.0% use some tobacco product,

https://doi.org/10.1037/0000380-007

Integrated Behavioral Health in Primary Care: Step-by-Step Guidance for Assessment and Intervention, Third Edition, by C. L. Hunter, J. L. Goodie, M. S. Oordt, and A. C. Dobmeyer

12.5% smoke cigarettes, 3.7% use e-cigarettes, 3.5% smoke cigars, 2.3% use smokeless tobacco, and 1.1% smoke pipes (Cornelius et al., 2022). Among adults who smoked daily, between 2005 and 2020, the prevalence of adults smoking up to 19 cigarettes per day significantly increased (1–9 cigarettes increased from 16.4% to 25%; 10–19 cigarettes increased from 36% to 40.7%), whereas those smoking 20 or more cigarettes per day significantly decreased (20–29 cigarettes, 34.9% to 27.9%; 30 or more, 12.7% to 6.4%; Cornelius et al., 2022). Among high school students, 34% reported ever using a tobacco product, with 9.3% reporting use of a tobacco product within the past 30 days (Gentzke et al., 2022), with other studies indicating that 14.1% of high school students reported current e-cigarette use (Cooper et al., 2022). Although a significant percentage of youth are using tobacco-related products, the trend has been toward a reduction in use, including of e-cigarettes (Gentzke et al., 2020). Most smokers (68%) want to quit smoking, with the highest rates being among those 25 to 44 years old (72.7%; Babb et al., 2017). The U.S. Preventive Services Task Force (USPSTF) recommended that clinicians ask all adults about tobacco use and advise them to quit (Krist et al., 2021). Although an increase from previous years, only 57.2% of tobacco-using adults report receiving tobacco cessation counseling (Babb et al., 2017).

Given the continued high prevalence of tobacco use, that most smokers want to quit, and that many do not receive tobacco cessation counseling, behavioral health consultants (BHCs) have many opportunities to become more involved in tobacco cessation efforts.

Cultural and Diversity Considerations

Tobacco use is greatest among men compared with women; those 25 to 44 years old compared with other age groups; people who earned GEDs compared with other education levels; people with incomes below $35,000 compared with other income levels; those living in rural areas compared with urban areas; and lesbian, gay, or bisexual adults compared with those describing their sexual orientation as heterosexual/straight (Cornelius et al., 2022). When comparing tobacco use between identified race and ethnicity groups, those describing themselves as American Indian/Alaska Native, non-Hispanic report the highest percent of tobacco use (34.9%), followed by "other," non-Hispanic (29.1%) and White, non-Hispanic individuals (21.1%). A greater percentage of Black (72.8%) and Asian adults (69.6%) and a lower percentage of American Indian/Alaska Native, non-Hispanic adults (55.6%) reported an interest in quitting compared with White adults (67.5%; Babb et al., 2017). Asian, non-Hispanic (69.4%) and Black, non-Hispanic adults (63.4%) reported the highest percentage of attempting to quit in the past year (Babb et al., 2017). It is important to consider possible environmental factors affecting differences in tobacco use. For example, there are often higher concentrations of stores selling tobacco and price promotions for tobacco products in lower income and higher ethnic minority communities (e.g., Jenkins et al., 2022; Ribisl et al., 2017).

Specialty Mental Health and Other Intensive Tobacco Cessation Programs

Intensive tobacco cessation programs often occur outside of traditional specialty mental health clinics. Interventions are typically focused on assisting with behavior change, pharmacology, or a combination of these interventions. Intensive tobacco cessation programs vary widely. These programs will incorporate extensive assessments (e.g., standardized measures of dependence, stress); use multiple providers and consultants (e.g., physicians, BHCs, nurses, pharmacists); meet for more than four sessions, often for an hour each session; and incorporate motivational interviewing (MI), behavioral, cognitive, pharmacological, and other interventions (DHHS, 2020; Fiore et al., 2008; Krist et al., 2021). The interventions may be provided individually or in groups, and there may be periodic contact between sessions. One example of an intensive program that is accessible broadly is the American Lung Association's Freedom From Smoking® group program, which includes in-person or online group sessions, support from tobacco cessation counselors, and community chats (American Lung Association, 2023).

Behavior Change Interventions

Based on a Cochrane systematic review, tobacco cessation counseling increases quit rates compared with no counseling, regardless of whether individuals are taking medicines to help quit smoking (Hartmann-Boyce et al., 2021). Another Cochrane systematic review found that providing behavioral interventions to those who are using pharmacotherapy increases quit rates from 10% to 20% (Hartmann-Boyce et al., 2019). Based on the most recent Cochrane systematic review focusing on MI, it is unclear whether MI, either by itself or when combined with other behavioral interventions, helps individuals quit smoking (Lindson et al., 2019). Overall, having at least four or more individual visits substantially improves abstinence rates, even if those appointments are brief (Krist et al., 2021). Therefore, brief and frequent contacts (e.g., multiple 10- to 15-minute appointments) with individuals who are quitting tobacco may provide the best results for successful cessation attempts. Based on Cochrane reviews, although more research is needed, the available evidence does not support the use of acupuncture, acupressure, laser therapy, or electrostimulation as effective smoking cessation treatments (White et al., 2014).

Pharmacological Agents

Pharmacological agents, including nicotine replacement therapy (NRT) and nonnicotine medication, are efficacious for tobacco cessation (Patnode, Henderson, et al., 2021). Current NRT agents, including chewing gum, transdermal patches, nasal spray, inhalers, and tablets, provide a 55% increase in cessation rates compared with placebo (Stead et al., 2012). Nonnicotine medications that have been found to assist with tobacco cessation include bupropion SR (e.g., Zyban, Wellbutrin), nortriptyline (e.g., Elavil), and varenicline tartrate (e.g., Chantix). These medications may more than double the likelihood of quitting successfully (Patnode, Henderson, et al., 2021). Therefore, it is important for behavioral health professionals to be familiar with these options, as pharmacological therapies are an important addition to behavior change strategies for tobacco cessation. Some have suggested that the use of e-cigarettes may be helpful for promoting quitting; however, the USPSTF has concluded that there is insufficient evidence to adequately assess the benefits and harms of this practice (Krist et al., 2021).

Behavioral Health in Primary Care

Providing counseling to quit tobacco use, cost-free tobacco cessation medications, and tailored printed materials improves rates of tobacco cessation based on a Cochrane review (Lindson et al., 2021). Although somewhat dated, the clinical practice guideline published by Fiore et al. (2008) remains one of the best guides for intervention strategies. This guideline, along with the Krist et al. (2021) recommendations, serves as the best guidance for behavioral health assessment and interventions for tobacco cessation. Very few studies have examined e-cigarette cessation interventions, but the existing limited studies have shown promise using techniques similar to those used for other forms of tobacco cessation (Huerne & Eisenberg, 2023). In addition to this chapter, there are multiple resources, including practical handbooks, that one can use to develop effective assessment and treatment plans in a primary care setting (e.g., Dollar et al., 2010; Peterson et al., 2011).

Primary Care Adaptation

Using established strategies in specialty mental health and in primary care, the BHC can adapt these strategies using the 5As to effectively target tobacco use.

Assess

Existing guidelines recommend that all patients entering a clinic be screened for tobacco use (Fiore et al., 2008; Krist et al., 2021). Brief interventions, even those that are 20 minutes or shorter in a single visit, can result in successful quit attempts. Incorporating screening questions into intake forms is one method of instituting a clinic-wide change. Asking tobacco users at every appointment about whether they are considering quitting is also important for a population health approach to decreasing tobacco use. Patients who have denied being ready for change at previous appointments may be ready to quit at the moment they are sitting with a provider. It is important to understand the situations that are conducive to tobacco use and why the person chooses to use tobacco. Successful tobacco cessation will often involve finding healthier alternatives that serve similar functions as tobacco. Multiple brief screening measures (e.g., the Readiness-to-Quit Ladder, Heavy Smoking Index, the Fagerstrom Test for Nicotine Dependence) are appropriate for use in primary care settings and were summarized by Peterson et al. (2015).

Establish a pattern of use. For tobacco cessation, it is important to establish the pattern of tobacco use. The BHC will need to determine what happens when patients use tobacco, what situations are associated with tobacco use, and the perceived benefits of tobacco use. Examples of questions to ask include the following:

- What kind of tobacco do you use?

- How much tobacco do you use?

- How often do you use tobacco?

- Do you use tobacco every day or on the weekends only?

The BHC should also attempt to find out what factors predispose the individual to use tobacco (i.e., the antecedents to use). Examples of questions to ask include the following:

- Are there situations, such as in the car, at home, or when you are with others, when you are more likely to use tobacco?

- How often do you use tobacco at work? What determines when you take a break to use tobacco?

- Are there certain emotions or thoughts that seem to be related to when you use tobacco? Stress? Sadness? Worry? Feeling overwhelmed?

- Physically, do you notice changes, such as your heart racing, muscle tension, or sweatiness, before you use tobacco?

- Are there other household members who smoke? Do your friends use tobacco? Do you have any friends who do not use tobacco?

- How does using tobacco help you?

- How do you feel when or just after you have used tobacco? Relaxed? Calmer? More stressed? What do you like about using tobacco? What do you dislike?

Establish a history of cessation attempts. Understanding whether someone has quit for a period of time in the past and what has and has not worked can be valuable for developing a treatment plan. These questions are examples of what a BHC might ask to establish a patient's history of quit attempts:

- How many times have you quit before?

- When was the last time you quit?

- What is the longest amount of time you have remained tobacco free? How did you stay tobacco free for that long?

- What contributed to you going back to tobacco use?

- Did you use the patch, gum, or any other nicotine replacement? Did you use any medication, such as Zyban, or any herbal supplements to help you quit?

Ultimately, a BHC's assessment should provide a brief understanding of why the individual chooses to use tobacco, what makes it difficult to quit, and what has and has not worked in the past. Individuals relapse for diverse reasons; however, higher levels of nicotine dependence, lower self-efficacy, and stress are common reasons cited for relapse (Smit et al., 2014; Vangeli et al., 2011). Therefore, in addition to knowing how much someone smokes, specifically determining methods for enhancing self-efficacy and potential alternatives for managing stress will be an essential component to a successful tobacco cessation plan. A BHC might ask the following:

- What could make it more likely that you will quit and stay quit?

- What do you do for enjoyment?

- When you are stressed, is there anything else that you do to manage the stress other than tobacco use?

- What do you do to relax? How effective is it in helping you to relax? Have you ever learned exercises or techniques to help you relax?

Advise

Consistent with tobacco cessation guidelines (Fiore et al., 2008; Krist et al., 2021), we inform patients that quitting tobacco is the most important change they can make for their long-term health, regardless of how much they are using. Even if the individual was not specifically referred for tobacco use, we advise them to consider quitting. For those individuals who demonstrate no interest in quitting, we say the following:

> It sounds like you are not interested in quitting right now, but if you ever change your mind and want to consider quitting, Dr. Smith [the patient's primary care provider (PCP)] and I would be happy to help you quit. We can help you right here in the clinic, or we can refer you to a more intense treatment program. We both consider quitting tobacco to be the most important change you can make for your health.

With patients who appear to be ambivalent or who are interested in change, we move to the agree phase, in which we discuss their motivations for change.

Agree

Like any behavior change, tobacco cessation requires a willingness to change. When attempting to initiate a health behavior change with a patient, it is necessary to determine the patient's motivation for change. Despite having multiple medical problems that are affected by health behaviors, individuals may still not be motivated to change those behaviors. The stages of change model (Prochaska & DiClemente, 1983; Prochaska & Velicer, 1997) is perhaps the most ubiquitous model for examining readiness to change. A central tenet of stages of change is that individuals are unlikely to change their behaviors unless they decide to make a change. MI strategies (W. R. Miller & Rollnick, 2013; Rollnick et al., 2022), which we discuss in Chapter 4, have been shown to increase the likelihood of behavior change across a broad range of behaviors and health outcomes (e.g., dental caries, death rate, quality of life, alcohol use; Lundahl et al., 2013), although the current data for tobacco cessation is mixed (Lindson et al., 2019).

In addition to assessing an individual's motivation to quit, it is important to establish whether the primary care setting is appropriate for the cessation attempt. For individuals who report that they participated in a tobacco group or more intensive treatments in the past and were successful, we discuss the possibility of using those treatment modalities again and also make them aware of the program that we can offer in primary care. After discussing the pros and cons of the more intensive program (e.g., more time commitment, a group of people supporting each other, past experience of success) and less intensive program (e.g., less time commitment, good success rates, no group support from other tobacco quitters), we allow the patient to choose which they prefer.

Assist

Helping patients quit tobacco use should involve establishing a plan that identifies when the patients are going to quit, working to prepare for that quit date, and developing skills to manage challenges the patients will face after they have quit. In Figure 6.1 we provide an example of a handout that we use to guide our tobacco intervention.

Preparing to quit. Consistent with the U.S. Surgeon General's recommendations (Fiore et al., 2008) for behavioral and cognitive interventions, a specific quit plan should be developed. To establish such a plan, tobacco users should be asked the following: "It is important to have a specific date and time when you will quit tobacco use. Considering your schedule, when would be the best time for you to use tobacco for the last time?" Elicit a specific date and time from the patient.

Once a date and time is established, discuss how the individual is going to facilitate the quit attempt by preparing their environment during the time before the quit date. We use the handout in Figure 6.1 to record the patient's

FIGURE 6.1. Tobacco Cessation (*continues*)

How to Change?

To effectively change your tobacco use, consider all of the factors that contribute to using tobacco. It can be helpful to group these factors into three main categories: physical, behavioral, and psychological (i.e., your thoughts and emotions).

Physically, nicotine is one of the most addictive substances on the planet. Your medical provider will tell you whether it is appropriate for you to use nicotine replacements, such as the patch or gum. Some medications, like Zyban, can help decrease cravings for tobacco.

Behaviorally, you will need to change your habits and the situations that you typically associate with tobacco. Undoubtedly you will experience situations that cause you to crave tobacco, but you can learn skills that will help you choose alternatives other than using tobacco.

Thoughts and emotions are some of the hardest aspects of tobacco use to change. Often individuals think that they need tobacco to get through a difficult situation. Changing these thoughts to cope with stress and negative emotions is an essential aspect of successful tobacco cessation.

FIGURE 6.1. Tobacco Cessation (*continued*)

Preparing to Quit

Your Quit Date

When is the last day and time that you are going to use tobacco?

Month_____   Day_____   Year_____   Time_____

What are the things that remind you to use tobacco? It is important to change your surroundings so that you won't be reminded about tobacco use as frequently. Before your quit date, consider the following recommendations:

- Don't buy tobacco in bulk (e.g., don't buy cartons).
- Find all of your hidden stashes of tobacco. Check in the couch, in the glove compartment, in your drawers at home, and at work—it is unwise to keep an emergency stash once you quit.
- Get rid of tobacco-related materials—things like ashtrays and lighters. You may need lighters for candles or fireplaces, but you likely don't need to carry lighters wherever you go.
- Prepare family and friends. Let them know that you are planning to quit and ask for their help. If you have friends and family who use tobacco, ask them to avoid using tobacco around you.
- Choose a quit method. There are several ways to consider quitting, but one of the most important considerations is to avoid romanticizing your last tobacco use. If you remember your tobacco fondly, then you may be more likely to go back to tobacco use when you perceive that you need it. Here are some ways to avoid romanticizing your last use of tobacco:
    - *Nicotine fading.* Gradually decrease the amount of tobacco you are using. You can do this by decreasing how often you use your current tobacco or switching to another brand of tobacco that has less nicotine.
    - *Brand switching.* On the day that you are planning to quit, use a different brand of tobacco, preferably a brand that tastes stronger or significantly different from the brand that you use today. Rather than the pleasant sensation you associate with your current brand, you'll remember the more unpleasant taste of the new brand.
    - *Aversive tobacco use.* The last time that you use tobacco, use a lot of it or use it quickly. Again, the idea is to have your last memory of tobacco be an unpleasant memory. So, you might decide to smoke your last cigarette very rapidly or use twice or three times as much chewing tobacco as you normally would.

Using the Four As to Outsmart Tobacco Urges

Avoid. What situations or places will you need to avoid over the next month?

1. _____
2. _____
3. _____

Alter. What situations will you need to change to help you be more successful?

1. _____
2. _____
3. _____

Alternatives. What can you put in your mouth or hands instead of tobacco?

1. _____
2. _____
3. _____

Action. When you get an urge, what can you do to be active or busy?

1. _____
2. _____
3. _____

quit date and to review strategies for quitting. Strategies include not buying tobacco in bulk; cleaning the areas where they are most likely to use tobacco, such as their house, garage, and/or car; and eliminating materials such as lighters and ashtrays. Patients may be reluctant to throw away ashtrays. If this is the case, BHCs could ask them the following:

> What can you do to make it harder for yourself to use tobacco if you suddenly got an urge to do so? If you are not willing to throw away your ashtrays, is there a place you can store them where they would be difficult to get to, such as at a neighbor's house?

Tobacco users should consider how they will live their lives differently after they quit and become nontobacco users. You could ask the following questions:

- Will you stop carrying lighters in your pockets?

- Will you be able to drink alcohol without using tobacco?

- Will you still take breaks at work without using tobacco?

Patients should decide whether they are going to enlist the support of people around them. Identifying individuals to serve as social supports can help facilitate the cessation attempt (Krist et al., 2021). BHCs can encourage patients to enlist the support of others by saying the following:

> It is often helpful to get the support of others when you are trying to quit. How would you feel about asking your significant other/spouse and coworkers to help you quit? Which of your friends or coworkers could you let know you are quitting?

Tobacco users should also examine whether there are certain individuals they should avoid, particularly other tobacco users. If others in the household smoke, they could be encouraged to smoke away from the patient or even to quit tobacco use at the same time as the patient. To accomplish this, patients might be asked the following:

- Could you ask your [significant other/spouse/housemate] to avoid you when they smoke?

- Could you ask coworkers not to invite you out to the smoking area?

The BHC should also assist the patient in effectively using medications for tobacco cessation when it is used. For example, if the patient will be using bupropion or varenicline, the BHC can reinforce the instructions for beginning the medication 1 week before their quit date.

Quitting. As they approach the quit date, patients can consider multiple behavioral techniques to help them quit. These methods include nicotine fading, aversive smoking, and brand switching. Nicotine fading involves gradually decreasing the amount of nicotine that is being consumed. Fading can be done by tapering the frequency of tobacco use over time or by switching to a different brand of tobacco that contains less nicotine. Aversive tobacco use and brand switching are intended to make the last experiences with tobacco unpleasant to decrease the likelihood that the patient will return to tobacco use. Aversive smoking (or aversive chewing) involves the rapid consumption of tobacco (e.g., rapidly smoking the last cigarette). Brand switching requires that the patient select a different brand of tobacco to consume on the last day of tobacco use. Any of these techniques and their rationale can be briefly described to the patient, who could then choose the preferred method of quitting. Ultimately, the BHC should work with the patient to decrease the likelihood that they will romanticize their last use of tobacco. Individuals who view quitting as "losing a good friend" and who remember that friend fondly may be more likely to return to the friend during a crisis period.

When patients reach their quit date, they should start using their nicotine replacements (i.e., patch, gum, and/or spray). The quit date, or shortly after, is a good time to meet with patients to discuss any concerns they may have about quitting.

Maintaining cessation. Once the patient has quit tobacco, the goal is to not have a single puff or chew. Withdrawal symptoms, negative affect, and cravings are three of the most significant reasons individuals return to tobacco use (Piasecki, 2006). Once individuals quit tobacco use, they will need to consider what they will do when they feel a strong urge to use tobacco again. NRT can help significantly with moderating withdrawal symptoms. Patients can use the mnemonic of the four As (not to be confused with the 5As) to help them to overcome tobacco urges. The four As guide the individual to consider ways to *avoid, alter*, use *alternatives*, or stay *active* to cope with urges to use tobacco. Patients should be encouraged to plan ahead for situations that are closely paired with tobacco use. Using the handout in Figure 6.1, BHCs can guide the patient by asking the following:

> What situations (e.g., bars, sporting events, smoking areas) do you need to avoid during the next month to limit your urges to use tobacco? How can you change situations that you can't avoid so that you'll be more successful with your quit attempt? When you feel an urge to put tobacco in your mouth, what could you use instead (e.g., gum, hard candies or mints, toothpicks, cinnamon sticks)? Are there activities (e.g., going for a walk, doing push-ups, running) you can do or ways you can keep busy if you feel an urge to use tobacco?

Cognitively, patients can be encouraged to consider themselves a nontobacco user and, when they encounter situations that result in increased urges to use tobacco, to ask themselves, "What would a nontobacco user do?" It will be important to ask patients what they will do when they believe that they must use tobacco. Briefly discuss methods to challenge these beliefs, such as telling themselves, "I'd *like* to have a cigarette, but I don't *need* to have one." We have found it helpful to use the metaphor of "riding the emotional wave" of the urge by using deep breathing and having the patients remind themselves that the urge is time limited and will subside.

The most common reason individuals return to tobacco use is negative affect (e.g., stress). Therefore, it can be valuable to talk specifically about what they can do in response to stressful situations. Ask what they currently do, besides using tobacco, to manage stress and whether they can use those techniques when they feel stressed. In addition, it may be useful to consider teaching brief relaxation methods and cognitive strategies (see Chapter 4) as well as increasing physical activity to manage stressors without tobacco.

Although the goal is for the patient to not use any tobacco, the likelihood that the individual will slip is very high; most lapses occur within the first 5 to 10 days after quitting, and 90% of lapses lead to a relapse (e.g., Piasecki, 2006). Therefore, it is important to consider a relapse prevention plan. Remind the patient as follows:

> The goal is to not use any tobacco, not a single puff/dip/chew, but if you do slip, what can you do to keep the slip from becoming a total collapse? A slip doesn't mean that you've failed. How can you recommit yourself to not using tobacco?

Despite the best relapse prevention plans, tobacco cessation attempts often are accompanied by relapses and return to previous tobacco use levels (Piasecki, 2006); it often takes multiple attempts for someone to successfully quit. Therefore, it is imperative that providers and patients do not become hopeless after a failed cessation attempt. Continuing to target tobacco use at all appointments is the best way to help patients return to their commitment to quit tobacco use and become nontobacco users. Even providing self-help print or internet material that is tailored to the patient can be effective for helping patients to quit tobacco (Livingstone-Banks et al., 2019).

The BHC can also provide the patient with a variety of additional resources that might be used in conjunction with BHC appointments or might be used by patients who will be following up with their PCP only. Patients might be interested in websites, mobile device applications, or self-help books to assist in managing their tobacco cessation efforts. Some of these resources are summarized in Figure 6.2.

Arrange
At a minimum, we recommend that BHCs meet with patients for 15 to 30 minutes at least four times during their quit attempt. A BHC's schedule might be arranged as follows:

- Appointment 1: Preparing for the quit attempt

- Appointment 2: On or around the quit date

- Appointment 3: Approximately 1 week after the quit date

- Appointment 4: Approximately 1 month after the quit date

BHCs may want to consider more frequent appointments because the number of contacts with the patient is positively associated with quitting (i.e., the largest effect was found in interventions providing eight or more appointments,

FIGURE 6.2. Resources for Patients Using Tobacco: Websites, Mobile Applications, and Books

Type	Location	Description
Websites	American Lung Association (https://www.lung.org/stop-smoking/)	Provides resources to patients to promote tobacco cessation
	Centers for Disease Control and Prevention (https://www.cdc.gov/tobacco/)	Provides information and resources for patients and providers about tobacco use, nutrition, physical activity, and obesity; free quit help is available at 1-800-QUIT-NOW
	National Cancer Institute (https://smokefree.gov)	Provides resources for patients to assist with smoking cessation, including quit lines
Mobile applications	QuitNow! (Apple iOS and Android)	Provides tools to support quitting smoking and connects users with a community
	quitSTART (https://smokefree.gov/apps-quitstart; Apple iOS and Android)	Serves as a complement to smokefree.gov
Book	*My Tobacco Cessation Workbook* (https://www.va.gov/vhapublications/ViewPublication.asp?pub_ID=2946)	Targeted toward veterans, provides evidence-based guidance and is easy to obtain

but the difference in effectiveness was small; Krist et al., 2021). However, the appointments do not have to be with the BHC. Instead, consider ways to incorporate the entire primary care team to facilitate tobacco cessation. Most patients can be appropriately targeted for cessation of tobacco use in primary care settings. However, individuals who have significant medical conditions or upcoming surgeries necessitating close monitoring of the patient during the quit attempt may be better served in the tertiary care setting. Individuals who have attempted to quit tobacco use through primary care in the past and have failed to remain tobacco free may also benefit from tertiary care treatments.

OVERWEIGHT AND OBESITY

In 2017 to 2018, 73.6% of the U.S. population 20 years and older was considered either overweight or obese, which was an increase from 56% in 1988 to 1994 (Fryar et al., 2020). Overweight and obesity are not only related to overeating. The primary causes for the recent increase in obesity are believed to be related to interactions between genetic predispositions; physiologic mechanisms; and complex behavioral, cognitive, emotional, and environmental factors (DHHS, 2013), including energy expenditure and increased food intake. In a national sample, patients were 2 times more likely to report a 5% weight loss in the past year if their medical provider addressed their weight (Pool et al.,

2014). As with tobacco use, the primary care environment may be an ideal place to start to target weight loss.

Cultural and Diversity Considerations

The obesity prevalence rate is highest among non-Hispanic Black adults (49.9%). Hispanic adults (45.6%) and non-Hispanic White adults (41.4%) have slightly lower obesity rates, and non-Hispanic Asian adults have the lowest rate (16.1%; Stierman et al., 2021). The reasons for these disparities are not completely clear but are likely related to a variety of biopsychosocial factors, including genetics, the prenatal environment, moving from one geographic area to another, racism and racial discrimination, and social attributions and cultural perceptions of weight (Candib, 2007; L. T. B. Carr et al., 2022).

Specialty Mental Health

The best current evidence-based recommendations for weight loss include creating a moderate energy deficit by reducing calorie intake (e.g., 1,200–1,500 kcal/day for women and 1,500–1,800 kcal/day for men; lowering calorie intake by restricting or eliminating certain foods), increasing physical activity to at least 150 minutes per week (i.e., 30 minutes or more per day), and using behavioral strategies to accomplish eating and physical activity goals (Curry, Krist, Owens, Barry, Caughey, Davidson, Doubeni, Epling, Grossman, Kemper, Kubik, Landefeld, et al., 2018; DHHS, 2013). Behavioral strategies usually include self-monitoring (e.g., food intake, physical activity, weight) and additional techniques (e.g., stimulus control, slowing eating rate, problem solving). Interventions with high (i.e., 14 or more contacts in 6 months) and moderate intensity (i.e., six to 13 contacts in 6 months) that incorporated behavioral change techniques (e.g., goal setting, self-monitoring), MI, and the 5As model (assess, advise, agree, assist, and arrange) were found to be effective for weight loss (Curry, Krist, Owens, Barry, Caughey, Davidson, Doubeni, Epling, Grossman, Kemper, Kubik, Landefeld, et al., 2018; DHHS, 2013).

Behavioral Health in Primary Care

Among those who have obesity and are seen in primary care, only 28.9% receive an obesity diagnosis and fewer than 26% receive counseling for weight reduction, diet, or exercise (Bleich et al., 2011). There are multiple reasons obesity and weight loss are not discussed more often, including trying to manage time, inadequate access to resources that would support weight interventions (e.g., psychologists, health educators, dietitians), and perceived lack of treatment effectiveness for weight loss (de Lannoy et al., 2021). Little is known about the most effective ways to target weight loss in primary care settings. Low- to moderate-intensity lifestyle interventions offered for weight loss have not been found to be effective (DHHS, 2013). The USPSTF recommends that individuals in primary care who are screened for obesity and those who are identified as overweight and demonstrate other risk factors (i.e., hypertension, dyslipidemia, abnormal blood glucose or diabetes) are offered intensive behavioral counseling interventions (Curry, Krist, Owens, Barry, Caughey, Davidson, Doubeni, Epling, Grossman, Kemper, Kubik, Landefeld, et al., 2018). LeBlanc et al. (2011) determined that interventions that could be offered in primary care are effective. Wadden et al. (2014), following their systematic review of behavioral treatment of obesity in primary care settings, also suggested that professionals who incorporate evidence-based strategies for targeting weight could improve the success of weight loss interventions in primary care. Integrating behavioral health providers into primary care may help physicians overcome some of the barriers to targeting weight loss and would expand the opportunities for targeting weight loss in primary care.

Primary Care Adaptation

The following recommendations are consistent with the recommendations by DHHS (2013) and focus on behavioral and cognitive assessments and treatments for weight loss, which will serve as the first step in a stepped-care approach, as encouraged by multiple researchers (e.g., Wadden et al., 2014). These approaches could be followed by more intensive treatments offered in specialty mental health settings, if necessary. The approaches may also be paired with medication management. The focus of these interventions is on adults. When working with children and adolescents, BHCs should review and adapt the American Academy of Pediatrics clinical guidelines for the evaluation and treatment of children and adolescents with obesity (Hampl et al., 2023).

Assess

Body mass index (BMI; BMI = [703 × weight in pounds] / [height in inches]^2) offers a fast, simple way to identify those who might benefit from weight loss interventions. BMI can be easily calculated using a smartphone app or online calculator such as the one available from the National Heart, Lung, and Blood Institute (n.d.-a). Posting a BMI chart in the area where patients are weighed encourages the medical personnel who weigh the patient to quickly identify patients who fall in the overweight (25 < BMI < 30) or obese (BMI > 30) category and then report that information to the patient's provider. It is also important to recognize that BMI is not perfect. In some cases, BMI may incorrectly identify an individual as overweight or obese (e.g., individuals with high muscle mass), and in other cases, BMI may underestimate a person's risk for disease (e.g., diabetes; Caleyachetty et al., 2021). Therefore, it is important to critically evaluate and discuss with the patient the appropriateness of overweight or obesity classification.

Once overweight or obesity is identified as a health concern for the patient, it can be valuable to review the medical record to gather relevant information about previous efforts to target weight and potentially weight-related medical conditions (e.g., hypertension, diabetes), which can help guide conversations about targeting weight. It is important to ask patients whether they are willing to discuss their weight and weight history; some patients may demonstrate reluctance or resistance to having this conversation. With patients who are willing to discuss their weight, it is useful to determine the patient's pattern of weight gain and weight loss to establish the learning history related to weight changes. If the individual has successfully lost weight in the past, they may have skills that can be built on when developing current recommendations. For instance, a BHC might ask the following:

> As an adult, what is the most you have weighed? What was the least? Have you lost weight in the past? Did you use a special program? What was it? Have you tried monitoring calories or increasing exercise? What has been your weight pattern over the last year? Have you been gaining, losing, or maintaining a steady weight?

Assessing thoughts associated with weight loss can be helpful for determining the individual's self-efficacy regarding controlling their weight and motivation for weight change.

Questions might include the following:

- Do you feel like you have control over your weight?

- Do you worry about gaining weight?

- What health effect has weight had on you?

- Are you concerned about the effect of weight on your appearance?

We recommend assessing current eating habits to include establishing where patients eat, whether they are distracted while they are eating, what situations tend to be associated with eating more, how much time elapses between meals or eating times, and what the individual typically eats and drinks. BHCs might ask the patient the following:

- Do you eat while you are watching TV or doing other things?

- How often do you eat out? Do you eat breakfast, lunch, and dinner?

- Do you snack during the day?

- Do you find that you are more likely to eat when you are upset or stressed?

Overweight and obesity is prevalent among those meeting criteria for bulimia nervosa (84.7%) and binge-eating disorder (78.9%; R. C. Kessler et al., 2013); therefore, it is important to rule out eating patterns that may be associated with an eating disorder (e.g., bingeing, purging) and symptoms related to negative moods (e.g., depression, anxiety). Ask short, clear questions to determine whether patients binge and engage in compensatory behaviors following a binge:

> Do you ever binge eat? That is, do you eat a lot at one sitting with a feeling that you have lost control over your eating?

If they say that they do, a BHC might ask the following:

How often do you binge? Once a month, once a week, every day? Do you ever make yourself vomit after you binge or do things soon afterward to try to eliminate the food you took in, such as exercise a lot or take laxatives? Do you feel guilty or disgusted after you binge? Are you secretive about your binges? Are you sad more days than not? Do you tend to eat more when you are sad? How often do you feel nervous or upset? Do you eat more when you are stressed?

Individuals engaging in bingeing and purging behaviors will need to be monitored closely for physical complications, such as damage to the teeth and throat, as well as electrolyte imbalances and may be better served in a specialty mental health clinic. However, if the patient is motivated to target these behaviors and the PCP is interested in managing the care in the primary care clinic, bingeing and, possibly, purging behaviors could be targeted in primary care (Klein et al., 2021).

Advise

When advising patients about losing weight, we emphasize that a relatively small amount of weight loss, such as losing 5% to 10% of their current weight, can have significant benefits for their health. We also discuss the recommendations that safe and effective weight loss strategies involve losing about 1 to 2 pounds per week. For some patients, this information can be disheartening, as they have been exposed to advertisements and television shows claiming rapid and large weight loss over the course of several weeks. We emphasize that to be able to sustain their weight loss they should lose the weight slowly. Thus, we would say the following:

To lose weight, and be able to keep the weight off, we recommend a plan in which you will lose weight at the rate of about 1 to 2 pounds per week. For some people this might not seem like it is fast enough, but we want you to be able to keep the weight off once you lose it, and we believe that this is the best way to do that. Over the course of about 6 months, we would expect that you would lose about 5% to 10% of your weight, which would significantly decrease the risk that your weight poses to your health.

Similar to other chronic conditions, overweight and obesity require regular follow-ups to ensure that they are being managed effectively. Therefore, we also let the patient know that, to maximize success, it will likely be important for them to follow up regularly (e.g., once per month) with us throughout their weight loss efforts.

It is common for patients to use self-help programs or diets (e.g., keto diets, intermittent fasting) or a more formalized commercial program (e.g., Jenny Craig, Noom, Weight Watchers). The available research suggests that these programs can help patients lose weight (Gudzune et al., 2015; Welton et al., 2020), at least in the short term (e.g., 6–12 months). Less is known about the effectiveness of these programs over the long term. We support patients using these programs if they find the program helpful. Unless it appears that they would benefit from additional help (e.g., they express difficulty implementing the program) or there are medical contraindications to their diet plan, we encourage patients to make a follow-up appointment within 3 to 6 months to evaluate whether they are continuing to be successful in their weight loss attempt.

The patient's PCP may also consider medications to help with weight loss. Common medications that have been used in the past (e.g., sibutramine [Meridia], orlistat [Xenical, Alli]) are effective for assisting with weight loss (Gray et al., 2012); however, these medications are associated with side effects that can contribute to discontinuation of the medication before achieving the desired weight loss. There are increasing data on and interests in the use of glucagon-like peptide-1 (GLP-1; e.g., dulaglutide [Trulicity], semaglutide [Ozempic], tirzepatide [Mounjaro]) receptor agonists, which were originally developed to treat diabetes, to promote weight loss. A systematic review found that weight loss of at least 5% to 10% was more common among those taking GLP-1 agonists when compared with those taking placebos (Vosoughi et al., 2022). A recent randomized controlled trial found that individuals taking 15 mg doses of tirzepatide lost a mean 20.9% of their weight, compared with a 3.1% weight loss among those taking a placebo (Jastreboff et al., 2022). The use of GLP-1 medications for weight loss is a relatively new development, and the medications can be expensive (e.g., $1,000/month). BHCs working to help patients lose weight should continue to monitor the development and use of the medications to promote weight loss.

Agree

Once a BHC has completed the assessment and advised patients about the benefits of losing weight, it is helpful to summarize for patients the understanding of their difficulties and concerns as well as their hopes and expectations for weight loss. Asking whether they are interested in developing a plan to start targeting weight loss can help to bridge the gap between the assess and assist phases. For example, a BHC might say the following:

> It sounds like you've struggled with weight loss for a long time. You've tried a variety of programs that helped you lose weight initially, but you have put the weight back on, which has been frustrating. Now that your doctor has suggested your weight might affect your health, you're concerned about your weight and want to do something about it. Are you interested in working with me to develop a plan that would help you lose weight and keep it off?

Again, the motivational enhancement questions that we discuss in Chapter 4 and in the tobacco cessation section of this chapter are important to ask when starting a weight loss program. DiLillo et al. (2003) presented specific examples of how motivational enhancement questions could be used to facilitate weight loss treatment. Such techniques have been shown to enhance adherence to weight control programs (R. D. Barnes & Ivezaj, 2015; DiLillo & West, 2011). For example, it is particularly important to elicit self-motivational statements associated with the patient's decision to lose weight. So a BHC could ask,

> What would make this weight loss attempt different from previous attempts? How would your life be different if you lost weight?

With this information, a BHC can then tailor the recommendations in the assist phase to enhance the motivators and decrease the barriers to maintaining weight loss behaviors.

Assist

Evidence-based interventions for losing weight and keeping weight off can be tricky in the primary care setting. Often, the patient has tried many methods and may have had some short-term success, but for most who struggle with weight problems, keeping the weight off in the long term is a challenge. Most individuals know the mantra of weight loss programs: "Eat less, exercise more." In the primary care setting, interventions are focused on putting this mantra into practice in a manageable way by providing specific, concrete recommendations that help patients adapt their behaviors to the specific situations they encounter. The primary focus of these interventions is to reduce the number of calories consumed and incorporate lifestyle changes, such as being mindful of portion sizes, which will help control the number of calories consumed. Because exercise can be a helpful addition to a weight loss regimen and is important in weight maintenance, we also encourage a gradual increase in physical activity. The details of these recommendations are addressed in the next section. It is critical to consider the feasibility of any recommendation and to ensure that BHCs are partnering with their patients to develop achievable goals. It can be important to consider environmental factors (e.g., walkability and safety of a neighborhood, access to healthier foods, financial limitations for purchasing foods or medicine) that could interfere with otherwise effective recommendations.

In addition, we recommend that being overweight and obese be conceptualized as chronic medical conditions. Therefore, like those for other chronic medical problems, such as hypertension and diabetes, intervention plans for weight loss are made both for the short term and for the long term. The best outcomes are typically consistent, with long-term follow-up care over years, not just months (Kirk et al., 2012). Unlike specialty care, in which an individual might be seen in a group setting for 16 consecutive weeks and then discontinue treatment, the goal in primary care is to establish a program that the individual understands and can self-manage with assistance from the primary care team. Although the visits may be less frequent, they often occur over a longer span of time.

Goal setting. Once patients are motivated to change behaviors, the first step for effective weight loss is to set realistic, doable goals. We set goals with patients that are consistent with the data from the DHHS (2013), which suggest that the best way for them to lose weight and maintain the loss is to lose 1 to 2 pounds per week, with the goal of losing no more than 10% of their current weight in a 6-month period. After those 6 months, they should focus on maintaining their weight loss for another 6 months. Although this may not be as appealing as the rapid weight loss promised in infomercials, patients are often reassured to know that this strategy can result in sustainable weight loss, whereas other plans likely will not. Questions to help patients set realistic goals might include the following:

If you were to lose 10% of your current weight, how many pounds would that be? Would it be realistic to lose 10% of your weight over the next 6 months?

Calorie education. The second step is to educate patients about the number of calories they need to consume to lose weight effectively. Although historically it has been recommended to use the 3,500 kcal rule (i.e., reducing kcal consumption by 500 kcal per day × 7 days = 3,500 kcal) to lose weight, more dynamic calculations are needed for effective weight loss (K. D. Hall et al., 2011) Using an evidence-based, online calculator, such as the Body Weight Planner, which is available from the National Institute of Diabetes and Digestive and Kidney Diseases (n.d.-a), can help to promote more weight loss. For health and safety reasons, we rarely recommend a goal of less than 1,200 kilocalories a day unless specifically prescribed and monitored by a physician.

Behavior change planning. Once the number of calories patients should consume is established, the next step is to help identify methods for meeting that calorie goal. One effective method is to encourage daily calorie monitoring using a food diary (Semper et al., 2016; Wadden et al., 2014). Using a simple food diary or calorie log and encouraging the purchase of a calorie guide can help patients start to monitor their calorie intake. We suggest patients complete a food diary for 1 week (see Figure 6.3) or use a mobile app and then return to discuss the contents to identify eating habits that could be changed.

FIGURE 6.3. Personal Food Diary

Date: _____

Time of day	Food or beverage item	Serving size	Estimated calories	Comments (e.g., stressors, eating due to boredom or emotions, high-risk eating situations)

Exercise and Activity Log

Type of exercise or activity	Total duration in minutes	Intensity (low, medium, high)	Estimated calories burned	Comments

Patients may find counting calories to be overwhelming or too time consuming. If they demonstrate a reluctance to monitor their calorie intake, reassure them that they can still lose weight by focusing on making behavior changes that will reduce their calorie intake. Reducing their intake of calorie-dense foods (e.g., meats) and increasing their intake of fruits, vegetables, and whole grains while reducing portion sizes will reduce their calorie intake. If the patient keeps a food diary, it can help the BHC to make recommendations for changes that are more specific.

The focus should be on simple changes related to what the patients ate. Suggesting dramatic changes or placing certain foods off-limits may decrease motivation for treatment and the likelihood that the patients will follow through with the changes. Focusing on small, concrete changes may contribute to the belief that sustained weight loss is possible. Using the information obtained during the assessment can be helpful to point out specific foods that patients could reduce, modify, or eliminate to reduce their calorie intake to the number of calories recommended using the online calculator. For example, by eliminating two nondiet sodas or two beers a day, patients could reduce their caloric intake by approximately 250 to 350 kilocalories. One way to target these changes is to discuss what foods to *cut, add, move, eliminate,* or *substitute* (i.e., the C.A.M.E.S. approach; McKnight, 2006). A handout to guide this discussion is presented in Figure 6.4. Some questions you can ask include the following:

- What foods could you eat less of or modify to help you meet your goal?

- Are there other foods that you could eat?

- Is there a sugar-free version of some of the foods that you enjoy?

- Are there foods you would like to eat more of?

In addition to recommending changes about what patients eat, it can be helpful to recommend changes to how they eat. Using a handout, such as the one in Figure 6.5, can help to highlight doable behavioral changes. Ultimately, patients should be encouraged to avoid distractions while eating (e.g., eat at a dining room table, avoid watching TV while eating). Distractions during eating may interfere with patients' awareness of how much is eaten and feelings of being full. Reeducating patients about standard serving sizes (e.g., a supersized drink is not a standard serving size) and suggesting the use of their fist or palm as a guide for the serving size of most foods provides a portable means for measuring how much they should eat, no matter where they are eating. Slowing eating rates (e.g., placing utensils down between bites) and making food less accessible (e.g., keeping serving dishes off the dining table) give patients more time to become aware of being full, meaning they will likely eat less.

Situations typically associated with unhealthy eating (e.g., buffets, parties) cannot be avoided completely, so identifying simple, concrete methods for modifying the situation may help to reduce unplanned eating. For example, eating at restaurants may be particularly difficult for some patients. Encouraging them to split their meals with someone, to place half of their meal in a

FIGURE 6.4. The C.A.M.E.S.™ Principle for Improvement

(CUT—ADD—MOVE—ELIMINATE—SUBSTITUTE)
Evaluate the foods in your diet. Make decisions about what you would like to do with
those foods in order to meet your calorie goals.

Top Ten Foods/Menus in My Diet

List of foods		C.A.M.E.S.
Example:	1. Donuts	1. C & S
	2. Vegetables	2. A
1.		1.
2.		2.
3.		3.
4.		4.
5.		5.
6.		6.
7.		7.
8.		8.
9.		9.
10.		10.

Note. From *Obesity Management in Family Practice* (p. 33), by T. L. McKnight, 2006, Springer. Copyright 2006 by Springer Publishing Company. Reprinted with permission.

FIGURE 6.5. Modifying Eating Habits

1. **Do Nothing Else While Eating.**
2. **Eat in the Same Place Each Time.**
3. **Do Not Clean Your Plate.**
4. **Eat on a Schedule.**
5. **Slow Your Eating Rate:** Put your fork down between bites. Pause during the meal.
6. **When Shopping for Food:** Shop on a full stomach. Shop from a list and get foods that require preparation.
7. **When Storing Foods:** Store high-calorie foods out of sight (out of sight, out of mouth). Keep healthy snacks available.
8. **When Serving and Dispensing Food:**
   - Remove serving dishes from the table.
   - Leave the table after eating.
   - Serve and eat one portion at a time.
   - Wait 5 minutes before getting second servings.
   - Avoid dispensing (serving) food.
9. **When Eating Away From Home:**
   - Order a la carte meals.
   - Watch the salad dressing.
   - Beware of the bread basket.
   - Be wise with dessert.
   - Share your meal with your friend/spouse/partner.
   - Take a portion of the meal home to eat at another time.

take-out container, and to avoid having bread on the table could reduce unwanted eating. Similarly, some may find that they eat more when they are stressed or when they experience heightened emotions, such as anxiety or depression. Discussing methods for delaying eating and engaging in alternative behaviors (e.g., relaxation techniques) may be helpful for decreasing the likelihood that they will eat as a way to distract themselves from unwanted emotions.

Physical activity, which is discussed more extensively in the next section, is another important component of an effective weight loss/maintenance program. Research suggests that although physical activity may be helpful but not necessary for initial weight loss, it plays an important role in the maintenance of weight loss (Butryn et al., 2022; Swift et al., 2014). In our experience, it has been helpful to encourage patients to modify their activity level throughout the day as an initial first step as opposed to developing a specialized exercise program.

The BHC can also provide the patient with a variety of additional resources that might be used in conjunction with BHC appointments or might be used by patients who will be following up with their PCP only. Patients might be interested in websites, mobile device applications, or self-help books to assist in managing their weight loss efforts. Some of these resources are summarized in Figure 6.6.

Arrange
After BHCs have met with patients one or two times to assess the problem and start a behavior change plan, determine how and when the patient will follow up. The purpose of these follow-up appointments is to assess progress, resolve difficult situations or lapses, and possibly introduce a new skill (e.g., communication). Initially (i.e., for the first 2–4 weeks), it may be helpful to meet with the patient on a weekly basis to assess progress and eliminate barriers to sticking to the established plan. At each appointment, the patient's weight should be recorded and compared with the previous weight. Throughout the remainder of the 6 months, monthly appointments may be helpful for maintaining weight loss progress. However, given the patient loads in primary care settings, it is impractical in terms of time and cost to maintain the frequency of such visits with the PCP or the BHC; therefore, consider health care extenders (e.g., nurses, medical technicians) and alternative methods (e.g., telephone contact, shared medical appointments) to help meet the needs of patients as they progress with their weight loss plan.

Once individuals have lost 10% of their initial weight, the focus of the plan should turn to maintaining their weight loss by continuing to implement the behavior changes they have found to be successful. Again, the primary care environment provides an ideal setting in which individuals can continue to monitor and maintain their weight loss. If weight is managed similar to other chronic illnesses, such as hypertension and diabetes, regular check-in appointments can be scheduled to ensure that individuals are maintaining their weight loss and help them deal with lapses. Each individual will have different require-

FIGURE 6.6. Resources for Patients Wanting to Lose Weight: Websites, Mobile Applications, and Books/Documents

Type	Location	Description
Websites	Centers for Disease Control and Prevention (https://www.cdc.gov/obesity/)	Provides information and resources for patients and providers about tobacco use, nutrition, physical activity, and obesity
	National Heart, Lung, and Blood Institute (https://www.nhlbi.nih.gov/health/educational/lose_wt/ and https://www.nhlbi.nih.gov/health/educational/wecan/)	Provides information and resources for patients and providers about weight loss for individuals and families
	Office of Disease Prevention and Health Promotion (https://health.gov/dietaryguidelines/)	Provides resources and guidelines for physical activity and diets
Mobile application	MyNetDiary (https://www.mynetdiary.com/)	Allows tracking of food and physical activity; determined to incorporate the highest number of evidence-based behavioral weight-loss strategies (Pagoto et al., 2013)
Books/ documents	*Managing Overweight and Obesity in Adults: Systemic Evidence Review From the Obesity Expert Panel* (https://www.nhlbi.nih.gov/sites/www.nhlbi.nih.gov/files/obesity-evidence-review.pdf)	Summarizes current evidence related to weight management for providers
	The Cognitive Behavioral Workbook for Weight Management: A Step-by-Step Program (Laliberte et al., 2009)	Helps patients reduce weight using evidence-based strategies

ments regarding the frequency of their follow-up appointments (e.g., monthly, quarterly, semiannually). To help patients recognize when they are having difficulty managing their weight, it may be useful to use a handout, such as the one in Figure 6.7, that establishes zones of care. If an individual is in the green zone, that is, they are at or below target weight, they should continue with their lifestyle. If they find that they are entering the yellow zone or the red zone (i.e., they are above their target weight), they may need to change their lifestyle or schedule an appointment with their PCP.

Individuals should be considered for management in specialty mental health care if bingeing and/or purging behaviors do not resolve or their BMI is equal to or exceeds 40 (or 35 if they are managing multiple, serious weight-related medical problems). Individuals in this weight range may be candidates for surgical interventions (Mechanick et al., 2013) or may need the closer contact that a specialty mental health care setting can provide. Individuals who do not lose weight after a primary care intervention should also be considered for specialty mental health referral.

FIGURE 6.7. Weight Maintenance

Zones for Timely Intervention Before Weight Is Regained

Green Zone: Minimal monitoring (within 4 lb of your target weight)
> If your weight is in the green zone, then simply monitor your weight periodically (e.g., once a week). Maintain your current eating and physical activity habits.

Yellow Zone: Adjust *either* eating behavior or physical activity (within 7 lb of your target weight)
> If your weight enters the yellow zone, then it is time to consider modifying your calorie intake or your physical activity levels to use more energy.

Red Zone: Adjust *both* eating behavior and physical activity; consider follow-up appointment with provider (more than 7 lb above your target weight)
> If your weight enters the red zone, consider modifying your calorie intake and your physical activity level. You may want to consider coming back to the clinic to get assistance if you have difficulty making these changes.

My Zones

Green	_____ to _____	(Maintain current eating and physical activity habits)
Yellow	_____ to _____	(Decrease calorie intake *or* increase physical activity)
Red	_____ or higher	(Decrease calorie intake *and* increase physical activity)

Note. Adapted from *Obesity Management in Family Practice* (p. 132), by T. L. McKnight, 2006, Springer. Copyright 2006 by Springer Publishing Company. Adapted with permission.

PHYSICAL INACTIVITY

Physical inactivity is not only a significant contributing factor to some of the most prevalent diseases, including cardiovascular disease (CVD), hypertension, obesity, and colon cancer, but also contributes to decreased cognitive functioning and increased anxiety, depression, and sleep impairment (Piercy et al., 2018). Overweight and obese individuals who engage in higher levels of physical activity have a lower risk of all-cause mortality and cardiovascular mortality compared with those who are normal weight and have poor aerobic fitness (Fogelholm, 2010). To improve the health of the nation, the DHHS (Physical Activity Guidelines Advisory Committee, 2018) recommended that adults engage in at least 30 minutes of moderate aerobic activity most days (i.e., 150 minutes [2.5 hours] a week) or 75 minutes a week of vigorous-intensity aerobic activity; adults should also engage in muscle strengthening activities two or more days a week. Only 24.2% of American adults achieve this combined level of activity, and 46.9% meet the aerobic activity guidelines. (Elgaddal et al., 2022).

Cultural and Diversity Considerations

Non-Hispanic White adults were more likely to meet the 2018 Physical Activity Guideline standards compared with their non-Hispanic Black adult and Hispanic adult counterparts (Centers for Disease Control and Prevention, 2013a). Additionally, men, those between 18 to 34 years of age, and those with higher incomes are more likely to meet the standards than their comparative groups (Elgaddal et al., 2022). Living in an urban area is associated with less sedentary time; factors such as neighborhood walkability, crime, and aesthetics have not been found to be consistently related to less sedentary time (Koohsari et al., 2015).

Specialty Mental Health

Stubbs and Rosenbaum's (2018) book *Exercise-Based Interventions for Mental Illness: Physical Activity as Part of Clinical Treatment* is an excellent resource summarizing the evidence base relating physical activity to a range of behavioral health concerns (e.g., depression, anxiety, stress disorders, bipolar, schizophrenia), populations (e.g., adolescents, older adults), and environments (e.g., secure and forensic settings) and discussing ways to promote physical activity interventions across mental health settings. Kahn et al. (2002) conducted a systematic review of interventions designed to increase physical activity, such as point-of-decision prompts (e.g., signs by elevators to encourage using the stairs), communitywide campaigns, mass media campaigns, classroom-based interventions, increased social support, individually adapted behavior change programs, and environmental and policy changes. Among the interventions that the authors determined had strong evidence supporting use were individually adapted behavior change programs, suggesting that working individually with patients is one important way to target physical activity levels in the population. Although more recent systematic reviews have not evaluated the breadth of interventions reviewed by Kahn et al. (2002), other reviews have found behavioral interventions across settings to be effective (e.g., Howlett et al., 2019). The Centers for Disease Control and Prevention indicates that individually adapted behavioral interventions have "strong evidence" for increasing physical activity (Community Preventive Services Task Force, 2022).

Behavioral Health in Primary Care

The USPSTF recommends that in adults *without* CVD risk factors, clinicians individualize the decision about whether to refer a patient to behavioral counseling to promote physical activity, as there is moderate certainty that such interventions have a small net benefit on CVD risk (Mangione et al., 2022). Among those *with* CVD risk factors, USPSTF recommends referring all adults for behavioral counseling to promote physical activity (Krist, Davidson, Mangione, Barry, Cabana, Caughey, Donahue, et al., 2020). Regardless of the other positive impacts of physical activity, targeting physical activity can be effective simply for managing CVD risk. Systematic reviews have found that counseling to increase physical activity in primary care increased self-reported physical activity and that interventions involving at least five contacts are associated with greater self-reported participation in moderate- to vigorous-intensity physical activity (Kettle et al., 2022).

Primary Care Adaptation

On the basis of the evidence that individual counseling using cognitive and behavioral strategies can help increase physical activity, we discuss ways that we have incorporated these skills into primary care settings. Before encouraging increases in physical activity, ensure that the patient's PCP has medically cleared the patient for increased activity levels. In addition to these recommendations, helpful resources are provided by the American College of Sports Medicine (see link provided in Figure 6.8).

FIGURE 6.8. Resources for Patients Who Want to Increase Physical Activity: Websites, Mobile Applications, and Books/Documents

Type	Location	Description
Websites	Office of Disease Prevention and Health Promotion (https://health.gov/paguidelines/)	Provides resources and guidelines for physical activity and diets
	Centers for Disease Control and Prevention (https://www.cdc.gov/physicalactivity/)	Provides resources for providers and patients to implement health behavior changes
	American College of Sports Medicine (https://www.exerciseismedicine.org/)	Provides resources for providers and professionals for supporting physical activity counseling
Mobile application	Sworkit Lite Personal Trainer (https://sworkit.com/)	Determined to be most consistent with existing evidence base for physical activity (Modave et al., 2015)
Book/document	*Physical Activity Guidelines for Americans*, 2nd ed. (https://health.gov/our-work/nutrition-physical-activity/physical-activity-guidelines/current-guidelines)	Serves as a patient and provider resource for physical activity guidelines

Assess

Individuals often equate physical activity and exercise. The term *exercise* may conjure up images of sweaty, burly men groaning as they lift hundreds of pounds in a smelly gym. This may not be an appealing image to many patients; therefore, we use the term *physical activity* when discussing ways to increase activity levels.

Unlike tobacco use and weight, which are parts of standard assessments in primary care, physical inactivity is not typically assessed as a routine measure of physical functioning. In addition, there are no medications or medical interventions that can increase an individual's physical activity. Most likely, patients will be identified as sedentary during the assessment of other chronic conditions, such as diabetes or hypertension, rather than receive a specific referral to help patients increase their physical activity. To begin assessing physical activity, a BHC could ask,

- What do you do for physical activity?

- Do you participate in any individual or team physical activities, such as basketball, running, tennis, or swimming?

- Do you go to the gym?

It can also be informative to assess whether the patient has ever engaged in physical activities. When we are developing the most effective ways to assist patients with increasing physical activity, it can be helpful to build on what they have already done. So a BHC could ask,

- Was there ever a time when you engaged in more physical activities?

- What activities did you participate in? Did you enjoy those activities?

Often patients will point to housecleaning or walking around at their job as evidence that they are engaging in sufficient physical activity. It is important to determine whether these activities would actually be classified as a moderate (i.e., the equivalent to walking at 3.0 miles per hour) or vigorous activity (e.g., race walking). Figure 6.9 includes additional examples of moderate and vigorous activities. The talk test may also help BHCs assess the rigor of the activity. The ability to talk, but not sing, is a sign of a moderate activity, and not being able to say more than a few words without taking a breath is a sign of a vigorous activity. BHCs could ask,

- What activities do you do that you would consider moderate or vigorous?

- Can you talk during those activities? Could you sing?

Once a BHC knows what activities individuals are engaging in, it is helpful to assess the duration and frequency of those activities. Patients may overestimate the amount of time that they engage in these activities or the distance involved, so it may be informative to ask how they know how much time they are engaged in the activity or how far they go. For example, a BHC could ask the following:

> How much time do you spend walking outside? When do you engage in moderate or vigorous activity? How long do you engage in that activity? Is there anything that you do to make sure that you engage in that activity (e.g., walk with a friend or family member, walk a pet)? Have you measured the distance? Do you keep track of the time on your watch?

Brief assessment measures are available to help obtain a standard assessment of physical activity, such as the Rapid Assessment of Physical Activity (RAPA; Topolski et al., 2006), which has been tested on older adults; a single question developed by Milton and colleagues (Milton et al., 2011, 2013); and the Physical Activity Vital Sign (Greenwood et al., 2010), which consists of two questions. Lobelo et al. (2018) used a 3-point scoring system to rate a range of criteria (e.g., concurrent criterion validity, assesses aerobic and muscle strengthening component of the physical activity guidelines) and found that the highest

FIGURE 6.9. Examples of Moderate and Vigorous Activities

	Moderate activity 3.0–6.0 METs[a] (3.5 to 7 kcal/min)	Vigorous activity > 6.0 METs (> 7 kcal/min)
Individual activities	Walking briskly (3–4.5 mph) Cycling 5 to 9 mph on level ground Yoga Home exercises Trampoline jumping Weight training	Jogging/running (> 5 mph) Cycling at > 10 mph Hiking uphill or with a heavy backpack Push-ups Pull-ups Karate Jumping rope Energetic dancing
Sports	Softball Basketball (shooting hoops) Golf Swimming (recreational) Canoeing/rowing < 4 mph	Tennis (singles) Football Basketball Soccer Lacrosse Squash Swimming (paced laps) Canoeing/rowing > 4 mph
Household activities	Pushing power lawn mower Shoveling light snow Scrubbing the floor/bathtub General household tasks Active playing with children	Pushing nonmotorized lawn mower Heavy/rapid snow shoveling Carrying heavy bags (25 lb or more) Vigorously playing with children
Occupational activities	Waiting tables/dishwashing Operating heavy vehicles Homebuilding tasks (e.g., electrical work) Farming (e.g., feeding and grooming animals, milking cows) Packing boxes Mail carrier duties Patient care (e.g., bathing, dressing, moving patients)	Heavy construction Firefighting Manually shoveling/digging Farming (e.g., forking straw, baling hay) Loading and unloading a truck

Note. Adapted from *Promoting Physical Activity: A Guide for Community Action*, by Centers for Disease Control and Prevention, National Center for Chronic Disease Prevention and Health Promotion, and Division of Nutrition and Physical Activity, 1999, Human Kinetics. In the public domain. List of physical activities adapted from *Activity Categories*, by Compendium of Physical Activities, n.d., Lippincott Williams & Wilkins (https://sites.google.com/site/compendiumofphysicalactivities/). Copyright Lippincott Williams & Wilkins.
[a]One metabolic equivalent of task (MET) is the energy expended when resting or sitting still (i.e., resting or basal metabolic rate).

scoring measures for measuring physical activity in medical clinics were the RAPA, the Milton single question, and the Physical Activity Vital Sign. The RAPA, in multiple languages, and scoring instructions can be downloaded for clinical use from the University of Washington Health Promotion Research Center (n.d.) website.

Advise

Usually, we advise individuals to increase their physical activity as a way of helping them to manage other conditions, such as depression, hypertension, insomnia, overweight, obesity, or stress management. A BHC's focus during the advise phase is to inform patients about recommended goals for physical activity and let them know that we are looking for ways that they may be able to build on what they already do. Therefore, BHCs could say the following:

> To help you improve your health and to help you avoid developing significant health problems, we know that it is important for you to engage in a moderate activity for 30 minutes at least five times per week or a vigorous activity for 20 minutes at least three times per week. In addition, for optimal health, it is important to discuss ways to engage in muscle strengthening exercises two times per week. We don't have to start at these levels, but we can work together to figure out a plan of how to get there. We want to build on what you are already doing and figure out ways to incorporate physical activity into your daily life.

It is also important to set realistic expectations. Physical activity, by itself, may not lower blood pressure, decrease weight, or improve glucose control, but it is an important aspect of managing health, so a BHC might say the following:

> We know that physical activity is one of the most important behaviors for overall health. Physical activity can help manage your [hypertension/diabetes/weight/etc.]. It will be important to choose an activity that you enjoy and gradually try to increase the amount of time that you engage in that activity. We may not see immediate changes in your [hypertension/diabetes/weight/etc.], but in the long run you will be healthier and you may help prevent this condition from getting worse.

Agree

In the agree phase, we evaluate whether patients accept that increasing physical activity would be important for them. As with tobacco use and weight, assessing importance, confidence, and patients' readiness to change are important aspects of determining whether patients are interested in changing their physical activity. Ultimately, BHCs want to know whether patients want to discuss a plan for targeting their physical activity. Thus, a BHC could ask the following:

> I've talked about how increasing physical activity could help you manage your blood pressure and weight. Do you think it would be valuable for us to take some time to discuss how you might be able to increase your physical activity?

Assist

Figure 6.10 can be used as a handout that might be useful when setting the patient's activity plan.

Identify the activity. The first step in the assist phase is to identify how the individual is going to increase their physical activity. We then discuss different options that we could consider for increasing physical activity. The individual may be engaging in an activity but not at the frequency or duration that is recommended, so we can easily discuss ways to increase the frequency or duration of those activities. If individuals have previously engaged in an activity or sport

FIGURE 6.10. Increasing Physical Activity

Do You Need to Change?

Overall, individuals who engage in at least 30 minutes of moderate physical activity at least 5 days a week are healthier overall compared with those who do less physical activity. If keeping extra weight off is important, then 60 to 90 minutes of moderate activity might be an important goal. Examples of moderate physical activities include brisk walking, riding a bicycle, and raking leaves. You might think it would be difficult to find 30 minutes, much less 90 minutes, to engage in physical activity or exercise.

How Do You Change?

Check with your physician. Make sure your physician has given you the okay.

Have fun. Choose an activity that you enjoy.

Set goals—short term and long term. Select specific days, times, activities, and durations.

Start slow and gradually increase. Generally, you don't want to increase by more than 10% each week.

Track your progress. Keeping track helps you know whether you are staying on your plan.

Have a plan B. If you are planning to do your physical activity outside, what are you going to do if the weather is bad? What about on vacation? How about during the holidays? Think ahead about the week and consider what you can do to meet your goals if something (e.g., bad weather) gets in the way.

Reward yourself. When you meet your goals, reward yourself.

or if they previously used a gym, then we might discuss how they could reinitiate that activity. Figure 6.10 is provided as an educational handout that can be used while developing the activity plan. We find it easiest to build on what someone is doing or what they have done in the recent past. Therefore, we might say, "You indicated that you used to play tennis with your neighborhood friend. Is that something you think you might be interested in starting again?" If the person has not regularly engaged in physical activity, we might say the following:

> It doesn't sound like you regularly engaged in a physical activity in the past. One of the easiest activities to start is walking. Is that something you might be interested in starting? If not, are there other physical activities you would consider increasing? We can talk about ways to integrate walking into your daily activities.

Some individuals may have difficulty leaving the home to engage in physical activities (e.g., a parent with a small child). In those situations, it is necessary to identify activities in the home, such as video or app-guided activities (e.g., home aerobics), that can be used to facilitate physical activity.

Set specific goals. Once a BHC has identified the activity or multiple activities in which the patient is going to engage, it is necessary to set specific goals about when and how long the patient will engage in the activities. We find it useful to establish the days when they will engage in the activity and then gradually increase the duration of the activity. We ask the following:

> To ensure that you get in 5 days of walking, which days of the week are generally going to be the best days for you to walk? What time during the day are you going to walk? How long are you going to walk?

Once a BHC establishes a plan for starting the activity, we discuss how the patient will gradually increase their activity level as follows:

> We've agreed that you will walk each weekday for 10 minutes at 7:00 a.m. It will be important to gradually increase the amount of time you are walking. Would it be reasonable to increase your walking by 2 minutes each week?

The rate of increase should be gradual and at a pace that the patient can sustain.

Measure progress. The simplest way to have patients measure their progress is to write down the days and the duration of their planned physical activity on a tracking form. Many individuals wear, or could wear, pedometers or other physical activity tracking devices (e.g., Fitbit, Apple Watch) or have phones that allow activity tracking. When appropriate (e.g., if financially feasible), it can be helpful to encourage the use of a physical activity tracking device. These devices can provide immediate and objective feedback regarding the number of steps taken by an individual. One method of attaining the recommended 30 minutes of physical activity is to accumulate 10,000 steps per day (Hatano, 1993; Wilde et al., 2001). Tracking step count with the feedback of a pedometer may be a more reliable method of increasing physical activity than suggesting individuals walk for 30 minutes. Although 10,000 steps may equate to 30 minutes per day, taking an additional 1,000 steps a day reduces risk for all-cause mortality, and there are also health benefits below the 10,000 step per day recommendation (K. S. Hall et al., 2020). Valid and reliable pedometers can be found for less than $100 (Fuller et al., 2020). Activity monitors embedded in smartphones and associated applications, which individuals may already own, have also been found to be valid and reliable for measuring activity and promoting increases in activity (Åkerberg et al., 2016; Romeo et al., 2019).

Prevent relapse. As with other behaviors, individuals are likely to lapse and not engage in their physical activity as they planned. We discuss with the patient foreseeable barriers to engaging in the physical activity and what the patient will do if they miss a day of the physical activity. In this case, we would say the following:

> Is there anything coming up that might get in the way of you walking when you are planning to walk? What will you do if you miss a day of walking? Sometimes it is useful to establish a makeup day, that is, a day when you would walk if you couldn't walk one day. So, for you, would it make sense to set Saturday as your makeup day? What time would be the best time for you to walk on Saturday if you missed a day during the week?

Alternatively, a BHC could establish another time during the day to walk, so if the patient did not walk at 7:00 a.m., they would plan to walk after work at 5:00 p.m. It is important to take time to discuss a plan to help prevent a lapse from become a total collapse of the physical activity plan.

The BHC can also provide the patient with a variety of additional resources that might be used in conjunction with BHC appointments or might be used by patients who will be following up with their PCP only. Patients might be interested in websites, mobile device applications, or self-help books to assist in changing their physical activity patterns. Some of these resources are summarized in Figure 6.8.

Arrange

As with other health behavior changes, following up with patients to assess progress is critical. We find it helpful to briefly meet with patients soon after starting an increase in physical activity (e.g., 1–2 weeks). If there are problems starting the program, we spend time discussing how to overcome those barriers. For individuals who appear to be doing well, we recommend following up in about a month with the primary care team to ensure that progress is continuing. We encourage the PCP to ask the patient about their physical activity levels at each follow-up appointment.

It is unlikely that most individuals will need specialty care to target physical activity. Of course, as we mentioned, other, more serious chronic medical conditions might necessitate referral to a specialty care setting. Patients who are interested in starting an exercise program would likely benefit from meeting with an exercise specialist who could help develop a specialized program.

SUMMARY

In the end, the time spent on targeting health behavior changes will likely save time in the future as chronic medical conditions may be avoided or more easily managed. Similar approaches to health behavior change can be used regardless of the health behavior. Informing patients of the need to change, assessing and enhancing patients' motivation to change, developing relapse prevention into the plan, tracking changes, and establishing follow-up appointments in the clinic to help monitor progress will likely help patients change a behavior, whether it is tobacco use, eating habits, or physical inactivity. Behavioral health professionals integrated into primary care can enhance the effectiveness of the primary care team in targeting the health behaviors that are the most significant contributors to morbidity and mortality.

7

Diabetes

Diabetes is a chronic disease characterized by high levels of blood glucose (i.e., blood sugar). In the United States, 37.3 million people (i.e., 11.3% of the entire population) and 29.2% of adults 65 years of age or older have diabetes (Centers for Disease Control and Prevention [CDC], 2022a). Additionally, 96 million adults 18 years and older in the United States have prediabetes (i.e., high blood glucose but not high enough to meet criteria for diabetes; CDC, 2022a). Among those with diabetes, 23% are undiagnosed (CDC, 2022a). Among those 18 years or older, the prevalence of diabetes is considerably higher for those who identify as non-Hispanic Black (17.4%), non-Hispanic Asian (16.7%), and Hispanic (15.5%) compared with those identifying as non-Hispanic White (13.6%; CDC, 2022a). Diabetes was the eighth leading cause of death in the United States in 2020, dropping one spot from seventh to eighth due in part to COVID-19 becoming the third leading cause of death in 2020 (CDC, 2021b). Diabetes is associated with multiple complications, including hyperglycemic crisis, heart disease, strokes, high blood pressure, blindness and other eye problems, kidney disease, nervous system disease, amputations, dental disease, and complicated pregnancies (American Diabetes Association Professional Practice Committee [ADAPPC], 2022h). In the United States, the estimated 1-year cost of diabetes is $327 billion, without considering the costs associated with pain and suffering, nonpaid caregivers, and undiagnosed diabetes (CDC, 2022a).

https://doi.org/10.1037/0000380-008

Integrated Behavioral Health in Primary Care: Step-by-Step Guidance for Assessment and Intervention, Third Edition, by C. L. Hunter, J. L. Goodie, M. S. Oordt, and A. C. Dobmeyer

A diabetes diagnosis is based on measuring blood glucose levels. Sugars and carbohydrates are broken down into glucose, which is the sugar cells use for energy. After one eats, pancreatic beta cells stimulate the secretion of insulin, which facilitates the transport of glucose into cells. The amount of glucose that stays in the blood is determined by how much insulin is available to transport glucose to the cells and whether there is a sufficient number of receptors on the cells to allow the glucose to enter. An insufficient number of available cell receptors results in *insulin resistance* and increases blood glucose levels.

There are multiple methods for determining blood glucose and estimating average blood glucose levels. As described by the ADAPPC (2022a), the A1C test, also called the hemoglobin A1C test (i.e., HbA1C), is based on the attachment of glucose to hemoglobin (i.e., the protein in red blood cells that carries oxygen). A1C test results reflect the average blood glucose over the past 3 months. Normal A1C levels are below 5.7%, and prediabetes A1C levels are between 5.7% and 6.4% in patients not previously diagnosed with diabetes. A1C levels of 6.5% or higher are diagnostic of diabetes. The A1C test does not require a person to fast and can be drawn at any time of the day. Other tests for diabetes include the Fasting Plasma Glucose Test, which requires a person to fast for 8 hours. If a person's fasting blood glucose level is at or above 126 mg/dL, the person is diagnosed with diabetes; a fasting blood glucose level between 100 mg/dL and 125 mg/dL indicates prediabetes. The Oral Glucose Tolerance Test requires a person to fast for 8 hours and then consume a special sugary drink. Individuals with prediabetes will have blood glucose levels between 140 mg/dL and 199 mg/dL, and those with diabetes will have levels at or above 200 mg/dL. Random blood glucose test (i.e., glucose measures taken any time of the day without fasting) results that are equal to or higher than 200 mg/dL indicate diabetes.

Diabetes is classified into four major groups: Type 1, Type 2, gestational, and other causes. Type 1 diabetes, previously known as insulin-dependent diabetes mellitus or juvenile-onset diabetes, accounts for approximately 5% to 10% of diabetes cases (ADAPPC, 2022a; CDC, 2022a). Type 1 diabetes is caused by the autoimmune destruction of beta cells in the pancreas. The destruction of beta cells can happen rapidly or quite slowly; therefore, although Type 1 diabetes is typically diagnosed in childhood or adolescence, it may not be diagnosed until much later in life (CDC, 2022a). Individuals with Type 1 diabetes typically require insulin injections for survival.

Individuals with Type 2 diabetes, previously referred to as noninsulin-dependent diabetes or adult-onset diabetes, demonstrate some insulin resistance but typically do not demonstrate absolute insulin deficiency in the early stages. These individuals represent 90% to 95% of all diagnosed diabetes cases (CDC, 2022a). People with Type 2 diabetes do not always need to take injectable insulin and can often manage their diabetes through healthy eating, weight loss, increased physical activity, and oral medications.

Gestational diabetes is diagnosed in women who demonstrate glucose intolerance after becoming pregnant (ADAPPC, 2022a, 2022f). Approximately 2%

to 10% of all pregnancies are associated with gestational diabetes (CDC, 2021a). There is evidence that maternal, fetal, and neonatal risks increase as maternal glycemia increases at 24 to 28 weeks of pregnancy (CDC, 2021a). For the fetus, the major risk is that it will grow to a larger than normal size and may experience hypoglycemia after it is born. Women with a history of gestational diabetes are at a greater risk of developing Type 2 diabetes later in life.

Other types of diabetes can result from genetic conditions, malnutrition, surgery, medication, and other illnesses. Although patients with all forms of diabetes may present in primary care, a behavioral health consultant (BHC) should be most familiar with Type 2 diabetes because of the high prevalence in primary care settings.

KEY BIOPSYCHOSOCIAL FACTORS

Considering the biopsychosocial factors that affect and are affected by diabetes can help BHCs more effectively use the 5As in assisting patients with diabetes management.

Physical Factors

Patients with diabetes must manage their blood glucose levels to avoid becoming hypo- or hyperglycemic. Hypoglycemia (i.e., blood glucose < 60 mg/dL) may result in increased heart rate, headaches, hunger, shakiness, sweating, decreased concentration, mood changes, and confusion. If untreated, it may lead to coma and death. Conversely, hyperglycemia (i.e., blood glucose > 140 mg/dL) results in increased thirst, increased urination frequency, and glucose in the urine. People with diabetes typically notice the symptoms of hypoglycemia and take corrective action to raise blood sugars to normal levels. However, symptoms of hyperglycemia may not be noticed. Unless the patient identifies hyperglycemia through monitoring of blood sugar, the levels may remain high for extended periods, leading to the development of future complications. Over the long term, the hyperglycemia associated with undiagnosed or inadequately managed diabetes can result in macrovascular and microvascular diseases. Macrovascular problems result in increased risk of heart disease, stroke, and high blood pressure. Microvascular problems contribute to the development of blindness, kidney failure, and neuropathy, which in turn contribute to pain, loss of feeling, and possibly paralysis. A1C levels are used to measure how well patients are managing their diabetes. Although the ADA recommends that patients maintain A1C levels below 7%, this may be challenging for some patients with diabetes (Qaseem et al., 2007).

Among those diagnosed with diabetes, 89.8% were overweight or had obesity (CDC, 2022a). The risk of diabetes is increased in overweight and obese individuals who are insulin resistant; however, weight loss is associated with decreased risk (Carbone et al., 2019). Diabetes is associated with other medical problems, including autoimmune diseases, cardiovascular disease, obstructive sleep apnea, fatty liver disease, cancer, cognitive impairment, low testosterone in men, pancreatitis, bone fractures, hearing impairment, hepatitis C infection, periodontal disease, and hearing impairment (ADAPPC, 2022b).

When health behavior changes do not adequately manage hyperglycemia in patients with Type 2 diabetes, it is recommended that patients be prescribed metformin. Long-term use of metformin may be associated with biochemical B_{12} deficiency, so it is recommended that B_{12} levels are periodically checked (ADAPPC, 2022h). If metformin is not sufficient, it is recommended that a second medication be added (ADAPPC, 2022g). Currently there are eleven types of oral medications or injectable medications used to treat diabetes, including sulfonylureas (e.g., Glucotrol, Micronase, Amaryl), biguanides (e.g., metformin [Glucophage]), meglitinides (e.g., Prandin, Starlix), thiazolidinediones (e.g., Avandia), DPP-4 inhibitors (e.g., Januvia, Nesina), SGLT2 inhibitors (e.g., Invokana, Farxiga), short- and long-acting glucagon-like peptide-1 receptor agonists (e.g., Trulicity, Bydureon, Ozempic), alpha-glucosidase inhibitors (e.g., Precose, Glyset), dopamine-2 agonists (e.g., Cycloset, Parlodel), amylin mimetic (e.g., pramlintide), and bile acid sequestrants (e.g., Welchol; ADAPPC, 2022g). These medications may affect insulin production, the body's sensitivity to insulin, or blood sugar absorption.

All individuals with Type 1 diabetes and approximately half of individuals with Type 2 diabetes need to take insulin (Davies et al., 2013). Insulin is injected into the fat under the skin to get into the blood stream. Insulin therapy adherence is poor; adherence rates range from 43% to 86% (Davies et al., 2013). Many factors contribute to poor adherence, including how insulin is injected (i.e., a pen device improves adherence over a syringe), high insurance copayments, low perceived self-efficacy, and lower perceived personal control (Davies et al., 2013). It is important to assess adherence to medication regimens and potential barriers.

Emotional and Cognitive Factors

There is a bidirectional relation between Type 2 diabetes and depression: Diabetes increases the risk of depression, and depression increases the risk of diabetes (Nouwen et al., 2019). Depression further contributes to treatment nonadherence among those with diabetes (Gonzalez et al., 2008). The evidence for a relation between anxiety and diabetes is less strong; however, some evidence suggests that those demonstrating anxiety are more likely to develop diabetes (K. J. Smith et al., 2018). Similarly, some evidence, based primarily on self-report data, suggests that those experiencing posttraumatic stress disorder are at greater risk for developing diabetes (Vancampfort et al., 2016).

Research has been conducted on diabetes distress, which is distinct from general depression and anxiety and is defined as a high-level negative emotional or affective experience associated with the day-to-day living with diabetes (Skinner et al., 2020). A meta-analysis found that the point prevalence of diabetes distress was 36% among those with Type 2 diabetes (Perrin et al., 2017). Those reporting diabetes distress have been shown to demonstrate lower levels of self-care and higher levels of A1C compared with those who do not demonstrate distress (S. Schmidt et al., 2020, 2023; Skinner et al., 2020).

Behavioral Factors

The development and course of diabetes, particularly Type 2 diabetes, is strongly related to multiple behavioral factors, including dietary habits, physical activity, blood glucose monitoring, and medication adherence. Regular blood glucose monitoring is necessary to maintain a healthy blood glucose range. Glucose content is usually measured in small amounts of blood, typically one drop, obtained through pricking a finger. Patients may need to test their blood sugar from one to seven or more times per day. According to the ADA (ADAPPC, 2022a, 2022c), managing nutritional intake is important for preventing and managing diabetes. There is no ideal percentage of calories from macronutrients, including carbohydrates, proteins, and fat, but managing the amount of carbohydrates with available insulin may be among the most important factors that influence glycemic response after eating (ADAPPC, 2022d). If an adult with diabetes consumes alcohol, total intake should be limited to moderate amounts (i.e., one standard drink per day or less for women; two standard drinks per day or less for men). Other health behaviors, including medication adherence, physical inactivity, and tobacco use, can affect blood glucose levels and the progression of diabetes.

In addition to health behaviors, patients with diabetes must monitor their feet, eyes, and renal function for complications related to the progression of the disease. Neuropathy and peripheral vascular disease place patients with diabetes at increased risk of ulcers and undetected wounds, particularly on their feet. Patients are asked to check their feet to identify cuts or sores that could become infected if they are not caught early. In addition, patients are instructed to always wear shoes that fit well, wash and dry their feet daily, maintain healthy nail care, and avoid skin removal. Diabetic retinopathy is the leading cause of blindness in patients 20 to 74 years of age. Damaged blood vessels associated with diabetic retinopathy can result in blood or fluid leakage in the eye, which can lead to impaired vision and blindness. Kidney functioning must also be regularly monitored for evidence of kidney disease. To accomplish these evaluations, patients with diabetes are often required to make multiple appointments with medical providers. As described previously, diabetes management may also require patients to adhere to multiple and sometimes complex medication and insulin regimens.

Environmental Factors

Social support is an important factor in the management of diabetes. Significant others in the patient's life may be overly critical or fail to support the patient in the multiple behavior changes necessary, particularly food choices. Lack of job flexibility and finances may limit the patient's ability to attend appointments, buy appropriate foods, or purchase glucose monitoring equipment and supplies.

Cultural and Diversity Considerations

Social determinants of health are critical to consider in the assessment and treatment of diabetes. In particular, the ADA recommends considering food insecurity; housing insecurity and homelessness; financial concerns, particularly those that may contribute to difficulty affording medication; living and working context (e.g., migrant and seasonal agricultural workers); language barriers; health literacy and numeracy; social capital; and community support (ADAPPC, 2022e). Often, patients do not express these concerns during the course of their medical care. One study found that half of adults with diabetes reported financial stress and one fifth reported food insecurity (ADAPPC, 2022e; Patel et al., 2016).

SPECIALTY BEHAVIORAL MEDICINE TREATMENT

Intensive lifestyle interventions that include dietary, physical activity, and behavioral interventions improve the management and decrease the risk of diabetes incidence in people identified with prediabetes (C. L. Gillies et al., 2007; Knowler et al., 2002; Nathan et al., 1993; Norris et al., 2005). Pragmatic prevention efforts focusing on lifestyle interventions are also effective (Dunkley et al., 2014). The Look AHEAD study, a multicenter, randomized controlled trial, examined whether lifestyle changes in a sample of patients with Type 2 diabetes reduced their cardiovascular morbidity and mortality. After 10 years, those in the intervention group maintained lower weights, smaller waist circumferences, higher levels of physical activity, and lower levels of glycated hemoglobin, but they did not show lower levels of cardiovascular morbidity or mortality (Wing et al., 2013). Although the primary desired outcomes were not achieved, other important functional outcomes were achieved, including reduced urinary incontinence, sleep apnea, and depression, as well as improvements in quality of life, physical functioning, and mobility (Wing et al., 2013). In addition to lifestyle modification interventions, cognitive behavioral therapy (Uchendu & Blake, 2017) and problem-solving therapy (Fitzpatrick et al., 2013) have both been shown to be effective at helping patients manage A1C levels.

The ADA recommends that individuals receive diabetes self-management education and support (DSMES), medical nutrition therapy, routine physical activity, smoking cessation counseling (when needed), and psychosocial care (ADAPPC, 2022c). DSMES includes coverage of the following core topics: (a) describing the diabetes process and treatment options, (b) healthy coping, (c) healthy eating, (d) being physically active, (e) taking medication, (f) monitoring, (g) reducing risk, and (h) problem solving and behavior change strategies (J. Davis et al., 2022). When DSMES is delivered, it should be person-centered and address the particular needs of the patient. DSMES should be discussed with patients (a) at diagnosis, (b) annually and/or when treatment goals are not met, (c) when complicating factors develop, and (d) following life or care transitions (Powers et al., 2020). The best outcomes occurred when individuals received 10 hours of DSMES over the course of 6 to 12 months (Powers et al., 2020).

Despite the demonstrated benefits of DSMES, fewer than 7% of eligible patients participate in DSMES (J. Davis et al., 2022). Integrating BHCs into primary care is one method for bringing behavioral interventions to more patients with diabetes.

BEHAVIORAL HEALTH IN PRIMARY CARE

Diabetes is the third most common chronic condition seen in outpatient medical settings (Santo & Okeyode, 2018). Medical management of Type 2 diabetes in primary care settings, even with the use of dietitians and diabetes educators, results in less than half of the patients with diabetes reaching targets for glycemic control (Spann et al., 2006). It is challenging for primary care providers (PCPs) to meet the standards of care necessary for patients with diabetes, particularly regarding promoting behavior change (Rushforth et al., 2016). Telemedicine has been found to be effective for helping to manage diabetes (Tchero et al., 2019).

The use of depression care managers improves health outcomes for a variety of chronic health conditions, including diabetes (Katon et al., 2010). Intensive primary-care-based interventions for depression have been shown to decrease death rates in diabetes patients over a 5-year period (Bogner et al., 2007) and are cost-effective (Katon et al., 2008; Simon et al., 2007). Brief interventions targeting medication adherence among patients diagnosed with depression and diabetes in primary care improved medication adherence, A1C values, and depressive symptoms compared with usual care (Bogner et al., 2012). Lifestyle interventions conducted in primary care and community settings have also been shown to be effective (Dunkley et al., 2014). Wolff et al. (2021) found that integrated care models, including the primary care behavioral health model, reduce depressive symptoms and A1C values among a low-income Latinx population. Based on self-report, the primary care behavioral health model has resulted in improved functioning among patients experiencing diabetes (Andrews et al., 2016). Diabetes interventions in primary care can be as effective as interventions provided in specialty mental health settings; however, primary care interventions affect more people and can be comparatively more cost-effective (Glasgow et al., 2006). Overall, good evidence suggests that the biopsychosocial factors that contribute to diabetes can be targeted effectively in primary care settings.

PRIMARY CARE ADAPTATION

BHCs can use evidence-based assessments and interventions to integrate behavioral science more effectively into primary care, as recommended by Fisher and Glasgow (2007). In addition, BHCs can facilitate ongoing contact with patients with diabetes to improve the long-term effectiveness of these interventions. We focus on how BHCs can help PCPs improve the management of physiological factors, reduce emotional distress, and facilitate positive health behaviors in their patients with diabetes. Although this chapter focuses on interventions for patients diagnosed with diabetes, the behavior change strategies discussed can be applied to patients who are prediabetic as well, to help them make lifestyle changes necessary to prevent diabetes.

Assess

Assessment of patients with diabetes ideally will begin with a review of the patient's electronic health record to gather relevant information such as use of diabetes medications and/or insulin, recent A1C lab values, problems with hypoglycemia, comorbid medical conditions, prior interventions for diabetes, and the current recommendations for treatment and self-management. The BHC's interview with the patient should then include questions regarding the key biopsychosocial factors relevant to diabetes, with a heavy focus on modifiable risk factors associated with poorer health outcomes. In addition, obtaining information regarding the patient's goals for change, as well as what the PCP believes is most important for the patient to change, helps guide the intervention process.

Modifiable Risk Factors

Assessing modifiable biopsychosocial factors associated with diabetes helps the BHC identify potential factors that patients could change to more effectively manage their diabetes.

Physical Factors
Potentially modifiable risk factors that are physical or biological in nature include the following:

- high blood pressure,

- problems with overweight or obesity,

- frequency of hyperglycemia and hypoglycemia, and

- A1C levels.

As mentioned previously, we recommend initially reviewing the electronic health record for information regarding relevant medical history. A brief discussion with the PCP about these items prior to seeing the patient, whenever possible, also typically yields valuable information. We then ask patients additional questions, such as the following:

- In a typical day, how many times do you measure your blood sugar level? When?

- In a typical week, how many times do your blood sugar levels run too high? What patterns have you noticed?

- In a typical week, how many times do your blood sugar levels get too low? What patterns have you noticed?

- Have you had any serious problems, such as car accidents or passing out because of low blood sugar?

- What medications are you taking? What difficulties are you having with your medications?

- Are you taking your medications/insulin as prescribed? What gets in the way of you taking these as prescribed?

- What complementary or alternative treatments are you using?

Emotional and Cognitive Factors

Assessing emotional and cognitive factors relevant to diabetes involves questioning the patient about the presence of problems with depression, anxiety, worry, stress, and anger. The Diabetes Distress Scale 2 (Fisher et al., 2008) is a two-item screening measure derived from the full-scale Diabetes Distress Scale 17 (W. H. Polonsky et al., 2005) and is useful for screening for emotional distress in patients with diabetes. The Diabetes Distress Scale 2 has a respectable 95% sensitivity and 87% specificity relative to the Diabetes Distress Scale 17 classification of patients reporting low or high distress (Fisher et al., 2008).

The Problem Areas in Diabetes Scale is another brief measure that may be useful for assessing diabetes-related distress (W. H. Polonsky et al., 1995). The original measure includes 20 items and uses 5-point response options (i.e., 0 [Not a problem] to 4 [Serious problem]); however, briefer versions, including a 5-item and a 1-item version, have been tested with good results (McGuire et al., 2010). The 5-item scale demonstrated a 95% sensitivity rate and an 89% specificity rate; the 1-item scale may be good for screening, with a sensitivity rate at 74% and a specificity rate at 86% (McGuire et al., 2010).

In the assessment of emotional factors, we focus most attention on depression, anxiety, and general distress because problems in these areas are most commonly associated with diabetes. In addition to gathering information about the presence of emotional problems, we ask questions to evaluate the effect these problems have on the management of diabetes. For example, we might ask the following:

> You described feeling quite a bit of sadness over the past few months. How has this affected your ability to stick with your plans to change your diet and to

exercise more? How else has it affected your management of your diabetes or your weight?

Alternatively, for a patient with high levels of worry about the consequences of diabetes, we might say the following:

> You mentioned that you worry a lot about your diabetes and the possible health complications that you might develop in the future. Some people find that this kind of thinking helps keep them on track with managing their diabetes. Others find that worry about diabetes leads to difficulty managing their health. They may avoid checking blood sugars for fear that they are too high or not follow up with medical appointments to avoid hearing bad news. How has worry affected your diabetes management?

Behavioral Factors

Assessment of behavioral factors focuses on the following major areas: eating patterns (i.e., particularly carbohydrate intake patterns, saturated fat, and cholesterol, as well as frequency and timing of eating), current and past strategies for managing weight, habits related to monitoring blood sugars (e.g., timing, frequency), response when blood sugar readings are too high or too low, medication adherence, physical activity, and use of tobacco and alcohol. In addition, we ask about adherence to recommendations regarding foot care and various medical appointments (e.g., eye checks). The Diabetes Self-Management Questionnaire (DSMQ) is a brief (i.e., 16 items), validated measure that can aid in the assessment of self-care activities among patients experiencing diabetes (Schmitt et al., 2013, 2016). A revision of the DSMQ (i.e., the DSMQ-R) was introduced in 2022 to reflect updates in technology (e.g., continuous glucose monitoring) and changes in terminology (Schmitt et al., 2022). The DSMQ-R uses 27 items, which may make it more challenging to deliver in primary care, but it demonstrated good validity and reliability, including significant associations with glycemic outcomes (Schmitt et al., 2022).

Chapters 6 and 11 contain suggestions for assessing diet and weight, physical activity, and tobacco and alcohol use. The following are some examples of questions we might ask to assess other behavioral factors specific to diabetes management:

- How often do you check your blood sugar level?

- What times of day do you typically check your blood sugar?

- How frequently does your PCP want you to check your blood sugar?

- What gets in the way of checking your blood sugar as often as your PCP recommends?

- Have you noticed any patterns related to high or low blood sugar levels (e.g., time of day, physical activity, eating habits, stress levels)?

- What do you do when your blood sugar reading is too high?

- What do you do when your blood sugar reading is too low?

- Has your PCP or diabetes nurse educator recommended a specific eating plan for you? If so, can you describe it for me (e.g., carbohydrate counting, exchange diet, low-fat diet, low-calorie diet)?

- What steps do you take before, during, or after physical activity to ensure your blood sugar levels remain in a safe range?

- When was the last time you checked your feet for cracks or sores?

- When was your last diabetic eye exam?

- What problems, if any, are you having with your medications? How difficult is it to take them as your PCP recommends?

Environmental Factors

Environmental risk factor assessment largely focuses on the presence and quality of social, family, and work factors that may support or interfere with management of diabetes. We gather information about the patient's perception of the amount and quality of the support they receive from their partner and family. We might ask, for example, how family members support their efforts to change their physical activity and eating patterns and whether they experience conflict over food issues (e.g., family member criticizing their eating behaviors, partner unhappy with the effects of meal changes on their own eating habits). We also inquire about whether the patient would be willing to involve their partner or another close family member in future medical or behavioral health appointments related to diabetes management in an effort to foster greater understanding of diabetes and the recommended lifestyle changes and perhaps to learn additional ways to support the patient in their diabetes management. For patients who are working, we assess whether work-related factors interfere with diabetes self-management behaviors (e.g., frequent work travel, difficulty taking breaks to check blood glucose levels). We also ask about any financial barriers that may affect their ability to manage their diabetes (e.g., affording medications).

Goals for Change

Finally, we want to understand the goals that the patient and the PCP have for better diabetes management. We review the PCP's referral question and, when necessary, speak with the PCP about their primary goals for the patient (e.g., keeping A1C below 6%–7%, decreasing blood pressure, reducing depression, losing 5%–10% of body weight). We ask patients what they believe their PCP wants them to change to determine whether they have an accurate understanding of their PCP's recommendations. We then assess the patient's goals. What do they want to change? Do they want to feel less depressed or less anxious about health problems? Do they want increased energy and ability to engage in physical activities? Do they believe that better managing their diabetes will help improve their quality of life? These broad, goal-oriented questions lead well into discussions of recommended changes and specific intervention strategies.

Advise

In shifting from assessment to advising, we begin with a summary of our understanding of the problem. Of particular relevance for many patients with diabetes is the large number of behavior changes required to best manage their illness compared with acute or many other chronic conditions. Therefore, if the patient has expressed feeling overwhelmed or discouraged by the multiple changes required for good management of diabetes, we reflect and validate this perception of multiple challenges inherent in the self-management of a chronic disease such as diabetes. Some of these changes may seem easy to the patient (e.g., checking feet daily), and others may seem quite difficult (e.g., regular blood sugar monitoring, insulin injections, eating changes, exercise). We balance this, however, with statements reflecting hope. Diabetes is one chronic disease that is quite responsive to behavioral changes over which the patient can exert control. Although some factors in diabetes cannot be changed, many factors that affect the course of the disease are modifiable. We then make a clear statement identifying which biopsychosocial factors are modifiable and the expected benefits from making such changes. We often describe diabetes as being more like a marathon than a sprint and discuss the need to pace how many changes are made at one time. Finally, we check to make sure the patient understands the advice and the rationale for the recommendations. Such an interaction might sound as follows:

> It sounds like you're feeling a bit overwhelmed by all the changes you've been asked to make to better manage your diabetes. You've been told by your health care providers that you should take your medicine regularly, check your blood sugar more often, lose weight, exercise daily, manage your stress better, and decrease your use of alcohol. That is certainly a lot of change, and it's not surprising that you feel overwhelmed at times. However, you're aware that not making changes can lead to some bad health complications in the future. One positive aspect is that many, if not most, of these negative outcomes can be prevented through changes in your behavior. Certainly, some aspects of diabetes are outside of your control. Nevertheless, there are many aspects that you can control—changes that you can make—that will help you stay healthier longer. Sometimes it is easier to treat diabetes like a marathon, rather than a sprint, and to pace how you make these changes in your life.
>
> Because of what you've told me today and what your health care providers have shared with me, I have some specific suggestions for changes we could work toward that can improve your management of diabetes and your long-term health. Two suggestions in particular stand out at this point. One is to increase how often you are checking your blood sugar, as a first step toward getting it under better control. Knowing your blood sugar levels will allow you to take steps needed to keep your blood sugar from getting (or staying) so high. These steps could involve taking medicine, cutting back on your carbs, or going for an extra walk, for example. Over the long term, keeping your blood sugars in a healthier range will help prevent some of the medical problems associated with diabetes. A second suggestion is to increase your physical activity. Results from research suggest that if you begin and maintain regular physical activity, you will gain better control of your blood sugar. Again, this should help to prevent many of the long-term complications of diabetes. Do these two recommendations make sense

to you? What questions do you have? Why do you think it might be important to focus on these areas?

This script should be tailored to make it applicable to the patient being seen by the BHC.

Agree

The agree phase of the interaction involves a shift from providing advice regarding general recommendations for change (described previously) to collaboratively setting specific goals related to these recommendations. In working jointly with the patient to negotiate a specific goal, BHCs should balance professional judgment with patient preference. It is often helpful to suggest several options and see whether the patient gravitates toward one. Although this standard approach is helpful in working with patients with a variety of behavioral health or medical conditions, it may be especially important for patients with diabetes, who frequently feel overwhelmed by the large number of changes they have been told to make in a short period of time. As an example of coming to an agreement on a specific plan for increasing physical activity, a BHC could propose several options, including increased walking through the use of planned short bursts (e.g., walking for 10 minutes three times per day), a more sustained period (e.g., walking 30 minutes a day with a partner), or lifestyle activity with the goal of specific increases in steps per day (measured by a pedometer).

As the BHC and the patient develop the specifics of the goal, the chances of success will be enhanced if the patient believes the changes are important and feasible. Sensitivity to the patient's level of motivation and efficacy may be especially important among patients with diabetes, given the high number of changes required to manage the illness well. Asking questions such as, "How likely is it, on a scale of 0% to 100%, that you will be able to make this change in the next month?" or "How confident are you that you can meet this goal?" can provide useful information for tailoring the difficulty level of the goal. The Readiness Ruler presented in Figure 4.6 may be helpful for guiding the patient through this discussion. Ultimately, BHCs want the patient to leave with a specific behavior change goal involving at least a moderate degree of self-efficacy and motivation to make the change. If the patient appears ambivalent about making the change, guiding a discussion about the advantages and disadvantages of making the change and of not making the change may help increase motivation (for additional guidance, see the discussion of motivational enhancement in Chapter 4).

Assist

Common interventions for better biopsychosocial management of diabetes include the following:

- addressing comorbid behavioral health problems (e.g., depression, anxiety, stress reactions),

- making health behavior changes (e.g., related to physical exercise, diet, medication adherence, blood sugar monitoring, response to high or low blood sugar readings, tobacco cessation, alcohol use reduction),

- assisting with building communication skills (i.e., particularly with health care providers and family members),

- performing interventions within the patient's primary support system (e.g., family, partner), and

- encouraging the use of community support organizations (e.g., religious organizations, local community centers, national diabetes organizations).

Approaches for addressing a number of these interventions are described in detail in other chapters of this volume. Strategies for addressing depression, anxiety, and stress reactions can be found in Chapters 4 and 5. Approaches for helping patients make health behavior changes such as modifying diet, exercise habits, and medication compliance are addressed in Chapters 6 and 11. We refer the reader to these other relevant chapters and focus here on diabetes-specific issues that may arise when addressing these areas, as well as on interventions not covered elsewhere. Figure 7.1 is an example of a form that can be used with patients to establish goals for managing their diabetes.

Blood Sugar Monitoring

Regular monitoring of blood sugar levels is a cornerstone of diabetes management for many patients. Appropriate monitoring provides the patient with information needed to make daily decisions regarding eating, exercise, and medication use to help keep blood sugar levels within healthy ranges. Regular monitoring also provides the health care team with valuable information for tailoring recommendations regarding these key areas. Most new glucose monitoring devices now store information regarding blood sugar levels that can be downloaded at the PCP's office. Although this information is helpful for the medical team, it may not provide the patient with much immediate information between medical visits regarding trends in blood sugar levels and related variables. Therefore, we encourage many patients to keep a personal monitoring log and record blood sugar levels as well as key factors (e.g., time of day, exercise, carbohydrate intake, medication). See Figure 7.2 for an example of such a form. We modify this form for patients, as needed, to address their specific behavioral health needs (e.g., add columns for tracking fat or calorie intake, eliminate medication section if not relevant, alter the mood type that is monitored). Mobile device applications are also available for recording blood glucose readings and monitoring trends (see Figure 7.3).

Assessment of barriers to blood sugar monitoring may reveal problematic beliefs or behaviors to target in intervention. For example, some patients feel embarrassed about checking blood sugars away from home (e.g., in a restaurant, during an afternoon of shopping, at a party). Cognitive interventions targeting thoughts contributing to embarrassment and subsequent avoidance of monitoring may then be indicated (see Chapter 4). Some patients may see the needle prick as a significant barrier to regular monitoring of blood sugar and may avoid or limit monitoring as a result. Guiding the patient through brief exposure-based interventions (see Chapter 4) can help increase comfort levels with drawing the small amount of blood, typically one drop, needed to check blood sugar. As technology continues to evolve, it may also be helpful to explore with patients and their PCP whether there are viable alternatives to daily finger pricks (e.g., continuous glucose monitors) to increase adherence.

FIGURE 7.1. Handout for Diabetes Goal Setting

Diabetes Goals

Checking Blood Sugar Levels
My health care provider recommends that I check my blood sugar levels _____ times per day, at these times:

_____ When I get up in the morning

_____ Before breakfast

_____ Before lunch

_____ Before dinner

_____ Before snacks

_____ Before exercise

_____ Other: _____

Physical Activity
I plan to exercise ___ times per week.

Days (circle):   M   Tu   W   Th   F   Sa   Su

Time(s) of day: _____

Type of activity: _____

Duration: _____ minutes

Location: _____

I can help myself meet my goal by: _____

Eating Patterns
Two achievable, specific changes I will make to improve my eating patterns and food choices over the next 2 to 4 weeks include:

1.   _____
     I can help myself meet this goal by: _____
2.   _____
     I can help myself meet this goal by: _____

Other Specific Goals for Managing Diabetes

1.   Goal: _____
     When, where, how often? _____
2.   Goal: _____
     When, where, how often? _____

FIGURE 7.2. Handout for Diabetes Self-Monitoring

Diabetes Self-Monitoring

Date _____

Eating (Carbohydrates)

Food	Time	Carb Count
_____	_____	_____
_____	_____	_____
_____	_____	_____
_____	_____	_____
_____	_____	_____
_____	_____	_____
_____	_____	_____
_____	_____	_____
_____	_____	_____
_____	_____	_____
_____	_____	_____
_____	_____	_____

Medication

Type	Amount	Time
_____	_____	_____
_____	_____	_____
_____	_____	_____
_____	_____	_____
_____	_____	_____
_____	_____	_____

Physical Activity

Type	Duration
_____	_____
_____	_____
_____	_____

Blood Sugar Readings

Blood Sugar	Time
_____	_____
_____	_____
_____	_____
_____	_____
_____	_____
_____	_____

Stress Level Today (0 to 10 scale; 0 = none, 10 = severe)

Rating: _____

Relevant Factors: _____

FIGURE 7.3. Resources for Patients With Diabetes: Websites, Mobile Applications, and Books (*continues*)

Type	Location	Description
Websites	American Diabetes Association (https://diabetes.org/)	Provides information about symptoms, diagnosis, and management of diabetes, as well as links to additional resources. Sections include strategies for living with diabetes; understanding complications and treatment options; and tips for food, fitness, and weight loss.
	National Institute of Diabetes and Digestive and Kidney Diseases (https://www.niddk.nih.gov/health-information/diabetes)	Contains information on a wide range of diabetes-related topics, informed by research and reviewed by physicians. Topic areas include (but are not limited to) symptoms, diagnostic tests, types and causes of diabetes, medications and other treatments, special populations, complications, and strategies for managing diabetes.
	Centers for Disease Control and Prevention (https://www.cdc.gov/diabetes)	Provides diabetes-related resources for professionals and patients. Includes a toolkit for diabetes self-management education and support.
Mobile applications	Honey Health: Conquer Diabetes (Apple iOS)	Connects user to expert creators and communities where the user can engage in topics related to improved self-management of diabetes.
	Glucose Buddy (Apple iOS and Android)	Provides a way to log blood glucose levels, medication use, eating behaviors, and exercise. Users can view charts that include blood sugar, medication, and food levels; customize their desired blood glucose target range; and see estimates of A1C test results based on logged blood sugar levels.
	MyFitnessPal (Apple iOS and Android)	Allows the user to input and track food consumption and physical activity. Includes tracking carbohydrate consumption as well as a recommended low carbohydrate diet. Requires payment for some features.

FIGURE 7.3. Resources for Patients With Diabetes: Websites, Mobile Applications, and Books (*continued*)

Type	Location	Description
Books	*The Official Pocket Guide to Diabetic Food Choices*, 5th ed. (American Diabetes Association, 2020)	Details the exchange list system to help plan meals, choose the healthiest foods, and estimate the right portions. By grouping similar foods into exchangeable portion sizes, people with diabetes can create meals specifically designed to help them control their blood glucose and lose weight. This proven system is the most popular approach to diabetes meal planning and has been used by dietitians, diabetes educators, and millions of people with diabetes for over 70 years.
	The Diabetes Carbohydrate & Fat Gram Guide: Quick, Easy Meal Planning Using Carbohydrate and Fat Gram Counts, 5th ed. (Holzmeister, 2017)	Provides complete nutrition information on 8,000 menu and food items. Contains complete nutrition information on calories, carbohydrates, fat/saturated fat, cholesterol, sodium, fiber, and protein, as well as diabetic exchanges for all entries.
	Mayo Clinic: The Essential Diabetes Book: A Complete Guide to Prevent, Manage and Live With Diabetes, 3rd ed. (Castro, 2022)	Includes information on the prediabetes stage and types of diabetes, symptoms, and risk factors. Covers treatments and strategies for managing blood sugar, how to avoid serious complications, insulin delivery, and new medications.

Response to Highs and Lows in Blood Sugar

Patients need to take appropriate corrective action in response to blood sugar levels that are too high or too low. Recommendations about the specific actions that they should take must come from the patient's PCP or other medical provider. For hypoglycemia, the typical recommendation involves eating or drinking a product with high glucose content. For hyperglycemia, there tends to be greater variability in recommendations, depending on patient characteristics, medication regimen, degree of hyperglycemia, and time of day. PCP recommendations may range from altering medication amount or timing, engaging in an immediate bout of exercise, delaying food intake, altering food intake, or seeking emergency medical care. Close coordination among the PCP, BHC, and patient ensures that all parties understand the recommended actions. The BHC and the patient may then work together to develop a plan for improved adherence to the corrective action plan.

Physical Activity

Regular physical exercise has multiple benefits for patients with diabetes, including improved glucose control, lowered weight and cardiovascular risk factors, and improved quality of life (ADAPPC, 2022c, 2022h). The ADAPPC (2022h) recommends that adults with diabetes accumulate at least 150 minutes of moderately intense physical activity (e.g., 50% to 75% of maximum heart rate; brisk walking) over the course of at least 3 days per week, with no more than 2 consecutive days without exercise. Additionally, because resistance training has been found to improve glycemic control, the ADA recommends that adults with diabetes should also engage in resistance training twice per week. These recommendations need to be tailored to the individual, particularly in identifying an initial manageable goal. Before helping a patient plan an individualized activity plan, however, it is important to check with the PCP to determine whether there are any medical contraindications to increasing physical activity or engaging in exercise that is more vigorous. The suggestions presented in Chapter 6 for helping patients increase physical activity are relevant for patients with diabetes.

Some additional considerations exist when working with this unique population. Given the risk of hypoglycemic episodes developing during the course of increased physical activity, patients should know the relationship between eating, exercise, and blood sugar changes and be vigilant in attending to any signs of hypoglycemia (e.g., shakiness, confusion, weakness, headache) that may develop during exercise. The PCP should be asked to provide guidance regarding precautions they recommend for the patient. Such recommendations may include eating 1 or 2 hours before increased physical activity or eating a small snack right before exercise to reduce the risk of hypoglycemia, determining whether or not to exercise when blood sugar is high, and determining whether to check blood sugar levels more frequently during exercise to ensure that levels do not become too low during periods of activity. When exercising away from home, it is wise for patients to wear identification with their personal information, emergency contact, and medical alert (i.e., indicating that they have diabetes) and to carry with them sources of sugar that are easy to access and absorb (e.g., glucose tablets, hard candy, fruit juice, soft drink). Finally, patients need to ensure they wear shoes and socks that fit well and check their feet for redness after exercise.

Eating Habits

The ADA does not recommend one type of dietary plan (e.g., low fat, low carbohydrate, low glycemic index, low calorie) over another for patients with diabetes; rather, they recommend that each patient collaboratively develop an individualized eating plan in conjunction with their health care provider, preferably with a registered dietician knowledgeable about medical nutrition therapy for diabetes (ADAPPC, 2022h). Thus, it is crucial that the BHC work closely with the patient's medical team when implementing interventions related to dietary changes. The BHC can then help the patient implement this individualized eating plan more successfully. The ADA (http://www.diabetes. org), the CDC (https://www.cdc.gov/diabetes), and the National Institute of Diabetes and Digestive and Kidney Diseases (https://www.niddk.nih.gov/health-information/diabetes) have resources related to the various types of diets followed by patients with diabetes. Some patients, particularly those with lower nutritional literacy or older adults, may be advised to follow simpler approaches to eating plans, such as healthy food choices or portion control (ADAPPC, 2022h). Monitoring of carbohydrates eaten remains an important factor in improving glycemic control (ADAPPC, 2022h); we recommend keeping a nutritional reference guide handy (e.g., Holzmeister, 2017) or using a mobile application, such as those listed in Figure 7.3, to help estimate the carbohydrate content of common foods.

Depression, Anxiety, and Emotional Distress

Helping patients with diabetes to decrease depression, anxiety, or stress is similar to helping nondiabetics develop these skills. Chapters 4 and 5 have more detailed discussions of working with these problem areas. One issue specific to diabetes, however, is the relationship between emotional functioning and blood glucose levels. The presence of depression or anxiety may interfere with healthy diabetes management behaviors through lowered motivation to eat healthy, exercise, and adhere to other recommendations. Therefore, in working with patients with diabetes who are also experiencing problems with mood management, we specifically assess and target health-related behaviors that are being negatively affected.

In addition to affecting diabetes-related health behaviors, emotional functioning can affect blood glucose directly. Many people with Type 2 diabetes find that emotional stress leads to higher blood sugars. Discussing this relationship between stress and blood glucose levels often provides additional incentive for patients to engage in stress- and mood-management strategies such as relaxation training or cognitive disputation (see Chapter 4).

Social Support

As with many other chronic illnesses, social support may help patients with diabetes cope better with the disease and with the many recommended lifestyle changes. To this end, we strongly encourage patients to identify someone (e.g., a partner, another family member, a friend) who might be willing to support them in their diabetes management. The patient may invite the support person to attend behavioral health, diabetes education, and other medical appointments. The BHC may work together with the patient and support person to increase helpful types of support (e.g., praising healthy food choices, joining the patient in exercise activities, agreeing on decisions regarding grocery shopping and restaurant choice) and to decrease unhelpful behaviors (e.g., overcontrolling food, eexcessively criticizing eating or exercise habits). The BHC may also work with patients to improve skills in assertive communication to help patients ask for what they need from family, friends, or medical providers. Community resources (e.g., local YMCA, community centers, diabetes support groups) and national diabetes organizations (e.g., ADA) may provide additional sources of support. Note that the ADA website (https://diabetes.org/) contains links to find local diabetes-related events and includes a chat function for diabetes-related questions available Monday through Friday. We recommend that BHCs become aware of local and national resources and encourage patients to use them.

Arrange

BHCs provide a key function in helping coordinate and arrange access to the numerous resources that may benefit patients with diabetes. For example, BHCs may be the first to identify a need for psychotropic medication evaluation, additional dietary guidance, education on how to use the blood glucose monitor correctly, or additional social support. Some clinics may have integrated dietitians and diabetes educators as part of the primary care medical team, which reduces the need to coordinate external referrals. Developing knowledge of available resources to meet needs that cannot be met within the primary care clinic, along with a willingness to coordinate referrals to psychiatry, nutritional medicine, diabetes education, and community resources, can help the BHC link patients with needed services.

We also recommend that BHCs develop explicit criteria with patients and medical providers about when the patient should revisit the BHC. For example, a BHC might recommend that the PCP refer the patient to the BHC again if their A1C level rises above 7%. BHCs could encourage a patient who has worked with them on weight loss to come back to see the BHC if they have gained 5 pounds. Alternatively, BHCs may decide that this patient needs to meet with someone on the medical team, including the BHC, at least once per month until the A1C level is at an acceptable level or while working on decreasing body mass index. Ultimately, the message to both medical providers and patients should emphasize that diabetes is a chronic disease requiring lifelong behavior changes; therefore, intermittent consultations with a BHC over the lifespan should be the norm for good diabetes care.

SUMMARY

Diabetes, a disease seen commonly in primary care environments, can often be managed with behavioral and cognitive changes. The chronic nature of diabetes requires that the primary care team remains involved with the patient. BHCs should be careful to screen for and help the PCP target the health behavior changes that affect the course of diabetes, as well as depressive, anxiety, and general distress symptoms. The BHC can play a vital role in helping the team develop the behavior and cognitive change plan that will work best for each patient and help to maintain the patient's involvement in effective self-management of diabetes.

8

Chronic Obstructive Pulmonary Disease and Asthma

Respiratory disorders include a wide range of acute and chronic conditions. Acute lower respiratory infections include pneumonia, influenza, and acute bronchitis. Other lower respiratory diseases, such as chronic obstructive pulmonary disease (COPD), asthma, cystic fibrosis, and bronchiectasis are chronic illnesses. This chapter focuses on two chronic respiratory diseases frequently seen in primary care clinics: COPD and asthma. Behavioral and psychosocial factors can complicate management of these diseases, presenting unique challenges to primary care providers (PCPs) and behavioral health professionals working in primary care.

Much of the literature on management of COPD focuses on intensive, specialty-level approaches. The effectiveness of multicomponent pulmonary rehabilitation programs in improving dyspnea, fatigue, emotional functioning, and quality of life in patients with COPD has been well established in numerous randomized controlled trials (RCTs; McCarthy et al., 2015), and pulmonary rehabilitation is included in clinical practice guideline (CPG) recommendations for the management of COPD (Global Initiative for Chronic Obstructive Lung Disease [GOLD], 2023). Smoking cessation is recommended to slow the progression of COPD (U.S. Department of Veterans Affairs and Department of Defense [VA/DoD], 2021), and recent practice guidelines support the use of guided self-management approaches with written action plans to decrease smoking, increase exercise, and manage symptom exacerbations for improved quality of life (VA/DoD, 2021).

https://doi.org/10.1037/0000380-009

Integrated Behavioral Health in Primary Care: Step-by-Step Guidance for Assessment and Intervention, Third Edition, by C. L. Hunter, J. L. Goodie, M. S. Oordt, and A. C. Dobmeyer

As with COPD, psychosocial and behavioral self-management interventions can also play a key role in successful management of asthma. Systematic reviews concluded that behavioral goal-setting interventions may be associated with improved asthma symptoms, self-efficacy, and quality of life (Liao et al., 2019) and that behavior change interventions decrease asthma symptoms and unscheduled health care use and increase appropriate use of preventive medications (Denford et al., 2014). Finally, cognitive behavioral interventions have shown promise in improving anxiety in patients with asthma (Pateraki & Morris, 2018). This chapter focuses specifically on how to adapt and apply evidence-based biopsychosocial assessment and intervention strategies with adult primary care patients diagnosed with COPD or asthma.

CHRONIC OBSTRUCTIVE PULMONARY DISEASE

COPD, a chronic lower respiratory disease, is defined as "a heterogeneous lung condition characterized by chronic respiratory symptoms (dyspnea, cough, sputum production and/or exacerbations) due to abnormalities of the airways (bronchitis, bronchiolitis) and/or alveoli (emphysema) that cause persistent, often progressive, airflow obstruction" (GOLD, 2023, p. 5). COPD is a leading cause of morbidity and mortality. In 2018, COPD was the fourth leading cause of death in the United States (Xu et al., 2020). Prevalence studies found that 6.4% of Americans reported that they have been diagnosed with COPD, with higher rates among current smokers (15%) and former smokers (10%; Biener et al., 2019). Prominent symptoms include dyspnea (i.e., airflow limitation or "shortness of breath," increased effort to breathe), chronic cough, chronic sputum production, wheezing, and chest tightness. COPD is one of the medical conditions known to increase risk of more severe illness from coronavirus disease-2019 (COVID-19; Lippi & Henry, 2020).

The functional impact of COPD can range from mild to severely debilitating. In more advanced stages, COPD often results in significant decreases in functioning and quality of life, including limitations in physical activity, work, self-care, recreation, and family routines; alterations in mood and cognitive functioning; social isolation; physical deconditioning; and declining economic status. Weight loss and fatigue are often seen in patients with more severe illness. The main environmental exposure risk factors for development of COPD are tobacco smoking and inhalation of toxic substances from indoor and outdoor air pollution (GOLD, 2023).

Key Biopsychosocial Factors

Understanding the biopsychosocial factors associated with COPD is important for successful consultation with medical personnel. The following sections highlight those important areas.

Physical Factors

COPD results from a complex interplay of genetic, biological, and environmental factors. Although cigarette smoking is a primary environmental risk factor, genetics (e.g., hereditary deficiency in alpha-1 antitrypsin) and other biological factors influence the development of this disease. Risk of COPD is impacted by age (increasing risk with age), gestational factors affecting lung development, history of early childhood respiratory infections, airway hyperresponsiveness, and history of asthma. The physiological changes responsible for the decreased lung function seen in COPD are considered largely irreversible. A more extensive summary of COPD pathophysiology is found in GOLD (2023).

Medical treatment of COPD primarily involves use of medications to decrease symptoms and complications. Medications have not been found to reverse the long-term decline in lung functioning but can result in reduction of symptoms and exacerbations and improvements in health status and exercise tolerance (GOLD, 2023). Several different classes of medications may be used depending on patient and disease characteristics. These include short-acting anticholinergics (SAMA), long-acting anticholinergics (LAMA), short-acting β2-agonists (SABA), long-acting β2-agonists (LABA), combination medications in one device (e.g., SABA/SAMA, LABA/LAMA), methylxanthines, combination of inhaled corticosteroids with LABA and/or LAMA, phosphodiesterase-4 inhibitors, and mucolytic agents. A number of vaccines (i.e., influenza, pneumococcal, COVID-19, Tdap, shingles) are recommended for patients with COPD to reduce the risk of exacerbations (GOLD, 2023; VA/DoD 2021). A subset of patients with COPD (those with severe resting chronic hypoxemia) may benefit from prescription of long-term oxygen therapy; however, patients with more stable COPD may not receive substantial benefit from oxygen therapy (GOLD, 2023). Surgical treatments (e.g., lung transplantation, lung volume reduction, bullectomy) are not recommended as first-line or routine treatments for COPD, although some evidence suggests that surgical approaches may be appropriate for certain patients with advanced COPD (GOLD, 2023).

Emotional and Cognitive Factors

Both anxiety and depression are associated with poorer COPD prognosis (GOLD, 2023). A meta-analysis of comorbidity rates found that approximately 25% of patients with COPD experience co-occurring depression (M. W. Zhang et al., 2011). Rates of anxiety disorders in patients with COPD range from 5% to 33% depending on the type of anxiety disorder and sample (Willgoss & Yohannes, 2013). Depression and anxiety may result from the decreased functioning, loss of roles, and decreased self-efficacy that can accompany the progression of COPD. The inactivity and anhedonia often seen in depressed individuals may lead to further physiological deconditioning, worsening the patient's ability to engage in physical activity. Anxiety symptoms may result from and compound the frightening symptom of dyspnea (i.e., shortness of breath) in an *anxiety–dyspnea* vicious cycle (e.g., dyspnea leading to decreased physical activity, leading to deconditioning, leading to worsening dyspnea on exertion, resulting in cognitive responses of alarming predictions, increasing anxiety and fear, leading to worsened dyspnea; see Figure 8.1). Breaking this cycle may require cognitive interventions as well as breathing retraining and relaxation skills. Given the increased risk of negative health and quality of life outcomes with these comorbidities, increased attention in the primary care setting to identify and treat anxiety and depression in patients with COPD is recommended (Yohannes et al., 2018).

Behavioral Factors

Nicotine use and physical inactivity are two primary behavioral factors exerting strong influence on the quality of life and symptom progression of those with COPD. Smoking cessation is critical in slowing the progression of COPD; practice guidelines (GOLD, 2023) recommend tobacco cessation counseling and pharmacotherapy for all tobacco users at risk of or diagnosed with COPD.

Individuals with COPD may reduce or eliminate physical exercise because of dyspnea. Unfortunately, lowered physical activity leads to physical deconditioning, resulting in worsened dyspnea on later exertion. Functioning and quality of life gradually decrease as ability to engage in activity progressively declines. Thus, interventions to increase physical exercise are considered key components of COPD treatment (GOLD, 2023; VA/DoD, 2021).

Environmental Factors

Although chronic exposure to tobacco smoke is the primary environmental risk factor for development of COPD, exposure to other toxic particles (e.g.,

FIGURE 8.1. Shortness of Breath Cycle for COPD and Asthma Patient Handout

Shortness of Breath Cycle for COPD and Asthma

Many people with COPD or asthma experience a shortness of breath cycle. In this cycle, shortness of breath from COPD or asthma leads to worry and panic, which in turn worsens shortness of breath. Here are the steps that often occur: Shortness of breath leads to . . .

- Worry (e.g., about breathing, passing out, dying), leading to . . .
- Anxiety or panic physical reaction, leading to . . .
- Increased breathing rate, leading to . . .
- Less effective (i.e., rapid, shallow) breathing, leading to . . .
- Increased oxygen use by, and less oxygen available for, muscles, leading to . . .
- More shortness of breath . . .
- And the cycle continues.

You can stop the shortness of breath cycle by following these steps:

1. When you first notice shortness of breath, STOP your activity.
2. Rest. Sit down or lie down, if possible.
3. Relax. Use diaphragmatic breathing or pursed-lip breathing techniques.
4. Reassure yourself. Tell yourself calming thoughts about your symptoms.
5. If possible, measure and record your peak flow and follow your action plan.
6. Take medications, if appropriate, following your PCP's recommendations.
7. After your breathing improves, gradually resume activity, in a paced manner.

Note. COPD = chronic obstructive pulmonary disease; PCP = primary care provider.

indoor air pollution; occupational hazards such as dust, gases, or fumes) also increases risk (GOLD, 2023). If present, interventions to reduce any ongoing exposures are warranted.

Cultural and Diversity Considerations

Age influences COPD risk, with higher rates of COPD found in older individuals. In terms of gender, earlier studies found higher rates of COPD in men, but more recent studies in developed countries have found equal or higher rates in women. It is thought that this change is likely due to gender differences in changes in rates of smoking. Of note, female smokers are more likely to develop COPD than male smokers (P. J. Barnes, 2016; GOLD, 2023). Lower socioeconomic status is a risk factor for a diagnosis of COPD, and poverty is associated with airflow obstruction; the causes of these relationships are unclear but may involve factors such as exposure to pollutants, low birth weight impacting lung development, infections, smoking, crowding, and poor nutrition (GOLD, 2023; Townend et al., 2017). Finally, individuals with lower health literacy and poorer cognitive abilities have decreased adherence to COPD self-management skills, such as correctly using an inhaler and adhering to medication recommendations (O'Conor et al., 2019). Those with lower health literacy are at heightened risk for depression and anxiety, increased emergency department visits, higher need for assistance with daily living activities, and poorer health outcomes, including higher mortality rates (Puente-Maestu et al., 2016).

Specialty Behavioral Medicine Treatment

Although physiological changes are largely responsible for COPD symptoms, treatment focused exclusively on modifying or addressing the biology of COPD is incomplete. Nonpharmacological and nonsurgical approaches to treatment of COPD, such as those found in multidisciplinary pulmonary rehabilitation programs and supported self-management approaches, are recommended components of care for COPD (GOLD, 2023; VA/DoD, 2021).

Most behavioral health interventions for COPD have been evaluated as components of multidisciplinary pulmonary rehabilitation programs, rather than as standalone psychological or behavioral interventions. The components of pulmonary rehabilitation typically include individualized assessment, supervised exercise training, education, psychological support, self-management interventions promoting behavior change, and dietary interventions (GOLD, 2023; McCarthy et al., 2015). A meta-analysis of 65 RCTs comparing pulmonary rehabilitation to usual care demonstrated that comprehensive pulmonary rehabilitation programs improve health-related quality of life and exercise capacity, reduce dyspnea and fatigue, and improve emotional functioning (McCarthy et al., 2015). Most programs last 8 to 12 weeks.

Supported self-management interventions focus on developing self-management plans, increasing motivation, and implementing skills to better manage COPD. A Cochrane systematic review found that self-management programs that include a written action plan component (e.g., steps to manage

COPD exacerbations) enhance a range of COPD outcomes, including decreased respiratory-related hospitalizations and improved health-related quality of life (Lenferink et al., 2017). CPGs endorse the use of supported self-management interventions in patients with COPD (GOLD, 2023; VA/DoD, 2021).

Primary Care Adaptation

An integrated primary care program involving brief cognitive behavioral therapy (BCBT) for depression and/or anxiety in patients with COPD or heart failure has been studied in the Department of Veterans Affairs (Cully et al., 2017). A pragmatic patient-randomized trial compared bCBT to enhanced usual care. The intervention, delivered by behavioral health providers in primary care, included up to six structured bCBT appointments followed by two telephone booster appointments over a period of 4 months. Intervention modules focused on chronic disease self-management, behavioral activation, cognitive restructuring, and relaxation training. Results indicated that individuals who received the bCBT intervention experienced greater improvement in symptoms of depression and anxiety and that these gains were maintained over the next year. Health-related quality of life also significantly improved during treatment but was not maintained at 12 months (Cully et al., 2017). A secondary analysis of the data found that mild to moderate physical functional impairment at baseline was associated with greater improvements in depression and anxiety. Patients with more severe functional impairment did not derive as much benefit from bCBT, suggesting that this subgroup may need more intensive behavioral health interventions. Interestingly, neither a measure of the treatment working alliance nor the number of appointments attended predicted response to treatment, suggesting that the benefits gained in bCBT may be less reliant on the therapeutic relationship than longer forms of specialty CBT (Hundt et al., 2018).

The following sections outline ways in which behavioral health consultants (BHCs) can support patients with COPD by providing evidence-based assessment and intervention within primary care clinics.

Assess

Perhaps the most important consideration to assess on referral of a patient with COPD is whether they smoke tobacco. Assessment and treatment of tobacco dependence in primary care is discussed more fully in Chapter 6. If the patient is willing to quit, focused tobacco cessation interventions often take precedence over other behavioral health interventions for COPD, given the potential for slowing the rate of progression of the disease through tobacco cessation. In addition, BHCs should evaluate other areas, including the following:

- peak flow (i.e., how fast air moves out of the lungs, from the electronic health record);

- severity and impact of dyspnea symptoms;

- medications and medication adherence;

- effects of COPD on physical functioning (including current patterns of physical activity);

- effects of COPD on work, social, and family functioning;

- effects of COPD on emotional and cognitive functioning;

- health-related behaviors (e.g., smoking tobacco, inadequate nutrition) affecting COPD;

- current or prior participation in pulmonary rehabilitation programs; and

- other behavioral interventions tried to date.

Figure 8.2 provides specific assessment questions that the BHC might ask about each domain.

Awareness of the overlap of COPD symptoms, medication side effects, and psychological symptoms is important to avoid overdiagnosis of mental health disorders. For example, symptoms of weight loss, fatigue, decreased concentration, and low energy may be due to physiological changes of COPD rather than depression. Similarly, chest pain, shortness of breath, and choking may be due to COPD rather than anxiety. Elevated heart rate and restlessness can be a side effect of certain COPD medications, rather than a symptom of an anxiety disorder (Labott, 2020). To distinguish between physical symptoms of COPD and depression or anxiety, BHCs should pay particular attention to cognitions consistent with a psychological disorder (e.g., negative or anxious thinking), the reported mood itself (e.g., feeling down or worried), and the timing of symptom onset in relation to medication use.

The COPD Assessment Test (Jones et al., 2009) can be used as part of a BHC's assessment of COPD. This eight-item self-report measure can be completed in less than 5 minutes and provides information on COPD symptom severity. Validation research has demonstrated good sensitivity in detecting change in symptom severity over time (Agustí et al., 2012).

Cognitive impairment may be present in patients with COPD because of hypoxemia and may negatively affect adherence to medical recommendations and quality of life. Administration of a brief cognitive screener, such as the Montreal Cognitive Assessment (Nasreddine et al., 2005), can help determine whether referral for more thorough neuropsychological evaluation is warranted.

Advise

The results of the functional assessment guide the recommendations provided to the patient. Given the clinical complexity of COPD in most patients, there will likely be more than one identified problem area that could be targeted for intervention. Common areas include tobacco cessation, increasing physical activity and exercise, relaxation training, breathing strategies (e.g., pursed-lip breathing), mood management, and adherence to medical recommendations.

FIGURE 8.2. COPD Assessment Questions

Sample Assessment Questions for COPD

Breathing Symptoms and Peak Flow

- How often do you have trouble breathing or feel you cannot get enough air?
- What kinds of activities lead to feeling out of breath?
- What affects your breathing the most (e.g., physical activity, stress, emotions)?
- What is your average peak flow? What is your best and worst peak flow?

Medications

- What medications do you take for COPD? When do you take them?
- Do you use oxygen at home for COPD?
- What side effects do you notice (e.g., tremor, anxiety, headache, shortness of breath)?
- Do you sometimes forget to take your medications or choose not to take them?
- Have you ever had treatment or medication for anxiety or depression?

Work, Social, and Family Functioning

- How has COPD changed what you do at work?
- Are you having trouble getting things done around the house? How so?
- What has changed, if anything, about what you do for fun? With friends?
- Describe what you do in a typical day.
- How has your family responded to your COPD? How has COPD affected your relationships?

Emotional and Cognitive Factors

- What changes have you seen in your mood as your COPD has gotten worse?
- How has your mood been lately? Have you been feeling more down or sad?
- How often do you feel worried or stressed?
- What goes through your mind when you have trouble catching your breath?
- What do you do when you feel you are having trouble getting enough air?

Health-Related Behaviors

- Do you smoke? What are your thoughts about quitting?
- What forms of exercise or physical activity are you getting?
- Do you believe you are being exposed to indoor air pollutants at work or home?

Interventions to Date

- Do you practice any form of relaxation (e.g., imagery, pursed-lip breathing, diaphragmatic breathing)?
- Have you ever participated in a pulmonary rehabilitation program?

Note. COPD = chronic obstructive pulmonary disease.

The following example illustrates how a BHC might advise a patient with COPD on options for change:

> It's great that you have already quit smoking. Congratulations! Staying tobacco-free is the number one thing you can do to help manage your COPD. Based on the other information you shared with me this morning, I think there are several more areas we could focus on that would help you feel and function better. One area is your physical activity. As you've had more trouble with your breathing symptoms, you've cut back on your physical activity. That makes sense in the short term because it doesn't feel good to be short of breath.

Unfortunately, in the long term, inactivity leads your body to become more deconditioned and out of shape. This makes it even harder in the future to do activities you'd like to do and worsens your breathing problems. If you'd like, we could work with your medical providers to help you develop and stick with a plan for gradually increasing your physical activity levels. A second area that really stood out in our discussion was your description of what happens when you notice your breathing symptoms worsening. You become worried that you won't be able to breathe and that you may pass out. This anxious thinking then worsens your breathing in a vicious cycle. I could teach you some breathing strategies to help control your breathing and promote relaxation. Are you interested in focusing on either or both of those options?

Agree

Often, patients select one of the areas that the BHC has just discussed and recommended. However, they may not always choose to address an area that the BHC believes is most in need of change. In this instance, it is often best to work with patients on goals that they have freely selected, with the hope that their motivation to make additional changes in other important areas will increase in the future as they experience success on initial goals. The following is an example of how a BHC might respond to a patient who appears to have a goal for treatment that differs from those recommended:

> It sounds like you're not too interested in working toward increasing your activity level or in making changes in how you manage your anxiety and breathing. You are concerned, though, about conflicts with your husband over sharing the household responsibilities, as you've been able to do less around the house. We can certainly focus on this. Learning new ways to communicate and negotiate responsibilities that have changed because of your COPD sounds important to you. Why don't we start there? Later, as your communication improves, you may find that you'd also like to focus on one of the other areas we discussed.

Assist

This section provides details on a number of frequently used interventions for patients with COPD, adapted for primary care. These include exercise training, breathing strategies, tobacco cessation strategies, and strategies for the anxiety–dyspnea cycle.

Exercise training. BHCs should closely coordinate with the patient's medical provider on any plan to increase exercise in patients with COPD. Before working on increasing exercise, BHCs should ensure the patient is medically cleared for home-based (i.e., rather than supervised) exercise and has received an exercise prescription. This may involve cardiopulmonary exercise testing to ensure that it is safe for the patient to exercise. BHCs may assist the patient in goal setting, motivation, tracking progress, and relapse prevention to support the recommended exercise plan. Typical recommendations for exercise training in patients with COPD include both cardiovascular and strength training. Although pulmonary rehabilitation programs may use cycling or treadmill walking, many patients initiating home-based exercise programs find walking programs easier. In addition, the exercise prescription may include upper extremity strength training because many COPD patients may experience fatigue when performing daily living tasks with their hands and arms. Chapter 6 contains additional information on working with primary care patients on increasing physical activity.

Diaphragmatic breathing and pursed-lip breathing. Training in relaxation methods is standard in most behavioral components of pulmonary rehabilitation programs. This training may involve teaching diaphragmatic breathing, progressive muscle relaxation, and other forms of relaxation. The resources available in Chapter 4 are certainly relevant for the patient with COPD who needs additional skills in relaxation. Several adjustments may need to be made for the patient with COPD because of the physiology of the disease. Patients with COPD have an obstructive airway disease, with trapped or residual air in the lungs worsening the feelings of breathlessness and dyspnea. For those with mild disease, standard training in diaphragmatic breathing may be appropriate to help manage physiological anxiety symptoms. For those patients with more advanced stages of COPD, however, a more controlled technique, pursed-lip breathing, can be an appropriate alternative. In pursed-lip breathing, patients more actively expel air from the lungs. The result is often similar to that of diaphragmatic breathing: lowered physiologic arousal and heightened awareness of body response. For a more detailed description of this exercise, see the handouts on pursed-lip breathing (Figure 8.3) and shortness of breath cycle (Figure 8.1).

An additional modification to standard relaxation training made for patients with COPD involves an expanded rationale for using breathing relaxation methods. Discussing with the patient that diaphragmatic breathing and pursed-lip breathing can not only lead to feelings of relaxation but can also increase oxygen saturation, decrease respiratory rate, and decrease dyspnea may help increase motivation to regularly use the techniques.

Tobacco cessation. Chapter 6 contains guidelines for helping individuals quit smoking in a primary care BHC practice. These strategies are appropriate to use with patients with COPD in primary care. With this population, it may be particularly helpful to focus on the ways that the patient's COPD symptoms and prognosis are closely linked to their current smoking behavior. Using motivational enhancement strategies can help the patient identify discrepancies between goals and hopes (e.g., live longer, do more, feel better) and current behavior (i.e., continuing to smoke despite its role in worsening COPD symptoms).

Breaking the anxiety–dyspnea cycle. For patients with COPD who demonstrate an anxiety–dyspnea cycle, described earlier, the first intervention often involves education about the relationship between physiology, thoughts, and emotions. The shortness of breath cycle handout (see Figure 8.1) often proves helpful in illustrating the way that shortness of breath can lead to anxiety or panic, which ultimately worsens dyspnea. Once patients have an understanding of this cycle,

FIGURE 8.3. Pursed-Lip Breathing Patient Handout

Pursed-Lip Breathing for Asthma and COPD

Pursed-lip breathing is one of the simplest ways to control shortness of breath in COPD and asthma. It provides a quick and easy way to slow your pace of breathing, making each breath more effective. Please note that this breathing technique *should not replace* the use of medications prescribed by your primary care provider for asthma or COPD but can be used in conjunction with them.

What Does Pursed-Lip Breathing Do?

- Improves ventilation and releases trapped air in the lungs, decreasing the feeling of breathlessness
- Helps keep the airways open for a longer time and prolongs exhalation to slow the breathing rate
- Helps improve breathing patterns by moving old air out of the lungs and allowing new air to enter the lungs
- Causes general relaxation and allows you to better control your symptoms

When Should I Use This Technique?

- During the difficult part of any activity like bending, lifting, or climbing stairs
- When you are finding yourself anxious or breathless
- Practice four to five times a day at first so you can get the correct breathing pattern

How Do I Use This Technique?

- Relax your neck and shoulder muscles and breathe in (inhale) slowly through your nose for two counts, keeping your mouth closed. Do not take a deep breath; a normal breath will do. It may help to count to yourself, "Inhale, one, two."
- Pucker or purse your lips as if you were going to whistle or gently flicker the flame of a candle.
- Breathe out (exhale) slowly and gently through your pursed lips while counting to four. It may help to count to yourself, "Exhale, one, two, three, four."

Note. COPD = chronic obstructive pulmonary disease.

interventions to stop the cycle can be introduced. These interventions may include stopping activity, resting, relaxing (e.g., diaphragmatic breathing, pursed-lip breathing), using reassuring thinking, taking medications if indicated, and ultimately resuming activity in a paced manner. Figure 8.3 may be useful for teaching about pursed-lip breathing in the context of breaking the anxiety–dyspnea cycle.

Arrange

Follow-up with the BHC, if indicated, ideally should be arranged before the patient leaves the clinic. Many patients with COPD will be able to make positive behavioral changes within a small number of appointments. Others may benefit from continuity consultation, meeting with the BHC monthly or quarterly over time to maintain progress in managing this chronic illness. Some patients may require referral to a specialty mental health provider or to a multidisciplinary pulmonary rehabilitation program (especially if they have not recently participated in one). These options may be considered if the patient's COPD is severe or if the patient does not show adequate progress in making changes through BHC intervention. Providers should ensure that patients are familiar with local resources for specialty mental health care and pulmonary rehabilitation programs. Potentially useful websites, mobile device applications, and books for patient education and self-management are included in Figure 8.4.

ASTHMA

The Global Initiative for Asthma (GINA; 2022) defines asthma as

> a heterogeneous disease, usually characterized by chronic airway inflammation. It is defined by the history of respiratory symptoms, such as wheeze, shortness of breath, chest tightness and cough, that vary over time and in intensity, together with variable expiratory airflow limitation. (p. 20)

Over time with more disease progression, airflow limitation may become persistent.

The respiratory symptoms in asthma may be present continuously or episodically and may vary from day to day. Symptoms often worsen during the night or early morning. Aggravating or triggering factors can include viral respiratory infections, indoor or outdoor environmental allergens, occupational allergens, exercise, change in weather, or other irritants (e.g., tobacco, air pollution, aerosols). Individuals with asthma may experience symptom exacerbations due to emotional expressions (e.g., hard crying, laughing), medications (e.g., aspirin, beta blockers, nonsteroidal anti-inflammatory drugs), and endocrine factors (e.g., pregnancy, menses). Severity of asthma is classified by the degree of treatment needed to control symptoms. Severity levels include severe, moderate, and mild. The severity category, along with current symptom patterns, influences decisions regarding medical treatment (GINA, 2022; National Institutes of Health [NIH], 2007; VA/DoD, 2019b).

Asthma affects a significant proportion of Americans. Prevalence estimates suggest that 7.7% of adults and 7.5% of children in the United States have received a diagnosis of asthma (Centers for Disease Control and Prevention [CDC], 2018). Rates are higher in women (9.1%) than men (6.2%) and in individuals below the poverty threshold. Racial and ethnic differences exist, with higher rates in Puerto Rican (14.0%), Black (10.7%), and Native American and Alaska Native (10.4%) populations compared with White non-Hispanic (8.0%) populations. Rates are lower in Hispanic (6.5%), Mexican (5.4%), and Asian (4.5%) populations in the United States (CDC, 2018).

Asthma poses a significant burden on the U.S. health care system. In 2016, asthma was the primary reason for seeking care in 188,968 urgent care visits, over 1.7 million emergency department visits, and nearly 9.8 million outpatient office visits (CDC, 2018). The total annual economic burden of asthma, including health care costs, mortality, and missed work and school, has been estimated at $81.9 billion, with an annual per-person medical cost of $3,266 (Nurmagambetov et al., 2018).

FIGURE 8.4. Resources for Patients With COPD: Websites, Mobile Applications, and Books

Type	Location	Description
Websites	National Heart, Lung, and Blood Institute (https://www.nhlbi.nih.gov/health/copd)	This website gives detailed information on COPD, including risk factors, overview of disease and treatments, and strategies for better managing COPD. It contains fact sheets in English and Spanish.
	American Lung Association (https://www.lung.org/)	This website offers information on a number of lung diseases, including COPD. It contains disease information, management tools to assist in coping with COPD, and tobacco cessation information and support, as well as links to an online support community for COPD patients and information and links to the American Lung Association's Lung Helpline (1-800-LUNGUSA).
	Global Initiative for Chronic Obstructive Lung Disease (https://goldcopd.org/)	This website offers medical information on COPD, a questionnaire for individuals to assess their risk for COPD, and a COPD informational guide for patients and their families.
	National Lung Health Education Program (https://nlhep.org/)	This website offers patient information on COPD diagnosis and treatment. It contains information on the anatomy of normal and obstructed airways, as well as tobacco cessation resources and information on spirometry testing.
Mobile application	myCOPDTeam (https://www.mycopdteam.com/)	This mobile app and website provide a social network for online peer support for individuals with COPD (MyHealthTeams Inc., 2020, 2.0.8 edition).
Books	*COPD: Answers to Your Most Pressing Questions About Chronic Obstructive Pulmonary Disease* (Mahler, 2022)	This patient education book provides answers to commonly asked questions about COPD. It includes information on the symptoms and causes of COPD, evidence-based treatments, strategies for management, guidance for smoking cessation, and the impact of COVID-19 on COPD, among other topics. Each chapter contains a patient vignette.
	Live Your Life With COPD: 52 Weeks of Health, Happiness, and Hope, 2nd ed. (J. M. Martin, 2020)	This patient education book, written by a respiratory therapist, provides a guide to living with and managing COPD. It provides information on a variety of topics, including medications, relaxation strategies, breathing techniques, and working with your physician, among others.

Note. COPD = chronic obstructive pulmonary disease.

The effects of asthma can range from minimal interference and near-normal functioning to high levels of impairment, including the need for frequent unscheduled medical care and emergency visits, missed work and school, limitations on physical activity and exercise, and nighttime awakening from symptoms. Long-term treatment goals focus on good control of asthma symptoms, maintaining normal activities, and reduction of persistent airflow limitation, medication side effects, and asthma-related death. Additionally, treatment goals should incorporate patient-specific preferences and goals (GINA, 2022).

Key Biopsychosocial Factors

Awareness of key biopsychosocial factors associated with asthma can help the BHC incorporate appropriate assessment variables, initiate relevant interventions, and effectively communicate with patients and providers.

Physical Factors

The inflammation of airways causes the hallmark symptoms of asthma (e.g., chest tightness, wheezing, breathing difficulty) as well as hyperresponsiveness of the airways to a variety of stimuli. Obstruction of airflow is often variable and may be reversible with treatment or may remit spontaneously. Labott (2020) provided an excellent summary for behavioral health professionals of the respiratory system, the physiological aspects of asthma, and the diagnostic tests used in the evaluation of asthma.

A primary physical factor routinely measured in asthma assessment and treatment is peak expiratory flow, commonly called peak flow. *Peak flow* is a measurement of how well patients can exhale air. As airways become narrowed, air becomes trapped in the lower segments of the lungs and peak flow values decline. Measurements of peak flow are not typically used for diagnosis but rather for ongoing monitoring of changes in the severity of airflow obstruction. Peak flow monitoring can be accomplished at home with an inexpensive peak flow monitor. To assess peak flow, individuals inhale deeply, place their lips around the mouthpiece of the monitor, and exhale as quickly and forcefully as possible. Providers may recommend patients check peak flow at home to monitor improvement after acute exacerbation of asthma symptoms, after changes in treatment, or to help identify triggers for exacerbation. Some patients may be asked to monitor peak flow on an ongoing basis. This is more typical in patients who have poor perception of symptoms, have a history of sudden severe symptom exacerbation, or have severe or difficult-to-control asthma (GINA, 2022).

Medications for asthma fall into several categories. Controller medications reduce airway inflammation, control symptoms, and reduce risk of future exacerbation and lung function decline. In patients with mild asthma, controller medication may be prescribed for use on an as-needed basis (e.g., before physical exercise, when symptoms increase). Individuals with more frequent symptoms may need to take controller medications daily. Inhaled corticosteroids, taken alone or combined with formoterol, are examples of frequently prescribed controller medications (GINA, 2022).

Asthma treatment guidelines recommend that all patients with asthma also be prescribed reliever (rescue) medications. These medications (often inhaled SABA) give quick relief of symptoms during asthma exacerbations. They also may be used to prevent exercise-induced asthma exacerbations. For optimal control of asthma, patients should use both controller and reliever medications correctly. Of note, a decreased need for the reliever medication is a common goal of asthma treatment, as decreased frequency of use can be a marker that symptoms are well controlled (GINA, 2022). Patients whose symptoms are not well controlled with a combination of controller and reliever medications may be prescribed add-on therapies. See GINA (2022) and NIH (2012) for additional information on commonly used controller, reliever, and add-on medications for asthma.

Despite the important role of medication in asthma treatment, the medications can have notable side effects, some of which mirror behavioral health symptoms. BHCs should be aware of potential side effects of asthma medications to prevent misdiagnosis of mental health conditions (e.g., depression, anxiety). For example, systemic corticosteroids taken to reduce asthma symptoms may lead to appetite changes, weight gain, and mood alteration; methylxanthines may lead to insomnia and gastrointestinal symptoms; and SABA may lead to tremor and heart rate changes (NIH, 2007). Other side effects that may affect patient willingness to adhere to certain medications include dysphonia, sore throat, and oral candidiasis (GINA, 2022).

Finally, obesity is a risk factor for development of asthma, and asthma symptoms are more difficult to control in obese patients (GINA, 2022). Thus, assisting a patient with weight loss could be part of a multifactorial treatment plan.

Emotional and Cognitive Factors
Depression and anxiety occur at higher rates in patients with asthma, and symptoms of depression and anxiety are associated with poorer asthma control, adherence to asthma medications, and quality of life (GINA, 2022). Anxiety or panic may further worsen respiratory symptoms through hyperventilation or constricted airways. At other times, panic symptoms may be mistaken for asthma exacerbations (GINA, 2022). Finally, inaccurate health beliefs about asthma, such as "no symptoms, no asthma," "I will not always have asthma," and "My doctor can cure asthma," are more prevalent in patients with asthma who report poor versus good adherence to medications (Sofianou et al., 2013) and influence adherence to use of corticosteroid medications, leading to poorer control of symptoms (Halm et al., 2006).

Health literacy, "the degree to which individuals have the capacity to obtain, process, and understand basic health information and services needed to make appropriate health decisions" (Ratzan & Parker, 2000, p. vi), also impacts asthma outcomes. Individuals with lower health literacy have higher rates of misconceptions about asthma, lower medication adherence, poorer asthma control, and lower quality of life (Apter et al., 2013; Soones et al., 2017).

Behavioral Factors

Certain modifiable behaviors may predispose the patient to asthma exacerbations. Smoking is a risk factor for asthma flare-ups, even in patients with few or mild asthma symptoms (GINA, 2022). Exercise-induced asthma symptoms also may be influenced by behavioral factors. Individuals who experience asthma symptoms during exercise may not engage in appropriate behaviors to manage these symptoms properly (e.g., lack of warm-up period, failure to use appropriate medications prior to exercise). As a result, they may limit or avoid exercise or other physical activity because of concerns about worsening symptoms. Other behavioral factors that may impair management of asthma include poor adherence to medical recommendations (e.g., failure to use daily peak flow monitoring or home-based action plans) or inappropriate use of medications (e.g., overuse of β2-agonists, taking less than prescribed dose, failure to fill initial or refill prescriptions). Rates of asthma medication adherence range from 30% to 70% and can be influenced by lack of knowledge about medications or asthma, forgetfulness, beliefs that the medication is not necessary, concerns regarding side effects, and complexity of treatment (Boulet et al., 2012).

Environmental Factors

Exposure to certain factors in the physical environment may contribute to asthma exacerbations. These may include animals; mold; pollen; cold air; and airborne smoke, chemicals, or dust.

Cultural and Diversity Considerations

As discussed earlier, rates of asthma are higher in African American, Puerto Rican, and Native American populations than non-Hispanic White populations in the United States. Significant asthma health disparities exist. Minority populations are less likely to receive corticosteroid prescriptions, are more likely to have frequent emergency department visits and inpatient hospitalization, have poorer control of asthma, and have higher mortality from asthma. Factors potentially contributing to these disparate rates and outcomes include living conditions (e.g., increased exposure to environmental triggers), reliance on nonbiomedical asthma management strategies, cultural variations in nutrition and obesity rates, and genetic variation (Ritz et al., 2013). A review of the relationship between asthma treatment and race and ethnicity noted that Latinx and African American populations are less responsive to asthma medications and may have poorer outcomes due to lower adherence and access to health care (Cazzola et al., 2018).

Some evidence suggests that culturally adapted and linguistically appropriate interventions may improve asthma management behaviors (e.g., appropriate inhaler use) and knowledge of asthma symptoms in specific populations (Poureslami et al., 2012). To reduce the impact of low health literacy, specific communication strategies are recommended, including discussing the most important information first; avoiding medical jargon; confirming understanding by asking patients to repeat key information; asking a second person to repeat the primary message; and using anecdotes, pictures, or graphs to enhance instructions (Rosas-Salazar et al., 2012).

Specialty Behavioral Medicine Treatment

A number of asthma treatment recommendations target psychosocial and behavioral factors to improve asthma outcomes and/or quality of life. Examples of nonpharmacological treatment recommendations (GINA, 2022) include

- smoking cessation for the patient and/or family members,

- weight reduction in patients with obesity,

- management of psychological problems such as anxiety and depression,

- avoidance of triggers (e.g., environmental smoke exposure) and indoor allergens,

- regular physical activity,

- adherence to recommendations regarding management of exercise-induced symptoms, and

- relaxation strategies and breathing exercises for stress management.

Specialty behavioral medicine providers have the expertise in behavior change and management of psychological conditions to effectively implement treatment targeting these factors, as well as to assist patients more generally with improving adherence to various aspects of the asthma treatment plan (e.g., peak flow monitoring, medications).

Asthma education is recognized as a valuable element of asthma treatment to enhance patients' ability to self-manage this chronic condition over time (GINA, 2022; VA/DoD, 2019b). Components of asthma education include (a) training in using inhalers correctly, (b) encouraging adherence to medications and other aspects of treatment, (c) information on asthma, and (d) self-management training (e.g., monitoring symptoms or peak flow, following written asthma action plans, regular review by health care provider; GINA, 2022). Although some aspects of asthma education fall within the domain of medical providers (e.g., developing the written asthma action plan), behavioral health providers may be involved in supporting a number of asthma education elements.

Behavioral Health in Primary Care

No studies directly examining the effects of BHC interventions in primary care settings on asthma outcomes could be found in the current literature. However, the integration of a BHC into primary care may help the clinic with implementation of a number of the evidence-based asthma CPG recommendations described in this chapter. BHCs can not only assist with assessment and intervention with patients with comorbid anxiety or depression but can work with patients and their PCPs on implementing self-management approaches to asthma control. For example, BHCs may assist with tobacco cessation, weight loss, and medication adherence in patients with asthma. BHCs may also play a useful role in helping patients adhere to recommendations regarding self-monitoring of peak flow, appropriately use written asthma action plans developed by the PCP and patient, modify behaviors to reduce exposure to factors that worsen asthma, learn relaxation and stress management skills, and increase physical activity levels.

Primary Care Adaptation

The following recommendations regarding behavioral interventions for patients with asthma in primary care are based on adaptations of specialty behavioral health approaches and the CPGs for asthma care summarized earlier (GINA, 2022; VA/DoD, 2019b). They describe strategies that the BHC can use within individual BHC appointments, as well as team-based strategies the BHC can implement to support the primary care team's ability to implement best practices for asthma management.

Assess

Assessment of asthma ideally starts with a brief discussion with the PCP to determine the specific reason the PCP wants to include the BHC in the patient's care. During this conversation, the BHC can also ask about the prescribed asthma medications, the asthma action plan, and any other specific recommendations the PCP has made for the patient's asthma self-management (e.g., peak flow monitoring, smoking cessation). If a discussion with the PCP is not possible, the BHC should review recent chart notes to gather relevant background information.

As with COPD, assessment of patients with asthma should include questions about breathing symptoms and functioning. See Figure 8.5 for examples of assessment questions to consider using for patients with asthma. Respiratory symptom and function questions include a focus on peak flow and/or symptom monitoring and whether the patient is using this monitoring to guide day-to-day decision making regarding home management of asthma.

Medication adherence proves difficult for many patients with asthma, so a close examination of medication use is warranted to determine whether they are either overusing or underusing medications. A common pattern is overuse of quick-relief medications and underuse of long-term control medications. This may be due to mistaken beliefs about the role of different types of medication or concerns about side effects from taking a medication daily. Medical data on the number of primary, urgent, or emergency care visits also should be

FIGURE 8.5. Handout for Asthma Assessment Questions

Sample Assessment Questions for Asthma

Breathing Symptoms and Peak Flow

- How often do you notice symptoms of worsening asthma?
- What affects your breathing the most (e.g., physical activity, stress, allergens)?
- Do you monitor your peak flow at home? How often?
- What is your average peak flow? What is your best and worst peak flow?
- Has your peak flow dropped below 80% of personal best since your last medical visit? What did you do?

Medications

- What medications do you take for asthma? When and how often do you take them?
- How long does it take you to go through a rescue inhaler?
- What side effects do you notice when you take your medication (e.g., tremor, anxiety, nausea, headache)? Have you stopped taking any regular doses for any reason?

Medical System Use

- When was your last hospitalization for asthma? How many have you had?
- How many visits have you had to the emergency room for asthma in the past year?
- What is your best estimate of how many primary care visits you have made in the past year? (Note: Obtain this through review of medical record, if available.)

Work, Social, and Family Functioning

- How has asthma changed what you do at work?
- Are you having trouble getting things done around the house due to breathing problems?
- What has changed, if anything, about what you do for fun? With friends?
- Describe what you do in a typical day.
- How many days of work/school have you missed due to asthma in the last year?
- How has your family responded to your asthma? How has asthma changed your relationships?
- What would you like to do that you can't do now or as well because of your asthma?

Emotional and Cognitive Factors

- Describe how your mood has been lately.
- How often do you feel anxious or panicky? When does this occur?
- What goes through your mind when you have an asthma attack?
- What do you do when you feel you are having trouble breathing?

Health-Related Behaviors

- Do you smoke? What are your thoughts about quitting?
- What forms of exercise are you getting? Are your symptoms worsened by exercise? Has your PCP advised you to use your inhaler or take other steps prior to exercising?
- What triggers have you identified (e.g., animals, mold, pollens, pollution, cold air, foods)? Which ones do you have most trouble avoiding?

Interventions to Date

- Are you monitoring your peak flow? How often?
- Do you have a written asthma action plan? Please describe it to me. When do you use the action plan?
- What kinds of problems do you have with following the plan?
- Do you practice any form of relaxation (e.g., visualization, imagery, diaphragmatic breathing)?

Note. PCP = primary care provider.

obtained during the assessment to help determine adherence to and effectiveness of current care plans. From these, the BHC can further assess whether current barriers to maintaining good health are the result of poor adherence to previously constructed care plans.

The CPG from the VA/DoD (2019b) suggests that primary care management of adults with asthma include an assessment of risk factors for asthma exacerbation, including the following:

- overweight/obesity,

- atopy,

- history of lower respiratory infection,

- depression,

- current smoking, and

- Operation Iraqi Freedom/Operation Enduring Freedom combat deployment.

Other guidelines also recommend screening for anxiety (GINA, 2022). Although some of these factors are best assessed by the medical provider (e.g., atopy, history of lower respiratory infection), relevant behavioral and emotional factors can be assessed by the BHC. Assessment of emotional functioning can include brief screening questions for anxiety and depression (see Chapter 5). Questions regarding tobacco use status and the patient's interest in making a quit attempt should be included. Assessment of the patient's exposure to factors that may exacerbate asthma, such as secondhand smoke, dust mites, mold, and other environmental factors at home or work, is warranted. Finally, obtaining information on what, if any, interventions the patient has tried can help guide decisions regarding future strategies.

Advise

The BHC's next step is to advise the patient on specific, evidence-based recommendations for change. The selection of particular recommendations may be based on what the BHC believes is the most important aspect to address (e.g., smoking cessation, regular use of controller asthma medication as prescribed); what the PCP believes is the most important aspect, on the basis of the referral question or issue (e.g., "Patient is not monitoring peak flow daily, which is part of their written asthma action plan. Please assist."); or what the BHC believes the patient might be most motivated or willing to try.

As with other types of patients, when working with individuals who have asthma, BHCs should ensure their advice does not overstep bounds of competence and stray into the practice of medicine. Rather than providing specific advice about medical interventions, BHCs provide consultation to the PCP and reinforce the medical treatment plans that the PCP and patient have jointly developed. For example, optimal medical treatment of asthma integrates home-based written action plans into the patient's care to promote regular monitoring of symptoms, early identification of exacerbations, and appropriate decisions regarding medication use and access of additional medical help. These plans need to be developed jointly between the patient and the PCP, not the BHC, because they involve specific recommendations about medication use and when to access urgent or emergency care. However, BHCs should be familiar with the format and content of the action plans used to assist patients in adherence. The following is an example of how a BHC might advise a patient with asthma on treatment options, without crossing over the line of inappropriately providing medical, rather than behavioral health, advice:

> I'm concerned by a few things you mentioned this morning. One is that you feel your asthma is getting worse. You've had more flare-ups and have been to the emergency room twice in the last 2 months, and you feel your asthma is getting out of control. Although Dr. Vasquez wants you to check your peak flow reading each morning, this is hard for you to remember. And you're not quite sure how to adjust your medications at home when you do get a peak flow reading that seems low or when you notice your asthma symptoms worsening. On the positive side, you're doing a great job remembering to use your daily asthma control inhaler.
>
> Based on what you've shared, I have a couple of recommendations. The first is that we set up an appointment with Dr. Vasquez to develop a written home action plan. Here is an example of the form she uses with most of her patients. [Show blank action plan.] If you'd like, I can attend the appointment too so that the three of us are on the same page. Dr. Vasquez will set guidelines for when you should take certain steps, such as using additional medication or going to the emergency room, based on your symptoms or peak flow readings.
>
> My second recommendation is that you and I work together to help you stay on track with daily checks of your peak flow, as Dr. Vasquez really thinks it is important in getting your asthma under control. We can develop some ways to help you remember to monitor each morning and tackle any other barriers that might be getting in the way. What do you think about these options?

Agree

Once the BHC has discussed with the patient their recommendations for change, the BHC and the patient need to come to an agreement on the specific direction they will take. We typically recommend that BHCs guide the patient to select just one or two areas to change at a time. Additional areas can be targeted later after initial progress has been made, if needed. Some amount of artful negotiation may be needed to come to mutually agreed-upon goals, as can be seen in the following example of a patient who is unwilling to monitor peak flow daily but wants to see improvements in their ability to be physically active with their children.

> Dr. Vasquez really wants you to monitor your peak flow every day. She and I both believe this is critical in helping keep you out of the emergency room, but it sounds like you really don't want to focus on this right now. You say you've done it before for a few weeks and didn't find it helpful and that you find it hard to remember to do it. What you're really concerned about is how your asthma has gotten in the way of being active, such as riding bikes and playing with your kids.
>
> In many ways, these two goals are linked. Regularly checking your peak flow can help you take your medications in a way that will keep your asthma under control. This will help you do more of what you want to do, like being active

with your kids. For now, why don't we begin by working on some ways for you to be more active with your kids, even if you're not ready today to commit to checking your peak flow every day. Then later, when you're ready, we can shift our focus back to peak flow monitoring, perhaps coming up with some ideas on how to make it easier for you. How does that sound to you?

An additional issue in the agree phase arises when family is involved in the management of asthma, whether in adults, adolescents, or children. Often, the proposed plan involves cooperation or action on the part of the family of the patient with asthma. For example, a partner might be asked to change their smoking behaviors in the home to minimize the amount of smoke exposure that the patient with asthma receives. Parents may need to assist with a complicated medication regimen for their child or with educating school personnel on actions to take if symptoms increase. Whenever possible, BHCs should elicit the agreement of all relevant parties (e.g., partner, parent, child) before moving on to the assist phase of the interaction.

Assist

Achieving the goals of good asthma management involves a number of complex choices and behaviors on the part of the patient. These can include monitoring lung functioning or symptoms, managing acute symptom exacerbations, using medications appropriately, identifying and modifying triggers, and safely engaging in regular physical activity. Interventions may also focus on management of depression or anxiety, when present (see Chapter 5), as well as weight loss in patients who are overweight or obese (see Chapter 6).

Monitor peak flow. PCPs may ask their patients with asthma to measure and record their peak flow on a daily basis. BHCs can help patients achieve this goal by working to increase motivation for this behavior change. This may be done through psychoeducation regarding the role that peak flow measures can play in providing early warning of exacerbations, even before physical symptoms may be noticeable to the patient. It may also be achieved through motivational interviewing strategies, such as highlighting discrepancies between the patient's overall asthma goals and current behavior or having the patient verbalize arguments for making the change. BHCs may also assist the patient in identifying and eliminating barriers to regular monitoring. Examples include providing a monitoring form that is easy to use and helping the patient identify cues to remember to monitor. The Asthma Monitoring Form (see Figure 8.6) provides one example of a self-monitoring log that patients may find helpful in recording their peak flow, along with several other relevant variables (i.e., asthma symptoms, effects of symptoms on activity, exposure to triggers, and quick-relief inhaler use).

Manage acute exacerbations. In accordance with clinical practice recommendations (GINA, 2022), medical providers should routinely use written asthma action plans to help patients recognize worsening asthma symptoms and make appropriate decisions about medication use and seeking medical help. An

FIGURE 8.6. Asthma Monitoring Form Patient Handout

Asthma Monitoring Form

Instructions: Please record your peak flow numbers in the spaces provided for each date. Rate your asthma symptoms of coughing, wheezing, and shortness of breath (SOB) on a scale of 0 to 3 (0 = no noticeable symptoms, 1 = mild, 2 = moderate, 3 = severe). List any activities that you restricted because of your symptoms. List any exposure to potential triggers or factors that worsen your asthma. Finally, record the number of puffs of your quick-relief ("rescue") inhaler (bronchodilator) you used to control your symptoms.

Date	Peak flow (a.m.)	Peak flow (p.m.)	Cough (0–3)	Wheeze (0–3)	SOB (0–3)	Activity restriction	Exposures	"Rescue" inhaler use

example asthma action plan template is available online from the National Heart, Lung, and Blood Institute (2020). Once the action plan is developed by the PCP, BHCs may play a role in helping patients adhere to the plan. Working with patients to identify and remove barriers to routine monitoring falls within the BHC's domain. For example, BHCs might help the patient plan a strategy to ensure that the action plan is available in various locations (e.g., work, car, home) through use of laminated copies, wallet cards, an image maintained in smartphones, and so forth. Finally, BHCs can assess whether psychological factors such as high anxiety are interfering with plan implementation when exacerbations occur. If so, assisting the patient in remaining calm during exacerbations may be indicated. This could take the form of teaching skills to rest, relax, and use reassuring thinking during exacerbations. The patient can learn and practice cognitive disputation skills and relaxed breathing, perhaps enlisting a significant other to help coach them. Information on the anxiety–dyspnea cycle (Figure 8.1) and the handout on pursed-lip breathing (Figure 8.3), discussed previously for use with COPD, may also be useful for these patients.

Use medications correctly. The referral question from a PCP may indicate concerns about medication use, such as "Patient is not regularly using her budesonide inhaler. Seen in urgent care last week. Please assist." or "Patient is using more than two canisters of albuterol a month. May be using for anxiety symptoms. Please evaluate." Alternatively, BHCs may discover inappropriate medication use patterns in their initial assessment or on review of self-monitoring forms. After ensuring that the BHC and the patient both know the type, dose, timing, and frequency recommended by the PCP, BHCs should identify barriers to appropriate adherence. For the patient underusing their control medications (e.g., budesonide inhaler), asking about their understanding of the role of this medication in asthma control may reveal an incorrect belief that this medication only needs to be taken when they experience symptoms. Effective interventions may include a discussion of how daily use of control medications (e.g., anti-inflammatories) is the most effective way to control their asthma. It may be helpful to provide behavioral strategies to assist in remembering to take medication as well as cognitive strategies for countering incorrect beliefs about the medication use. For patients who have decreased adherence due to medication side effects, BHCs can support adherence to recommendations for managing side effects (e.g., using a spacer with the inhaler and rinsing the mouth after inhaler use to minimize sore throat, hoarseness, or thrush; GINA, 2022).

Overuse of reliever medications may result from a number of factors. Some patients may not have their symptoms well controlled by their current controller medication or may not be effectively avoiding factors that exacerbate their asthma. These reasons could necessitate another appointment with the PCP to evaluate whether medications need adjusting, or they may require renewed efforts to identify and modify potential triggers. Additionally, some patients with anxiety symptoms may overuse their reliever medications in response to physical symptoms of anxiety (e.g., increased heart rate, rapid shallow breathing, tightness in chest) rather than to symptoms of an asthma exacerbation. BHCs should consult with PCPs if this pattern is suspected, and if this behavior is occurring, the patient may benefit from modifying symptom perception and learning anxiety management and breathing retraining strategies (e.g., deep breathing, pursed-lip breathing, reassuring thinking).

Recognize and minimize triggers. Reducing exposure to factors that exacerbate asthma can be useful for certain patients. Although avoiding indoor and outdoor allergens is not recommended as a general strategy for all patients with asthma, sensitized patients may benefit from avoiding or minimizing exposure to a specific allergen when feasible (GINA, 2022). Having the patient complete a checklist of factors they may be exposed to can provide a starting point for developing a behavioral plan to minimize exposure. Figure 8.7 contains a sample checklist that may prove helpful. Alternatively, some patients benefit from 1 to 2 weeks of self-monitoring, tracking exposure to potential triggers along with changes in asthma symptoms or peak flow readings. If warning indicators are discovered, BHCs should bring this to the attention of the PCP, who can evaluate whether allergy testing or medical interventions for allergies are warranted. Once factors that exacerbate asthma have been identified, the BHC can work with the patient to develop strategies to reduce exposure (for additional details, see GINA, 2022, pp. 79–80).

Stop smoking. Smoking worsens lung function in patients with asthma and decreases the effectiveness of many asthma medications. Therefore, quitting

FIGURE 8.7. Asthma Allergen and Exposure Checklist Patient Handout

Factors That May Worsen Asthma

Some people with asthma find that their symptoms are worsened or triggered by identifiable factors or situations. Sometimes these are allergies; other times they are simply sensitivities or reactions to environmental factors. Please review the following list of factors that may worsen asthma and check the items that you believe might affect your symptoms. If you are unsure about a given item, place a question mark on the line.

_____	Pets or other animals	_____	Sulfites in food or beverages
_____	Pollens	_____	Tobacco smoke
_____	Mold	_____	Outdoor air pollution
_____	Dust mites	_____	Wood fire smoke
_____	Dust	_____	Physical exercise
_____	Cockroaches	_____	Cold air
_____	Airborne chemicals	_____	Other (List: _____)

smoking may be the most important change that patients can make to improve their asthma management. For more information, see the discussion earlier in this chapter on smoking cessation for patients with COPD as well as the more detailed information on tobacco cessation in primary care found in Chapter 6.

Increase physical activity and minimize exercise-induced bronchospasm. CPGs suggest that all patients with asthma should be encouraged to engage in regular physical activity to improve general health, quality of life, and asthma control (GINA, 2022; VA/DoD, 2019b). Patients who experience exercise-induced bronchoconstriction may also be advised by their provider to use asthma reliever medications in a preventive manner before exercise and to engage in an adequate warm-up period prior to exercise (GINA, 2022). BHCs can assist patients in adherence to these physical activity recommendations. Those without asthma-induced symptoms may still struggle, like many Americans, to develop patterns of regular physical activity. BHCs can apply the information in Chapter 6 to working with these patients to increase activity. For those with exercise-induced bronchospasm, BHCs can help patients adhere to medical recommendations for safer exercise, such as remembering to take the reliever medication prior to exercise or having the medication accessible at the time of exercise (e.g., pack an extra inhaler in gym bag in advance). BHCs can work with patients to regularly incorporate a 6- to 10-minute period of gradual warm-up, typically walking, before exercise that is more vigorous.

Arrange

Some patients with asthma may show improvement in self-management behaviors within a few appointments. Others may benefit from meeting periodically with the BHC over time to maintain progress. If a patient does not show improvement with BHC interventions, a referral for specialty mental health treatment could be considered. The need for a referral may be higher when significant mental health disorders are affecting the self-management approach to asthma care. For example, patients with comorbid panic disorder may need a more intensive level of treatment.

Alternately, some patients may be interested in accessing web-based patient educational material to improve their understanding of or management of their respiratory problems. These resources may be used by the patient independently or as part of a guided self-help approach in conjunction with BHC appointments. A number of these resources are summarized in Figure 8.8. Of note, the VA/DoD (2019b) CPG concluded that there was insufficient evidence to recommend for or against the use of mobile applications for management of asthma. Interested readers are referred to a systematic review of 12 RCTs investigating mobile application use on asthma outcomes (Hui et al., 2017).

SUMMARY

Pulmonary disorders, particularly COPD and asthma, are a major cause of disability and health care burden. These diseases often have a significant negative impact on physical functioning, psychosocial functioning, and quality of life. COPD and asthma are among the most common chronic illnesses seen at primary care medical clinics and are often difficult for PCPs to manage in an allotted 15- to 20-minute medical appointment because of the complex interactions between physical, behavioral, emotional, and environmental factors often seen in these patients. BHCs can assess and intervene with appropriate evidence-based strategies to address behavioral, emotional, cognitive, and environmental factors (e.g., smoking, physical inactivity, inappropriate use of medication) that may be making symptoms and functioning worse. BHCs can also assist the PCP in identifying which patients are not benefiting from intervention at the primary care level and can recommend referrals to specialty mental health providers when indicated. Overall, through team-based primary care, BHCs can help patients with COPD and asthma experience improved management of their disease, better functioning, and increased quality of life.

FIGURE 8.8. Resources for Patients With Asthma: Websites, Mobile Applications, and Books

Type	Location	Description
Websites	National Heart, Lung, and Blood Institute (https://www.nhlbi.nih.gov/health/asthma)	This website offers patient information on asthma, including specific symptoms and diagnosis, medications, treatment options, and self-management materials. It also includes an asthma action plan and asthma wallet card to assist patients in tracking information such as medications, peak flow, and their doctor's contact information. Patient education materials are available in English and Spanish.
	American Lung Association (https://www.lung.org/lung-health-diseases/lung-disease-lookup/asthma)	This website offers patient guidance on managing asthma and living a healthy life, including information on understanding asthma medications, creating an asthma management plan, monitoring asthma control, and reducing exposure to asthma triggers.
	United States Environmental Protection Agency (https://www.epa.gov/asthma)	This website aids patients in noticing asthma triggers while gaining control and reducing exposure to those triggers. It also contains basic asthma information and information on how to improve asthma health in communities and schools. Some resources are available in Spanish.
	Centers for Disease Control and Prevention (https://www.cdc.gov/asthma/)	This website offers tools for asthma control, such as asthma action plans and information on the National Asthma Control Program. Patient education materials cover information on symptoms and management, use of inhalers, and avoidance of triggers. Materials are available in multiple languages.
Mobile applications	Ask Me, AsthMe! (https://apps.apple.com/app/ask-me-asthme)	This mobile app provides asthma education for pediatric patients and families. The app provides a place to keep a log of asthma symptoms and triggers. It is available in English and Spanish (New York City Health and Hospitals Corp.: Ask Me, AsthMe! 2021, 1.1.2 edition).
	AsthmaMD (https://www.asthmamd.org/)	This app provides patients with tools to log asthma symptoms, triggers, and medications. Data shown in graphs can be shared with their provider (Mobile Breeze: AsthmaMD. 2017, 3.35 edition).
Book	*Asthma for Dummies, Pocket Edition* (Berger, 2010)	This brief patient education book provides an overview of asthma symptoms and diagnosis as well as key aspects of asthma management, including self-monitoring, appropriately using medications, and avoiding allergens and other asthma triggers.

9

Cardiovascular Disease

Cardiovascular disease (CVD) is an umbrella term that refers to diseases of the heart and blood vessels. Some of the more common conditions and diseases that fall under this umbrella include coronary artery disease, cardiomyopathy, valvular heart disease, pericardial disease, arteriosclerosis, atherosclerosis, aneurism, high blood pressure, stroke, and peripheral artery disease. Since 1900, except for 1918, CVD has been the number one cause of death in the United States. Although the number of deaths attributable to CVD declined 13.2% between 2007 to 2009 and 2017 to 2019 (Tsao et al., 2022), CVD still accounts for approximately one of every three deaths in the United States across sex and race (e.g., White, Black, Asian, Hispanic or Latinx). On average, a person dies every 36 seconds from CVD (Tsao et al., 2022). Over one third of the United States population has some form of CVD, contributing to an estimated $378 billion in direct and indirect costs (Tsao et al., 2022).

Allan and Fisher (2012), whose book remains as a useful resource for behavioral health professionals working with CVD, categorized CVD into three major areas, namely coronary heart disease, valvular heart disease, and cardiomyopathy. *Coronary heart disease*, also referred to as coronary artery disease, results from the buildup of fatty deposits (i.e., atherosclerosis) on the arterial walls that supply the heart with blood. It can result in transient chest discomfort (i.e., angina pectoris), heart attacks (i.e., acute myocardial infarctions), and sudden cardiac death. *Valvular heart disease* affects one to four heart valves and results in insufficient blood flow or backward leakage through the heart valves.

https://doi.org/10.1037/0000380-010
Integrated Behavioral Health in Primary Care: Step-by-Step Guidance for Assessment and Intervention, Third Edition, by C. L. Hunter, J. L. Goodie, M. S. Oordt, and A. C. Dobmeyer

Valvular heart disease generally results from rheumatic heart disease, age-related degeneration, or congenital abnormalities or may be related to intravenous drug abuse. *Cardiomyopathy* refers to a weakening of the heart muscle and most commonly results in heart failure, an inability of the heart to pump sufficient amount of blood throughout the body.

KEY BIOPSYCHOSOCIAL FACTORS

The development of CVD has been linked to a variety of biopsychosocial factors. Although certain risk factors, such as age, sex, race, and heritable risk, cannot be modified, the risk of developing CVD, particularly coronary heart disease, can be decreased by targeting physical, behavioral, and emotional factors. In this chapter we discuss the factors that contribute to the development and progression of CVD. Familiarity with these factors can help behavioral health consultants (BHCs) more effectively assess and facilitate change among patients with CVD. The interventions recommended in this chapter rely heavily on those described in Chapters 4, 5, and 6.

Physical Factors

The development and progression of CVD is often related to diabetes, high blood pressure, and high cholesterol. Diabetes, which we discuss more extensively in Chapter 7, is associated with the development of coronary heart disease, peripheral arterial disease, and potentially cardiomyopathy. Figure 9.1 lists the classification of blood pressures. The American College of Cardiology/American Heart Association (ACC/AHA) Task Force on Clinical Practice Guidelines (Whelton et al., 2018) redefined categories of blood pressure in adults from previous definitions. Among those 40 to 70 years old, the risk of CVD doubles for every 20-mmHg increase in systolic blood pressure and 10-mmHg increase in diastolic blood pressure starting at 115/75 mmHg (Lewington et al.,

FIGURE 9.1. Classification of Blood Pressure for Adults

	Blood pressure classification			
	Normal	Elevated	Stage 1 hypertension	Stage 2 hypertension
Systolic blood pressure (mmHg)	< 120	120–129	130–139	≥ 140
Diastolic blood pressure (mmHg)	and < 80	and < 80	or 80–89	or ≥ 90

Note. Data from Whelton et al. (2018).

2002). Essential hypertension is the most common primary diagnosis in primary care settings (Santo & Okeyode, 2018).

Cholesterol travels through our blood stream in two major forms of lipoproteins, low-density lipoproteins and high-density lipoproteins. Excess low-density lipoproteins cholesterol, referred to as hypercholesterolemia, contributes to atherosclerosis (i.e., hardening of the arteries), whereas higher levels of high-density lipoproteins are largely protective. Guidelines for treatment of high cholesterol are based on an individual's overall risk for heart disease, which can be calculated using the risk calculator link available in Figure 9.2. Lifestyle changes remain the foundation for lowering cholesterol; however, if these changes are not sufficient for reducing risk, then statin therapy may be recommended (Grundy et al., 2019). In patients that tolerate them, statins are the only class of medications currently recommended for reducing cholesterol and reducing the risk of CVD.

Behavioral Factors

In addition to tobacco use, obesity, and physical inactivity, which we discuss in Chapter 5, dietary nutrient and alcohol consumption, as well as medication adherence, affect the course of CVD.

Dietary Nutrients

The ACC and the AHA published guidelines for reducing cardiovascular risk (Arnett et al., 2019). The committee recommended diets that (a) emphasize the intake of vegetables, fruits, legumes, nuts, whole grains, and fish; (b) replace saturated fats (e.g., butter, cheese, red meat, whole milk) with dietary monounsaturated fats (e.g., avocado, olive oil, almonds) and polyunsaturated fats (e.g., flaxseed, walnuts, salmon, tuna); (c) reduce cholesterol and sodium; (d) reduce sugar-sweetened and artificially sweetened beverages, processed meats, and refined carbohydrates; and (e) avoid trans fats (e.g., fried foods, margarine, nondairy creamer, pastries). By following the Dietary Approaches to Stop Hypertension (DASH) eating plan, the U.S. Department of Agriculture food pattern (U.S. Department of Agriculture & U.S. Department of Health and Human Services, 2020), or the AHA diet, patients can reduce their blood pressure and cholesterol (Arnett et al., 2019; Lichtenstein et al., 2021). The recommendations of the DASH eating plan are presented in Figure 9.3. DASH-consistent dietary alternatives are available on the National Heart, Lung, and Blood Institute (2021) website. An increasing body of well-established evidence indicates that the Mediterranean diet reduces blood pressure and cholesterol and reduces the risk of major cardiovascular events (e.g., Bazzano et al., 2013; Delgado-Lista et al., 2022; Lichtenstein et al., 2021).

FIGURE 9.2. Resources for Patients With Cardiovascular Disease: Websites, Mobile Applications, and Books

Type	Location	Description
Websites	American Heart Association (https://www.heart.org/)	Provides information and resources for patients and providers about heart disease and risk factors (e.g., cholesterol, hypertension); particularly useful for patients
	Centers for Disease Control and Prevention (https://www.cdc.gov/heartdisease/)	Provides information and resources for patients and providers about heart disease and risk factors (e.g., cholesterol, hypertension)
	U.S. Food and Drug Administration (https://www.fda.gov/forconsumers/consumerupdates/ucm327369.htm)	Provides information about reducing sodium intake
	National Heart, Lung, and Blood Institute (https://www.nhlbi.nih.gov/health/educational/hearttruth/)	Provides information and resources for patients and providers about heart disease and risk factors (e.g., cholesterol, hypertension)
Mobile applications	My Life Check (https://mlc.heart.org/)	Patient-oriented app and website assists with monitoring and behavior change
	ASCVD Risk Estimator (https://tools.acc.org/ascvd-risk-estimator-plus/#!/calculate/estimate; Apple iOS and Android)	Helps providers and patients estimate 10-year and lifetime risk for ASCVD
Books/documents	*Dietary Guidelines for Americans* (USDA & DHHS, 2020)	Summarizes dietary recommendations for Americans
	Your Guide to Lowering Blood Pressure (DHHS, 2003)	Provides patient guide for lifestyle and medication management of blood pressure
	Your Guide to Lowering Your Blood Pressure With DASH (DHHS, 2006)	Provides patient guide for the DASH eating plan
	Heart and Mind: The Practice of Cardiac Psychology (Allan & Fisher, 2012)	Provides overview of biopsychosocial assessment and treatment of cardiovascular disease for behavioral health professionals

Note. ASCVD = atherosclerotic cardiovascular disease; USDA = U.S. Department of Agriculture; DHHS = U.S. Department of Health and Human Services; DASH = Dietary Approaches to Stop Hypertension.

Alcohol Consumption

Alcohol consumption has a J-shaped curve relation with mortality. Individuals consuming a moderate amount of alcohol (i.e., daily consumption of one standard drink for women and two standard drinks for men) have a lower risk of

FIGURE 9.3. Components of the DASH Eating Plan

Food group	Daily servings
Grains	6–8
Meats, poultry, fish	6 or less
Vegetables	4–5
Fruit	4–5
Low-fat or fat-free dairy	2–3
Fats and oils	2–3
Sodium	2,300 mg[a]
Food group	**Weekly servings**
Nuts, seeds, dry beans, and peas	4–5
Sweets	5 or less

Note. DASH = Dietary Approaches to Stop Hypertension. From *DASH Eating Plan*, by National Heart, Lung, and Blood Institute, 2021, National Institutes of Health (https://www.nhlbi.nih.gov/education/dash-eating-plan). In the public domain.
[a]1,500 mg sodium was found to be more effective for lowering blood pressure, particularly among middle-aged and older adults, African Americans, and those diagnosed with high blood pressure.

death from all causes, including coronary heart disease, compared with individuals who do not drink alcohol and individuals who consume three or more drinks a day (Ronksley et al., 2011; Xi et al., 2017). However, beyond moderate intake, alcohol begins to have a negative impact on cardiovascular health.

Medication Adherence

Among individuals with CVD, adherence to lifestyle and medication recommendations is a significant problem. For example, approximately one quarter to one half of hypertensive patients fail to adhere to a recommended treatment regimen (Ho et al., 2009; Tomaszewski et al., 2014). Multiple factors that predict decreased adherence, including psychological problems (e.g., depression), asymptomatic conditions, and negative side effects of medication (Osterberg & Blaschke, 2005), may account for the poor adherence to medication regimens among patients with CVD. A systematic review (Hong et al., 2022) found that effective interventions for improving adherence included (a) education programs, (b) daily reminders, (c) regular follow-ups, and (d) use of blister packs to deliver medication. Educating patients, establishing readiness for self-care, setting specific goals, self-monitoring, and using cues are some of the behavioral strategies that could be incorporated into a primary care environment to assist patients with adherence. However, no method reliably increases adherence to medication regimens over the long term in individuals with chronic medical conditions (Nieuwlaat et al., 2014). Therefore, it is important to recommend to PCPs that they regularly assess and target adherence to medications.

Emotional and Cognitive Factors

Stressors, depression, anxiety, and posttraumatic stress disorder (PTSD) have been related to the development of CVD. Both acute (e.g., bereavement, natural disasters, terrorist activities) and chronic stressors (e.g., work-related, marital, and caregiving stress) have been linked to the development of CVD and hypertension (Cohen et al., 2015). The treatments for CVD can also lead to the development of emotional distress. For example, 14.5% of patients demonstrated new anxiety onset and 11.3% demonstrated the new onset of depression following the insertion of an implantable cardioverter defibrillator (ICD; i.e., a device placed in the chest that delivers electric shocks to restore a normal heart rhythm; Pedersen et al., 2021). Interventions that reduce stress responses have demonstrated short-term benefits for reducing cardiovascular responses (e.g., lower heart rate, lower blood pressure), but there is not well-established evidence that decreasing stress independently reduces risk for CVD (Sara et al., 2022).

Depression

There is a bidirectional relation between depression symptoms and CVD (Harshfield et al., 2020; Ogunmoroti et al., 2022). Those diagnosed with depression are more likely to develop CVD, and those who develop CVD are more at risk of demonstrating depressive symptoms. Those individuals who are diagnosed with both CVD and depression have worse prognoses. It is particularly important to carefully screen for depressive symptoms in patients with CVD. Some evidence indicates that treating depression before the patient develops symptomatic CVD will decrease the risk by half (Stewart et al., 2014). However, most evidence suggests that treating depressive symptoms may not reduce risk for future cardiac events or reduce risk for early mortality (Cohen et al., 2015). Targeting depression, for those with and without CVD, is important for reducing depressive symptoms and improving quality of life.

Anxiety

Based on a meta-analysis of 37 studies, anxiety symptoms are associated with a 52% increased incidence of CVD (Batelaan et al., 2016). However, other studies have found that when controlling for depressive symptoms and other potential confounders, these relations diminish (Cohen et al., 2015). Among those with CVD, anxiety disorders occur in 16% of this population (Tully et al., 2016). Similar to treating those with depressive symptoms, despite the mixed evidence regarding the relations between anxiety and CVD, it is important to help patients manage anxiety symptoms to improve quality of life. Identifying anxiety in those with known CVD can be challenging, as many symptoms may overlap (e.g., chest pain, palpitations, arrythmias; Tully et al., 2016), so BHCs should work closely with PCPs when identifying and treating anxiety symptoms in this patient population.

Posttraumatic Stress Disorder

Increasingly, researchers are examining the relations between PTSD and CVD. Existing data have suggested that PTSD is associated with the development of CVD and early mortality, risk factors for CVD (e.g., hypertension, diabetes), and the risk of CVD events (e.g., heart attacks, strokes; O'Donnell et al., 2021). Whether PTSD is an independent risk factor for CVD remains to be determined; however, PTSD may involve systemic changes that contribute to the development of CVD (Krantz et al., 2022). PTSD may also develop following a cardiac event or due to treatments associated with CVD (e.g., ICD; Vilchinsky et al., 2017).

Environmental Factors

Environmental factors, including social support and socioeconomic status, influence CVD. Small social support networks, low levels of perceived support, loneliness, and social isolation are associated with increased risk of developing coronary heart disease, independent of other risk factors (Bu et al., 2020; Freak-Poli et al., 2021; Golaszewski et al., 2022). In 2002, Hogan et al. reviewed the literature and found that although some evidence suggests social support interventions improve a variety of problems (e.g., cancer, weight loss, surgery, birth preparation), this research is often conceptually and methodologically flawed (Hogan et al., 2002) and efforts to improve social support do not reduce the frequency of coronary heart disease events (Lett et al., 2005). A more recent review (Clayton et al., 2019) largely supported these findings for CVD, with the exception that there is some support for caregiver-oriented interventions. Similar to social support, low socioeconomic status and other social determinants of health (e.g., employment status, access to medical care) are related to the development and progression of CVD (Havranek et al., 2015). Socioeconomic status, food insecurity, structural racism, and targeted marketing of unhealthy foods and beverages can determine the food consumption affecting CVD rates among individuals and should be considered in the development of interventions for individuals (Lichtenstein et al., 2021).

Cultural and Diversity Considerations

Heart disease is the leading cause of death for non-Hispanic White, Black, Native American or Alaska Native, and Native Hawaiian or Pacific Islander adults and is second to cancer among non-Hispanic Asian/Pacific Islander and Hispanic adults (Heron, 2021). At least 30% of individuals identifying as Hispanic or non-Hispanic White, Black, or Asian demonstrated total cholesterol levels above 200 mg/dL, with non-Hispanic White women demonstrating the highest prevalence (i.e., 41.8%; Tsao et al., 2022). Black men and women 20 years old and older have the highest prevalence of hypertension (men = 58.3%, women = 57.6%) compared with their White (men = 51.0%, women = 40.5%) and Hispanic counterparts (men = 50.6%, women = 40.8%; Tsao et al., 2022). The reasons for these differences are linked to multiple biopsychosocial factors. Some of the observed differences are related to physical factors (e.g., Black adults have higher levels of aldosterone, which is associated with obesity-related high blood pressure), access to care, and health behaviors

(Graham, 2014). Even within ethnic groups, CVD risk varies significantly based on geographic origin (e.g., European Spanish-speaking vs. Central American vs. South American; Graham, 2014). It is critical for the BHC to be mindful of health-related disparities to enhance equity and work to avoid disparities in treatment. The National Heart, Lung, and Blood Institute (n.d.-b) maintains resources related to CVD for diverse populations to reduce health disparities and inequalities.

SPECIALTY MENTAL HEALTH

Providers in outpatient clinical health psychology settings often see patients following a significant cardiac event (e.g., myocardial infarction) or cardiac surgery (e.g., bypass surgery, placement of a stent) and may participate in comprehensive cardiac rehabilitation programs, which have been found to reduce subsequent cardiac mortality, hospitalizations, and risk factors (e.g., blood pressure, smoking, weight; Dalal et al., 2015; Dibben et al., 2021). Multiple studies (e.g., Blumenthal et al., 2021; P. Chu et al., 2016) have demonstrated that high-intensity treatments for changing health behaviors can have an impact on physical factors that are risk factors for disease. The impact of changing health behaviors on mortality was assessed by Iestra et al. (2005). The results of their study estimated mortality reductions for those with CVD of 35% with smoking cessation, 25% with increased physical activity, 20% with moderate alcohol use, and 45% with dietary changes. These risk reductions are similar to or greater than the risk reduction associated with preventive medication interventions (e.g., low-dose aspirin, statins, beta blockers, angiotensin-converting enzyme inhibitors; Iestra et al., 2005). Although treatment of depression with medication or cognitive behavioral interventions in those with CVD may improve quality of life, it is unclear whether there are reductions in cardiac-related events or in early mortality (Fernandes et al., 2021; Reavell et al., 2018). Physical activity interventions (e.g., 30 minutes, three times per week) decrease depressive symptoms, improve risk factors for CVD (e.g., hypertension, high cholesterol), and reduce CVD morbidity and mortality (Kraus et al., 2019; Oja et al., 2018). A Cochrane systematic review and meta-analysis (Whalley et al., 2014) found that compared with usual care, psychological interventions were associated with fewer deaths due to cardiac causes but were not associated with reduced all-cause mortality, risk of revascularization, or nonfatal infarctions in patients with CHD.

BEHAVIORAL HEALTH IN PRIMARY CARE

In Chapter 6 we discuss the data supporting interventions in primary care for the three most important health behaviors related to CVD, namely tobacco use, obesity, and physical inactivity. The effectiveness of targeting multiple CVD health behaviors simultaneously in primary care settings is unclear. A systematic review and meta-analysis examining multiple health behavior change interventions in primary care for preventing CVD found no significant effects (Alageel et al., 2017). Similarly, although we discuss the effectiveness of emotional management strategies in primary care in Chapter 5, we do not have extensive data that tell us whether these interventions work in patients with CVD in primary care. Therefore, in our primary care clinical practice, we adapt our assessments and interventions on the basis of the available evidence to target the behaviors, thoughts, and emotions we know affect and are affected by CVD.

PRIMARY CARE ADAPTATION

Working in the primary care clinic places BHCs on the front lines of CVD prevention and treatment. Target areas may include achieving a healthy weight (i.e., a body mass index < 25 kg/m²), being physically active, and avoiding tobacco, which we discuss in Chapter 6. The ACC/AHA Task Force also advised that individuals maintain recommended blood pressure levels (Whelton et al., 2018). Even small reductions in blood pressure in the population (e.g., a 5-mmHg reduction of systolic blood pressure) are believed to reduce mortality due to coronary heart disease by 9% and all-cause mortality by 7% (Whelton et al., 2002). Weight loss, healthy diets (e.g., DASH), reduction in dietary sodium, physical activity, and moderation in alcohol content are each associated with a 4- to 11-mmHg reduction in blood pressure in those with hypertension (Whelton et al., 2018). The U.S. Preventive Services Task Force concluded that behavioral counseling interventions are likely to have a "moderate net benefit" (Krist, Davidson, Mangione, Barry, Cabana, Caughey, Donahue, et al., 2020, p. 2,069) on reducing CVD risk in adults.

Common medications used in the treatment of CVD can be found on the AHA website presented in Figure 9.2. BHCs need to be familiar with these medications and their effects to communicate effectively and assess primary care patients with CVD. When assessing adherence to these medical treatments, it is helpful to be familiar with the side effect profiles (e.g., increased urination with diuretics) to help patients adhere to their medical regimens.

In primary care, BHCs are likely to start seeing a patient because they have been diagnosed with some physical condition associated with CVD, such as high blood pressure or diabetes. As BHCs conduct assessments and develop interventions, it is important to be mindful of how these factors affect their physical condition and long-term risk for CVD.

Assess

CVD is complex; therefore, it is important to understand the basic underlying pathology and the factors that may contribute to the presenting problems. Often, BHCs fail to target important risk factors for CVD and miss opportunities

236 Integrated Behavioral Health in Primary Care

to improve a patient's health (Wilfong, 2021). BHCs need to consider ways to identify and target individuals with known risk factors. Assessments of primary care patients at risk for or diagnosed with CVD should include an evaluation of the following:

- their knowledge of their current condition,

- health behaviors potentially impacting their cardiovascular system,

- cognitive and emotional functioning, and

- environmental factors known to influence CVD.

The BHC's assessment should occur only after the individual has been evaluated medically and only when the medical provider is requesting assistance with managing the patient's CVD. It is also important to review the electronic health record for relevant medical and behavioral health history.

Figure 9.4 presents a broad range of questions to consider asking in the assessment. As we have emphasized throughout this volume, BHCs should

FIGURE 9.4. Assessment Questions for Patients With Cardiovascular Disease

The following questions represent a guide for the assessment of those referred for the reduction of risk or management of cardiovascular diseases. Depending on the responses of the patient, you may want to ask questions that are more detailed.

Health Behaviors

- Do you use tobacco? How much? How often do you use it?
- What do you typically do for physical activity? How long do you do that activity? How often?
- What is your current weight? Height? [Determine BMI.]
- Describe what you typically have for breakfast, lunch, dinner, and snacks.
- How often do you eat red meat? How often do you eat out? Where do you usually eat?
- Do you monitor the amount of sodium and fat in the food you eat? How much do you typically eat in a day?
- How much alcohol do you drink each day? Each week?

Emotional Responses

- During the past 2 weeks, have you often been bothered by feeling down, depressed, or hopeless?
- During the past 2 weeks, have you often been bothered by little interest or pleasure in doing things?
- How overwhelmed would you generally rate yourself, if 0 is not overwhelmed and 10 is the most overwhelmed you could imagine?
- Have you had any recent major life changes, such as beginning or ending a relationship, moving, or changes in your financial status?
- Are the demands of your job difficult to manage? Would you describe your job as stressful?
- How do you manage stress? Whom do you lean on for support? Do you easily lose your cool? Do you get frustrated quickly?
- Some people feel afraid, worried, sad, and/or angry about their heart disease and the impact it has on their life. Others don't feel those emotions. How would you describe your reactions to your CVD diagnosis?

Note. BMI = body mass index; CVD = cardiovascular disease.

select the questions most pertinent to the referral problem. For example, if someone is referred for assistance with management of hypertension, it may be more important to focus on sodium content of their food compared with someone referred for assistance with managing their weight, which would require more focus on calorie intake. In addition to evaluating the factors that affect and are affected by CVD, motivation for change is especially important to assess. Someone who has undergone a surgery or had a heart attack may be more motivated to change their behaviors than someone diagnosed with hypertension because those diagnosed with the latter condition often do not feel sick. When motivation to change is low, BHCs may find it worthwhile to spend time on motivation enhancement strategies prior to implementing an intervention.

Physical Factors

The patient's experience with physical symptoms will vary significantly depending on their CVD. Questions associated with physical factors should focus on assessing the patient's experience with physical symptoms, medications and side effects, surgical procedures and interventions, and the patient's understanding of their medical condition.

If the patient has been diagnosed with a physical precursor to CVD, consider asking the following:

- What physical symptoms, if any, have you noticed associated with your condition?

- What medications have you been prescribed? What side effects have you noticed since starting that medication? Has your medication affected how you live your life?

- Have you noticed changes in your sleep?

If the individual has had a surgical procedure or significant cardiac event (e.g., heart attack), consider asking the following:

- What physical symptoms do you notice that affect your daily living?

- Are you experiencing pain? If so, what does your pain keep you from doing?

- Do you get fatigued more easily? Have you participated in a cardiac rehabilitation program?

- How important is it for you to get back to doing the activities you have given up as a result of your symptoms? How confident are you that you can get back to being more active?

- What is your plan for becoming more active?

Behavioral Factors

Health behaviors are some of the most important areas to assess because of their independent and direct impact on the cardiovascular system and the benefits associated with changing these behaviors. We cover some of the relevant health behaviors, including tobacco use, weight, and physical inactivity in Chapter 6; sleep in Chapter 5; and alcohol use in Chapter 11. In addition to these behaviors, we recommend BHCs spend time evaluating whether the patient consumes high-sodium and/or high-fat foods and is taking medications as they are prescribed.

Unlike assessments associated with weight (when the primary focus is on calories) assessing sodium and fat intake is important for those referred for consultation related to CVD. If a highly detailed analysis of their food is necessary, they should be referred to a specialist in nutrition. The intent of the assessment is to identify foods that may be high in sodium or fat that could be decreased in the patient's diet, as well as determine whether the patient is eating adequate amounts of foods high in potassium. Significant sources of sodium include processed foods and condiments. Saturated fats are commonly found in dairy, red meat, butter, and some vegetable oils. High amounts of potassium are found in potatoes, spinach, bananas, and legumes (e.g., soybeans, lentils, kidney beans).

Some examples of questions include the following:

- What foods do you typically eat for breakfast, lunch, and dinner?

- How often do you eat red meat?

- How often do you eat out? Where do you usually eat?

- Do you monitor the amount of salt and fat in the food you eat? How much sodium do you typically eat in a day? Do you add salt to your food? How much?

- How often do you eat processed/luncheon meats (e.g., turkey, ham)? Canned meats, fish, vegetables, or soups? Processed cheese? Frozen dinners or entrees? Mexican food? Foods with soy sauce? Salted snacks like pretzels, chips, crackers, or popcorn?

- Have you been advised to change your diet? How important is it to you to make dietary changes? How confident are you that you can successfully make changes in your diet to improve your health?

In addition to food consumption, it is important to assess how patients are taking their medications. To assess medication adherence, consider asking the following:

- How many medications are you taking? Do you take them as prescribed? How often do you miss taking a medication?

- What side effects concern you? How often do you not take your medication due to concerns about side effects?

- Do you feel overwhelmed by the number of medications that you are taking?

- On a scale of 0 to 10, how important is it to you that you take your medications regularly, with 0 being not important at all and 10 being very important?

Emotional Factors

Patients with CVD will typically be at higher risk for some form of negative mood. Therefore, it is particularly important to screen these patients for depression, anxiety, anger, hostility, and stress. Targeting these emotional responses may improve their quality of life, but there is no consistent evidence that reducing these symptoms will necessarily reduce their risk for CVD. Chapters 4 and 5 provide more detailed descriptions of methods for assessing and targeting these emotions. If the patient experienced a particular cardiac event, such as a myocardial infarction, or if there have been invasive treatments, such as an ICD, BHCs will want to spend some time asking how the patient's functioning has changed since that event. Collaborate with the physician to determine reasonable limitations on functioning. Negative mood may be assessed as follows:

- Since your heart attack, what has changed in your daily functioning?

- Do you feel down more often?

- What activities have you taken out of your life? Are you interested in restarting them?

In addition, pain, particularly chest pain, may be a trigger for increased anxiety symptoms. Assess how thoughts about pain affect functioning, as follows:

- Do you worry when you experience pain? Do you think it is a sign of a heart attack?

- Because of your worry, do you avoid activities that might increase pain?

- How would you tell the difference between cardiac-related pain and other pain?

Patients often hear of links between stress and CVD, but they may be less familiar with how other emotions relate to their cardiovascular problem. Similarly, obesity and sedentary behaviors are commonly cited as causes of heart disease, but individuals may be less familiar with the relations between tobacco use and heart disease. Based on their assessment, BHCs can offer the patient a list of choices of which behaviors or emotions they would be most interested in targeting. An example might sound like the following:

> On the basis of what you've told me, it sounds like you may be experiencing a more negative mood and may be depressed at times. The more depressed you are, the less you feel like doing physical activity and the more you eat as a way to comfort yourself. You find that you get yourself much more stressed at work than you would like, and recently you've started smoking again as a way to manage stress. Is my understanding of your current situation accurate, or have I missed something important?

The patient may be interested in targeting multiple behaviors or just one. Focus on what the patient is interested in changing but be realistic about the impact of the changes that the patient makes. Decreasing depressive symptoms may not significantly lower blood pressure but may improve their daily functioning and their motivation to make other changes in the future.

Advise

Quitting tobacco, increasing physical activity, losing weight, changing eating habits, and improving medication adherence are often the most important lifestyle changes for patients referred for CVD-related concerns. Following the assessment, BHCs can list possible areas that could be targeted. We have developed a handout that could be used with patients with high blood pressure to guide this discussion (see Figure 9.5). One review of randomized controlled trials that examined the impact of counseling, educational interventions, and/or medications targeting multiple cardiovascular risk factors (e.g., blood pressure, smoking, physical activity) found limited or no significant changes in outcome measures for mortality, blood pressure and cholesterol changes, and smoking status (Ebrahim et al., 2011). These data may suggest that it is most beneficial to individually target behaviors or problems rather than trying to change multiple behaviors simultaneously. Review the possible areas that could be addressed while advising the patient about which areas would be most beneficial to target for their present condition. For example, a BHC could say,

> Your weight is high enough that it may be impacting your blood pressure, and you are relatively sedentary. Decreasing your stress response, reducing your weight by 10%, increasing your physical activity, or stopping your smoking may help to reduce your blood pressure, whereas targeting your depressed mood may help you to enjoy more aspects of your life and improve your life satisfaction. Which of these things are you most interested in targeting?

Agree

Once a BHC has advised patients on what they could possibly change, elicit from them what they want to target. Despite the known impact of tobacco cessation and weight loss on the risk and progression of CVD, patients may not be motivated to make the necessary changes at the time of the referral. Determine which behavior changes patients are motivated to make and develop a set of recommendations that reflect the patient's current goals. Provide directions for continuing to assess the patient's interest in making additional changes. For example, a patient diagnosed with hypertension who is overweight and smoking one pack of cigarettes per day may agree to focus on medication adherence and fail to demonstrate interest in changing other health behaviors. The following are examples of recommendations a BHC could make for the patient:

- Buy a pill box that includes separate day and time slots.

- Put a reminder in your calendar to prompt you to take your medicine each day.

- On Sunday evening, place medications in the appropriate time slot for each day.

- Take your medications each day.

- Make a list of the benefits, for you personally, of continuing to use tobacco, and then list the negatives or harms.

- Consider implementing a weight loss plan.

FIGURE 9.5. High Blood Pressure Handout (*continues*)

High Blood Pressure

Blood pressure is defined by two numbers, your systolic blood pressure and your diastolic blood pressure. Your *systolic blood pressure* is the pressure in your arteries when your heart is squeezing blood out to your body. The systolic blood pressure is represented by the top number of your blood pressure. Your *diastolic blood pressure* is the pressure in your arteries when your heart is relaxed; it is represented by the bottom number of your blood pressure reading.

What was your last blood pressure? Systolic = _____ Diastolic = _____

Often, you don't feel sick when you have high blood pressure. Except for the numbers on the blood pressure monitor, there may not be any other indication your blood pressure is high. Below is a table we can use to classify your blood pressure. How would you classify your blood pressure?

Blood pressure classification	SBP mmHg	DBP mmHg
Normal	< 120	and < 80
Elevated	120–129	and < 80
Stage 1 hypertension	130–139	or 80–89
Stage 2 hypertension	≥ 140	or ≥ 90

Making Changes
Many different factors can affect your blood pressure. Some of these factors you may be able to change; other factors you cannot change. By making changes where you can, you can lower your blood pressure. The following is a list of some of the factors that you can change.

How important is it to you to make these changes? If it doesn't apply or if it is not important, rate it a 0. If it is important, what are steps you can take to make changes?

Tobacco Use
Quitting tobacco use is one of the most important health behavior changes you can make. If you are not a tobacco user, great! If you currently use tobacco, have you considered quitting?

How important to you is it to quit tobacco use?

0   1   2   3   4   5   6   7   8   9   10
Not Important   *Most Important*

If tobacco cessation is important to you, what is your plan to quit tobacco?

_____

_____

_____

FIGURE 9.5. High Blood Pressure Handout (*continues*)

Weight Loss

If you are overweight or obese, even small reductions in your weight (e.g., 10 pounds) can have a significant impact on your blood pressure. Weight loss requires a reduction in the number of calories you eat or drink and an increase in your physical activity.

How important is it to you to lose weight?

0   1   2   3   4   5   6   7   8   9   10

Not Important   *Most Important*

If weight loss is important to you, what can you do to start making changes in your eating, drinking, and physical activity habits?

_____

_____

Dietary Changes

Beyond weight loss, it is important to consider changing what you eat to reduce your blood pressure. A special diet called the DASH diet is often encouraged for individuals with high blood pressure. The DASH diet encourages you to decrease the amount of salt and fat in your diet while increasing the amount of potassium and fiber you consume. Often these changes require simple substitutions in your diet, such as replacing salt with other spices and choosing lower fat alternatives to your typical foods.

How important is it for you to change your diet?

0   1   2   3   4   5   6   7   8   9   10

Not Important   *Most Important*

If dietary changes are important to you, what are some of the foods that you are willing to substitute or eliminate from your diet?

_____

_____

Physical Activity

To improve cardiovascular health, it is recommended that you engage in 30 minutes of moderate-intensity activity at least 5 days a week or vigorous-intensity activity for 20 minutes at least 3 days a week.

How important is it for you to meet these activity recommendations?

0   1   2   3   4   5   6   7   8   9   10

Not Important   *Most Important*

If physical activity changes are important to you, how can you incorporate moderate or vigorous activities into your daily life?

_____

_____

Medication Adherence

If your blood pressure is in the hypertensive range, you may have been prescribed a medication to help you lower your blood pressure. However, the effectiveness of the medications depends on individuals taking them as they were prescribed.

FIGURE 9.5. High Blood Pressure Handout (*continued*)

How important is it for you to change the way you take your medications?

0   1   2   3   4   5   6   7   8   9   10

Not Important   *Most Important*

If medication adherence is important to you, what are some of the techniques you can use to manage your medications more effectively?

_____

_____

Stress Management

The stressors that we experience can contribute to higher blood pressure levels. You can manage stressors differently by changing the way you think or what you do and by using relaxation techniques.

How important is it for you to manage your stress response?

0   1   2   3   4   5   6   7   8   9   10

Not Important   *Most Important*

If stress management is important to you, what are some of the techniques you can use to manage stressors more effectively?

_____

_____

Note. SPB = systolic blood pressure; DBP = diastolic blood pressure; DASH = Dietary Approaches to Stop Hypertension.

The following are examples of recommendations for the primary care provider:

- Continue to assess patient's motivation to quit tobacco or change eating habits.

- Consider asking whether patient is ready to change or ask patient to rate importance of change on a scale from 0 (not important) to 10 (very important). For example, the patient may rate the importance of quitting smoking as a 3 and changing diet as a 4. Knowing that dietary changes are of greater importance to the patient can guide the care team in determining where to start making changes by capitalizing on the higher motivation.

Assist

Based on the assessment, the BHC's knowledge of the relative impact of health behaviors and emotional responses on an individual patient's CVD will help guide appropriate behavior change recommendations. The form of CVD may also alter the interventions that would be offered to a patient. Interventions may focus on a single biopsychosocial factor or a combination of several.

Behavioral Factors

To assess whether the patient is moving in the right direction, it is important for the patient and all members of the health care team to set specific goals for any behavior change.

Tobacco use. We discuss methods for targeting tobacco use in Chapter 6. It can be useful to spend some time discussing the impact of tobacco use on cardiovascular risk. It may even be helpful to demonstrate the impact of smoking on blood pressure by comparing blood pressure values immediately after smoking and then after a couple of hours of abstinence. Assuming that the patients are motivated to quit, it is important to develop a plan that includes a quit date, steps patients will take to prepare to prepare for their quit date, medications and/or nicotine replacement, and methods for dealing with cravings and high-risk situations.

Excess weight. Methods for reducing weight are also discussed in Chapter 6. As mentioned earlier, 10 pounds of weight loss can significantly reduce risk for CVD and result in lowered blood pressure, lowered cholesterol, and improved diabetes management. Some individuals may find it overwhelming to monitor calories and make significant dietary changes. For individuals interested in losing weight, BHCs can relate their cardiovascular health to reductions in their weight. As we discuss in Chapter 6, establish a specific plan for how to reduce calories. Consider obtaining pre- and postintervention blood pressure and cholesterol readings to help the patient and medical team see the changes that weight loss can have on objective measures of cardiovascular risk.

Diet. Changing dietary behaviors will require collaboration to identify foods that patients could substitute for their typical dietary choices. Use a handout like the one in Figure 9.6 to help patients consider and identify diet alternatives. It may be necessary to briefly educate the patient about how to read a nutrition label and to discuss the areas on the nutrition label to focus on. The most important changes will likely be reductions in salt and fat. Often patients are not aware of the salt and fat content in the foods they consume and how much they should be eating. As BHCs develop a specific plan with the patient, assess what foods the patient could eliminate or substitute to make the necessary changes. For example, patients may not realize how much salt can be contained in canned soups. Discussing alternatives (e.g., low-sodium soups) or decreasing the amount of canned soup they consume could represent a significant change in their sodium intake.

Physical activity. Physical activity changes are discussed in Chapter 6. Specific goals to increase activity or start exercise programs will increase the likelihood that patients will follow through with the plan. Particularly with exercise plans, it is important to collaborate with the patient's medical provider to make decisions about the intensity and duration of their exercise program. Discuss with

FIGURE 9.6. Diet Change Handout

Diet Change

To help reduce blood pressure, it is recommended that individuals reduce their sodium content to 2,300 mg or to 1,500 mg if they have high blood pressure, diabetes, or chronic kidney disease; are African American; or are at least 51 years old. To reduce cardiovascular disease risk, it is recommended to avoid foods high in fat. Below are foods high in sodium and fat that individuals should consider avoiding or replacing with low-sodium or low-fat alternatives.

Reducing Salt Content

Top 10 foods typically consumed by Americans that are high in salt (sodium)

- Breads and rolls
- Cold cuts and cured meats (deli and packaged meats)
- Pizza
- Poultry (fresh and processed)
- Soups
- Sandwiches (hot dogs, hamburgers)
- Cheese (natural and processed)
- Mixed pasta dishes (lasagna, spaghetti)
- Mixed meat dishes (meat loaf, chili, beef stew)
- Snacks (chips, pretzels, popcorn)

Reducing Fat Content

Food category	Foods high in fat	Lower fat alternatives
Dairy	• whole milk • ice cream • cheese	• skim, 1%, 2% milk • sorbet, sherbet, frozen yogurt • low- or reduced-fat cheese
Pasta	• ramen noodles • pasta with cream sauce • granola	• rice • pasta with tomato sauce • reduced-fat granola
Meat, fish, poultry	• ground beef • chicken or turkey with skin • hot dogs • bacon, sausage • oil-packed tuna • whole eggs	• low-fat, extra-lean meats • skinless chicken or turkey • low-fat hot dogs • turkey bacon • water-packed tuna • egg whites, egg substitutes
Baked goods	• croissants • donuts • muffins • party crackers • cake, cookies	• hard rolls, English muffins • bagels • reduced-fat muffins • low-fat crackers • angel food cake
Snacks and sweets	• nuts • ice cream	• popcorn, fruits, vegetables • frozen yogurt, pudding bars
Fats, oils, and salad dressings	• butter, margarine • mayonnaise • salad dressings • oils, shortening, lard	• light margarine • light mayonnaise, mustard • fat-free salad dressing • nonstick cooking spray

What are the changes that you plan to make in your diet?
Reduce salt by: _____
Reduce saturated fat by: _____

Note. Reducing salt content data from U.S. Food and Drug Administration, 2022. Reducing fat content data from U.S. Department of Health and Human Services, 2000.

the patient ways that they can increase their physical activity. For reducing the risks associated with CVD, individuals are recommended to engage in at least 30 minutes of moderate-intensity activity most, if not all, days of the week. Help the patient define moderate-intensity activities (e.g., brisk walking). We find that simply prescribing a change is less effective than working collaboratively with the patient to figure out what physical activity changes will fit into their life (e.g., walking during work, taking the stairs, playing with children).

Alcohol. We address ways to target excess alcohol use in Chapter 11. If patients are medically cleared to consume alcohol and there is no concern or risk for alcohol misuse (e.g., substance misuse history), then individuals should not be discouraged from drinking one (for women) to two (for men) standard alcohol-containing drinks per day.

Medication adherence. To improve medication adherence, identify the barriers that interfere with taking medications as prescribed. Sometimes the regimen of medications is overly complex, and discussing a simpler regimen with the patient's medical provider may improve adherence. Simple tools, such as a medication box/organizer with days and times during the week for each medication, can be used to organize pills according to the time of day that they should be taken. Consider using some external cue to remind patients to take their medications. Multiple consumer products, including mobile device applications and alarms, clocks, and computer software, can be used to provide external prompts. Consider ways of enlisting the support of other individuals (e.g., spouse/significant other) to help improve adherence. Discuss situations that could lead to slips in their medication regimen (e.g., traveling) and how the patient could plan to reduce the chances of nonadherence to the medication. If the patient is not motivated to take the medications (e.g., concerned about side effects), then consider methods of improving motivation, such as those presented in Chapter 4.

Emotional Factors

Patients diagnosed with a CVD often report some emotional distress. Identifying and targeting this distress can improve the patient's functioning.

Stress and emotional reactivity. If the individual struggles with stress management, consider teaching brief relaxation strategies (e.g., deep breathing, progressive muscle relaxation, guided imagery) and methods to change stressful thinking as described in Chapter 4. It may be useful to measure blood pressure before and after the relaxation exercise to demonstrate the effect of relaxation. If patients are taking medications that lower blood pressure, relaxation exercises may result in some difficulty, with blood pressures becoming so low that patients experience difficulty moving from a seated to standing position. Therefore, carefully monitor such individuals as they make such changes and ask about lightheadedness. Interestingly, we have often found that individuals with

CVD do not perceive themselves as being stressed. Therefore, consider using other terms for stress, such as distress, frustration, or overwhelm.

Depression. Interventions for depression and anxiety are usually not different for this population, so BHCs should find the strategies in Chapter 5 helpful with these patients. It is often useful to relate the changes to their cardiovascular functioning when appropriate. However, it would *not* be appropriate to state, "By decreasing your depressive symptoms we will reduce your risk for having a heart attack." Instead place the focus on improving their functioning, such as "By decreasing your depressive symptoms, we can help you live your life more the way that you want to."

Incorporate behavioral activation with other potentially beneficial activities, such as increasing social support and physical activity. Patients may have depressive thoughts focused on how their CVD has changed their life or their outlook on life. Again, helping patients to focus on current functioning and methods of improving that functioning using methods from cognitive behavioral therapy or acceptance and commitment therapy may help to decrease negative thinking related to their disease.

Anxiety. Although the physical aspects of anxiety may not be different among CVD patients, the content of alarming or distressing thoughts may be unique. Individuals may have had life-threatening situations (e.g., heart attacks) and therefore may have a fear of death associated with pain, which can be difficult to distinguish from benign pain. BHCs should encourage the PCP to discuss with the patient the specific symptoms that they should be concerned about when distinguishing cardiac-related chest pain (e.g., pressure, tightness, squeezing, which may be associated with shortness of breath, nausea or vomiting, and dizziness) from other pain (e.g., sharp, knifelike, associated with coughing, lasting a short period of time; Harvard Health Publishing, 2020). Teaching relaxation strategies, targeting negative thinking by developing alternative reassuring thoughts, using acceptance-based techniques, and increasing physical activity as discussed in Chapters 4, 5, and 6 may help to reduce anxiety symptoms in those with CVD (Farquhar et al., 2018).

Posttraumatic stress disorder. Although there is increasing evidence on the relations between PTSD and CVD, no studies have examined specific interventions for PTSD in this population. It is important to screen for PTSD in those with CVD, as these symptoms may contribute to and complicate other interventions (Krantz et al., 2022; Meinhausen et al., 2022); however, the best evidence for targeting PTSD in primary care settings is reviewed in Chapter 5.

Environmental Factors

Social support is an important factor to consider in assisting patients with CVD. To improve social support, examine how people found support in the past. Consider encouraging patients to spend more time with family, plan outings with friends, join a social club or group that has a shared interest (e.g., running groups), become more active with a religious organization, or join a volunteer organization. Physical activity is such an important aspect for good health that it is suggested to combine physical activity and social support interventions. Often patients may demonstrate reluctance to engage in an activity that is designed to facilitate enjoyment, but relating the activity back to their functioning and to helping them live a more enjoyable life may improve the likelihood that they will participate in the activity.

Arrange

The frequency of follow-up appointments will depend on the behaviors that are targeted, just as with other patient populations discussed throughout this volume. BHCs will find most patients require a small number of appointments (i.e., one to two) to begin making behavior changes in their lives. Others may benefit from periodic consultation (e.g., bimonthly or quarterly) to help them maintain behavior change. It is important to be aware of specialty groups or clinics that may be a resource for helping those patients who have a more difficult time initiating behavior changes. Nutritionists, exercise physiologists, cardiac rehabilitation services, diabetes care clinics, and clinical health psychology specialty clinics can provide necessary support to the medical team for helping to manage patients with CVD.

SUMMARY

Primary care environments offer unique opportunities to work with patients across the spectrum of CVD. BHCs can have a tremendous impact on cardiovascular risk factors, particularly health behaviors. BHCs could fill their entire schedule simply by targeting patients who have elevated blood pressures, have blood pressures in the hypertensive range, or are at higher risk of CVD. Working with these patients usually does not require specialized skills because the behavior changes and emotional responses are similar to many other patient populations. However, taking the time to develop a more in-depth knowledge of the cardiovascular system and how behavior, thoughts, and emotions affect and are affected by changes in the cardiovascular system will likely contribute to more effective assessments and interventions for these populations.

10

Pain Disorders

In the United States, 20.9% of adults suffer from chronic pain, and 6.9% experience chronic pain that limits life or work activities (Rikard et al., 2023). Chronic pain impacts all age groups but is highest for those over age 65, with 30.8% of that age group reporting chronic pain and 11.8% reporting high-impact chronic pain in the previous 3 months. Both chronic pain and high-impact chronic pain are slightly more prevalent in women than men. Prevalence of chronic pain also varies by race and ethnic origin, with non-Hispanic White adults (23.6%) being more likely to report chronic pain than individuals identifying as non-Hispanic Black (19.3%), Hispanic (13%), and non-Hispanic Asian (6.8%). Adults who live in rural settings also report more chronic pain than those in urban settings, with 28.1% of rural residents reporting chronic pain compared with 16.1% of urban residents.

Most people first report pain to a health care provider in the primary care setting (Dobkin & Boothroyd, 2008), putting it at the forefront of pain treatment delivery. In the United States, approximately 52% of chronic pain treatment is delivered by primary care practitioners (Mills et al., 2016).

Assessment and treatment of pain have changed over the past decades. In the traditional medical model, pain was viewed as a purely physiological phenomenon. The objective in pain assessment was to identify its biological cause. Treatment could then be accomplished by eliminating or blocking that cause. From this perspective, when a physical cause could not be identified, the pain was assumed to be psychologically generated; this was known as *psychogenic*

https://doi.org/10.1037/0000380-011
Integrated Behavioral Health in Primary Care: Step-by-Step Guidance for Assessment and Intervention, Third Edition, by C. L. Hunter, J. L. Goodie, M. S. Oordt, and A. C. Dobmeyer

pain. This model is no longer widely accepted. Newer understandings of pain and pain management have recognized the role that various other factors, beyond physiology, play in pain.

The gate control theory of pain, first proposed by Melzack and Wall in 1965, and later the biopsychosocial model developed by Engel in 1977, provided essential frameworks for better understanding the role of nonphysiological factors in the experience of pain. Melzack's (1999) neuromatrix theory of pain advanced these early theories based on growing knowledge about the brain. His work proposed a network of neurons consisting of loops between various brain components labeled the neuromatrix. Repeated nerve impulses through the neuromatrix can develop a characteristic pattern for pain through which the brain generates pain sensations. This occurs when the brain perceives body tissue is in danger and action must be taken to avoid it (Moseley, 2003), even without a triggering stimulus from an injury or disease process. In this model, sensory input plays only a part in the experience of pain; it is not solely a triggering stimulus that causes the pain to occur. Therefore, clinical intervention can focus on modulating or reducing factors that tell the brain that body tissue is in danger, with the goal of preventing the pain neuromatrix from activating its pain output. Each of these models seeks to explain the multifaceted and complex experience of pain and help those experiencing pain find ways of improving their quality of life.

With these more comprehensive understandings, the role of behavioral health professionals in the assessment and treatment of pain conditions has expanded. In the old model, psychiatrists' and psychologists' role was to address conditions where the problem was judged to be imaginary or psychogenic. Now behavioral health providers collaborate with physicians to address multiple contributing and restorative factors; these include affect, beliefs and expectations, coping resources, sleep quality, physical function, and pain-related interference with daily activities (Turk et al., 2016).

Misuse of pain medications, which may involve psychological and physical addiction, is also a significant concern for patients with chronic pain. Individuals can develop tolerance to opioid pain medications, which results in a need for increasing doses for the desired analgesic effect (Volkow & McLellan, 2016). Problems can also occur when individuals with past or current unhealthy substance use problems are prescribed medication for chronic pain. Chapter 11 addresses this issue in more detail and provides guidance on the assessment and intervention for unhealthy opioid use and nonpharmacological strategies to assist patients with pain management while tapering opioids.

The fifth edition of the *Diagnostic and Statistical Manual of Mental Disorders, Text Revision* (*DSM-5-TR*; American Psychiatric Association, 2022) provides a classification system regarding the interaction of psychological factors in pain conditions. Pain-related diagnoses fall in the category of "somatic symptom and related disorders." *Somatic symptom disorder* is a diagnosis used to describe when patients experience persistent distressing somatic symptoms that result in significant disruption of functioning and abnormal thoughts, feelings, and behaviors regarding their symptoms. "Psychological factors affecting other medical conditions" (American Psychiatric Association, 2022) is another diagnosis that may apply to patients with pain. The key criterion for this diagnosis is one or more clinically significant psychological or behavioral factors that adversely affects a medical condition by increasing the risk for suffering, death, or disability.

Another useful classification differentiates between acute pain, recurrent pain, and chronic pain. Specific definitions vary in the literature; however, they are distinguished by the duration over which the pain occurs. *Acute pain* generally occurs with an injury or illness and resolves with healing or resolution of the illness. *Recurrent pain* is episodic, such as with migraines. *Chronic pain* is persistent pain, lasting at least 3 to 6 months.

CULTURAL AND DIVERSITY CONSIDERATIONS

As noted, recent data from the Centers for Disease Control and Prevention (Rikard et al., 2023) showed disparities exist in the pain prevalence and seriousness of pain across population groups. A comprehensive review of the literature by the Institute of Medicine (IOM; 2011) also showed differences in rates of undertreatment across groups. Vulnerable populations, such as older adults, children, and ethnic and racial minority groups, are more often inadequately treated for pain than other population groups. Although pain treatment is highly guideline driven in primary care, research indicates that socioeconomic status can be a factor in the care patients receive. Gebauer et al. (2017) found that patients from lower socioeconomic neighborhoods were 63% more likely than higher socioeconomic patients to receive only opioid treatment for chronic pain in primary care versus a combination of opioid and nonpharmacological approaches. These groups can be discouraged from seeking appropriate care for pain by poor access to health care services and lack of trust in medical providers, low expectations for treatment outcomes, and language/communication barriers. Differences in pain and pain perception are related to gender, education, and economic status across a broad range of health conditions (IOM, 2011). Screening for social needs can help the primary care provider (PCP) and the behavioral health consultant (BHC) understand social determinants that may be relevant for each patient and help mitigate these disparities when delivering care for pain disorders. The Accountable Health Communities Health-Related Social Needs Screening Tool, developed by the Centers for Medicare and Medicaid Innovation (2019), is one of many available screening tools.

SPECIALTY MENTAL HEALTH

Behavioral and cognitive behavioral interventions are essential to the successful treatment of chronic pain and are typically integrated into multidisciplinary chronic pain treatment programs (Gatchel et al., 2014). Standalone cognitive behavioral treatments also result in significant changes in pain experience, cognitive coping and appraisal, and reduced behavioral expression of pain. A review of research studies on cognitive behavioral interventions by Ehde et al. (2014) illustrated the success of these treatments. Hughes et al. (2017) found evidence for effectively using acceptance and commitment therapy for chronic pain. Broderick et al. (2016) additionally found that patients benefited from cognitive behavioral treatment regardless of gender, race, ethnicity, and body mass index. Patients with greater disease severity benefited more than those with lower disease severity. They also found that patients who are interpersonally distressed in their pain benefit relatively little from cognitive behavioral interventions and suggested that interventions more directly focused on interpersonal skills (e.g., assertiveness training, interpersonal problem solving) may be necessary.

BEHAVIORAL HEALTH IN PRIMARY CARE

The literature on behavioral and psychological treatments for chronic pain in primary care has grown substantially (e.g., Beehler et al., 2019; Goodie et al., 2020; Hooker et al., 2020; Hughes et al., 2017). Primary care is often the first place patients with pain go for care. Unfortunately, however, primary care is structured in ways that seldom allow health care providers time to perform comprehensive assessments of pain complaints (IOM, 2011). Nevertheless, it is becoming more widely recognized that within primary care clinics, commonly seen problems such as pain are optimally managed through interdisciplinary collaborations that include behavioral health specialists (Bholat et al., 2012). BHCs can help significantly in bridging this gap.

Guidelines for chronic pain treatment have been developed (Bair et al., 2005; Chou et al., 2009; North American Spine Society, 2020; Pangarkar et al., 2019), and although they are often pharmacologically focused, these guidelines increasingly include nonpharmacological forms of care. For example, the U.S. Department of Defense (DoD) has implemented a care pathway for patients with chronic pain that includes nonpharmacological treatments, including brief cognitive behavioral therapy for chronic pain (BCBT-CP), which is available from BHCs in primary care clinics (Beehler et al., 2018). BCBT-CP has seven modules covering key pain management components, such as education regarding chronic pain, relaxation training, time-based activity pacing, increasing of pleasant activities, cognitive coping strategies, and relapse prevention methods. Consistent with the primary care behavioral health model, the BCBT-CP recommends a minimum of three visits with the BHC to implement the treatment plan and monitor progress, although many patients may benefit from the full intervention, which is seven visits. Depending on the patient's needs, follow-up appointments are typically scheduled at

2-week intervals. The Defense and Veterans Pain Rating Scale (Polomano et al., 2016) is administered at each visit to monitor progress. Patients requiring greater intensity are referred for specialty chronic pain and/or mental health care.

The DoD's stepped care model for treating chronic pain is one approach to standardizing care of patients with chronic pain in primary care to overcome some of the barriers that exist in the primary care structure. The pathway capitalizes on a collaborative team-based approach to permit a psychosocial assessment of pain. PCPs are trained to assess biopsychosocial components to assist in the collaboration of clinical team members. This approach also incorporates a broad range of interventions likely to be beneficial to chronic pain patients while maintaining the constructs of primary health care.

At the time of this writing, the BCBT-CP is being evaluated through a randomized pragmatic clinical trial (Goodie et al., 2020). Preliminary data revealed a dose-dependent response to BCBT-CP, as indicated by improved scores on the Defense and Veterans Pain Rating Scale, with patients who attended more modules reporting better outcomes at the 3-month assessment. It is still unknown whether these benefits will be sustained in the long term. Beehler et al. (2019) evaluated a similar modular brief cognitive behavioral treatment in Veterans Health Administration primary care clinics using integrated behavioral health providers to deliver care. Their analysis found significant improvement on a composite measure of pain intensity and function by the third session. Modules focusing on psychoeducation and goal setting, pacing, and relaxation training were associated with the most significant improvements. Other studies have evaluated primary-care-based treatment for pain disorders and found them to be effective in reducing dysfunction and improving quality of life (Ahles et al., 2006; Brensilver et al., 2012; Dobscha et al., 2009; Kanzler et al., 2022; S. E. Lamb et al., 2010; Sveinsdottir et al., 2012; van Hooff et al., 2012; Vitiello et al., 2013).

PRIMARY CARE ADAPTATION

The following section reviews how to adapt behavioral and psychological assessment and intervention for pain complaints in the primary care setting. Handouts and scripts are provided to facilitate interventions and suggest ways of discussing pain-related topic areas with patients. It must be noted here that behavioral health interventions for pain should be done only in collaboration with a medical workup. Because pain can be a symptom of serious illness or injury requiring medical intervention, a thorough evaluation by a physician should be obtained before proceeding with assessments and interventions from a behavioral health perspective. A thorough review of the electronic health record will provide the biological/physiological findings and diagnosis needed to build on in the biopsychosocial assessment.

Assess

A functional assessment by the BHC is appropriate for all patients referred by a PCP who might benefit from primary care cognitive and behavioral pain interventions. The assessment can help identify factors that contribute to initiation, exacerbation, or maintenance of pain, as well as identify factors that lead to excessive suffering from pain. Key areas for assessment include pain variability, what increases or decreases pain, the effect of pain on activities, how an individual copes in response to pain, and how social interactions and environments affect the individual. The following areas are recommended to address when conducting an assessment:

- variability in pain intensity and factors that contribute to increases or decreases in intensity, such as thoughts, emotions, behaviors, environments, or social interactions;
- functional impact of pain on daily activities;
- adaptive coping in response to pain, including emotional distress, cognitions, and behaviors; and
- the effects of social and environmental contingencies.

The following questions are recommended for primary care assessment of chronic pain:

- general description of the pain: "Where is the pain located, and what is its quality (e.g., aching, shooting, stabbing, binding, pinching, squeezing, throbbing)?";
- onset of pain: "When did the pain start? What was going on when the pain started?";
- frequency of the pain: "How many times per day, week, or month does it occur?"; and
- duration of the pain: "How long does the pain last when it occurs?"

Several methods can be used to determine the intensity of the pain; however, the most common is a numerical rating of 0 to 10 with 0 representing no pain and 10 representing excruciating pain. Obtain ratings for the pain at its worst, least, and most common, as follows:

- On a scale of 0 to 10, 0 being no pain and 10 being excruciating pain, what is your pain level right now? Where is it on that scale at its worst? When is it at its best?
- What can you do to decrease the pain?
- What makes the pain worse? What makes it better?
- Why do you think you are experiencing pain?

- What has your PCP told you about the cause of the pain? [Although your review of the electronic health record will provide this information, asking will help ascertain the patient's understanding of the causes.]

- Describe a typical day, including home, work, and leisure time activities.

- How does the pain limit you? What would you be doing differently if you didn't have pain? Have you lost any functioning due to your pain?

- Are there activities or settings you avoid because of fear that the pain might increase? How often? How important are these activities to you?

- How has the pain affected you emotionally? [Assess depression, anxiety, and anger.]

- How have others responded to the pain? Family? Friends? Coworkers?

- How would you like others to respond?

- What have you done to help deal with the pain? [Include medical treatments, procedures, and self-management strategies. Assess for unhelpful medication use, alcohol or illicit substance use (see Chapter 11), and excessive sleep or inactivity.]

- In what other ways has the pain affected your life? [Listen for extreme or catastrophizing language.]

Advise

Popular understandings of pain in which pain is viewed exclusively as either a physical problem or a psychological problem continue to be prevalent. Therefore, a primary goal of the advise phase is to help patients understand the interaction of biopsychosocial domains in their pain problem and to increase motivation to address components such as emotions, thoughts, behaviors, and interpersonal issues as part of their approach to manage pain more effectively.

Providing the patient with a framework for understanding the role of psychological factors in pain may be helpful. The following script is one way of describing this framework:

> Pain is a complex problem; medical science is finding this to be truer all the time. Our old understanding of pain such as yours was that pain was a direct reflection of an injury or disease and that the only way to address pain was to identify the physiological cause and remove it or block it. The problem with that model is that it didn't account for pain very well. In other words, sometimes there is a great deal of physical abnormality with little pain, and at other times, there can be minimal or no physical disease but significant pain.
>
> Let me give you a couple of examples of how physical injury and the experience of pain don't always correspond well. One is the phenomenon of pain blocking. Take as an example a soldier who might fight bravely and assist his injured buddy to get to a helicopter for medical evacuation in the midst of a battle. The soldier realizes that he too has been injured only after his buddy is

safe. Because of situational demands, mental distraction, and the flow of adrenaline, he didn't recognize his own injury or feel the pain. In this situation, these other factors played more of a role in pain and perception of pain than did the actual physical injury.

Another example is a phenomenon called phantom pain, which sometimes occurs when people have a limb amputated. These individuals sometimes feel pain in the location of the amputated limb even though that limb is no longer there. If pain were purely a physiological issue, phantom pain could not occur. These are just a couple of examples that show the role of psychological factors in pain perception. Let me be clear, this does not mean people make up their pain or that it is not real. Pain is real, as you know. Understanding and targeting these other factors, however, gives people more control over their pain.

One way scientists have conceptualized how these nonphysical factors contribute to pain is that the brain develops a characteristic pattern or signature for pain over time. This pattern of neurological firing in the brain can generate pain sensations when your brain registers that body tissue is in danger and can occur even without any physical stimulus from your body. This pain signature connects various parts of the brain, including the limbic system, which controls emotions. Negative emotion is one factor that can trigger the brain to increase pain sensations. People feel more pain when they are depressed, angry, or anxious. Reducing the intensity of these emotions is one way to limit the activation of the pain signature and thus reduce pain. This is important because chronic pain and its effect on one's life can contribute to feelings of depression, helplessness, anxiety, and frustration.

Negative thinking is also a factor that can trigger pain activation. People tend to hurt more when they are focused on the pain than they do when they are distracted from it. Parents use this with children; if a child is distressed over falling and skinning a knee, they will kiss it to make it better and send the child off to play. The kiss did not heal the injury but changed the child's mental focus, reducing the pain. Because the sensation of pain automatically draws one's mental focus, it can require real skill to distract oneself successfully.

There are also behavioral and physical factors that affect activation of the pain signals. For example, if a person is inactive because it hurts to walk or exercise, their muscles will become weak, which in turn adds to the pain. Lack of involvement in enjoyable activities contributes to depression and frustration, boredom, and more focus on the pain, which in turn increases pain signals.

Another helpful concept is the distinction between pain and suffering. Pain is the sensation caused by neurological signals from the site of an injury or disease to the brain; suffering is the sum total of the emotional, mental, behavioral, social, occupational, and lifestyle effects of the pain. As a behavioral health provider, I am limited in what I can do to help you with injury in your body; that's the role of your primary care provider. I can work with you and your primary care provider on some of those other components that play a role in how much you suffer from the pain. In other words, I can help you learn to take more control of your life so you are living more as you would like to rather than letting the pain have so much control in your life. That may or may not result in less pain; however, many patients report better quality of life after this kind of treatment. Is that something you would be interested in working on together?

Now discuss the skills and changes that the BHC can use to help the patient learn and describe how those changes would directly affect symptoms, functioning, and suffering. Figure 10.1 provides a handout that summarizes the

FIGURE 10.1. Understanding Chronic Pain Handout

Chronic pain is best understood as an interaction of numerous factors. Many aspects of these factors can be addressed to help manage chronic pain conditions.

Factor	What you can do to improve pain management
Physical	Keep muscles toned through physical activity. Take prescribed pain medication. Use relaxation techniques to relax muscles and manage the stress response.
Emotional	Use relaxation to manage anxiety. Stay involved with relationships and enjoyable activities to protect against depression and other negative moods.
Cognitive	Recognize unhealthy thinking patterns that interfere with adaptive coping with pain (e.g., catastrophizing). Challenge unhelpful thinking; replace it with more helpful thoughts. Focus thoughts on what you can control.
Behavior	Stay physically active. Pace your activities; avoid a cycle of overactivity and underactivity. Adhere to medical recommendations (including medications and physical therapy).
Social	Discuss what you find helpful and not helpful with family and others who are close to you. Stay socially connected and involved.

factors contributing to pain and what can be done to address them. The discussion might transpire as follows:

> One thing that seems to increase your pain is your stress level. One way to help you manage that would be to help you learn how to turn on your body's natural relaxation response by learning how to use slow, relaxed breathing. Another thing we might do is to help you learn how to question your thoughts. You said that sometimes you have a variety of unhelpful thoughts that run through your mind and, in reaction to those, you choose not to do things you enjoy, you withdraw from others, and you notice your pain more. By not reacting to those thoughts and instead stepping back and questioning them, you can choose how you want to respond to the situation. This can make it easier to choose to do the things you enjoy and not make your pain intensity increase.

Agree

Behavioral health approaches to pain management are based on a self-management model of care. Improvements in pain management will not be the result of a procedure done by the provider on the patients but will come through changes patients make themselves. This requires a shift in thinking for many pain patients who want to be cured. The agree phase is critical so that both the patient and provider have a common framework for moving forward.

Agreement should be reached in several areas before moving on to treatment. The first area is whether the patient desires a behavioral approach to treatment. If the patient's only agenda is to obtain pain medications, more exploration, education, and motivational approaches may be necessary before moving on. If agreement on this cannot be reached, the BHC may conclude that the patient is not a good candidate for a behavioral pain management approach. A second area for agreement is the goals of treatment. Ensure the patient understands that the likely outcome of many pain management approaches is enhanced function, decreased distress, and improved quality of life rather than a cure for their pain disorder. It is important to clarify that this may not include freedom from pain. Further discussion of goal setting can be found in Chapter 4 of this volume. In the third area, the provider and the patient should agree on the practical aspects of care. This may include homework assignments, frequency of visits, commitment to self-monitoring, and involvement of family members.

Assist

Numerous clinical practice guidelines exist for addressing pain in primary care (Ernstzen et al., 2017; Oliveira et al., 2018); however, most focus on pharmacological intervention and do not address nonpharmacological aspects of care (Ernstzen et al., 2017). Newer guidelines increasingly incorporate nonpharmacological approaches, such as relaxation training, biofeedback, and mindfulness-based stress reduction. For example, the American Academy of Family Physicians' clinical practice guideline for low back pain (Qaseem et al., 2017) recommended a stepped care approach, starting with nonpharmacological interventions. Along with superficial heat and nonsteroidal anti-inflammatory drugs (if desired), family practitioners are advised to begin by recommending exercise, relaxation training, biofeedback, mindfulness-based stress reduction, and cognitive behavioral therapy. BHCs can play an essential role in delivering the initial interventions for patients with pain in primary care.

If lower levels of intervention are not adequate, the PCP may advance care to the next level, including the use of synthetic opioids, antidepressant medication, or opioids. Multidisciplinary chronic pain rehabilitation is also an option when lower levels of care have failed. This type of rehabilitation program may be appropriate for patients who do not respond to less intense interventions and those at risk of significant and permanent disability. Specialists in these programs can address complicating factors such as psychiatric comorbidity, family dynamics, and unhealthy substance use that could, depending on unique patient circumstances, be beyond what can be effectively addressed in primary care.

The following approaches are suggested for working with pain issues during an office visit.

Challenging Unhealthy Beliefs About Pain

During an assessment, patients will often reveal attitudes and beliefs about pain that are unrealistic, are unhealthy, and may contribute to disability and distress. The term "pain catastrophizing" has been used to describe the cognitive–emotional response to actual and anticipated pain that significantly impacts pain experience and outcomes (Quartana et al., 2009). Bringing these beliefs to patients' attention and helping them, through education and information, to develop more accurate and realistic beliefs and thoughts can be beneficial. Figure 10.2 is a patient education handout the BHC can use to help patients question faulty beliefs related to pain.

Pacing Activities

Individuals with chronic pain often fall into an unhealthy cycle of overactivity and underactivity. They get frustrated because their activities are limited by pain; therefore, when pain decreases sufficiently, they engage in physical

FIGURE 10.2. True or False: Common Pain Beliefs

True or False: Common Pain Beliefs

- "Pain must be a sign of serious physiological disease or injury."

  FALSE: *Pain is a neurological event that is not highly related to severity of harm.*

- "The best intervention for pain is rest and inactivity."

  FALSE: *For acute injuries, a short period of rest to allow healing to occur is helpful. When pain lasts beyond a normal healing period, it is best to be active to build strength and maintain full use of your body.*

- "Other people must understand how much I hurt."

  FALSE: *Making a point to ensure everyone around you knows how much you hurt and expecting them to really understand is likely to keep you focused on your pain and may lead you to feel disappointed, angry, resentful, and unsupported. It may be better to let a few key individuals know, those who can support you in coping adaptively with your condition, and let the others in your life continue to be unaware.*

- "Having chronic pain means I am broken and a flawed human being."

  FALSE: *Thinking about yourself in unrealistic, negative terms will likely make coping more difficult. It is best to find ways to live life with meaning, grace, and dignity and to find ways to adapt to the pain.*

- "Pain is ruining my life and will ruin my future."

  FALSE: *Pain is a difficulty you have in your life; however, whether it ruins your life or your future is up to you.*

- "I can't be happy as long as I have pain."

  FALSE: *Pain can certainly impact your mood, but it doesn't control it. Happiness is a choice and mindset. You can choose to engage in meaningful activities while adapting to the pain.*

- "If my doctor is recommending nonmedical intervention for my chronic pain, it must mean she does not believe me or thinks I'm exaggerating my pain."

  FALSE: *The state-of-the-art treatment for chronic pain is to use a multidisciplinary approach that combines the expertise of many medical specialties to address multiple factors contributing to pain, such as emotions, thoughts, behaviors, social interactions, learning, and environment. This gives you the best chance of improvement.*

- "The only worthwhile goal is to be pain free."

  FALSE: *Although it is desirable to eliminate the pain, this may be an unrealistic goal. There are other worthwhile goals for improving your quality of life without eliminating the pain.*

behaviors as if they did not have a pain problem. This overuse, in turn, makes the pain worse again, resulting in another period of prolonged inactivity. This cycle increases pain severity and significantly interferes with maximal functioning. The following script presents one way of discussing this with patients and offers a strategy for better pacing of activities:

> People without chronic pain have an alarm system to tell them when something is wrong. If they feel pain, it can be taken as a signal to stop doing whatever they are doing to avoid harming themselves, such as walking on a sprained ankle. However, when you have chronic pain, this alarm system no longer works well. Because you have pain frequently or constantly, it no longer reliably serves to help you tell the difference between harm and hurt. If you stop doing everything when you feel pain, you will end up doing nothing. The fact that the pain is no longer a symptom of harm means that stopping activity is not necessary or helpful.
>
> Because the "pain equals harm" message is well-engrained in most of us, people with chronic pain often needlessly continue to use pain as a signal in this manner. As a result, they remain inactive, sitting or lying for extended periods. Because pain tends to fluctuate in a natural cycle, the pain will typically decrease. Being tired, bored, and frustrated with not having been doing anything, people often will become active, trying to make up for lost time and engaging in activities they could not do while they were experiencing higher levels of pain. As a result, these individuals frequently will be overly active, which increases their pain. This cycle of underactivity and overactivity continues as a pattern.
>
> Learning to pace your activities can break this pattern. Pacing involves doing a reasonable level of physical activity for a period of time you have determined to be appropriate, followed by a period of rest or sedentary activity that is long enough to allow you to be active again shortly. By deliberately pacing yourself, you can become more functional while avoiding the consequences of being overly active or inactive.
>
> One pacing strategy I encourage you to use is called time-based pacing. Start by estimating how long you can safely do one of your regular activities, such as housework or yardwork, without causing a severe pain flare. Subtract 1 minute from that time and set that as your "active" goal time for the activity. Next make a best guess on the amount of resting time you will need in order to safely resume activity or continue your day. Those times will now become your schedule for pacing yourself, rather than working until pain becomes too intolerable to continue. It is okay to adjust your schedule after pacing begins. The goal, however, is to stick to your time-based pacing goals whether you are having a good or a bad pain day to avoid the crash–burn/overactivity cycle or the avoidance/inactivity cycle. Moderation is the key!
>
> Spread out activities during the week and be reasonable with the schedule so you can succeed. This handout (see Figure 10.3) has a chart for you to record how you pace activities this week.

Relaxing for Pain Control

Muscle tension can contribute to pain in several ways. First, muscle tension is a direct contributor to some pain conditions. Examples include tension headaches and some forms of temporomandibular disorder. Second, people with chronic pain sometimes develop habits of muscle overuse in response to pain, which includes bracing behaviors in anticipation of pain or for protection of injured areas. These habits also may include overuse of certain muscles to

FIGURE 10.3. Pacing Activities Handout

Pacing Activities

People who live with chronic pain may try to push through pain to complete rigorous activities, especially when they are experiencing lower levels of pain, only to wake up with increased pain levels the next day. They will then avoid activity and spend a significant amount of time resting to recover. This *overactivity/underactivity cycle* may happen on a recurring basis and can lead to negative consequences, such as increased stress and anxiety, decreased efficiency, lowered self-esteem, and avoidance of any activity.

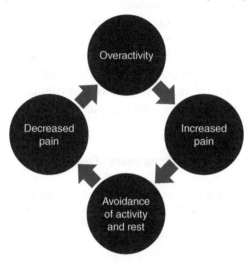

Engaging in a moderate, safe level of activity on a regular basis is key to avoiding this cycle. Using the skill of pacing, where time is the guide for activity engagement, can be a helpful strategy.

How to Pace

Estimate how long you can safely do one of your regular activities (e.g., yardwork, dishes) without causing a severe pain flare. Subtract 1 minute from that time and set that as your "active" goal time for the activity. Approximate the amount of "resting" time you will need in order to safely resume activity or continue your day. Times may need to be adjusted after pacing begins. Stick to time-based pacing goals whether you are having a good or a bad pain day to avoid the crash–burn/overactivity cycle or the avoidance/inactivity cycle. Moderation is the key! Spread out activities during the week and be reasonable with the schedule so you can succeed.

Use the table below to record how you pace activities this week. Use the sample as your guide, where each period of activity and rest equals one cycle. In the examples provided, 10/15 (1) indicates *working for 10* minutes and *resting for 15* minutes for *one cycle* of pacing.

	Sample	Activity 1	Activity 2	Activity 3
Activity	Cleaning house			
Active goal	10 minutes			
Rest goal	15 minutes			
Day 1	10/15 (1)			
Day 2	10/15 (2)			
Day 3	10/15 (3)			
Day 4	15/15 (1)			
Day 5	15/15 (2)			
Day 6	15/15 (3)			
Day 7	20/15 (2)			

compensate for weak or painful muscles. Third, generalized tension in response to pain can further exacerbate the pain condition. A variety of relaxation techniques can be used for managing chronic pain, including deep breathing, progressive muscle relaxation, and visual imagery. These techniques are reviewed in Chapter 4. Patients are recommended to use relaxation both on a routine basis to prevent development of cumulative tension as well as in response to the onset or exacerbation of pain.

Coping With Intense Pain Episodes

For patients who experience acute episodes of intense pain, learning strategies for coping with pain can improve their quality of life. These strategies will not alleviate the pain but can help increase a sense of personal control and mitigate distress. A five-step model for teaching management of intense pain episodes is recommended (see Figure 10.4). Acceptance and commitment therapy techniques may also be useful for helping patients manage distress through

FIGURE 10.4. Five Steps for Managing Intense Pain Episodes

1. **Manage your thinking.** What do you think before pain episodes? What do you think during pain episodes? What do you think following pain episodes? Which of these thoughts are helpful in managing your pain? Which are unhelpful? How can you alter your thinking to make it more helpful?

Unhelpful Self-Talk	Helpful Self-Talk
I can't stand this pain. (*This is an example of underestimating your ability.*)	I've dealt with it before; I can get through it again. (*This is an example of acknowledging your ability to tolerate pain.*)
This pain is horrible/awful/terrible. (*This is an example of an emotional evaluation.*)	This pain is an 8 on a 0 to 10 scale. (*This example uses a concrete, unemotional evaluation method.*)
This pain is ruining my life. (*This is an example of a global assessment.*)	This is a difficult time for me. (*This is a more specific assessment.*)
I can't do anything to make this stop. (*This is an example of all-or-nothing thinking.*)	There are things I can do to get through this. (*This example avoids all-or-nothing thinking.*)

2. **Stay as relaxed as possible.** Use deep breathing when you first feel an increase in pain; continue using deep breathing throughout the pain episode.
3. **Use imagery and distraction.** Use relaxing imagery, watch television, listen to music, or do a mentally challenging puzzle or game.
4. **Use medications effectively.** Recognize early warning signs of increased pain; take medication early to help manage pain episodes better.
5. **Use your support network.** Talk to your family members or others about what they can do or say to help during a pain episode; let them know what is not helpful during a pain episode.

increased acceptance of pain (Hughes et al., 2017). These techniques are summarized in Chapter 4.

Managing Your Thinking

Patients' thoughts about their pain can contribute to how well the pain is tolerated and can affect the consequences of the pain. Coach patients to recognize thoughts that work for or against them during pain episodes by using the following steps:

- Assess your self-talk before, during, and after the pain episode.

- Evaluate whether your self-talk was helpful or unhelpful. Review the common unhealthy pain beliefs in Figure 10.2 to assist patients in recognizing false or extreme catastrophic thought patterns and how they can be unhelpful.

- Practice replacing unhealthy thinking with more helpful thoughts.

Staying as Relaxed as Possible

During an intense pain episode, people are likely to become tense as a way to brace against the pain. Efforts to relax during pain episodes will often help increase the person's sense of self-efficacy, reduce emotional distress, and sometimes mitigate the pain intensity. Deep breathing (see Chapter 4) can be a useful strategy. Recommend that patients use deep breathing when they first feel an increase in pain. The technique should be used throughout the pain episode. The goal of the breathing exercise should not be to reduce or eliminate the pain. If patients perceive this as the goal, they are likely to discontinue its use as the pain increases. Instead, discuss relaxation as a strategy for distraction and for coping with and successfully enduring the pain episode.

Using Imagery or Distraction

Individuals with pain tend to suffer more when they are focusing on their pain than when they are distracted. Helping patients learn to distract themselves effectively by identifying and practicing specific activities or stimuli can be helpful. Examples include mental imagery of relaxing scenes, watching television, listening to music, playing video games, or performing mentally challenging activities such as puzzles or games (e.g., sudoku, crossword).

Using Pain Medications

Effective use of pain medications is also helpful for staying relaxed during intense pain episodes. Encourage the patient to discuss optimal pain medication management with their PCP. Some patients will wait until the pain episode is severe before taking prescribed medications. Sometimes this is because they want to minimize medication use; other times, they have become habituated to the pain and are not aware of the early signs of a severe pain episode. Recognizing early warning signs and taking medication at that point may help the patient manage pain episodes better.

Using a Support Network

Often people will withdraw from others during pain episodes and, in doing so, do not receive the benefits that their support network can give. One of these benefits is moral support and encouragement for getting through the pain episode. Supportive words from a significant other can encourage adaptive coping, discourage unhelpful thinking, and decrease distress. We frequently hear from patients just how helpful a significant other was in helping them deal with an intense pain episode. Furthermore, family members or friends who understand the principles of coping with pain can help patients mentally distract themselves and effectively pace activities. This kind of support often requires education and training for the support person. Encourage patients with pain to bring their partner or other supporters to their medical visits to receive this education. Patients should be encouraged to identify what type of support does and does not help; they can then be encouraged to share that information with significant others. It is best to share this information when the patient is at a baseline level of pain and not during an acute pain episode.

Patients might be interested in websites, mobile device applications, or self-help books to assist in managing their chronic pain. Some of these resources are summarized in Figure 10.5.

Arrange
Stepped Care Models

Many patients with acute, recurrent, and chronic pain have never been exposed to behavioral or cognitive pain management principles and approaches. Therefore, stepped care models that gradually integrate these principles into their care can be most beneficial. It might be helpful to have patients monitor their pain and their responses to their pain to determine the effects of the interventions. A pain monitoring form such as the one in Figure 10.6 could be used for this purpose. Provide follow-up consultation appointments over 1 to 4 weeks to assess the effects of the interventions and resolve problems. Outcome measures such as the PEG scale (Krebs et al., 2009) and the two-item short form of the Pain Self-Efficacy Questionnaire (M. K. Nicholas et al., 2015) may be helpful for tracking patient progress.

It is vital for those who benefit from the interventions to discuss when further medical evaluation or care for pain is indicated. Generally, this would occur when there is new pain or significant changes to the nature of the pain, location of the pain, or intensity or character of the pain. Those who do not benefit from these primary care approaches and display significant functional impairment may need to be referred to higher level care. Consider a referral to a specialty-trained clinical health psychologist to address coexisting mental disorders, unhealthy substance use, family conflict, and other relevant factors if it appears they cannot be adequately addressed in primary care over time. Patients and family members may benefit from a chronic pain support group focusing on enhancing coping and increasing function. Referral to a multidisciplinary chronic pain program will be helpful for others.

FIGURE 10.5. Resources for Patients With Chronic Pain: Websites, Mobile Applications, and Books

Type	Location	Description
Websites	American Pain Society (https://americanpainsociety.org/)	Multidisciplinary organization of scientists, clinicians, and other professionals dedicated to increasing knowledge of pain, transforming public policy related to pain, and enhancing clinical practice to reduce pain-related suffering
	International Association for the Study of Pain (https://www.iasp-pain.org/)	Largest multidisciplinary international association in the field of pain
Mobile applications	Pain Care (Google Play store, Android and Apple iOS)	Free mobile application helps users manage chronic pain. It is designed to help users regain control of their lives from pain through calming meditations, evidence-based training strategies, breathing tools, and functions for tracking pain.
	BioZen (Google Play store, Android and Apple iOS)	Free mobile application developed by the U.S. Department of Defense's National Center for Telehealth and Technology (now renamed Connected Health), with a variety of commercially available physiological sensors and Bluetooth technology helps manage pain and improve health through biofeedback. It is compatible with sensors measuring brainwave activity, cardiac activity, muscle tension, galvanic skin response, respiratory rate, and skin temperature.
Books	*Managing Pain Before It Manages You*, 4th ed. (Caudill, 2016)	Details 10 steps that can change the way pain sufferers feel, both physically and emotionally. Includes treatments for coping with flare-ups, solving everyday problems, and using power of relaxation techniques. It has content on mindfulness, a "Quick Skill" section in each chapter with simple exercises, supplementary reading and resources (including smartphone apps), and more. Practical tools include MP3 audio downloads and easy-to-use worksheets that purchasers can now download and print.
	The Pain Management Workbook: Powerful CBT and Mindfulness Skills to Take Control of Pain and Reclaim Your Life (Zoffness, 2020)	Uses a biopsychosocial approach rooted in CBT, mindfulness, and neuroscience. It also addresses improving sleep, nutrition for pain, and methods for resuming desired activities.

Note. CBT = cognitive behavior therapy.

FIGURE 10.6. Monitoring Pain Handout

Monitoring Pain

Date/ time	Pain intensity (0 = none; 10 = excruciating)	Duration (hr/min)	Precipitating factors	Thoughts related to pain	Emotional reactions	Pain behaviors

Opioid Use Disorder and Medication-Assisted Treatment

Although most clinical practice guidelines for treating pain in primary care caution against unnecessary and premature use of opioid prescriptions (Ernstzen et al., 2017), opioid prescription rates remain high in the United States. An estimated 20% of patients seeking care for noncancer chronic and acute pain receive a prescription for opioid medications (Dowell et al., 2016). Studies show that 21% to 29% of patients develop problematic opioid use following prescriptions for pain, with rates of unhealthy use averaging between 8% and 12% (Vowles et al., 2015), indicating physician-prescribed opioids are a factor in the development of substance use disorders. The *DSM-5-TR* (American Psychiatric Association, 2022) has 11 criteria for opioid use disorder (OUD), of which two or more criteria must be met within a 12-month period for a diagnosis.

BHCs should assess patients who are prescribed opioids for signs of OUD and communicate findings and impressions with the PCP. Guidance on assessment of substance use disorders is covered in Chapter 11. Medication-assisted treatment (MAT) may be indicated when patients are diagnosed with OUD and the medications need to be discontinued. Three medications have been approved in the United States for MAT to control the physical withdrawal symptoms and psychological cravings. These are buprenorphine, naltrexone, and methadone. Patients needing MAT are often referred to a comprehensive unhealthy substance use program that has integrated behavioral health, medical, and other services to provide a holistic approach to care. BHCs can play an essential role in preparing the patient to benefit from the MAT program through education, motivation enhancement, and brief cognitive interventions to address barriers to following through on the referral. In some cases, MAT medications will be prescribed in primary care. Regardless of the setting, patients will benefit from counseling and other behavioral health interventions as an integral part of MAT (Substance Abuse and Mental Health Services Administration, 2021b). Interventions that generally apply to substance use disorders can be used (see Chapter 11). Furthermore, approaches to pain management discussed in this chapter can be beneficial to support the patient's OUD recovery.

CONSIDERATIONS FOR SPECIFIC PAIN CONDITIONS
Headaches

Primary headaches are one of the most common pain conditions seen in primary care. Roughly one out of every six Americans and one in five women experience a migraine or other severe headache in a 3-month period (Burch et al., 2018). Migraines are ranked as the sixth greatest cause of disability worldwide (Global Burden of Disease Study 2013 Collaborators, 2015). Tension-type headaches are even more common, with an estimated global prevalence rate of 42% (Ferrante et al., 2013). Although effective medications are available to prevent and abort both tension and migraine headaches, some patients do not tolerate medications well or may prefer not to use a pharmacological approach. Studies have shown that triggers such as menstruation, skipping meals, alcohol consumption, caffeine withdrawal, sleep problems, psychological stress, and environmental conditions are common factors in bringing on headaches (Lee et al., 2019). BHCs can assist patients in recognizing their triggers by using monitoring logs as shown in Figure 10.7. Cognitive behavioral interventions can address triggers such as sleep problems, stress, and alcohol use. Moderate empirical support has been found for relaxation training, biofeedback, and cognitive behavioral therapy for helping patients with migraines (Ha & Gonzalez, 2019). These approaches are more useful for migraine prevention than for reducing headache pain after onset. Therefore, they are most applicable for patients with frequent headaches and more significant disability than for those who experience them infrequently. The evidence for psychological therapies to reduce migraines is not strong when treatment aims to reduce stress, change interpretations about the migraine experience, or cope with migraine symptoms once they occur (Sharpe et al., 2019). Relaxation training, biofeedback, and cognitive behavioral treatment aimed at improving stress management may be more effective for reducing tension-type headaches, although studies have mixed results and the study designs are somewhat weak (Harris et al., 2015).

Fibromyalgia

Fibromyalgia is a condition involving widespread pain throughout the body. Patients with fibromyalgia are more sensitive to pain than other people, and they typically experience fatigue, sleep disturbance, memory issues, and psychological distress. The etiology and nature of the syndrome are still debated, and there is not an established course of treatment that applies well to all patients. Thus, many individuals with fibromyalgia have interacted with medical providers who believe the condition is psychogenic or even involves malingering, which can contribute to the psychological distress patients feel. Because of this, patients need to understand that the involvement of a BHC in providing care does not mean fibromyalgia is a mental health condition. It can be helpful for the BHC to educate patients on the range of medical conditions with which they help provide care to normalize behavioral or psychological treatment approaches for medical conditions. Systematic reviews of the research have

FIGURE 10.7. Headache Monitoring Form

Date	
Time headache started	
Duration of headache	
Where did it hurt?	
Type of pain? (e.g., throbbing, tight band, dull ache)	
Intensity at its worst (0–10 scale)	
Any sensations before the pain began (aura)?	
How much sleep did you have last night?	
When was your last meal before the headache?	
How much caffeine did you have today?	
How much alcohol did you have today? What type?	
How much water have you consumed today?	
How much stress were you feeling (0–10 scale)? What were you stressed about?	
Did you consume any of the following? • Aged cheese • Red wine • Peanuts or peanut butter • Chocolate • Soy • Smoked fish • Soda • Hot dogs • Processed lunch meat • Bread • Dried fruit • Potato chips • Pizza	
Any other foods you feel might be triggers	
What did you do to address the headache? Did it help?	

found that cognitive behavioral therapy is effective for addressing the psychological distress related to fibromyalgia and also pain relief, health-related quality of life, fatigue, and disability (Bernardy et al., 2018). Cognitive behavioral therapy is also effective for addressing pain catastrophizing, which in turn improves quality of life (Alda et al., 2011). Evidence also shows benefits from progressive muscle relaxation training, mindfulness-based approaches (Hassett & Gevirtz, 2009), guided imagery, and hypnosis (Zech et al., 2017).

Gastrointestinal Disorders

Irritable bowel syndrome (IBS) and Crohn's disease are two gastrointestinal disorders that are chronic and involve pain as a predominant symptom. IBS is common, with an estimated prevalence rate of 14.1%, although most people who meet diagnostic criteria go undiagnosed (Hungin et al., 2005). A diagnosis of IBS is made when recurrent abdominal pain or discomfort has occurred at least 3 days per month in the last 3 months and is associated with two or more of the following symptoms: (a) improvement with defecation, (b) onset associated with a change in frequency of stool, and (c) onset associated with a change in form (i.e., appearance) of stool (Longstreth et al., 2006). Stress has a significant effect on IBS, and there is often a co-occurrence of depression and anxiety. Therefore, recommended interventions include relaxation training, cognitive behavioral therapy, assertive communication training, motivational enhancement, and problem-solving approaches to improve physician or nutritionist dietary change recommendations. Crohn's disease is a type of chronic inflammatory bowel disease. Patients likely will experience periods of flare-ups followed by periods of remission. Pain is experienced as abdominal cramping, and other common symptoms include persistent diarrhea, rectal bleeding, an urgent need to move bowels, a sensation of incomplete bowel evacuation, and constipation. These symptoms reduce quality of life and can contribute to depression, anxiety, and other emotional distress (Mikocka-Walus et al., 2017). Positive evidence exists showing that cognitive behavioral therapy, including relaxation and mindfulness approaches, is helpful for managing the psychological components of inflammatory bowel disease, such as depression and anxiety (C. A. Lamb et al., 2019). However, little evidence exists for impact on the bowel symptoms, including pain (Mikocka-Walus et al., 2017).

SUMMARY

Pain is one of the most common problems in primary care. Behavioral health assessment and interventions are now recognized as essential components for helping patients manage pain, especially when it is chronic or causes significant functional impairment. Critical areas for assessment include variability in the patient's experience of pain, factors that increase or decrease pain intensity or frequency, the effect of pain on the individual's activities, how effectively an individual copes when experiencing pain, and how the individual's social interactions and environments affect the pain. It is essential to provide the individual with a framework to understand various psychosocial factors and their effects on pain perception and functioning. Encouraging the individual to shift from pursuing a cure to focusing on management is important. Primary treatment may involve returning to daily activities as soon as possible or increasing physical activity. Questioning unhelpful thoughts, learning relaxation techniques and imagery, and drawing on social support can be effective components of a primary care pain management intervention. Integrated BHCs in the primary care setting have a rich opportunity to help the PCPs and their patients use effective nonpharmacological pain management strategies to improve functioning and quality of life.

11

Unhealthy Substance Use
Alcohol, Illicit Drugs, and Prescription Medication

Unhealthy substance use and substance use disorder (SUD) are prevalent among patients seen in primary care (L. T. Wu et al., 2017). Having a team approach to screening and intervention and providing acute and chronic care that actively leverages the behavioral health consultant's (BHC's) expertise can have a significant impact. This chapter provides a launching point for BHCs for screening and intervention strategies that might prove useful.

UNHEALTHY ALCOHOL USE

Unhealthy alcohol use is a significant chronic public health problem in the United States (U.S. Department of Health and Human Services, 2016). In 2017, more than 140 million people 12 years of age and older reported using alcohol in the past month (Substance Abuse and Mental Health Services Administration [SAMHSA], 2018a). Almost 67 million of them reported binge drinking in the past month, and 14.5 million met alcohol use disorder (AUD) diagnostic criteria. What is even more concerning is that nearly half of the 18.7 million individuals 18 years old and older who met criteria for unhealthy alcohol use also experienced a comorbid behavioral health condition such as anxiety or depression (SAMHSA, 2018a).

Unhealthy alcohol use (previously referred to as alcohol misuse) was defined by the United States Preventive Services Task Force (USPSTF; O'Connor et al.,

https://doi.org/10.1037/0000380-012

Integrated Behavioral Health in Primary Care: Step-by-Step Guidance for Assessment and Intervention, Third Edition, by C. L. Hunter, J. L. Goodie, M. S. Oordt, and A. C. Dobmeyer

2018) as a spectrum of behaviors from risky drinking to AUD. Risky or hazardous alcohol use occurs when an individual drinks more than the recommended daily, weekly, or per-occasion amounts, resulting in increased risk for health consequences but not meeting criteria of AUD (National Institute on Alcohol Abuse and Alcoholism [NIAAA], 2007). Risky use as defined by the NIAAA (2007) is eight or more drinks per week or four or more drinks per occasion for women and 15 or more drinks per week and five or more drinks per occasion for men. Unhealthy use also includes *harmful alcohol consumption*, defined by the tenth edition of the *International Statistical Classification of Diseases and Related Health Problems* (*ICD-10*) as a pattern of use that causes damage to physical or mental health (World Health Organization, 2016). Adults who drink at elevated risk levels have a greater chance of developing diabetes, neuropsychiatric conditions, cardiovascular and circulatory diseases, digestive diseases, and cancer (Shield et al., 2014). Epidemiological data also suggest that those who engage in risky, hazardous, or harmful alcohol consumption are at increased risk of alcohol-related problems, such as increased psychological and financial burden on coworkers, families, and friends and impaired interpersonal functioning and productivity (Rehm et al., 2009).

Cultural and Diversity Considerations

In the 2017 National Survey on Drug Use and Health (SAMHSA, 2018b), risky alcohol consumption levels for those aged 21 years or older were reported at 25.6% for Black or African Americans, 30.3% for American Indians or Alaska Natives, 27.1% for Whites, 29.3% for Hispanics or Latinx individuals, 28.4% for Native Hawaiians or other Pacific Islanders, 14.1% for Asians, and 26.0% for Not Hispanic or Latinx individuals. When looking at gender alone, for those aged 21 years or older, men (31.7%) engage in risky alcohol consumption at a greater rate than women (21.7%). Although risky drinking behavior can occur in anyone, male individuals are most likely to be engaged in risky alcohol consumption.

Specialty Mental Health

A great deal of research has been conducted regarding mental health treatment for risky, hazardous, or harmful alcohol consumption in specialty mental health and addiction treatment settings. In sum, a variety of strategies have been found effective, including but not limited to cognitive behavioral treatment, motivational interviewing, brief interventions, social skills training, community reinforcement, behavior contracting, behavioral marital therapy, case management, and pharmacotherapy. For details of approaches and effectiveness, see W. R. Miller et al. (2005) and Witkiewitz et al. (2019).

Primary Care Adaptation

It is common for primary care providers (PCPs) to see individuals who engage in risky, hazardous, or harmful levels of alcohol consumption. Prevalence estimates from a variety of primary care settings and populations suggest that approximately 7% to 30% of individuals consume alcohol in an unhealthy manner (Rehm et al., 2016; Saitz 2005; Vinson et al., 2010). To best identify those who might benefit from additional assessment and intervention, the USPSTF (O'Connor et al., 2018) recommends screening for unhealthy alcohol use in primary care settings in adults 18 years or older. They also recommend providing those engaged in risky or hazardous drinking with brief behavioral counseling interventions to reduce unhealthy alcohol use, consistent with the components of screening, brief intervention, and referral to treatment (SBIRT). At its core, SBIRT comprises three components (Cimini & Martin, 2020):

- efficient and effective screening and assessment of the severity of alcohol and other substance use with the goal of identifying the appropriate level of treatment;

- brief intervention focused on helping the patient understand their unhealthy alcohol and other substance use and comorbid behavioral health conditions, with the goal of enhancing motivation to change consistent with the patient's goals and values; and

- referral of those who need more extensive treatment to specialty care and assisting them in attaining that care.

The evidence-based recommendation for those who appear to have a clinical presentation consistent with AUD is referral to specialty substance treatment, as they are not as likely to benefit from brief intervention (American Academy of Family Physicians [AAFP], 2017; Centers for Disease Control and Prevention [CDC], 2014; Moyer, 2013; NIAAA, 2007). More recent reviews of the literature, however, point to the effectiveness of brief interventions in the primary care setting. In their meta-analytic review, O'Connor et al. (2018) indicated that adult patients identified through screening who received brief counseling interventions reduced unhealthy alcohol use by an average of 1.6 drinks a week and reduced the odds of exceeding recommended drinking limits by 40% and heavy use episodes by 33% at 6- and 12-month follow-ups. They also found no evidence to suggest that patients of different race/ethnicity or lower socioeconomic status would have a lower likelihood of benefit from interventions. These strategies are consistent with the 5As approach to effective behavioral counseling interventions in primary care and with SBIRT screening and intervention components (O'Connor et al., 2018). The best evidence for effectiveness was with brief (each contact is 6–15 minutes), multicontact (i.e., two to five contacts) behavioral counseling. From a population health perspective, these data are critical because a greater number of patients with AUD may be exposed to a brief intervention than would be willing to accept an intensive specialty referral, thus resulting in a greater impact on the population of patients in the practice.

PCPs have been encouraged to identify and treat those who are engaging in risky, hazardous, and harmful drinking, and specific tools, strategies, and recommendations are available for doing so effectively (e.g., AAFP, 2017; CDC,

2014; NIAAA, 2007). Despite this, few PCPs use recommended screening treatment protocols (9.4%–40% depending on the study; Chan et al., 2021) or even offer any other kinds of treatment intervention within primary care (Mitchell et al., 2012). Working in primary care, a BHC has the ability to affect how clinics screen, assess, and intervene with unhealthy alcohol use by changing patients' behaviors through education and training or by providing support for assessment and intervention within primary care.

The NIAAA (2007) publication *Helping Patients Who Drink Too Much: A Clinician's Guide*; the CDC (2014) publication *Planning and Implementing Screening and Brief Intervention for Risky Alcohol Use: A Step-by-Step Guide for Primary Care Practices*; the AAFP (2017) publication *Addressing Alcohol Use Practice Manual: An Alcohol Screening and Brief Intervention Program*; and Cimini and Martin's (2020) publication *Screening, Brief Intervention, and Referral to Treatment for Substance Use: A Practitioners' Guide* are excellent sources of information and contain useful clinical tools to help assess, treat, and appropriately refer individuals in the primary care setting who engage in unhealthy alcohol consumption patterns. The SAMHSA (2022) website on SBIRT also has a wealth of information and tools that might be useful in one's practice.

The following sections draw on selected pieces from the NIAAA (2007), CDC (2014), AAFP (2017), and Cimini and Martin (2020) publications as well as adapted evidence-based strategies we use in our own clinical work to efficiently and effectively screen; intervene; and, when necessary, refer to specialty services for patients engaging in unhealthy alcohol consumption patterns.

Assess

BHCs should develop methods for screening, assessing, and diagnosing patients who may have unhealthy alcohol use. BHCs may also want to introduce these methods to other medical staff to enhance the consistent identification of patients with alcohol consumption problems. Because unhealthy alcohol use screening is recommended in primary care for patients 18 years of age and older (O'Connor et al., 2018), clinics might also start screening every patient 18 years old and older at most appointments as part of a standard clinical pathway (see Chapter 18). Having a BHC in the clinic may help the rest of the team have more confidence in being able to effectively treat or refer individuals who screen positive for unhealthy alcohol use.

Screening. Whether screening is done by other team members or the BHC, screening questions may be ideally placed within the context of general health screening questions, like those concerning tobacco use. This might help the patient feel less stigma than if the questions were asked in a standalone manner. Good evidence indicates that screening can accurately identify individuals who are drinking in a risky, hazardous, or harmful manner. The USPSTF (O'Connor et al., 2018) has determined that one-item to three-item screening measures are most accurate for assessing unhealthy alcohol use in patients 18 years of age and older. These measures include the abbreviated Alcohol Use

Disorders Identification Test-Consumption (AUDIT-C; Dawson et al., 2005) and the NIAAA-recommended Single Alcohol Screening Question (SASQ; P. C. Smith et al., 2009): "How many times in the past year have you had X or more drinks in a day?" where X is five for men and four for women. Although either would be fine to use as a screen for unhealthy alcohol use, we suggest using the AUDIT-C, which consists of the first three questions of the AUDIT (Saunders et al., 1993). The AUDIT-C is identified as having "good" sensitivity and specificity, whereas the SASQ is identified as having "adequate" sensitivity and specificity (O'Connor et al., 2018). A score on the AUDIT-C of 4 or more for men and 3 or more for women has been recommended as a positive cutoff that yields optimal balance for sensitivity and specificity of the measure (Moyer, 2013). However, O'Connor et al. (2018) showed optimal cutoff scores (best sensitivity and specificity) for adults could be 5 or 6 for men and 4 or 5 for women, depending on the study.

It is recommended that the full AUDIT be administered if the patient is positive on the SASQ or AUDIT-C (CDC, 2014; O'Connor et al., 2018). The AUDIT is sensitive to a broad spectrum of alcohol consumption problems and can help determine who may benefit from a referral to specialty substance treatment. When the AUDIT manual was published in 2001, the authors suggested using a score of 8 for men and 7 for women to identify those who might be engaged in unhealthy alcohol consumption. In 2013, Johnson et al. reported that data regarding the use of the AUDIT in primary care suggested an optimal score for identifying those who engage in unhealthy alcohol consumption is 5 for men and 3 for women to better identify the full spectrum of unhealthy alcohol use. Similar recommendations were made by USPSTF (O'Connor et al., 2018), suggesting that if the AUDIT is used as an initial screening test, providers might use a lower cutoff such as 3, 4, or 5 to balance sensitivity and specificity in screening for the full spectrum on unhealthy alcohol use.

If the individual's AUDIT score meets or exceeds a positive screening score, consider further assessment to determine whether referral to specialty substance treatment may be warranted. We discuss this further in the section on AUD diagnosis.

Alcohol use disorder diagnosis. To help determine the best treatment course, it is important to determine whether the patient's alcohol consumption is at a severity level that might warrant referral to specialty substance misuse treatment services. An AUD diagnosis is made on a continuum of mild (two or three criteria), moderate (four or five criteria), and severe (six or more criteria). One approach might be to consider those who meet moderate and severe levels of AUD as more likely to benefit from specialty services outside of primary care. At the same time, it is important to take into consideration the context, which includes but is not limited to patient preferences, patient strengths and weaknesses, social and community support, comorbidities, and availability of specialist and primary care clinic resources. Spithoff and Kahan (2015), after conducting a nonsystematic review of the literature, recommended PCPs offer patients with AUD counseling; ongoing regular follow-ups; medications (for individuals with moderate or severe AUD); and encouragement to attend counseling, day or residential treatment programs, and support groups. However, this may be more than some PCPs are able to do without additional team support. Oslin et al. (2014), in their single-blind randomized clinical trial with veterans, examined what impact additional support from a BHC might produce. Their study demonstrated that treatment for an AUD can effectively be delivered in primary care, leading to better rates of treatment engagement and reductions in heavy drinking compared with a control group that received treatment in a specialty outpatient addiction treatment program. Treatment intervention focused on pharmacotherapy (Naltrexone) and relied on a BHC trained to deliver personalized measurement-based addiction care. Patients met weekly with the BHC, and if they were unable to attend appointments in person, appointments were conducted by phone covering the same content. As patients improved, the frequency of appointments could be reduced to two times per month after the first 3 months. The BHC provided information to help them learn about AUD as a treatable problem, possible benefits of medication, side effects to look for and manage, and medication adherence. BHCs were trained in motivational interviewing techniques (see Chapter 4) and the use of action plans focused on achievable goals. Participants set their own drinking reduction goals, with abstinence as one option.

To help assess for an AUD, one could ask the following questions to help determine whether a patient is positive on any AUD criteria (NIAAA, 2015): "In the past 12 months have you . . ."

- Had times when you ended up drinking more, or longer, than you intended?

- More than once wanted to cut down or stop drinking, or tried to, but couldn't?

- Spent a lot of time drinking? Or being sick or getting over other aftereffects?

- Wanted a drink so badly you couldn't think of anything else?

- Found that drinking, or being sick from drinking, often interfered with taking care of your home or family? Or caused job or school problems?

- Continued to drink even though it was causing trouble with your family or friends?

- Given up or cut back on activities that were important or interesting to you or gave you pleasure in order to drink?

- More than once gotten into situations while or after drinking that increased your chances of getting hurt (e.g., driving, swimming, using machinery, walking in a dangerous area, having unsafe sex)?

- Continued to drink even though it was making you feel depressed or anxious or adding to another health problem? Or having had a memory blackout?

- Had to drink much more than you once did to get the effect you wanted? Or found that your usual number of drinks had much less effect than before?

- Found that when the effects of alcohol were wearing off, you had withdrawal symptoms, such as trouble sleeping, shakiness, restlessness, nausea, sweating, a racing heart, or a seizure? Or sensed things that were not there?

If the individual answers yes to two or three of the criteria, they meet criteria for AUD mild severity. These individuals may be appropriate for further primary care intervention. If they meet four or five of the criteria, they are at the moderate severity level. These individuals might be appropriate for primary care treatment or might be better served by specialty substance use treatment outside of primary care, depending on the criteria for which they are positive and other contextual factors. For example, if a patient experiences tolerance or withdrawal and has low social support and comorbid depression, they might be more appropriate for specialty care than someone who, by comparison, is in the moderate severity range but is not positive for tolerance or withdrawal, has good social support, and has mild to moderate anxiety symptoms. Those who meet six or more of the criteria are at the severe level and might benefit more from specialty services if they are interested in those services. As discussed previously, however, multiple factors should be considered in order to get the best treatment match for that patient given clinic and community resources as well as patient motivation and preferences.

Additional questions. There are several other areas one might assess, in addition to standard BHC initial appointment functional assessment questions (see Chapter 1), because the patient's answers can influence treatment recommendations and skill building during the advise and assist phases of the appointment:

- What are the benefits of consuming alcohol?

  For example, if patients identify benefits such as winding down, relaxing, improving sleep, or decreasing anxiety, the BHC might provide an intervention designed to increase other healthy activities that can provide similar benefits. See Chapters 4 and 5 for examples of interventions to teach these skills.

- Is there anything associated with an increase or decrease in use?

  For example, if patients identify drinking more with friends versus alone and drinking less or more when out of town, then the BHC might provide an intervention designed to minimize thoughts, behaviors, and environments associated with increased drinking and to increase thoughts, behaviors, and environments associated with decreased drinking. See Chapter 4 for examples of interventions to teach these skills.

- How do others respond with increased or decreased use?

  For example, if the patient says, "Friends say I am not as fun when I don't drink or drink less," "My husband says I am easier to be around when I drink more," and "My children say they like me better when I don't drink beer," then the

BHC might use these responses to evaluate patient's motivation to decrease drinking. See Chapter 4 for motivational enhancement interventions.

Advise

The goal of this phase is to increase readiness to change alcohol use patterns by informing individuals that their drinking rate places them at increased risk of medical problems and showing them how their current drinking pattern compares with other individuals in the United States. One may want to use the patient education material in the NIAAA (2022) publication *Rethinking Drinking: Alcohol and Your Health*. The following is an example of providing advice:

> Based on your current drinking pattern, you're drinking at a level that is higher than what we consider to be medically and behaviorally safe. This is putting you at increased risk for death, specifically through fatal injury, cancer, stroke, and high blood pressure. It could also lead to driving under the influence of alcohol or other risky or unsafe behaviors you might not engage in if you were drinking at a different level. If it's okay with you, I'd like to take just a moment to review with you what a standard drink is and how your current alcohol use compares with people in the United States. After that, I'd like to discuss whether now is a good time to commit to changing your alcohol intake. If you decide that it is a good time, we can review your options and design an individual plan for you that will meet your needs and lifestyle.

This may serve as a good time to gauge the individual's receptivity to change, and it might also be a good time to discuss common mistakes and assumptions people have about alcohol consumption. See Figure 11.1 for a handout one can use to dispel any misconceptions the patient might have regarding alcohol consumption.

Agree

Before moving to the assist phase with a specific plan to change alcohol consumption, it is important to determine whether the patient agrees that a change is necessary. One way to do this is to gauge readiness to change. If the individual seems ambivalent about changing, consider using motivational enhancement strategies to decrease ambivalence and increase willingness and motivation to change. See Chapter 4 for a discussion of motivational enhancement strategies, such as reviewing risks and benefits of change, importance of change, and confidence in being able to change. The following are some specific questions using a motivational interviewing approach that might be helpful in enhancing motivation to change:

> On a scale of 0 to 10, with 0 being not important at all to alter drinking amount and 10 being extremely important to alter drinking amount, how important is it to you to alter your drinking amount? How confident are you that you can alter your drinking habits, with 0 being not at all confident and 10 being extremely confident?

If the answer is less than 7 on importance or confidence, ask what the patient would have to change or what would need to be different to move the importance or confidence to a 7 or higher. One might say,

It is not unusual for people to see changing their drinking as relatively unimportant. There are clearly significant benefits to drinking alcohol such as relaxation and stress reduction. What would have to change in order for drinking less to be important to you at this point in time?

If the answer is 7 or higher, ask what factors led them to have that much confidence or for it to be that important.

Once one has assessed importance and confidence and they seem to be at a reasonable level to move forward (e.g., 5–7+ on confidence and importance) one might gauge the patient's willingness to change. One might then ask, "Are you willing to commit to changing your drinking pattern at this point in time?" If patients answer yes, discuss options for helping them change. If they answer no, ask about major barriers to change and deal with these as you are able. If they are still not willing to change, let them know that assistance is available when they decide they are ready.

Advise

It is important to review options for change. For those with AUD who are motivated for change, regardless of severity level, one might discuss options for primary care interventions and for specialty services so the patient has a clear idea about what each option includes. This includes allowing them to partner

FIGURE 11.1. Common Mistakes and Assumptions About Alcohol Patient Handout

Common Mistakes and Assumptions About Alcohol

Drinking beer is safer than other drinks, so I only drink beer.
The belief that beer and wine are less intoxicating and safer compared with hard liquor is false. It may take longer to get intoxicated with beer and wine because of the volume that has to be consumed, but the percentage of alcohol per volume from beer and wine will make someone as intoxicated as the same percentage of alcohol per volume of a drink that contains hard liquor.

Drinking with others is safer, so I never drink alone.
The belief that people who drink alone are the only individuals who may have problems is false. Drinking alone or with others does not determine intoxication level or problems associated with alcohol consumption.

Mixing types of drinks will increase intoxication, so I stick to drinking the same thing.
The belief that sticking with one type of drink will decrease intoxication is false. Mixing types of drinks has no differential impact on intoxication; intoxication is related to the total amount of alcohol consumed.

Eating a meal before drinking helps to avoid getting drunk, so I never drink on an empty stomach.
The belief that eating prior to drinking will prevent an individual from getting intoxicated is false. Eating will slow down the absorption rate of alcohol into the bloodstream but not stop it.

Consuming caffeinated (e.g., coffee) or energy drinks (e.g., Monster, Red Bull) after drinking reduces the impact of alcohol.
Although caffeinated and energy drinks may increase alertness, they do not "sober you up" or reverse the impairments associated with alcohol use.

for a shared decision about the next step. Options will vary depending on the patient's unique presentation, but in primary care the following might be common options:

- reduce the number of drinks consumed (e.g., daily, weekly, in high-risk situations such as driving);

- abstain from drinking for a particular period of time;

- improve depression-, anxiety-, and stress-coping skills;

- develop a plan to minimize situations where unhealthy drinking is likely to occur;

- develop a plan to increase social support while making changes;

- address other comorbid behavioral health or physical challenges; and

- as appropriate, use medications such as naltrexone along with the other nonmedication interventions.

It is generally useful for the BHC to seek out information about what specialty treatment for AUD involves in one's community/health system. Ideally, it would involve the evidence-based interventions discussed in this chapter. In some cases, it may look similar to what one might do as a BHC, with greater frequency (e.g., one appointment a week), intensity (e.g., 60-minute appointments), and duration (e.g., 8–12 weeks). Being able to help the patient know the specialty treatments they could receive might help increase willingness to engage in that referral. Despite being confident and motivated for treatment, patients may not be willing or able to go to a specialist or inpatient treatment for a variety of stigma, financial (no insurance or underinsured), or time constraints and/or geographical barriers with no treatment available close to home. If that is the case, being flexible and working with the patient, the PCP, and the rest of the team with treatments much the same way as one would for someone who is engaged in risky, hazardous, or harmful drinking may be beneficial with the following additions:

- The drinking goal recommendation might be abstinence for most, but if the patient is unwilling to abstain, negotiating a reduction may be helpful. It can reduce resistance to change and open the door for consideration of abstinence in the future. It can also be a good way to work with individuals who do not want to stop drinking but want to avoid some of the consequences (e.g., being caught driving under the influence, having trouble at work). These early steps in high-risk situations are usually more beneficial than an all-or-nothing approach with patients who are reluctant to stop alcohol consumption.

- Recommend a helping group or agency (e.g., Alcoholics Anonymous) and provide local contact information or resources (e.g., a website with local meeting information) to make it easier for the patient to follow through.

- For those with alcohol dependence, include medical management of withdrawal (for more guidance, see Hoffman & Weinhouse, 2021; NIAAA, 2007).

A significant number of patients with AUD are likely to have no desire to change even after one has discussed importance and confidence and the pros and cons of ongoing consumption at current levels. For these individuals, having a patient-centered approach in which one acknowledges and understands they have no desire to change at this time might leave the door open for future engagement. Perhaps say,

> Based on our discussion, it sounds like you are comfortable with your frequency of alcohol consumption; you see significant benefits and little or no downside. If you decide in the future that changing your alcohol consumption is something you'd like to do and would like some assistance with that, I'm/we're happy to assist as desired.

These individuals might also be flagged in the electronic health record for being at high risk for alcohol consumption consequences, and a team-based plan might be developed on how to reengage the patient in the alcohol use discussion in follow-up primary care appointments.

Assist

The ways one can assist patients with reducing or stopping their alcohol consumption will vary depending on their goal and the individual factors involved in their alcohol consumption. To this end, we list a variety of options that one might use:

Increase awareness of alcohol consumption recommendations. Educate on what a standard drink is, focusing on the type of drink the patient typically consumes.

Determine their drinking goal. As a way to reduce their risk of alcohol-related problems, we recommend encouraging patients to stay within moderate drinking limits: no more than two drinks a day for a man and one drink a day for a woman (U.S. Department of Agriculture & Department of Health and Human Services, 2020). If patients are unwilling to adhere to these standards, work with them to set some type of a decrease from their current level. Set a plan for the days they want to drink and how many drinks they will have on those days.

Tracking drinks. Keep track of the number of drinks consumed using a method (e.g., spiral notebook, a Post-It note, calendar, mobile device, Excel spreadsheet) that is easiest for the individual. Another method involves having a list of drinks per day that can be consumed and having the individual mark each drink off the list before it is consumed. It might look like this for a given 2-day period for a man: Monday. 1, 2; Tuesday. 1, 2. It is important to define what constitutes a drink for tracking purposes using standard drink measures. For example, a 3-ounce pour of whiskey should be marked as two drinks, and a 16-ounce pint of beer should be marked as 1.3 drinks (see Figure 11.2).

FIGURE 11.2. What Is a "Standard Drink"?

Although the drinks pictured here are different sizes, each contains approximately the same amount of alcohol and counts as one U.S. standard drink or one alcoholic drink-equivalent.

Standard Drink in the United States

  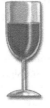

12 fl oz of regular beer	=	8–9 fl oz of malt liquor (shown in a 12 oz glass)	=	5 fl oz of wine	= 1.5 fl oz shot of distilled spirits (e.g., gin, rum, tequila, vodka, whiskey)
about 5% alcohol		about 7% alcohol		about 12% alcohol	about 40% alcohol

The table below shows the approximate number of standard drinks (or alcoholic drink-equivalents) found in common containers.

Regular beer (5% alc/vol)	Malt liquor (7% alc/vol)	Wine (12% alc/vol)	80-proof distilled spirits (40% alc/vol)
12 fl oz = 1 16 fl oz = 1⅓ 22 fl oz = 2 40 fl oz = 3⅓	12 fl oz = 1½ 16 fl oz = 2 22 fl oz = 2½ 40 fl oz = 4½	750 ml (a regular wine bottle) = 5	A shot (1.5 oz glass/50 ml bottle) = 1 A mixed drink or cocktail = 1 or more 200 ml (a "half pint") = 4½ 375 ml (a "pint" or "half bottle") = 8½ 750 ml (a "fifth") = 17

The examples shown on this page serve as a starting point for comparison. For different types of beer, wine, or malt liquor, the alcohol content can vary greatly. However, some differences are smaller than you might expect. Many light beers, for example, have almost as much alcohol as regular beer—about 85 percent as much, or 4.2 percent versus 5.0 percent alcohol by volume (alc/vol), on average.

Note. Adapted from *Rethinking Drinking: Alcohol and Your Health* (NIH Publication No. 21-AA-3770, p. 3), by National Institute on Alcohol Abuse and Alcoholism, 2022, National Institutes of Health (https://www.niaaa.nih.gov/sites/default/files/publications/NIAAA_RethinkingDrinking.pdf). Copyright 2022 by National Institutes of Health. Adapted with permission.

We recommend giving some suggestions on how individuals might track consumption and then asking whether any of those would work or whether they have additional ideas.

Reducing alcohol consumption. The following strategies might be useful in helping the patient reduce their alcohol consumption:

- Review ways to pace drinking.
  - Put glass or bottle down between drinks (i.e., do not hold it in your hand).
  - After you have finished half your drink, wait 5 minutes before you take another sip.
  - Drink a nonalcoholic drink between your alcoholic drinks.
  - Have no more than one drink per hour.
  - Delay when drinking starts (e.g., wait 1.5 hours after getting home to have a drink).

- Review ways to avoid or manage situations in which it may be a challenge for the individual to stay within their goals. See the Four As handout in Figure 11.3 to help plan for difficult situations. We recommend using this in an interactive fashion, with you filling in the form. Our experience suggests that the individual is able to solve problems more effectively and be more collaborative if you are the one writing things down through this process.

- Review assertive communication skills to be able to refuse drinks when appropriate (see Chapter 3).

- Review stress and anxiety management skills to take the place of drinking for relaxation (see Chapters 4 and 5).

Stopping alcohol consumption. If stopping all alcohol consumption is the goal, then focus on avoiding or managing situations, assertive communication, and stress and anxiety management skills in the same manner as for reducing consumption. Because alcohol consumption is a pleasurable activity for most drinkers, we recommend setting a plan to incorporate alternative pleasurable activities into the days and periods when individuals typically consume alcohol. See Chapter 4 for instructions on goal setting to help produce a plan to increase enjoyable activities.

The BHC can also provide the patient with a variety of additional resources that might be used in conjunction with BHC appointments or might be used by patients who will be following up with their PCP only. Patients might be interested in websites, mobile device applications, or self-help books to assist in managing their risky alcohol consumption. Some of these resources are summarized in Figure 11.4.

Arrange

For those cutting down as well as those who are stopping alcohol consumption, we suggest the following:

- Make a follow-up appointment to assess adherence to the plan.

- Support and encourage the individual to continue with the plan if it is working well. Ask whether anything has occurred that the individual sees as a

FIGURE 11.3. Four As for Managing Alcohol Consumption Patient Handout

Four As for Managing Alcohol Consumption

Avoid
What are the highly tempting situations in which you might drink more than you plan? Avoid these situations if possible over the next month.

1. _____
_____

2. _____
_____

Alter
For situations you can't avoid, how can you alter them to make them easier?

1. _____
_____

2. _____
_____

Alternatives
What can you do with your mouth and hands when you want to drink and it is a day you are not drinking or have already reached your limit?

1. _____
_____

2. _____
_____

Action
When you get the urge to drink and it does not fit with your drinking plan, what can you do to be active or busy until the urge passes?

1. _____
_____

2. _____
_____

Are there situations in which it will be a challenge to stay within your drinking limits? If so, list them and what you will do to effectively manage those situations.

1. _____
Plan: _____

2. _____
Plan: _____

FIGURE 11.4. Resources for Patients With Unhealthy Substance Use: Websites, Mobile Applications, and Books (*continues*)

Type	Location	Description
Websites	National Institute on Alcohol Abuse and Alcoholism (https://www.niaaa.nih.gov/alcohol-health)	Provides patient materials on a range of health consequences of risky drinking and a selection of pamphlets and brochures on finding help, changing drinking behavior, effects of alcohol, alcohol use and different groups (e.g., women), and engaging with family members
	Centers for Disease Control and Prevention (https://www.cdc.gov/alcohol/fact-sheets.htm)	Provides patient fact sheets on alcohol use and health, binge drinking, men's and women's health, and moderate drinking
	National Council on Alcoholism and Drug Dependence (https://ncadd.us/)	Provides a range of resources including how to get help; information about alcohol use; and information targeted for parents, youth, those in recovery, and family and friends
Mobile applications	Saying When (Android and Apple iOS)	Enables self-assessment with a few quick questions to set a baseline for success. Includes tools to help patients understand when and why they drink to help them know when to "say when" and links to additional support. Prompts patients to set their own goals to fit their lifestyle with tips for success. Includes a personal dashboard that lets the patient know how they are doing based on goals. Patients can track when they have a drink or an urge to drink, view daily stats, and monitor progress.
	Stop OD NYC (Android and Apple iOS)	Developed by the New York City Department of Health and Mental Hygiene, application provides detailed information on opioids (e.g., heroin, fentanyl) and naloxone administration instructions in the event of an overdose. Includes risk-reduction content, including (a) a *find naloxone* option that links users to mapped pharmacies, harm reduction programs, and health care centers providing free naloxone; (b) intramuscular, intranasal, and autoinjector formulations of naloxone administration instructions; (c) tools to recognize those suspected of an overdose; and (d) legal protection information for individuals administering naloxone. Uses text messaging, cartoons, and YouTube-based videos for multimedia educational instructions. Users can access other health resources within the Department of Health and Mental Hygiene platform (e.g., cardiovascular health, reducing glucose intake, smoking cessation).

FIGURE 11.4. Resources for Patients With Unhealthy Substance Use: Websites, Mobile Applications, and Books (*continued*)

Type	Location	Description
Books	*Controlling Your Drinking: Tools to Make Moderation Work for You*, 2nd ed. (W. R. Miller & Muñoz, 2013)	Includes tools to evaluate alcohol consumption and determine changes to make in a manner that fits with goals and lifestyle. Covers topics like enjoying social events, defusing tension and stress, and coping with difficult emotions—with or without a glass in hand.
	Alcohol and You: 21 Ways to Control and Stop Drinking: How to Give Up Your Addiction and Quit Alcohol (David, 2017)	Covers a range of topics including but not limited to making a decision to alter consumption; understanding alcohol use disorder; addressing myths; choosing abstinence or moderation; and understanding medication, withdrawal, motivation, cravings, solution-focused thinking, social support, cognitive behavioral therapy, and relapse prevention
	How to Change Your Drinking: A Harm Reduction Guide to Alcohol, 2nd ed. (Anderson, 2010)	Written for the patient who wants to drink more safely, reduce drinking, or quit alcohol altogether. Contains detailed selection of harm-reduction tools and strategies from which to build an individualized alcohol harm reduction program.

future problem and determine whether the plan can be modified to adapt to the change. Collaboratively determine whether additional plans for follow-up would be helpful or whether checking on the plan at the next medical appointment might be the best option.

- If the patients do not meet their goal, encourage them to learn from this experience (i.e., what went well, what did not, how they might plan differently for the future).
  - Suggest that change can be difficult and may take a while.
  - Evaluate barriers to the plan.
  - Consider engaging the patient's social network for assistance.
  - If unable to abstain or cut down, reassess for AUD.
  - Negotiate a follow-up appointment to assess the plan and resolve difficulties.

Summary

Unhealthy alcohol use has numerous health and social consequences. With up to a third of the individuals in primary care engaged in drinking patterns that increase their risk for physical and social consequences, primary care is ripe for unhealthy alcohol use screening and intervention. Despite the data supporting the effectiveness of screening and brief interventions for risky, hazardous, or harmful drinking, few PCPs use recommended screening or treatment protocols or offer any other kind of treatment within primary care. You can help to change this practice. Increasing unhealthy alcohol use screening with standardized instruments, discussing with a patient their drinking rate in comparison with U.S. drinking norms, tailoring interventions to the patient's goals, and arranging for appropriate follow-up care will help you to effectively help PCPs and their patients manage unhealthy alcohol consumption.

ILLEGAL DRUGS AND UNHEALTHY PRESCRIPTION MEDICATION USE

Unhealthy drug use is using illegal drugs or using prescription medication in a manner or dose other than that intended by the prescribing PCP; taking someone else's prescription, even if for a legitimate health problem such as pain; or taking medication to feel euphoria (i.e., get buzzed or high; Krist, Davidson, Mangione, Barry, Cabana, Caughey, Curry, et al., 2020; National Institute on Drug Abuse [NIDA], 2020). This might also include problematic use of legal drugs (e.g., marijuana in some locations) and using prescription medication in greater amounts, more frequently, for other symptoms, or with different administration routes, all of which might lead to adverse consequences. Use of illicit substances is a growing problem, with over 59 million individuals 12 years of age or older reporting using illicit drugs in the past year. Marijuana was most commonly used (49.6 million; legal in 18 states), followed by hallucinogens (7.1 million), cocaine (3.3 million), methamphetamine (2.5 million), inhalants (0.9 million), and heroin (0.9 million; SAMHSA, 2021a). Unhealthy use of prescription medications occurs in over 16 million people 12 years of age and older (SAMHSA, 2021a). The most common prescriptions used in an unhealthy manner are opioids (9.3 million), which are normally used to treat pain (e.g., oxycodone [OxyContin], combined hydrocodone and acetaminophen [Vicodin]); tranquilizers or sedatives (6.2 million), which are used to treat anxiety and sleep problems (e.g., diazepam [Valium], alprazolam [Xanax], zolpidem [Ambien]); and stimulants (5.1 million), which are commonly used to increase attention, energy, and alertness (e.g., methylphenidate [Ritalin], dextroamphetamine [Dexedrine]; SAMHSA, 2021a). Factors associated with unhealthy drug use include being aged 18 to 25 years; being male; having a behavioral health condition, including nicotine or alcohol SUD; having a history of sexual or physical abuse, childhood adversity, or parental neglect; and having a history of alcohol or other SUD in a first-degree relative (SAMHSA, 2021a). Those who might be at greater risk for unhealthy prescription use are those with a history of depression and anxiety, acute and chronic pain, other health problems that include fatigue and headaches, and heightened physiological reactions (subjective euphoria) to certain types of drugs (SAMHSA, 2016). Those who have a history of other substance use or misuse are also at greater risk for unhealthy prescription use.

The USPSTF recommends screening for unhealthy drug use in adults 18 years of age or older. They recommend screening be implemented when services for accurate diagnosis, effective treatment, and appropriate care can be offered or referred (Krist, Davidson, Mangione, Barry, Cabana, Caughey, Curry, et al., 2020).

Cultural and Diversity Considerations

The rate of current illicit drug use by those 12 years of age or older varies by racial/ethnic groups (Patnode, Perdue, Rushkin, & O'Connor, 2020). The highest rates of use are found in Alaska Natives or American Indians (17.6%) and those identifying themselves as being two or more races (17.1%). They are followed by Black (13.1%), White (11.6%), and Pacific Islander or Native Hawaiian individuals (10.4%). Latino or Hispanic (9.8%) and Asian individuals (4.5%) report the lowest rates of use (Patnode, Perdue, Rushkin, & O'Connor, 2020).

Specialty Mental Health

Research literature suggests that cognitive behavioral interventions can be moderately effective for treating illicit drug use and unhealthy prescription use in specialty settings (Darker et al., 2015; Gates et al., 2016; NIDA, 2020; Patnode, Perdue, Rushkin, et al., 2020; Zamboni et al., 2021). Although there is certainly variability regarding type, intensity, and duration of specialty setting interventions, in general they tend to consist of identifying and changing unhelpful thought patterns; altering exposure or response to high-risk environments; and altering social, emotional, physical, and behavioral contingencies that increase or decrease unwanted illicit drug or unhealthy prescription use. Strategies that appear to be effective include motivation interventions targeting ambivalence, relapse prevention that focuses on cues for use and developing alternative responses to those cues, psychoeducation focused on helping the patient make more informed choices in situations where they might be at greater risk to use, engaging in alternative behaviors that reinforce and are consistent with values, questioning thoughts about benefits of use, and cognitive and behavioral strategies that target unpleasant physical and emotional responses associated with unwanted use.

Primary Care Adaptation

In their review of the literature, Patnode, Perdue, Rushkin, and O'Connor (2020) found that for a range of illicit and unhealthy prescription use, provided interventions and intensity were generally similar.

Most consisted of one or two appointments ranging in length from 3 to 60 minutes per appointment. Most interventions were conducted in person by trained peers, health educators, or behavioral health specialists, and one third of the studies had phone booster appointments. Study intervention content was similar, including personalized normative feedback; motivational interviewing techniques to establish rapport; and discussion focused on the association between unhealthy use, potential health consequences, discrepancies between unhealthy use and patient-valued goals, and behavior change options that could enhance patient self-efficacy (Patnode, Perdue, Rushkin, et al., 2020).

Assess

Consistent with our recommendations regarding assessment of unhealthy alcohol use, we believe BHCs should develop methods for screening, assessing, and diagnosing patients who may have illicit drug or unhealthy prescription use. BHCs may also want to discuss with clinic leadership the pros and cons of implementing universal screening for all patients in primary care as part of a standard clinical pathway (see Chapter 18).

Screening. Patnode, Perdue, Rushkin, et al. (2020) reported that screening tools that ask questions about illegal or unhealthy prescription use are available for identifying one or more classes of unhealthy use. Interviewer-administered tools and self-administered tools appear to have similar accuracy. The USPSTF (Krist, Davidson, Mangione, Barry, Cabana, Caughey, Curry, et al., 2020) recommends primary care clinics consider selecting brief screening tools like the NIDA Quick Screen (NIDA, 2011; see Figure 11.5), which asks about alcohol, tobacco, nonmedical use of prescription drugs, and illegal drugs in the past year on a scale from "never" to "daily or almost daily," as it might be more feasible to use in a busy primary care clinic. A yes to any response but "never" on the prescription drugs or illegal drugs use question might then prompt continued screening with the eight-item Alcohol, Smoking and Substance Involvement Screening Test (NIDA, 2011; see Figure 11.6), which assesses risks associated with unhealthy drug use or comorbid conditions and might produce additional information suggesting the need for further diagnostic assessment (Krist, Davidson, Mangione, Barry, Cabana, Caughey, Curry, et al., 2020). If the individual's Alcohol, Smoking and Substance Involvement Screening Test score meets or exceeds a positive screening score (0–3 [lower risk], 4–26 [moderate risk], 27+ [high risk]), consider further assessment to determine whether referral to specialty substance treatment may be warranted. We discuss this in the section on SUD diagnosis. Similar to alcohol-use-only screening, screening questionnaires like these may be more ideally placed within the context of general health screening questions than asked in a standalone manner.

Substance use disorder diagnosis. To help determine the best treatment course, it is important to determine whether the patient's illicit drug use or unhealthy prescription use is at a severity level that might warrant referral to specialty substance misuse treatment services. Consistent with the criteria for an AUD diagnosis, other SUDs (e.g., illicit drug use and unhealthy prescription) are categorized on a continuum of mild (two to three criteria), moderate (four to five criteria), and severe (six or more criteria). One approach might be to consider those who meet moderate and severe levels of SUD as more likely to benefit from specialty services outside of primary care. At the same time, it is important to take into consideration the context, including but not limited to patient

FIGURE 11.5. NIDA Quick Screen V1.01

Name: _____   Sex: ( ) F ( ) M   Age: ____

Interviewer: _____   Date: ____/____/_____

Introduction (Please read to patient)

> *Hi, I'm _____ , nice to meet you. If it's okay with you, I'd like to ask you a few questions that will help me give you better medical care. The questions relate to your experience with alcohol, cigarettes, and other drugs. Some of the substances we'll talk about are prescribed by a doctor (like pain medications). But I will only record those if you have taken them for reasons or in doses* other than prescribed. *I'll also ask you about illicit or illegal drug use—but only to better diagnose and treat you.*

Instructions: For each substance, mark in the appropriate column. For example, if the patient has used cocaine monthly in the past year, put a mark in the "Monthly" column in the "Illegal drugs" row.

NIDA Quick Screen Question: *In the past year*, how often have you used the following?	Never	Once or twice	Monthly	Weekly	Daily or almost daily
Alcohol • For men, five or more drinks a day • For women, four or more drinks a day					
Tobacco products					
Prescription drugs for nonmedical reasons					
Illegal drugs					

- If the patient says **"No"** for all drugs in the Quick Screen, reinforce abstinence. **Screening is complete.**
- If the patient says **"Yes"** to **one or more days of heavy drinking**, *patient is an at-risk drinker.* Please see the NIAAA guide *Helping Patients Who Drink Too Much: A Clinician's Guide* (NIAAA, 2007a), for information to **Assess, Advise, Assist, and Arrange** help for at risk drinkers or patients with alcohol use disorders.
- If patient says **"Yes"** to **use of tobacco:** *Any* current tobacco use places a patient at risk. Advise *all tobacco users to quit.* For more information on smoking cessation, please see *Helping Smokers Quit: A Guide for Clinicians* (Public Health Service, 2008).
- If the patient says **"Yes"** to **use of illegal drugs or prescription drugs for nonmedical reasons**, proceed to **Question 1** of the NIDA-Modified ASSIST.

Note. This guide is designed to assist clinicians serving adult patients in screening for drug use. The NIDA Quick Screen was adapted from the single-question screen for drug use in primary care by P. C. Smith et al. (2010) and the NIAAA's (2007) screening question on heavy drinking days. NIDA = National Institute on Drug Abuse; NIAAA = National Institute on Alcohol Abuse and Alcoholism; ASSIST = Alcohol, Smoking and Substance Involvement Screening Test.

preference, patient strengths and weaknesses, social and community support, comorbidities, and availability of specialist and primary care clinic resources. To that end, Logan et al. (2019) reported on an integrated primary care addiction medicine program in which they evaluated a treatment approach for patients who met criteria for moderate or severe opioid use disorder. Approximately

FIGURE 11.6. Questions 1–8 of the NIDA-Modified ASSIST V2.0 (*continues*)

Instructions: Patients may fill in the following form themselves, but screening personnel should offer to read the questions aloud in a private setting and complete the form for the patient. To preserve confidentiality, a protective sheet should be placed on top of the questionnaire so it will not be seen by other patients after it is completed but before it is filed in the medical record.

Question 1 of 8, NIDA-Modified ASSIST 1. In your *LIFETIME*, which of the following substances have you ever used? *Note for physicians: For prescription medications, please report nonmedical use only.*	Yes	No
a. Cannabis (e.g., marijuana, pot, grass, hash)		
b. Cocaine (e.g., coke, crack)		
c. Prescription stimulants (e.g., Ritalin, Concerta, Dexedrine, Adderall, diet pills)		
d. Methamphetamine (e.g., speed, crystal meth, ice)		
e. Inhalants (e.g., nitrous oxide, glue, gas, paint thinner)		
f. Sedatives or sleeping pills (e.g., Valium, Serepax, Ativan, Xanax, Librium, Rohypnol, GHB)		
g. Hallucinogens (e.g., LSD, acid, mushrooms, PCP, Special K, ecstasy)		
h. Street opioids (e.g., heroin, opium)		
i. Prescription opioids (e.g., fentanyl, oxycodone [OxyContin, Percocet], hydrocodone [Vicodin], methadone, buprenorphine)		
j. Other, specify:		

- Given the patient's response to the Quick Screen, the patient *should not indicate* "**No**" for all drugs in Question 1. If they do, remind them that their answers to the Quick Screen indicated they used an illegal or prescription drug for nonmedical reasons within the past year and then **repeat Question 1**. If the patient indicates that the drug used is not listed, please mark "**Yes**" next to "Other" and continue to **Question 2** of the NIDA-Modified ASSIST.
- If the patient says "**Yes**" to any of the drugs, proceed to **Question 2** of the NIDA-Modified ASSIST.

Question 2 of 8, NIDA-Modified ASSIST 2. *In the past 3 months,* how often have you used the substances you mentioned (e.g., first drug, second drug)?	Never	Once or twice	Monthly	Weekly	Daily or almost daily
a. Cannabis (e.g., marijuana, pot, grass, hash)	0	2	3	4	6
b. Cocaine (e.g., coke, crack)	0	2	3	4	6
c. Prescription stimulants (e.g., Ritalin, Concerta, Dexedrine, Adderall, diet pills)	0	2	3	4	6
d. Methamphetamine (e.g., speed, crystal meth, ice)	0	2	3	4	6
e. Inhalants (e.g., nitrous oxide, glue, gas, paint thinner)	0	2	3	4	6
f. Sedatives or sleeping pills (e.g., Valium, Serepax, Ativan, Xanax, Librium, Rohypnol, GHB)	0	2	3	4	6
g. Hallucinogens (e.g., LSD, acid, mushrooms, PCP, Special K, ecstasy)	0	2	3	4	6
h. Street opioids (e.g., heroin, opium)	0	2	3	4	6
i. Prescription opioids (e.g., fentanyl, oxycodone [OxyContin, Percocet], hydrocodone [Vicodin], methadone, buprenorphine)	0	2	3	4	6
j. Other, specify:	0	2	3	4	6

FIGURE 11.6. Questions 1–8 of the NIDA-Modified ASSIST V2.0 (*continues*)

- For patients who report "**Never**" having used any drug in the past 3 months: **Go to Questions 6 through 8.**

For any recent **illicit or nonmedical prescription drug use**, go to **Question 3.**

3. *In the past 3 months*, how often have you had a strong desire or urge to use (e.g., first drug, second drug)?	Never	Once or twice	Monthly	Weekly	Daily or almost daily
a. Cannabis (e.g., marijuana, pot, grass, hash)	0	3	4	5	6
b. Cocaine (e.g., coke, crack)	0	3	4	5	6
c. Prescription stimulants (e.g., Ritalin, Concerta, Dexedrine, Adderall, diet pills)	0	3	4	5	6
d. Methamphetamine (e.g., speed, crystal meth, ice)	0	3	4	5	6
e. Inhalants (e.g., nitrous oxide, glue, gas, paint thinner)	0	3	4	5	6
f. Sedatives or sleeping pills (e.g., Valium, Serepax, Ativan, Xanax, Librium, Rohypnol, GHB)	0	3	4	5	6
g. Hallucinogens (e.g., LSD, acid, mushrooms, PCP, Special K, ecstasy)	0	3	4	5	6
h. Street opioids (e.g., heroin, opium)	0	3	4	5	6
i. Prescription opioids (e.g., fentanyl, oxycodone [OxyContin, Percocet], hydrocodone [Vicodin], methadone, buprenorphine)	0	3	4	5	6
j. Other, specify:	0	3	4	5	6

4. *During the past 3 months*, how often has your use of (e.g., first drug, second drug) led to health, social, legal, or financial problems?	Never	Once or twice	Monthly	Weekly	Daily or almost daily
a. Cannabis (e.g., marijuana, pot, grass, hash)	0	4	5	6	7
b. Cocaine (e.g., coke, crack)	0	4	5	6	7
c. Prescription stimulants (e.g., Ritalin, Concerta, Dexedrine, Adderall, diet pills)	0	4	5	6	7
d. Methamphetamine (e.g., speed, crystal meth, ice)	0	4	5	6	7
e. Inhalants (e.g., nitrous oxide, glue, gas, paint thinner)	0	4	5	6	7
f. Sedatives or sleeping pills (e.g., Valium, Serepax, Ativan, Xanax, Librium, Rohypnol, GHB)	0	4	5	6	7
g. Hallucinogens (e.g., LSD, acid, mushrooms, PCP, Special K, ecstasy)	0	4	5	6	7
h. Street opioids (e.g., heroin, opium)	0	4	5	6	7
i. Prescription opioids (e.g., fentanyl, oxycodone [OxyContin, Percocet], hydrocodone [Vicodin], methadone, buprenorphine)	0	4	5	6	7
j. Other, specify:	0	4	5	6	7

FIGURE 11.6. Questions 1–8 of the NIDA-Modified ASSIST V2.0 (*continues*)

5. *During the past 3 months*, how often have you failed to do what was normally expected of you because of your use of (e.g., first drug, second drug)?	Never	Once or twice	Monthly	Weekly	Daily or almost daily
a. Cannabis (e.g., marijuana, pot, grass, hash)	0	5	6	7	8
b. Cocaine (e.g., coke, crack)	0	5	6	7	8
c. Prescription stimulants (e.g., Ritalin, Concerta, Dexedrine, Adderall, diet pills)	0	5	6	7	8
d. Methamphetamine (e.g., speed, crystal meth, ice)	0	5	6	7	8
e. Inhalants (e.g., nitrous oxide, glue, gas, paint thinner)	0	5	6	7	8
f. Sedatives or sleeping pills (e.g., Valium, Serepax, Ativan, Xanax, Librium, Rohypnol, GHB)	0	5	6	7	8
g. Hallucinogens (e.g., LSD, acid, mushrooms, PCP, Special K, ecstasy)	0	5	6	7	8
h. Street opioids (e.g., heroin, opium)	0	5	6	7	8
i. Prescription opioids (e.g., fentanyl, oxycodone [OxyContin, Percocet], hydrocodone [Vicodin], methadone, buprenorphine)	0	5	6	7	8
j. Other, specify:	0	5	6	7	8

Instructions: Ask Questions 6 and 7 for all substances *ever used* (i.e., those endorsed in Question 1).

6. Has a friend or relative or anyone else *ever* expressed concern about your use of (e.g., first drug, second drug)?	No, never	Yes, but not in the past 3 months	Yes, in the past 3 months
a. Cannabis (e.g., marijuana, pot, grass, hash)	0	3	6
b. Cocaine (e.g., coke, crack)	0	3	6
c. Prescribed Amphetamine type stimulants (e.g., Ritalin, Concerta, Dexedrine, Adderall, diet pills)	0	3	6
d. Methamphetamine (e.g., speed, crystal meth, ice)	0	3	6
e. Inhalants (e.g., nitrous oxide, glue, gas, paint thinner)	0	3	6
f. Sedatives or sleeping pills (e.g., Valium, Serepax, Xanax, Ativan, Librium, Rohypnol, GHB)	0	3	6
g. Hallucinogens (e.g., LSD, acid, mushrooms, PCP, Special K, ecstasy)	0	3	6
h. Street opioids (e.g., heroin, opium)	0	3	6
i. Prescribed opioids (e.g., fentanyl, oxycodone [OxyContin, Percocet], hydrocodone [Vicodin], methadone, buprenorphine)	0	3	6
j. Other, specify:	0	3	6

FIGURE 11.6. Questions 1–8 of the NIDA-Modified ASSIST V2.0 (*continues*)

7. Have you ever tried and failed to control, cut down, or stop using (e.g., first drug, second drug)?	No, never	Yes, but not in the past 3 months	Yes, in the past 3 months
a. Cannabis (e.g., marijuana, pot, grass, hash)	0	3	6
b. Cocaine (e.g., coke, crack)	0	3	6
c. Prescribed Amphetamine type stimulants (e.g., Ritalin, Concerta, Dexedrine, Adderall, diet pills)	0	3	6
d. Methamphetamine (e.g., speed, crystal meth, ice)	0	3	6
e. Inhalants (e.g., nitrous oxide, glue, gas, paint thinner)	0	3	6
f. Sedatives or sleeping pills (e.g., Valium, Serepax, Ativan, Xanax, Librium, Rohypnol, GHB)	0	3	6
g. Hallucinogens (e.g., LSD, acid, mushrooms, PCP, Special K, ecstasy)	0	3	6
h. Street opioids (e.g., heroin, opium)	0	3	6
i. Prescribed opioids (e.g., fentanyl, oxycodone [OxyContin, Percocet], hydrocodone [Vicodin], methadone, buprenorphine)	0	3	6
j. Other, specify:	0	3	6

Instructions: Ask Question 8 if the patient endorses any drug that might be injected, including those that might be listed in the other category (e.g., steroids). <u>Circle appropriate response</u>.

8. Have you ever used any drug by injection (nonmedical use only)?	No, never	Yes, but not in the past 3 months	Yes, in the past 3 months

- Recommend to patients reporting any prior or current intravenous drug use that they get tested for HIV and hepatitis B/C.
- If patient reports using a drug by injection in the past 3 months, ask about their pattern of injecting during this period to determine their risk levels and the best course of intervention.
  - If patient responds that they inject once weekly or less OR fewer than 3 days in a row, provide a brief intervention including a discussion of the risks associated with injecting.
  - If patient responds that they inject more than once per week OR 3 or more days in a row, refer for further assessment.

Recommend to patients reporting any current use of alcohol or illicit drugs that they get tested for HIV and other sexually transmitted diseases.

FIGURE 11.6. Questions 1–8 of the NIDA-Modified ASSIST V2.0 (*continued*)

Tally Sheet for Scoring the Full NIDA-Modified ASSIST

Instructions: For each substance (labeled a–j), add up the scores received for questions 2–7 above. This is the SI score. Do not include the results from either the Q1 or Q8 (above) in your SI scores.

SI score	Total (SI score)
a. Cannabis (e.g., marijuana, pot, grass, hash)	
b. Cocaine (e.g., coke, crack)	
c. Prescription stimulants (e.g., Ritalin, Concerta, Dexedrine, Adderall, diet pills)	
d. Methamphetamine (e.g., speed, crystal meth, ice)	
e. Inhalants (e.g., nitrous oxide, glue, gas, paint thinner)	
f. Sedatives or sleeping pills (e.g., Valium, Serepax, Xanax, Ativan, Librium, Rohypnol, GHB)	
g. Hallucinogens (e.g., LSD, acid, mushrooms, PCP, Special K, ecstasy)	
h. Street opioids (e.g., heroin, opium)	
i. Prescription opioids (e.g., fentanyl, oxycodone [OxyContin, Percocet], hydrocodone [Vicodin], methadone, buprenorphine)	
j. Other, specify:	

Use the resultant SI Score to identify patient's risk level.

To determine patient's risk level based on his or her SI score, see the table below:

Level of risk associated with different SI score ranges for illicit or nonmedical prescription drug use	
0–3	Lower risk
4–26	Moderate risk
27+	High risk

Note. The NIDA-Modified ASSIST was adapted from *The Alcohol, Smoking and Substance Involvement Screening Test (ASSIST) Manual for Use in Primary Care*, World Health Organization, 2010 (https://www.who.int/publications/i/item/978924159938-2). Copyright 2010 by World Health Organization. NIDA = National Institute on Drug Abuse; ASSIST = Alcohol, Smoking and Substance Involvement Screening Test; SI = substance involvement.

three quarters of these patients used tobacco, had at least one other SUD, and had a comorbid behavioral health condition such as depression or anxiety. The integrated program combined medication-assisted treatment with buprenorphine and either a weekly, biweekly, or monthly 16- to 30-minute appointment with a BHC followed by a 5- to 15-minute appointment with the BHC and prescribing provider together. BHC appointments were individualized and included at least one of the following:

- motivational enhancement strategies to improve readiness to change, resolve ambivalence, and support the patient in action and maintenance stages;

- relapse prevention to include identification of apparently irrelevant decisions that ultimately increase risk of relapse, understanding the difference between a lapse and relapse, and mindfulness strategies;

- cognitive behavioral skills geared to addiction, including living life without substances, increasing social contact, and practicing assertiveness;

- cognitive behavioral treatment for comorbid behavioral health conditions, including depression and anxiety symptom management, behavioral activation strategies, challenging unhelpful thoughts, Socratic questioning, and relaxation training; and

- crisis assessment and intervention with safety assessments and plans and referral to crisis services and higher levels of care as needed.

At 1 month, 92% of the patients were retained in treatment; 64% had follow-up through 3 months. Inconsistent urine drug tests, meaning tests that were sometimes positive, were more common at treatment initiation (74%) than with the most recent sample (43%), which was statistically significant. There was also a significant decrease in depression and anxiety symptoms for those who were retained in treatment for at least 3 months. This study suggests that patients who are traditionally challenging to treat in primary care (as a result of the severity of their use and other comorbidities) may have successful initial primary care treatment when it involves BHC services.

The remaining assess, advise, agree, and assist components parallel what we detailed earlier in the chapter for AUD. Context, motivation for change, use of evidence-based interventions, and collaborative treatment planning with respect toward patient values and goals and a nonjudgmental approach focusing on achievable goals are likely to prove valuable in helping patients stop illicit and unhealthy prescription use or decrease the frequency, duration, and impact of unhealthy use.

Arrange

For those cutting down, as well as those who are stopping unhealthy drug use, we suggest the following:

- Schedule multiple follow-up appointments, with the BHC and other team members, to assess adherence to the plan and problem solve barriers.

- Depending on severity and chronicity, it might be helpful to take a chronic disease approach. Ongoing future appointments, whether by telehealth or in person, regardless of whether the patient is doing well or not, might become a good long-term plan to maximize success, similar to the approach if the patient had another chronic condition, such as diabetes.

Our experience suggests that BHCs may be relied on in the following ways:

- as an informal consultant for the PCP,

- to help the PCP and patient improve communication and work out an agreed solution for appropriate use of medication to continue receiving medication (this may be especially relevant if the individual is hoarding medication because symptoms such as pain or anxiety are not being adequately treated and they are concerned about running out of medication when it is needed most), and

- to support the PCP with their stance on stopping a prescription that is no longer medically needed.

We believe the following information is important, particularly for effectively informing and assisting the PCPs in your clinic with screening, recognition, and intervention for unhealthy prescription use. Helping the PCP be aware of the potential for unhealthy prescription use so that they can assess and intervene effectively improves the chances of preventing unhealthy use or catching it early. This may enhance the opportunity for better care and better satisfaction with care for both the patient and the PCP.

For effective team-based care, it may also be important for BHCs to learn what their PCPs are doing with regards to reducing opioid risk and, if opportunities exist, what the BHC can do to support or enhance those efforts. Some examples of what PCPs might be doing to decrease risk include the following (American College of Preventive Medicine, 2011; Patnode, Webber, et al., 2021):

- checking the Prescription Drug Monitoring Program electronic database prior to prescribing;

- using low-dose opioids;

- conducting a risk assessment prior to and during long-term opioid use;

- having a group practice policy for after-hours prescriptions;

- informing individuals about the prescription regimen and the refill policy before giving medication;

- carefully documenting the diagnosis, the reason for using medication, the prescription policy, and individual education;

- when prescribing multiple substances, carefully considering the benefit and risk of prescribing more than one controlled substance at a time;

- maintaining a refill flowchart for easy access to prescription refill history; and

- having use agreements to specify the PCP's and patient's roles and the consequences of breaching the agreement (highlight that the relationship is consensual and that there is room for negotiation).

BHCs might also provide in-service training to PCPs on potential warning signs of unhealthy use and steps to take if identified. Some of those warning signs might include the following:

- losing medication,

- running out of medication earlier than expected based on number prescribed and dose per day,

- seeking new or multiple physicians or calling the clinic for a refill when the PCP is not in the clinic,

- showing more concern about obtaining medication than the comprehensive management of the problem,

- playing one PCP's opinion against another's,

- threatening to get medication from a more caring or knowledgeable PCP, and

- claiming that the PCP is the only one who can help by providing the prescription.

Assist

The BHC can suggest the following strategies to the PCP for when and how to implement treatment (American College of Preventive Medicine, 2011; Patnode, Webber, et al., 2021).

- Provide specific instructions about how to take the medication and emphasize that it is to be used only for the problem for which it was prescribed. The BHC might assist the patient and PCP with a medication agreement to ensure that there is an understanding of terms, implementation strategies, and identification of ways of working with violations of the agreement that improve relationships with the PCP and team.

- Explain to the patient that learning new skills with the assistance of the BHC might help the patient achieve desired outcomes with less or no medication.

- Remain empathetic and direct concern in a nonjudgmental way. The following is an example for a patient with chronic pain:

  I understand you are concerned about the treatment and management of your pain. I want to work with you so we can manage it in the best way possible. At the same time, I'm concerned about the way you are using your medication and that you are having difficulty taking it in the way in which it is designed to be used. I'm also concerned about the short- and long-term consequences of that type of use, which can include addiction, liver problems, and tolerance to the medication so that it no longer works for you.

- When a potentially addictive medication is not indicated, communicate this in a straightforward manner, explaining to the individual why this is the case and what the options are. If the patient is pressuring the PCP to fill the prescription, the patient should be told the medication cannot be prescribed. It can be useful for the PCP to express to the patient that it feels like they are being pressured to write a prescription that is not medically indicated. This could then be used by the PCP as a transition to discuss concerns about the patient's medication use and the potential unhealthy pattern that might be starting.

SUMMARY

Millions of individuals in the United States use illicit drugs and engage in unhealthy prescription use. PCPs are under pressure by an ever-increasingly informed public to prescribe a variety of medications that relieve symptoms and decrease suffering and to screen for and address illicit substance use. Illicit drugs and unhealthy use of prescriptions can negatively affect health, affect functioning, and lead to substance dependence. In addition to the skills you can offer, which can help manage a variety of problems that may lead to the discontinuation or reduction in unhealthy substance use, you can proactively help PCPs be aware of, assess, and intervene effectively with unhealthy substance use. Assisting your clinic in setting standards for screening and assessment and/or diagnosis of unhealthy substance use is a valuable role for the BHC.

12

Sexual Problems

exual dysfunctions involve clinically significant problems in sexual response or in experiencing sexual pleasure. They may be lifelong or acquired and may be generalized or limited to specific situations, partners, or stimulations. The etiology of sexual dysfunction is often multifactorial and may include psychological factors (i.e., emotional, cognitive, or behavioral factors), partner or relationship problems, religious or cultural factors, effects of a drug or medication, medical conditions, or a combination of these (American Psychiatric Association, 2022). Sexual dysfunctions may contribute to psychological symptoms, increased distress, and decreased sexual and relationship satisfaction (Frost & Donovan, 2021; Jern et al., 2020; Rowland & Kolba, 2018; Stephenson et al., 2018). This chapter focuses specifically on three of the more common sexual dysfunctions: male erectile disorder (ED), premature ejaculation (PE), and female orgasmic disorder (OD). Evidence-based specialty mental health interventions exist for each disorder; less is known about behavioral health interventions offered within the primary care setting.

ERECTILE DISORDER

ED is characterized by "a marked difficulty in obtaining or maintaining an erection or a marked decrease in erectile rigidity in all or almost all occasions of sexual activity" that has been present for at least 6 months in almost all sexual

https://doi.org/10.1037/0000380-013
Integrated Behavioral Health in Primary Care: Step-by-Step Guidance for Assessment and Intervention, Third Edition, by C. L. Hunter, J. L. Goodie, M. S. Oordt, and A. C. Dobmeyer

activities; causes significant distress; and is not due to a nonsexual mental disorder, significant relationship problems or other stress, another medical condition, or the effects of a substance or medication (American Psychiatric Association, 2022, p. 482). In some individuals, the primary cause of ED may be organic factors. In many men, however, ED may be caused or worsened by an interplay of factors, including relationship or partner variables, psychiatric comorbidity, cultural factors, and medical conditions.

The prevalence of ED increases with age, particularly after age 50. In younger men (< 40 years), prevalence rates appear to be lower than 10%, whereas 20% to 40% of men in their 60s and over half of men aged 70 and older meet criteria for ED (American Psychiatric Association, 2022).

Key Biopsychosocial Factors

Understanding the biopsychosocial factors in ED is important for the behavioral health consultant (BHC) to conduct an effective assessment and intervention. The following are areas of particular importance.

Physical Factors

Multiple organic or biological factors increase risk for ED, including age (risk rises with increasing age), genetics, medical conditions, and certain medications. Conditions of the vascular, nervous, or endocrine systems can lead to ED, including Type 2 diabetes, heart disease, high blood pressure, multiple sclerosis, chronic kidney disease, obesity, and nerve injury. See Allen and Walter (2019) for additional information on medical conditions and genetic markers that have been identified as risk factors for ED. Medications that may contribute to ED include antihypertensives, antiandrogens (used for prostate cancer), antidepressants, prescription sedatives, appetite suppressants, and medications for ulcers, among others (National Institute of Diabetes and Digestive and Kidney Diseases [NIDDK], n.d.-b). If the erectile problems are fully explained by medical conditions, a diagnosis of ED based on the fifth edition of the *Diagnostic and Statistical Manual of Mental Disorders, Text Revision* would not be given (American Psychiatric Association, 2022); however, as mentioned previously, the majority of erectile problems results from a complex interplay of multiple factors.

Several oral medications approved by the Food and Drug Administration are available for the treatment of ED, including sildenafil (Viagra), vardenafil (Levitra, Staxyn), avanafil (Stendra), and tadalafil (Cialis). Testosterone may be beneficial if levels are low and the ED is not primarily caused by nerve or circulatory problems. Some patients may benefit from medical interventions such as surgical prostheses or implants, penile injections or suppositories, external vacuum pump devices, and constriction rings (NIDDK, n.d.-b). Additional patient information on medical treatments for ED is available through the NIDDK (n.d.-b).

Emotional and Cognitive Factors

In some individuals, emotional or cognitive factors may be primary causes of ED. In many others, thoughts and emotions serve as perpetuating factors once ED has developed for other reasons. Kalogeropoulos and Larouche (2020) noted that cognitive distraction and anxiety during sexual activity can interfere with arousal, contribute to ED, and lead to behavioral avoidance of sex. Depression has emerged as a predictive factor for the onset of ED in middle-aged and older men (S. A. Martin et al., 2014). In young men (18–40 years), depression and anxiety occur at higher rates both prior to and following a diagnosis of ED (Manalo et al., 2022). In men with diabetes, ED occurs at significantly higher rates when comorbid depressive symptoms are present (74.2% vs. 37.4%; Wang et al., 2018).

Behavioral Factors

Lifestyle behaviors play a role in ED in some individuals. Current and past tobacco use, low physical activity, excessive alcohol use, use of certain illegal drugs, and being overweight all may contribute to ED risk. Poor control of diabetes and hypertension also increases risk for ED (Allen & Walter, 2019; NIDDK, n.d.-b).

Environmental Factors

Partner relationship problems, other relationship factors, and interpersonal distress are associated with erectile problems (American Psychiatric Association, 2022; Shaeer & Shaeer, 2012). These interpersonal problems may be a cause, an effect, or both of erectile dysfunction. Although early research suggested those who experienced sexual abuse as children have an increased risk of developing problems with erectile dysfunction (e.g., Laumann et al., 1999), a recent literature review found inconsistent results in the relationship between history of childhood sexual abuse and later problems with male sexual arousal (Gewirtz-Meydan & Opuda, 2022).

Cultural and Diversity Considerations

As noted earlier, older age is a predictive factor for ED. There does not appear to be ethnic/racial differences in rates of ED in the United States, although rates do vary across countries. Prevalence of ED does not differ in older men who have sex with men versus those who have sex with men and women (American Psychiatric Association, 2022).

Specialty Mental Health

A review of randomized treatment trials found behavioral interventions to be effective in the treatment of ED, with some indication of benefit in combining behavioral and medication treatments (Allen & Walter, 2019). A meta-analysis of eight randomized controlled trials of combined treatment (phosphodiesterase-5 inhibitors plus cognitive behavioral therapy) found that combined approaches yielded better outcomes in ED symptoms than either treatment alone and led to improved levels of sexual satisfaction compared with medication alone (H. M. Schmidt et al., 2014). A combination approach (medical and psychological) to treatment of ED has been recommended by international sexual medicine organizations (e.g., European Society of Sexual Medicine; Dewitte et al., 2021).

Specialty mental health interventions for ED may include a number of psychosocial components, including psychoeducation, enhancing relationship and communication skills, improving sexual technique, learning cognitive change skills (e.g., fostering realistic expectations, restructuring cognitions), using structured behavioral techniques (e.g., sensate focus, start–stop method), and addressing modifiable lifestyle risk factors (e.g., weight loss, tobacco cessation, increasing physical exercise, improving glycemic control). Of note, a review of treatment meta-analyses concluded that interventions to increase physical activity were the most effective behavioral approaches for ED (Allen & Walter, 2019).

Behavioral Health in Primary Care

We have not found any published studies of behavioral or psychological treatment of ED in integrated primary care settings by behavioral health professionals. The following section, therefore, is based on our clinical experiences in adapting evidence-based specialty mental health treatments for ED to approaches that are consistent with a primary care behavioral health (PCBH) consultation model of service delivery.

Primary Care Adaptation

To adapt approaches from specialty mental health, we often focus on education and brief behavioral and cognitive interventions, supplemented by handouts to assist patients in home-based practice. The 5As model provides a useful structure for guiding BHC discussions about ED.

Assess

BHCs should begin with a review of information in the electronic health record (EHR) and information from the primary care provider (PCP) regarding potential biological factors and treatments attempted to date. The BHC's biopsychosocial assessment for ED should include questions to assess timing and factors related to the onset of the problem, the specific context(s) in which ED occurs, thoughts and behaviors that make erectile functioning better and worse, and the effect of ED on functioning and quality of life (Dewitte et al., 2021; Kalogeropoulos & Larouche, 2020; Urology Care Foundation, 2014). Relevant assessment questions could include the following:

- Was the onset of your problem with erections gradual or sudden? What factors do you believe may have contributed to the start of the problem?

- Do you have naturally occurring erections in the morning?

- Can you get an erection by yourself (i.e., via masturbation)?

- Are your problems with erections specific to one particular partner or situation?

- During sexual intercourse, how difficult is it to maintain your erection to complete intercourse?

- Do you have to concentrate to maintain an erection?

- Can you identify any thoughts you have during sex that seem to make it more difficult to keep an erection?

- What medical problems do you have? [Information may be obtained from medical record.]

- What medications are you taking? [Information may be obtained from medical record.]

- Do you use tobacco? If so, how much?

- How many drinks containing alcohol do you consume in a typical week?

- Have you had any injury, surgery, or radiation therapy in the pelvic area?

- Are you experiencing problems with your mood, such as depression, anxiety, or stress?

- Some people have feelings of guilt or anxiety about sex. Tell me how this is for you.

- Have you experienced any sexual trauma, either as a child or as an adult?

- How is your relationship with your partner? Have there been any recent changes in your relationship or changes around the time your erectile problems began?

- How have your problems with erections affected your sex life? Your relationship (if in one)? Your mood or stress level?

- Have the erectile problems led you to avoid or cut back on sexual activity?

- Do you believe your partner would be interested in being involved in this treatment?

Assessing the patient's interest in or history of medical treatments for ED provides useful information for treatment planning. We recommend always reviewing the patient's medical record for medical diagnoses and medications that may affect ED because this typically yields more detailed information than patient self-report of medical history. Discussions with the patient's PCP may also yield useful information regarding potential medical and psychosocial factors impacting erectile functioning, as well as treatment approaches tried.

The Erectile Performance Anxiety Index (Telch & Pujols, 2013), a 10-item validated self-report measure of performance-related anxiety related to erectile dysfunction, may also provide useful information for understanding the potential contribution of anxiety to ED and for tailoring intervention strategies.

Advise

After conducting the assessment, we advise the patient on intervention approaches that might be effective. At this point, we typically introduce two concepts. First, we discuss that it is often not helpful in treatment to draw a sharp line between organic and psychogenic ED and that even ED that is primarily organic in origin has a psychological effect that may perpetuate and worsen the problem. This discussion may decrease concerns about being seen by a behavioral health provider for what the patient may see as a purely physical problem. Second, we share our belief that, in most cases, it is helpful to involve the patient's partner in future appointments. Finally, if patients have a history of being sexually abused or if there is significant dysfunction in the partner relationship, we consider recommending a referral for specialty mental health individual or couples treatment.

Agree

With the proliferation of medical treatments for ED, including medications such as sildenafil (Viagra) and tadalafil (Cialis), patients may be hesitant to engage in behavioral health treatments for ED, preferring a medical management approach to the problem. Sharing with the patient a biopsychosocial conceptualization of the problem, highlighting not only the relevant biological factors influencing ED but also the ways that thoughts, emotions, and behaviors may cause or worsen their experience, may help decrease reluctance to try behavioral health approaches, either alone or in conjunction with medical management.

Assist

The following section describes the interventions we commonly use in primary care for ED, including education, support of medical interventions for ED, sensate focus, communication training, cognitive restructuring and anxiety management, and changing lifestyle habits. As mentioned earlier, we generally prefer to work jointly with the couple rather than with the individual alone.

Education. Many patients experiencing erectile problems may benefit from education regarding general sexuality and ED in particular. Discussing and providing written materials (i.e., handouts or books) on ED definition, risk factors, and treatments; the sexual response cycle; the role of sexual stimulation; male and female sexual anatomy; and specific behavioral strategies for ED is a foundational intervention. Figure 12.1 contains a sample psychoeducational handout for general information about ED. Figure 12.2 lists books and websites we frequently recommend to patients experiencing a variety of sexual problems, including ED. Within this list, the books by McCarthy and McCarthy (2012, 2020) include significant focus on ED and incorporate information and strategies for patients and their partners.

Support of medical intervention. With the increased availability of medical treatment options for ED, BHCs can help patients succeed with treatments that are not as easy as an oral medication, such as penile injections, a urethral suppository, or a vacuum device. BHCs may work with couples on ways to integrate

FIGURE 12.1. Erectile Dysfunction Handout

Erectile Dysfunction

What Is Erectile Dysfunction?
Erectile dysfunction (ED) is a condition in which you are unable to get or keep an erection firm enough for sexual intercourse. ED can be a short-term or long-term problem. Health care professionals, such as primary care providers and urologists, often can treat ED.

How Common Is ED?
ED is very common. It affects about 30 million men in the United States. Although ED is very common, it is not a normal part of aging; talk with your health care professional about treatment.

What Causes ED?
Many different factors affecting your vascular system, nervous system, and endocrine system can cause or contribute to ED.

- The following diseases and conditions can lead to ED: type 2 diabetes; heart and blood vessel disease; atherosclerosis; high blood pressure; chronic kidney disease; multiple sclerosis; Peyronie's disease; injury from treatments for prostate cancer; injury to the penis, spinal cord, prostate, bladder, or pelvis; or surgery for bladder cancer.
- ED can be a side effect of many common medicines, such as blood pressure medicines, antiandrogens, antidepressants, tranquilizers or prescription sedatives, appetite suppressants, or ulcer medications.
- Psychological or emotional factors may make ED worse. You may develop ED if you have one or more of the following: fear of sexual failure, anxiety, depression, guilt about sexual performance or certain sexual activities, low self-esteem, stress about sexual performance, or stress in your life in general.
- The following health-related factors and behaviors may contribute to ED: smoking, drinking too much alcohol, using illegal drugs, being overweight, or not being physically active.

How Is ED Treated?
You can work with health care professionals to treat an underlying cause of your ED. Choosing an ED treatment is a personal decision. However, you also may benefit from talking with your partner about which treatment is best for you as a couple.

- *Lifestyle changes*: Your health care professional may suggest that you make lifestyle changes to help reduce or improve ED. You can quit smoking, limit or stop drinking alcohol, increase physical activity and maintain a healthy body weight, and stop illegal drug use.
- *Counseling*: Talk with your doctor about going to a counselor if psychological or emotional issues are affecting your ED. A counselor can teach you how to lower your anxiety or stress related to sex. Your counselor may suggest that you bring your partner to counseling sessions to learn how to support you. As you work on relieving your anxiety or stress, a doctor can focus on treating the physical causes of ED.
- *Changes to your medicines*: If a medicine you need for another health condition is causing ED, your doctor may suggest a different dose or different medicine. Never stop taking a medicine without speaking with your doctor first.
- *Medicines you take by mouth*: A health care professional may prescribe an oral medicine, or medicine you take by mouth, such as one of the following, to help you get and maintain an erection: sildenafil, vardenafil, tadalafil, or avanafil. A health care professional may prescribe testosterone if you have low levels of this hormone in your blood.
- *Injectable medicines and suppositories*: Some men get stronger erections by injecting a medicine called alprostadil into the penis, causing it to fill with blood. Instead of injecting a medicine, some men insert a suppository of alprostadil into the urethra.
- *A vacuum device*: A vacuum device causes an erection by pulling blood into the penis.
- *Surgery*: For most men, surgery should be a last resort. Talk with your doctor about whether surgery is right for you. A urologist performs surgery to implant a device to make the penis erect, or to rebuild arteries to increase blood flow to the penis.

Note. Adapted from *Erectile Dysfunction* (*ED*), by the National Institute of Diabetes and Digestive and Kidney Diseases, n.d. (https://www.niddk.nih.gov/health-information/urologic-diseases/erectile-dysfunction/all-content). In the public domain.

FIGURE 12.2. Resources for Patients With Sexual Problems Handout: Websites and Books (*continues*)

Type	Location	Description
Websites	American Urological Association: Urology Care Foundation (https://www.urologyhealth.org/)	Urology Care Foundation website provides patients with information in English and Spanish on urologic conditions and sexual conditions, including ED and healthy lifestyles for urologic health. A urology care podcast is also available.
	American Association of Sexuality Educators, Counselors and Therapists (https://www.aasect.org/)	Website primarily designed for use by sexual health professionals. Patients may benefit from the "Locate a Professional" feature to identify sex therapists and counselors certified by the AASECT.
	NIDDK (https://www.niddk.nih.gov/health-information/urologic-diseases/erectile-dysfunction)	Contains information for both health professionals and patients on ED. Detailed patient information focuses on definitions, causes, diagnosis, and treatment of ED. Information is available in English and Spanish.
Books	*The Elusive Orgasm: A Woman's Guide to Why She Can't and How She Can Orgasm* (Cass, 2007)	Written by a clinical psychologist and sex therapist, book provides information on female sexual anatomy, stages of arousal, causes of orgasmic difficulty, and strategies for increasing sexual satisfaction and orgasm.
	Rekindling Desire, 3rd ed. (McCarthy & McCarthy, 2020)	Now in its third edition, book written for couples struggling with low sexual desire includes recommended exercises and strategies for improving relationship and sexual communication, as well as sexual skills, to increase sexual desire and intimacy. It includes clinical case study examples and illustrations.
	Are You Coming? A Vagina Owner's Guide to Orgasm (Hiddinga, 2021)	Aims to assist women in understanding anatomy, orgasm, how to talk about sex, and strategies to achieving orgasm.
	Sexual Awareness: Your Guide to Healthy Couple Sexuality, 5th ed. (McCarthy & McCarthy, 2012)	Now in its fifth edition, book aims to help couples improve their sexual satisfaction. Focus is given to strategies to increase sexual awareness, improve sexual communication, and enhance desire. Psychosocial skill exercises are described.
	Coping With Erectile Dysfunction: How to Regain Confidence and Enjoy Great Sex (Metz & McCarthy, 2004)	Contains information on the nature of ED; physical, social, and psychological factors related to ED; overview of treatment options; and cognitive behavioral treatment strategies. It received a "Self-Help Seal of Merit" from the Association for Behavioral and Cognitive Therapies for its incorporation of evidence-based, cognitive behavioral principles and strategies.

FIGURE 12.2. Resources for Patients With Sexual Problems Handout: Websites and Books (*continued*)

Type	Location	Description
Books (cont'd)	*Coping With Premature Ejaculation: How to Overcome PE, Please Your Partner, and Have Great Sex* (Metz & McCarthy, 2003)	Provides an overview of PE from a biopsychosocial perspective. It provides guidance for couples by using evidence-based strategies to decrease problems with PE.
	Women's Anatomy of Arousal: Secret Maps to Buried Pleasure (Winston, 2010)	Book on female sexuality that won the 2010 "Book of the Year Award" from the AASECT focuses on women's sexual anatomy and strategies/techniques for sexual pleasure and orgasm.
	Sex and Love at Midlife: It's Better Than Ever (Zilbergeld & Zilbergeld, 2010)	Focuses on sexuality and intimacy in couples in midlife. It describes approaches for couples in their 40s and beyond to continue to have satisfying sexual experiences. It includes sections on the sexual effects of physical changes related to aging and health conditions.

Note. ED = erectile dysfunction; AASECT = American Association of Sex Educators, Counselors and Therapists; NIDDK = National Institute of Diabetes and Digestive and Kidney Diseases; PE = premature ejaculation.

these interventions into their sexual behavior in ways that feel comfortable to both partners. Assisting couples in openly discussing their concerns or embarrassment about the treatments may be a first-line intervention. For other couples, discussing ways to have the partner be involved with the intervention (e.g., having the partner give the injection or help with the vacuum device) as part of foreplay can enhance sensuality and arousal.

Sensate focus. Sensate focus, originally developed by Masters and Johnson (1970), continues to receive empirical support and has been increasingly used with diverse populations for both sexual dysfunction and optimizing intimacy (Avery-Clark et al., 2019). Implementing sensate focus interventions with patients in primary care first relies on psychoeducation. Initially, BHCs should ensure that the couple understands the rationale for the proscription on sexual intercourse (i.e., creating a relaxing environment free from demands and expectations for an erection and intercourse), the purpose of the exercise (i.e., to give and receive sensual pleasure in a nondemanding, nonsexual context, to focus on sensations rather than performance), and its progressive nature (i.e., over time, gradually moving from sensual touch to sexual touch of the breasts and/or genitals, to an eventual transition to intercourse). In addition to a discussion of these topics during the appointment, BHCs may want to provide written materials that describe the approach in more detail. Figure 12.3 describes an initial behavioral exercise that we have found useful as a starting point with couples who can then further develop and tailor their

FIGURE 12.3. Sexual Problems and Self-Management Interventions Handout (*continues*)

Sexual Problems and Self-Management Interventions

Sexual problems occur for many people and result from both medical and nonmedical reasons. Sexual problems can include things such as reduced interest in sex, difficulty feeling aroused, not being able to have or keep an erection (for men) or become lubricated (for women), difficulty staying aroused, and/or difficulty having an orgasm.

Medications Can Cause Sexual Side Effects
Medications can affect desire, arousal, and orgasm. The following are some medications that can affect sexual functioning:

- Antidepressants, mood stabilizers, tranquilizers, and other drugs given for anxiety
- Oral contraceptives and hormonal therapies
- Chemotherapy medications
- Alcohol, narcotics, and other controlled substances
- Some medications for treatment of allergies, hypertension, and glaucoma
- Anticonvulsant medications

Medical Problems Can Cause or Worsen Sexual Problems

- Diabetes
- Cardiovascular disease
- Thyroid conditions
- Emphysema
- Sleep loss (i.e., insomnia)
- Chronic pain
- Recent surgery (e.g., mastectomy, hysterectomy, removal of ovaries, prostatectomy)
- Cancer

Relationship Difficulties Can Affect Sexuality

- Dissatisfaction, resentment, or struggles for power or control within the relationship
- Poor communication
- Having different value systems
- Lack of intimacy, emotional expression, or physical affection
- Discrepancies in sexual preferences

Personal and Psychological Factors Can Affect Sexual Functioning

- Fatigue
- Depression
- Anxiety and stress
- Age: As we get older, sexual response slows and we need more stimulation and time.
- Performance anxiety (i.e., fears about sexual response, performance, or loss of control)
- Negative beliefs about sex or certain sexual practices
- Low self-esteem and poor body image
- Narrow or unrealistic standards for sexual interactions

Strategies That Can Help Sexual Problems
On your own:

- Self-exploration and stimulation: This can help you increase awareness of your own body and make it easier to communicate likes and dislikes to your partner.
- Change negative thoughts and assumptions about sex with more positive and realistic thoughts about what feels good and right for you.
- Challenge negative thoughts about your partner by focusing on what is attractive and positive about them.

FIGURE 12.3. Sexual Problems and Self-Management Interventions Handout (*continued*)

- Challenge negative thoughts about yourself by focusing on what is attractive and positive about you.
- Physical exercise: This increases blood flow, reduces tension, enhances body image, and can improve other conditions that hinder sexual functioning.

With your partner:

- Rebuild or establish emotional intimacy.
- Schedule time together when you simply talk to each other. Use the time to share feelings and get reacquainted with what is attractive and unique about your partner.
- Share leisure activities.
- Increase small expressions of affection back into your daily routine (e.g., an affectionate note, phone call, or email; hugs or holding hands).
- Discuss sexual interests, desires, needs, and difficulties when you are *not* engaged in sexual activity.
  - Talk about what is going well and what you would like to be different in the relationship overall, then work together to come up with solutions.
  - Add something new to sexual encounters (e.g., place, position, clothing, erotica).
  - Allow more time for foreplay and provide more partner-guided stimulation.
  - During sexual encounters, focus on sensations rather than thoughts, performance, expectations, and appearances.

Behavioral Exercise

This exercise is designed to help you and your partner learn more about what types of stimulation you like. It also encourages physical intimacy and provides a way for you to give as well as receive pleasure. It is not a prelude to sex and does not include intercourse or orgasm, so there are no sexual performance demands.

- Pick a time and place for you and your partner to be together. Allow at least 1 hour. The place should be private, comfortable, and free of distractions.
- Both partners should, at most, wear comfortable, light underclothes, although you may find being nude more comfortable.
- Without touching genitals, take turns giving and receiving stimulation (e.g., massaging, fondling, caressing). Take about half an hour per partner.
- Each partner should focus on the sensations of touching and being touched.
- The receiving partner should direct the giving partner by providing feedback about what is pleasurable or not or what could be done differently. The giving partner should adjust their stimulation accordingly. Use various strokes (e.g., long, short, soft, hard). Try using the palms, fingertips, and so forth.
- Partners should do only what is comfortable for them and let the other person know when something feels pleasurable or becomes uncomfortable.

Remember, this exercise is designed to increase intimacy and decrease performance expectation, pressure, and anxiety, so NO SEX!

specific activities. We also encourage additional reading to further guide this sensate focus approach (e.g., McCarthy & McCarthy, 2012; Weiner & Avery-Clark, 2017).

Communication training. Some couples may benefit from improving their ability to communicate in an appropriate manner, either on general topics or on those specific to sexuality. Chapter 16 describes PCBH approaches to enhancing couples' communication, and Chapter 4 reviews specifics on developing assertive communication skills. Examples tailored for couples who have difficulty talking about sexual topics appropriately might include statements such as the following:

- I feel unloved when you rush right into sex without cuddling first. I'd like it if you would spend a few minutes snuggling and holding me before we take off our clothes.

- I feel aroused when you gently stroke me right here.

- When you are completely silent during sex, I feel isolated. I'd prefer if you would be a bit more vocal, such as sighing and telling me what feels good.

- When I lose my erection, I feel anxious and embarrassed when you try to directly stimulate my penis right away. I'd like it if you would kiss me and stroke my thighs instead.

- I feel irritated when you approach me for sex so late at night. I'm tired and worry about getting up for work the next morning. I'd really like it if we could agree on some other times of the day for sex, before 11 p.m.

If couples have more severe relationship or communication problems that do not improve with brief intervention, referral for couples therapy and/or sex therapy may be warranted.

Cognitive restructuring and anxiety management. When the evaluation suggests that performance anxiety may be causing or worsening ED, we initiate interventions to change anxious thought patterns. Identifying and modifying inaccurate beliefs about sexual functioning may help decrease unrealistic expectations and performance anxiety. Introducing strategies to identify and change unhelpful thinking can be used when patients describe thoughts that are counterproductive (e.g., "I must be 100% hard to satisfy my partner," "If I lose my erection again, I'll disappoint my partner," "If I can't get an erection soon, my partner will leave me"). Encouraging the patient to focus on sensations or sexual behaviors, rather than alarming thoughts, may also prove beneficial. Finally, we also include training in general relaxation methods (see Chapter 4) to help decrease anxiety and tension and promote relaxation before sexual activity.

Changing lifestyle habits. Use of tobacco and alcohol and poor control of diabetes, weight, and hypertension can cause or worsen problems with erectile dysfunction. A focus on changing problematic health behaviors may be warranted for some patients with ED. Current evidence suggests that losing weight (for individuals with a body mass index greater than 30), increasing exercise, and quitting tobacco may be helpful in improving erectile function (Allen & Walter, 2019; Glina et al., 2013). For those with diabetes or hypertension, strategies to assist with improved control of blood sugar and blood pressure may be warranted (Glina et al., 2013). Specific strategies to assist patients with these health behavior changes can be found in other chapters of this book.

Arrange

Patients with significant partner relationship dysfunction or severe psychological comorbidity affecting ED may not experience improvement from brief PCBH intervention. The BHC may assist in linking them to specialty behavioral health services for continued care. Other patients with less complex presentations may desire to address their ED through accessing self-help materials or online resources. Figure 12.2 includes resources that may be useful. For patients who show improvement with PCBH intervention, we recommend arranging one to two relapse prevention appointments over the course of the ensuing 6 to 12 months to help minimize recurrence of ED.

PREMATURE EJACULATION

PE is characterized by ejaculation that persistently occurs during sexual activity with a partner, shortly after penetration (within approximately 1 minute), earlier than desired, and causes significant distress. The problem must occur during nearly all (approximately 75%–100%) sexual occasions with a partner and persist for at least 6 months. PE should not be diagnosed if the problem is due to severe relationship distress; other significant stressors; another nonsexual mental disorder; or a medical condition, medication, or other substance (American Psychiatric Association, 2022). Although a large percentage (up to 30%) of men worldwide report some concerns with early ejaculation, only approximately 1% to 3% of men meet formal criteria for a diagnosis of PE (American Psychiatric Association, 2022). A distinction is typically made between lifelong and acquired PE.

Key Biopsychosocial Factors

Understanding the biopsychosocial factors associated with PE improves the BHC's ability to assess and treat this disorder. The following review highlights these important factors.

Physical Factors

There exists growing recognition of biological factors in the etiology of PE. Genetic and epigenetic factors appear primary for many patients with lifelong PE. In acquired PE, there is likely a complex interplay of genetic, endocrine, urologic, and psychological factors resulting in the disorder. Biogenic factors can include hyperarousability, penile hypersensitivity, genetic predisposition, and alterations in dopamine and serotonin, among others (American Psychiatric Association, 2022; El-Hamd et al., 2019). Medical conditions that may cause problems with PE include multiple sclerosis, epilepsy, hyperthyroidism, chronic prostatitis, chronic renal insufficiency, and pelvic or neurologic injury. Additionally, side effects of certain medications (e.g., desipramine, cold medications with ephedrine or pseudoephedrine) and withdrawal symptoms from medications or drugs (e.g., trifluoperazine, opiates) may also contribute to PE. More detailed summaries of the literature on PE etiology can be found in El-Hamd et al. (2019) and Althof et al. (2014).

Pharmacological approaches are often used as first-line treatments for PE. Medications prescribed off-label for PE may include topical anesthetics, selective serotonin reuptake inhibitors (SSRIs), and tricyclic antidepressants, taken either daily or on an as needed basis (Althof et al., 2014). A recent Cochrane review of SSRI effectiveness concluded that SSRIs improve a number of meaningful outcomes, including PE symptoms, satisfaction with sex, and perceived control over ejaculation (Sathianathen et al., 2021). Surgical approaches (e.g., cryoablation) and injections are used infrequently due to limited evidence of effectiveness for PE combined with risk of negative outcomes (Althof et al., 2014).

Emotional and Cognitive Factors

Individuals with anxiety, particularly social anxiety, may be more prone to problems with PE (American Psychiatric Association, 2022). Similarly, correlations exist between PE; relationship distress; and psychological problems, including depression, low self-confidence, poor body image, and anxiety (Althof et al., 2014; American Psychiatric Association, 2022; Rowland & Kolba, 2018). The causal direction of these relationships remains unclear, however, and it is likely that they often exert reciprocal influences.

Behavioral Factors

Deficits in psychosexual skills may contribute to PE. Some standard behavioral treatments for PE, such as the stop–start technique (Semans, 1956) and the squeeze technique (Masters & Johnson, 1970), are based on the assumption that individuals with PE do not adequately recognize signs of, or exert control over, ejaculation. A systematic review of controlled clinical trials concluded that these behavioral approaches are effective for PE (Berner & Günzler, 2012).

Environmental Factors

Earlier literature has suggested that male victims of child sexual abuse have twice the risk of developing problems with PE compared with men without an abuse history (Laumann et al., 1999); however, a recent review of studies examining the impact of child sexual abuse on sexual functioning (including ODs) concluded that the literature is inconclusive and that additional, higher quality studies are needed (Gewirtz-Meydan & Opuda, 2022). Problems in current relationships are correlated with PE, although as discussed earlier, it is unclear to what extent these problems cause or result from the problems with PE.

Cultural and Diversity Considerations

The prevalence of PE may increase with age. Cultural differences exist in what is considered normative latency for ejaculation. Additionally, there are measured differences in ejaculatory latency across countries. These differences may be related to cultural, religious, or genetic differences (American Psychiatric Association, 2022).

Specialty Mental Health

The International Society for Sexual Medicine (Althof et al., 2014) guidelines on the treatment of PE recommend inclusion of psychological/behavioral interventions, both to improve the symptoms of PE and to address relational and psychological aspects or consequences of the problem. Psychological treatments for PE may include behavioral approaches to increase ability to delay ejaculation (e.g., stop–start technique, squeeze technique) as well as interventions to address performance anxiety, sexual self-confidence, and interpersonal/relationship issues. The authors noted, however, that the research literature is relatively weak and additional well-designed studies are needed.

Behavioral Health in Primary Care

Despite growing recognition of the value of managing PE with an interprofessional team approach including behavioral health professionals (e.g., Crowdis et al., 2019), interventions for PE through PCBH services have not yet been empirically studied or described in the professional literature. The following discussion represents our adaptation of specialty mental health treatment for PE into our PCBH practices.

Primary Care Adaptation

Adapting the evidence-based techniques for PE to a primary care setting requires the BHC to have knowledge and experience in applying specialty behavioral approaches to PE, skill in educating the patient, and ability to translate specialty behavioral health approaches into effective self-management interventions. Using the 5As structure can be useful in organizing contacts with these patients.

Assess

Review of information in the EHR provides a starting point for assessment of PE. Assessment of relevant biopsychosocial factors for PE in primary care then continues with questions to determine whether problems with PE are lifelong or acquired. This distinction may be helpful in selecting appropriate interventions because consensus guidelines recommend medication use for lifelong PE. Assessment could begin as follows:

> Dr. Jones referred you to me because of some concerns about sexual functioning. Is that your understanding of why you are meeting with me today? [Patient responds affirmatively.] Dr. Jones said that you spoke with him specifically about trouble with premature ejaculation—or "coming" earlier than you would like—when you're having sex with your partner. Is this right? How long has this

been a problem for you? [Patient responds that PE only has been a problem for about 6 months.] What changes can you think of that happened in your life or in your relationship around the time the problem started? Did you have any changes in your health or medications around that time?

Other relevant questions could include the following:

- How much control do you feel you have when you ejaculate?

- Does PE occur in all situations (e.g., with different partners, with masturbation)?

- Do you usually ejaculate before entering your partner, as you enter, or after? How much time passes between when you enter your partner and when you ejaculate? [Modify question as needed on the basis of the response to prior question.]

- What thoughts go through your mind when you are having sex? What do you focus on?

- Have you had difficulty getting erections or getting as hard as you would like during sex?

- What strategies have you tried to help yourself "last longer"?

- How would you describe your relationship with your partner?

- How has PE affected your sex life?

- How has PE affected your relationship?

- What health problems do you have? What medications do you take? [Information may be obtained from the EHR.]

- How has your mood been lately? Have you felt down or depressed much of the time? Anxious or stressed?

BHCs may wish to supplement their clinical interview with the use of a standardized measure. The Premature Ejaculation Diagnostic Tool (Symonds et al., 2007) is a brief, self-report inventory measuring severity of problems with PE that can quickly be completed by patients before the behavioral health consultation.

Advise

If a medical evaluation has not been conducted, particularly if the onset of PE is recent, we advise the referring provider to rule out any medical problems or medications that may be contributing to problems with controlling ejaculation. We also discuss with the PCP whether any medications have been considered or tried with the patient. We typically advise that the patient and their partner attend several BHC appointments to learn specific behavioral skills that may help improve control over ejaculation, as well as communication and relationship skills that may decrease distress and negative impact of PE. We discuss that although there is some evidence that behavioral methods might be helpful in reducing PE, effectiveness is not guaranteed, and we encourage the patient to continue working with their PCP on potential medication approaches that might also help. We strongly encourage partners to attend the appointments. Although the patient can complete some aspects of the intervention themselves, other aspects require cooperation from the sexual partner (e.g., transitioning from use of the squeeze technique, discussed later, during masturbation to using the method during intercourse).

Agree

Reaching agreement on the goals of the intervention may be hampered by unrealistic expectations. It is common for patients with PE to believe that they should be able to have complete control over the timing of their ejaculation or that they should always be able to postpone it indefinitely, even during long periods of intense stimulation. Identifying these unhelpful beliefs and working to develop more reasonable goals and measures of success may help prevent early discouragement and subsequent abandonment of efforts to change.

Assist

The intervention components we use with patients experiencing PE include education, sensate focus, stop–start and squeeze techniques, and relationship interventions, consistent with International Society for Sexual Medicine recommendations (Althof et al., 2014).

Education. We typically begin work with a patient and partner, if available, by providing psychoeducation regarding sexual functioning, behavior, and attitudes. Normalizing problems with PE (i.e., by emphasizing that they are not alone, that PE is the most common sexual problem men experience) can help reduce embarrassment and reluctance to talk about their experiences. We routinely discuss the nature and physiology of the sexual response cycle. We highlight the differences between the two stages of ejaculation, emission (i.e., when seminal fluid enters the urethra) and expulsion (i.e., when seminal fluid is expelled from the penis), and discuss whether the patient can recognize the sensations that immediately precede emission, as the ability to identify precursors to emission is key in using the stop–start technique described later. Finally, we highlight the role thoughts play in the sexual response cycle, with mental focus influencing arousal. Metz and McCarthy's (2004) self-help book for PE, although an older publication, can still provide patients with greater depth of information, as well as a series of home-based strategies for PE.

Stop–start and squeeze techniques. The goal of the stop–start and squeeze techniques, described initially by Semans (1956) and Masters and Johnson (1970), is to learn to recognize signs of impending emission and then do something different to decrease the physical and/or mental stimulation leading to ejaculation and hence improve control over its timing. We rely on an approach initially described by D. C. Polonsky (2000). Figure 12.4 is the handout we use with patients. In implementing this approach, we initially advise the patient to masturbate without lubrication. When the patient notices sensations indicating they are close to emission, the patient should stop masturbating and, if helpful, firmly squeeze the penis at the juncture between the head and the shaft or at the base. After waiting for the sensations to lessen (about 1 minute), the patient should begin masturbating again. This cycle is repeated several times. With practice, the patient will learn more about their own sensations as well as how to control them through changes in stimulation. The patient may then progress to exercises involving continuous stimulation (i.e., rather than stopping or squeezing) but at varied or lower levels (e.g., slowing down the masturbation

FIGURE 12.4. Gaining Control Over Premature Ejaculation Handout

Improving Premature Ejaculation

Many men experiencing problems with premature ejaculation (PE) see improvements after learning and practicing specific behavioral skills alone and with their partner. These skills can be broken down into four steps:

Step One: "Stop/Start" Masturbation Without Lubrication

- Masturbate without lubrication until you feel close to ejaculating.
- STOP. Wait 1 minute and allow sensations to subside. You may find that squeezing your penis (at the base or where the shaft meets the head) between your thumb and forefinger helps delay ejaculation.
- Resume masturbation. Repeat cycle several times before allowing yourself to ejaculate.
- Practice several times per week until you find greater control over delaying ejaculation.

Step Two: Masturbation Without Lubrication

- Masturbate without lubrication until you feel close to ejaculating.
- Rather than stopping, experiment with varying the types of stimulation (e.g., slow down or lighten strokes) to delay ejaculation. Keep arousal high but still controlled.
- Repeat cycle several times before allowing yourself to ejaculate.
- Practice several times per week.

Step Three: Masturbation With Lubrication

- Practice Steps 1 and 2 above, but with the addition of lubrication (which typically increases sensations of pleasure).

Step Four: Intercourse With Partner

- Use the same basic steps learned earlier for controlling ejaculation, while progressing to intercourse with your partner.
- When you feel you are close to ejaculating, stop thrusting or moving.
- Wait a minute for arousal level to decrease. Squeeze the base of your penis if this is helpful. Repeat the cycle several times before ejaculating.
- Ask what you can do for your partner.

Remember: Practice is needed to help develop skills in controlling ejaculation. Even with practice, it is not realistic to expect successful control 100% of the time. Keep a balanced perspective, remember that setbacks are expected, and return to practicing these exercises when needed.

rhythm) to keep arousal levels high but still controlled. After the patient has achieved greater control over ejaculation with the prior exercises, they may add a lubricant while masturbating, which typically increases pleasurable sensations. We advise the patient to practice these exercises at least three times per week.

The final phase involves intercourse between the patient and their partner. If the partner has not yet attended an appointment with the patient, we encourage the patient to allow the partner to come in for joint consultation at this point in the intervention. We stress the need for open communication about PE and the behavioral techniques being used. The couple is advised to initially continue to use the stop–start or squeeze techniques during intercourse. When the patient feels sensations indicating emission is close, the patient either stops thrusting or squeezes the base of the penis until sensations decrease. When movement is resumed, it should be slow. This cycle is repeated several times before the patient allows themself to ejaculate. The couple should then discuss what the partner would like in terms of sexual stimulation before ending the encounter.

Relationship interventions. Communication skills between partners, particularly regarding sexuality, may need to be improved. The couples communication strategies discussed in Chapters 4 and 16 may be useful for couples with PE. One theme unique to PE that may need to be addressed involves the partner's perception of the cause of the PE. It is common to find that the partner harbors the belief that the PE is somehow due to the patient's selfishness and lack of concern for the partner's pleasure. This may lead to resentment and further relationship problems. In this situation, we work with couples to openly communicate their beliefs about the cause of PE and the effect PE has on the partner. We discuss the complex interplay of biopsychosocial factors contributing to PE, and we also may provide recommendations for the couple to enhance the partner's pleasure during sexual interactions.

Arrange

As mentioned previously, not all patients benefit from brief psychoeducation and behaviorally based interventions in the primary care setting. Patients whose PE involves more complex etiology (e.g., significant comorbid psychological or relationship problems) may require more intensive specialty mental health services (e.g., sex therapy, cognitive behavioral therapy, relationship counseling). BHCs will want to develop an awareness of local resources for these services and recommend referral if it becomes apparent that a higher level of care is necessary for improvement of PE.

FEMALE ORGASMIC DISORDER

Female OD is defined as marked delay, infrequency, or absence of orgasm. The problem must occur for approximately 6 months in nearly all (75%–100%)

sexual occasions and cause significant distress. OD should not be diagnosed if it is directly caused by medical conditions, medications or substances, or a mental disorder or if it is associated with severe relationship distress (e.g., partner violence). Reports of orgasmic difficulty in women vary widely, ranging from 8% to 72%. Prevalence rates using strict diagnostic criteria of OD may be in the lower range given the diagnostic criterion for significant distress (American Psychiatric Association, 2022).

Key Biopsychosocial Factors

As with ED and PE, understanding the biopsychosocial factors that contribute to female OD help the BHC operate more effectively in the primary care environment. This knowledge can help improve patient education and communication with PCPs.

Physical Factors

Medical problems (e.g., spinal cord injury, multiple sclerosis, pelvic nerve damage, vulvovaginal atrophy) and medications (e.g., SSRIs) can impair ability to achieve orgasm. Genetic factors may also play a role in vulnerability to OD, whereas menopausal status is not consistently associated with orgasmic problems (American Psychiatric Association, 2022). There currently are no medications approved by the Food and Drug Administration for female OD, although a limited number of small studies and case reports have suggested possible benefit from testosterone, bupropion (i.e., Wellbutrin), and sildenafil citrate, which may be prescribed off-label (see summary by Wheeler & Guntupalli, 2020).

Emotional and Cognitive Factors

Negative attitudes about sex, high levels of guilty feelings about sex, sexual inhibition, and fears of performance failure are associated with orgasmic difficulty and should be assessed when a patient presents with possible OD (Laan et al., 2013; Tavares et al., 2018). In a summary of contributing factors, Marchand (2021) similarly noted that psychosocial factors play a significant role in many cases of OD. Such factors may include negative views of female sexuality, limited information or inaccurate beliefs about sexuality and orgasm, depression, anxiety/stress, poor body image or self-esteem, and feelings of shame or guilt regarding sex, among others.

Behavioral Factors

Lack of appropriate sexual stimulation from a partner, limited experience with masturbation, and limited skill with specific sexual techniques that may enhance arousal and orgasm have been cited as potential contributors to female orgasmic difficulty (Laan et al., 2013; Marchand, 2021).

Environmental Factors

Women who have experienced sexual abuse or trauma may be more likely to experience problems with orgasm (American Psychiatric Association, 2022; Marchand, 2021). Current intimate relationship problems, poor communication, low sexual skills in a partner, and family attitudes toward sexuality also may contribute to orgasmic difficulty (Marchand, 2021).

Diversity Factors

Cultural factors influence the extent to which orgasmic difficulty is seen as problematic or causes significant distress. Additionally, gender role expectations, religious factors, and generational differences may affect a patient's expectations and experiences regarding orgasm (American Psychiatric Association, 2022; Laan et al., 2013). Studies have found that lesbian women report experiencing fewer difficulties with orgasm in comparison with heterosexual women (Frederick et al., 2018; Garcia et al., 2014).

Specialty Mental Health

A recent review of behavioral and psychological treatment approaches for female OD (Marchand, 2021) indicated that lifelong OD can successfully be treated with directed (or guided) masturbation training. Directed masturbation training yielded significant positive outcomes, with 50% to 100% of women with lifelong OD achieving orgasm with masturbation and 33% to 85% achieving orgasm with a partner (Marchand, 2021). Based on these outcomes, directed masturbation training was recommended as a first-line intervention.

Other approaches that may yield success (with lower efficacy) include systematic desensitization and sensate focus. Orgasmic difficulties that appear primarily related to anxiety about sexual situations and activities may respond to systematic desensitization using a hierarchy of feared sexual situations, although outcomes and study quality vary considerably. Sensate focus included as an adjunct to other approaches may also yield positive results for some patients, particularly those experiencing difficulty achieving orgasm with a partner (Marchand, 2021).

Finally, it should be noted that acquired (vs. lifelong) OD may be more difficult to treat. If onset appears related to complex problems such as sexual trauma or significant relationship difficulties, interventions may need to focus on these areas.

Behavioral Health in Primary Care

No studies examining the effect of brief behavioral health consultation in primary care settings on female OD could be identified. However, a number of effective specialty-based approaches, including behavioral techniques such as psychoeducation, sensate focus, directed masturbation training, and cognitive approaches, may be readily adapted for brief primary care consultative interventions.

Primary Care Adaptation

Structuring the assessment and intervention using the 5As format can promote efficiency in information collection and effectiveness in intervention for this potentially sensitive subject. Next, we detail how to use the 5As for successful BHC–patient interaction.

Assess

Functional assessment of female OD should include assessment of the ways in which physical, emotional, cognitive, behavioral, and environmental factors may contribute to the onset or maintenance of the orgasmic difficulties. Figure 12.5 summarizes recommended assessment questions for female OD. Inquiring about medications (e.g., antidepressants, antihypertensives, benzodiazepines, neuroleptics, opioids), use of substances (e.g., alcohol), and medical problems (e.g., back problems, nerve damage, multiple sclerosis, diabetic neuropathy, history of abdominal surgery, hysterectomy, vascular disease) can help determine whether physical factors may be contributing to problems achieving orgasm. A review of the EHR and discussion with the patient's PCP may provide information on many of these areas. Particularly close attention to the

FIGURE 12.5. Sample Assessment Questions for Female Orgasmic Disorder

- Have you ever experienced an orgasm?
- When did your problems with having an orgasm develop?
- Were there changes in your health, relationships, or other areas when the problem began?
- During what types of sexual activity have you had orgasms (e.g., masturbation, intercourse, oral sex)?
- Do you always have trouble achieving orgasm or just in specific situations?
- Do you experience any pain with intercourse?
- Have you had any unwanted sexual experiences? (If so, how do you believe this has affected your sexuality?)
- What are your views or thoughts on masturbation?
- How often do you do or experience the following?
  - Feel sexual desire? Find you are interested in sex?
  - Engage in sexual activity, including masturbation?
  - Become aroused with a partner? Through masturbation?
  - Experience orgasm with a partner? Through masturbation?
  - Feel satisfied by your sexual experience?
- What medications or substances do you use?
- What medical conditions do you have?
- Are you aware of any concerns or thoughts that might be interfering with having orgasms?
- Are you having conflicts or problems in your relationship?
- Do you feel down or sad much of the time? Have you lost interest in activities you enjoyed?
- How often do you feel anxious or stressed?
- What do you think is contributing to your difficulties with achieving orgasm?

possible role of physical factors should be given when a patient's OD is acquired rather than lifelong. Similarly, close assessment of environmental factors (e.g., current relationship problems, recent sexual trauma) is warranted when a patient who previously was able to achieve orgasm presents with new orgasmic difficulties.

Advise

The advice given to patients regarding treatment options varies on the basis of information gathered in the assessment, particularly the evaluation of which biopsychosocial factors are most relevant in the onset and maintenance of the orgasmic difficulties. If it appears that health problems or medications may be involved but this has not yet been medically evaluated, we advise patients and the PCP to assess the extent to which physical factors are playing a significant role in the orgasmic dysfunction before working with these patients further. If the etiology seems largely related to significant relationship problems, we typically advise that the patient participate in interventions that initially focus on improving the couple's relationship, either BHC-provided services or through a specialty mental health referral if the severity of the relationship distress is high or if improvements do not occur with BHC interventions. If significant psychological problems such as posttraumatic stress disorder or depression appear largely responsible for the OD, as may be the case with acquired OD, we often advise the patient to receive treatment for these problems before explicitly focusing on treatment of OD. Depending on the nature of the problem, we again would either recommend follow-up with BHC services (e.g., in the case of mild to moderate depression) or advise that the PCP consider a referral for specialty mental health treatment (e.g., in the case of posttraumatic stress disorder or severe depression or if symptoms do not approve with BHC interventions). Patients presenting with lifelong OD that appears related to a lack of sexual knowledge, skills, or experience seem to be the best candidates for brief psychoeducational and behavioral interventions that can be accomplished in primary care. We typically advise these patients to continue services through the BHC.

Agree

The core intervention for female OD, as discussed previously, involves masturbation training. The degree to which patients feel comfortable with an approach founded on masturbation varies greatly. Personal, cultural, and religious beliefs may influence whether a patient is open to this form of intervention. Therefore, as BHCs are attempting to reach agreement with patients on the goals of intervention and the specific strategies used to reach these goals, it is critical to assess a patient's views on masturbation and their willingness to engage in this type of intervention. Providing detailed rationale for how masturbation training may help with the problem can be helpful in many instances. Treatment approaches need to be modified for patients who strongly oppose masturbation. For example, if a patient is unwilling to masturbate, BHCs might work with the couple to increase skills and comfort with sexual experimentation and communication (e.g., open discussion about what types of sexual touch are most stimulating), to minimize thoughts that interfere with sexual assertiveness or that increase anxiety, or to increase use of sexual fantasy.

Assist

The interventions we use most frequently with female patients with OD include psychoeducation, masturbation training, sexual communication, and sensate focus.

Psychoeducation. We provide psychoeducation aimed at increasing knowledge about physiology, the sexual response cycle, types of stimulation that often produce pleasure, and the role of cognition in enhancing arousal and orgasm. Exploring myths that patients may hold about orgasm can provide an opportunity to develop helpful beliefs about sexuality. Figure 12.6 is a handout that we use to facilitate discussion with patients about beliefs they may hold that might perpetuate their problems with OD. Having anatomical models or diagrams available in the clinic can aid in educating patients about relevant anatomy and ensuring that patients and partners are communicating accurately about anatomy. We also routinely recommend that patients engage in additional psychoeducational reading about female OD, which we can then incorporate in a guided self-help format. The list of readings in Figure 12.2 contains material specifically written for improving female sexuality and OD.

FIGURE 12.6. Developing Helpful Beliefs for Enhancing Arousal and Orgasm Handout

Developing Helpful Beliefs for Enhancing Arousal and Orgasm

Unhelpful belief	Helpful belief
It is my partner's job to give me an orgasm.	I can take control of my own sexuality and pleasure.
The only acceptable method of reaching an orgasm is through intercourse.	Intercourse is just one way to have an orgasm. An orgasm through rubbing, oral sex, or using a vibrator has the same physiological response and can give me pleasure.
An orgasm is the most important aspect of sexuality.	An orgasm is one aspect of my sexuality. I can enjoy desire and emotional satisfaction without an orgasm.
I should be able to have an orgasm every time I have sex.	It is not realistic to expect an orgasm every time. The majority of women do not have an orgasm each time they have sex. Sexuality is complex and variable. I can enjoy the sexual experience even without an orgasm.
If I tell my partner what I want, I'll be seen as "pushy" or "slutty."	My partner wants to give me pleasure. By talking about our desires, we can both increase our arousal and pleasure.

Masturbation training. A core intervention, guided masturbation training gives patients the opportunity to learn about their own sexual preferences and responses and to discover what types of stimulation may lead to orgasm. We typically begin with a discussion of the patient's prior history of how or if the patient has masturbated in the past. We encourage patients to consider various approaches to masturbation, including using different pressures, rhythms, and speeds with manual stimulation; using a vibrator; or experimenting with rhythmically tightening and relaxing the pelvic floor muscles (i.e., as in Kegel exercises) and the leg muscles. We often encourage the patient to incorporate sexual fantasy during masturbation, particularly if anxiety or self-consciousness is present. Self-help books for female sexuality and orgasm (see Figure 12.2) can provide patients with more detailed exercises and can be integrated into BHC interventions in a guided self-help approach.

Sexual communication. As patients transition from masturbation to sexual activity with a partner, communication about sexual preferences is essential. Some patients may benefit from interventions to increase their ability to discuss sexual matters and preferences openly. Assertive communication training (see discussion earlier in this chapter and in Chapter 4) can be incorporated to increase patient comfort in telling their partners the types of sexual stimulation they like and do not like or the types of sexual behavior they might like to try.

Sensate focus. Sensate focus exercises may be a helpful adjunct to treatment with certain subsets of patients with OD, particularly those who experience sexual anxiety or who may have more difficulties with orgasm in partnered sexual situations (Marchand, 2021). If these factors appear to play a role in the maintenance of OD, we incorporate sensate focus as an intervention. See the discussion of sensate focus earlier in this chapter, as well as Figure 12.3, for additional information.

Arrange

As discussed previously, we are more likely to initially coordinate a referral for specialty mental health treatment of female OD when the patient presents with acquired (vs. lifelong) problems achieving orgasm. Patients with lifelong OD who do not benefit from the PCBH intervention described earlier are considered for referral to specialty care.

SUMMARY

Sexual dysfunctions affect the functioning and quality of life of substantial numbers of individuals. With greater availability of medical treatments for some of the sexual dysfunctions (e.g., medication for ED), primary care medical providers are seeing larger numbers of individuals presenting with sexual dysfunction concerns. However, medical providers may not feel adequately prepared to offer treatment that incorporates more than medication or surgery. BHCs can offer a unique service by conducting a biopsychosocial evaluation and tailoring recommendations for intervention to target underlying cognitive, emotional, behavioral, and environmental factors that may be causing or maintaining sexual dysfunction. As outlined in this chapter, evidence-based specialty mental health interventions can be tailored to be consistent with a brief, structured PCBH model. Additional research is needed to better understand the impact of PCBH approaches for these sexual dysfunctions.

13

Special Considerations for Older Adults

American adults aged 65 years and older (i.e., older adults) accounted for 16% of the U.S. population in 2019 and are expected to represent 21.6% of the U.S. population by 2040 (Administration on Aging, 2021). The vast majority (96%) of older adults have a usual place for medical care (Administration on Aging, 2021). Although it is commonly assumed that older adults are seen in internal medicine clinics, family medicine physicians provide care from "cradle to grave," and as many as 25% of patients seen in family medicine clinics are over 65 years old. Often older age is associated with illness and poor functioning; however, only one quarter of older adults rate their health as "fair" or "poor" (Martinez & Clarke, 2021). For those older adults who require medical care, this care can become quite complex. Over 60% of older adults are diagnosed with at least two chronic medical conditions (Santo & Okeyode, 2018). Among older adults in the United States, 20% meet criteria for a mental health diagnosis; 13% reported taking medicine for worry, nervousness, or anxiety; and 12% reported taking medication for depression (Administration on Aging, 2021; B. D. Carpenter et al., 2022). Suicide is higher for men aged 70 years or older compared with any other demographic, and suicide rates for women between 45 and 74 years old are rising the fastest (B. D. Carpenter et al., 2022). When working in primary care settings, it is essential to have the breadth of knowledge and resources available to provide appropriate recommendations for helping to successfully manage the health care of older adults.

https://doi.org/10.1037/0000380-014

Integrated Behavioral Health in Primary Care: Step-by-Step Guidance for Assessment and Intervention, Third Edition, by C. L. Hunter, J. L. Goodie, M. S. Oordt, and A. C. Dobmeyer

CULTURAL AND DIVERSITY CONSIDERATIONS

The older adult population in the United States is expanding in diversity. In 2019, 24% of older adults belonged to racial or ethnic minority groups (Administration on Aging, 2021); it is expected that over 28% of the U.S. older adult population will belong to a racial or minority group by 2030, and 42% will belong to these groups by 2050 (Centers for Disease Control and Prevention [CDC], 2013b). Among those 65 and older in 2019, 9% were non-Hispanic African Americans, 9% were of Hispanic origin, 5% were Asian American, 0.6% were Native American or Alaska Natives, 0.1% were Native Hawaiian or Pacific Islanders, and 0.8% identified as being of two or more races (Administration on Aging, 2021). Although poverty rates among older U.S. adults are lower than among the 18- to 64-year-old population, many older adults (8.9% in 2019) live below the poverty level, especially non-White older adults. In comparison with 6.8% of White older adults who live below the poverty line, 17.1% of Hispanic, 18% of African American, and 9.3% of Asian American older adults live below the poverty level (Administration on Aging, 2021). Currently and in the future, it will be critical for individuals working with older adults to be aware of the cultural as well as financial factors that may affect assessments and the delivery of health care.

SPECIALTY MENTAL HEALTH

Over a third of psychologists report that they see older adults in their practice "frequently" or "very frequently"; however, only 1.2% of these psychologists describe their primary specialty as geropsychology (Moye et al., 2019). The American Psychological Association (APA) updated its guidelines to assist practitioners in their evaluation of their skills and readiness to work with an older adult population (APA, 2014). These 21 guidelines address areas including competence and attitudes about older adults; knowledge about adult development, aging, and older adults; clinical issues (e.g., cognitive changes, problems in daily living, psychopathology); assessment; interventions and consultations; and continuing education (APA, 2014). Although most psychologists work in specialty mental health settings, these guidelines are useful for any behavioral health provider working in primary care. The Pikes Peak Geropsychology Knowledge and Skill Assessment Tool (Karel et al., 2012) can help behavioral health practitioners self-assess their competence and learning needs. Links to this tool and other resources for clinicians and older adults are available at https://gerocentral.org/.

BEHAVIORAL HEALTH IN PRIMARY CARE

Integrating behavioral health providers into primary care increases the likelihood that older adults will engage in behavioral health services (Bartels et al.,

2004). Primary care clinicians indicated that the integration of behavioral health professionals into the primary care setting enhances the behavioral health care of older adults (Gallo et al., 2004), and others have highlighted the value of using the primary care behavioral health model to target the needs of older adults, particularly in rural settings (Ogbeide et al., 2016). In this chapter, we highlight some of the presenting problems seen more frequently in primary care settings, such as problems with cognitive impairment and incontinence. These concerns are not unique to older adults but tend to be more common among this cohort. We briefly discuss special considerations for caregiver burden, depression and anxiety, sexual functioning, and social role changes and bereavement. Finally, we discuss practical adaptations for the care of older adults in primary care. Anytime a behavioral health consultant (BHC) is working with an older adult, regardless of the presenting problem, it is important to be mindful of signs of elder abuse (e.g., depressed, withdrawn, isolated, unexplained bruising, changes in spending) and mistreatment (e.g., physical, neglect, financial, emotional, abandonment). Among cognitively intact older adults, 9.5% experience mistreatment each year, and this number is likely higher among those with poorer health, racial and ethnic minorities, and those changing from coresiding with someone to living alone (Burnes et al., 2021). Additional information on elder abuse is available from the National Institute on Aging (n.d.) and the CDC (2021c).

COGNITIVE IMPAIRMENT

Among those 65 years of age and older, it is estimated that 5 million experience dementia and that this number will climb to 14 million by 2060 (CDC, 2019). Although concern about dementia among older adults is common, between 26% and 76% of cases go undiagnosed in primary care (Aldus et al., 2020; Holsinger et al., 2007). Alzheimer's disease is commonly cited as the reason for dementia; however, other medical conditions, including cerebrovascular diseases (e.g., strokes) and Parkinson's disease, can be associated with impaired cognitive functioning. In addition, mild cognitive impairment, which may not affect instrumental activities of daily living (IADLs) but may help to predict dementia, is important to detect. It is estimated that 10% to 20% of older adults experience mild cognitive impairment. Aside from dementia and mild cognitive impairment, normal aging is often associated with a decline in cognitive abilities, including processing speed, reasoning, and memory (Salthouse, 2019).

Assess

One challenge associated with memory complaints is distinguishing whether problems with memory are associated with dementia, depression, delirium, and medication side effects or reflect normal aging. A variety of standardized measures can help providers assess the extent of cognitive impairment; however, many of these measures are not easily adaptable to the context of a primary care visit. Often the main goal when assessing memory problems in primary care is to determine whether the patient is experiencing a significant cognitive impairment that needs further assessment in a specialty clinic by a neuropsychologist, neurologist, or geriatrician.

A systematic review of brief screening measures for dementia found that the Montreal Cognitive Assessment (MoCA), Mini-Mental State Examination (MMSE), and Clock Drawing Test have good sensitivity and specificity for distinguishing between normal cognition and Alzheimer's-type dementia (Fink et al., 2020). Although the U.S. Preventive Services Task Force concluded that there is insufficient evidence to determine the benefits and harms among community-dwelling, asymptomatic adults (Owens et al., 2020), these brief screenings can be useful for guiding assessments in primary care for those concerned about cognitive impairment.

The MoCA assesses visuospatial/executive functioning, naming, memory, attention, language, abstraction, delayed recall, and orientation domains. Scores of 26 or higher out of 30 are considered normal; the test takes approximately 10 minutes to administer. Although the MoCA is available for no cost at https://www.mocatest.org in a variety of languages, including versions for blind individuals and administration by phone, there is a fee for training, certification, and then recertification every 2 years to administer the MoCA. The MoCA can also be administered using an electronic tablet. Systematic reviews of evidence related to the MoCA confirm that it has high sensitivity (90%) for detecting Alzheimer's and other dementias but lower rates of specificity (60%; D. H. Davis et al., 2015; Ozer et al., 2016). Comparisons between the MoCA and the MMSE have found that the MoCA is more sensitive for detecting neurocognitive declines (Siqueira et al., 2019)

The MMSE (Folstein et al., 1975) is one of the most widely used measures for screening for cognitive functioning in older adults. The test consists of 30 questions assessing orientation, registration, attention and calculation, recall, and language. The MMSE is brief (i.e., it takes approximately 5–10 minutes to administer) and has extensive research examining its use. Overall studies have shown the MMSE to have a sensitivity of 88.3% and specificity of 86.2% using cutoffs of 23/24 or 24/25 for detecting dementia (Lin et al., 2013). Nasreddine et al. (2005) examined the validity and reliability of the MoCA for assessing mild cognitive impairment and Alzheimer's disease. The MoCA demonstrated 90% and 100% sensitivity for detecting mild cognitive impairment and Alzheimer's, compared with the 18% and 78% sensitivity of the MMSE. Specificity was 87% for the MoCA and 100% for the MMSE. The MMSE can be ordered from Psychological Assessment Resources Inc. (http://www.minimental.com/).

The Clock Drawing Test is a measure of executive functioning (e.g., how well an individual can plan behaviors). According to Shulman (2000), the most common method of conducting the Clock Drawing Test includes the following steps:

1. Hand the patient a predrawn 4-inch diameter circle.

2. State, "This circle represents a clock face. Please put in the numbers so that it looks like a clock and then set the time to 10 minutes past 11."

There are a variety of ways to score the Clock Drawing Test and a wide range of sensitivity (67%–98%) and specificity (69%–94%) estimates for dementia (Lin et al., 2013). One of the quickest scoring methods is to divide the clock into four quadrants by drawing a line between the 12 and the 6 and then a perpendicular line between the 3 and the 9 to divide the circle into four equal quadrants. Errors in the first through third quadrant are assigned a 1, and an error in the fourth quadrant is assigned a 4. Scores of 4 and higher are considered clinically significant and indicate that more extensive testing should be performed. Essentially, a clock drawing with any significant abnormalities is a cue that more testing is needed. Harvan and Cotter (2006) recommended the combined use of the MMSE and the Clock Drawing Test, which has demonstrated the best sensitivity (100%) and specificity (91%) to screen for dementia in primary care settings (Yamamoto et al., 2004).

In addition to these measures, the Saint Louis University Mental Status Exam (Tariq et al., 2006), the Short Portable Mental Status Exam (Pfeiffer, n.d., 1975), and the Short Blest Exam (Katzman et al., 1983) are cognitive functioning screening measures that are easy to administer and demonstrated good validity and reliability.

When screening for cognitive problems, clinicians often ask the patient about the changes that they have noticed. However, asking patients to remember what they are forgetting may not be the most effective method to screen for cognitive decline. It can be helpful to review the electronic health record for any history of problems related to cognitive functioning. Asking family members about a patient's memory problems is more likely to elicit accurate information about decline than a patient's self-report (D. B. Carr et al., 2000; Holsinger et al., 2007). The 16-item Informant Questionnaire on Cognitive Decline in the Elderly (Jorm, 1994) may assist with guiding a brief assessment with family members. Behavioral and emotional problems (e.g., depressive symptoms, social withdrawal, paranoia, sleep disturbance) may be present before changes in memory are evident (Jost & Grossberg, 1996). To screen for memory problems, talk with family members and ask the following:

- What have you noticed your dad forgetting? Does he forget your name? The names of people he knows well? What are some examples?

- Does he get lost easily, including in places that he has been to before?

- Does he have difficulty operating common appliances? Has he left the stove on? Is this a change for him?

- Does his mood change frequently? Is this unusual for him?

- Have you noticed changes in his behavior or thinking, such as not spending time with others, hopelessness, or paranoia? Have you noticed changes in his sleeping patterns?

It is also valuable to ask about activities of daily living (ADLs; Katz et al., 1963), those activities that are essential for self-management (e.g., bathing, walking, climbing stairs), and IADLs (Lawton & Brody, 1969), which are higher level skills (e.g., shopping, managing money, using public transportation). Some questions BHCs can ask about ADLs include the following:

- Can they bathe themselves?

- Do they brush their teeth?

- Can they dress themselves?

- Can they use the bathroom on their own?

- Do they have any difficulties feeding themselves?

- Do they walk on their own without assistance?

- Can they climb stairs on their own?

  Some questions you could ask about IADLs include the following:

- Do they do their own cooking? Shopping?

- Do they keep their living area or home clean?

- How do they get around when they want to go somewhere?

- Have they had difficulties managing their money? Do they pay bills on time?

- Do they take their medication on their own?

With these questions, BHCs are looking for changes in functioning. Dementia is usually associated with gradual changes, unless there has been a sudden event, such as a stroke. Loss of ADLs implies that a significant dementia may be present. Skill deficits may become suddenly apparent when a caregiver becomes incapacitated or dies. For example, an individual who relied on their spouse to cook and clean may not be able to prepare their own meals and maintain their living space.

When assessing cognitive functioning, it is important to consider possible contributions of depressive symptoms. Depression can be an early sign of cognitive decline (S. Bennett & Thomas, 2014), and it can be difficult to distinguish whether changes in cognitive functioning are associated with depression or dementia. Typically, individuals who are depressed rather than showing signs of dementia are less likely to be disoriented and are less likely to have impairments with writing, speaking, or motor skills. The onset of cognitive decline is more rapid in depression, and those who are depressed are more likely to notice and remember their memory lapses (Harvard Health Publishing, 2022).

Increases in apathy (i.e., decreased motivation and goal-directed behavior) have been found to be associated with increased dementia severity and an overall poorer prognosis compared with depressive symptoms (Connors et al., 2022). Integrating questions about orientation, skills deficits, progression of symptoms, examples of what has been forgotten, and apathy may be helpful for guiding how BHCs advise and assist patients. We discuss depression among older adults later in this chapter. Additionally, medical problems can result in cognitive impairments. For example, urinary tract infections can cause sudden and unexplained changes in cognitive functioning and behavior. Therefore, it is always important to collaborate with the primary care provider (PCP) to rule out possible medical factors that may contribute to cognitive impairment.

Impairments in cognitive and behavioral functioning can affect an individual's ability to make decisions that are necessary to sustain an independent lifestyle (e.g., managing health and finances). Determining someone's capacity to make decisions requires balancing clinical, legal, and ethical concerns because the consequences of finding someone incapacitated may result in the appointment of a surrogate decision maker (Moye et al., 2006). Although in the past a distinction was made between competence (i.e., a legal determination) and capacity (i.e., an informal evaluation), the legal system has increasingly adopted the term "capacity" (Moye et al., 2006). Formal capacity evaluations are unlikely to be performed in the primary care setting, but BHCs should be aware of the factors that are important in the determination of capacity because many informal decisions about capacity are made in this setting. Information about formal capacity evaluations can be found in the publication by the American Bar Association (ABA) and APA (ABA & APA, 2008). This handbook includes a variety of resources for individuals working with older adults, including a list of legal and social interventions to consider if someone is demonstrating diminished capacity. Determinations about capacity are increasingly more specific (i.e., rather than global) and can include a variety of areas, including medical consent, sexual consent, financial, testamentary (i.e., the capacity to make a will), driving, and independent living (ABA & APA, 2008). It is also recommended that capacity assessments include consideration of legal standards, functional elements (e.g., IADLs, ADLs), cognitive underpinnings, psychiatric or emotional factors, values and preferences, risk of harm, means for enhancing capacity, and clinical judgment.

Informal (i.e., nonlegal) decisions about capacity are more common in primary care, wherein decisions are made through evaluations of functioning and discussions with the patient and family member(s). Although clinical judgment remains the gold standard for determining capacity because measures for assessing capacity are not well studied, clinical judgment tends to overestimate a patient's health care decision-making capacity (Amaral et al., 2022; Moye et al., 2006). Coupling clinical judgment with standardized decision-making capacity instruments, such as the Aid to Capacity Evaluation, Hopkins Competency Assessment Test, or the MacArthur Competence Assessment Tool, along with cognitive assessments, provides a systematic approach for the assessment of capacity (Amaral et al., 2022; Barstow et al., 2018).

Advise

The possibility of significant cognitive impairment can be overwhelming for patients and their families. Again, in primary care settings, BHCs are not making the diagnosis of a dementia but may play an important role in alerting patients and their family members to the possibility of a dementia process. We advise patients, their family members, and the PCP when there appears to be a sufficient reason to pursue a more detailed evaluation of the patient's cognitive functioning. The Alzheimer's Association (2013), in conjunction with the American College of Physicians Foundation, posted a video about how a provider might discuss the possible diagnosis of a dementia. It is important to communicate the importance of further testing to determine the best course of action. BHCs could say the following to patients and their family members:

> Based on your responses and the screening measure we used, I recommend we work with your PCP to set up additional testing to gain a better understanding of the difficulties that you are having. A lot of factors can contribute to memory problems, including stress, depression, sleep problems, and even diet. We won't know what is going on until we get those tests and consult with additional medical experts. I'll go speak with your PCP now, and we'll work on developing a plan and setting up referrals.

For those individuals who do not screen positive for significant memory decline, we may recommend that the patient return in 6 months for a reevaluation. In addition, regardless of whether we believe that an individual may meet criteria for a dementia diagnosis, we discuss techniques that could be used to manage memory concerns. For example, we might say,

> There are multiple things you can do that may improve your ability to remember, including using reminder devices, memory exercises, physical exercise, and relaxation. Would you be interested in spending some time learning how to use these techniques?

We also advise patients about available resources. An important resource for older adults and their families is the local Area Agency on Aging (https://www. n4a.org/), which consolidates community resources for older adults. Depending on the level of functioning, we may also encourage patients and caregivers to contact community organizations that serve older adults, such as the Alzheimer's Association (https://www.alz.org), the state's department of human services, or local senior centers. If we know that a patient may have difficulty managing their meals, then we may encourage the use of a group such as Meals on Wheels (https://www.mealsonwheelsamerica.org/). If the patient belongs to a religious or spiritual organization, we encourage the patient and the family to explore what services that group might offer. Additional resources are provided in Figure 13.1.

Agree

When individuals need more testing, we discuss with the patients and their family members the purpose of the testing and help schedule appointments

FIGURE 13.1. Resources for Older Adults: Websites and Mobile Applications

Type	Location	Description
Websites	Alzheimer's Association (https://www.alz.org/; https://www.alz.org/care/overview.asp)	Provides resources for patients and families (e.g., caregivers) who are coping with Alzheimer's disease
	American Association of Retired Persons (https://www.aarp.org/; https://secure.aarp.org/home-family/caregiving/)	Provides resources for patients and families of "older adults" (i.e., 50 years or older)
	Family Caregiver Alliance (https://caregiver.org/)	Community-based nonprofit organization addresses needs of those providing care at home
	USAging (https://www.usaging.org/)	Represents Area Agencies on Aging; helps patients and providers connect with local resources for older adults
	National Council on Aging (https://www.ncoa.org/; https://www.ncoa.org/center-for-healthy-aging/)	Partners with nonprofit organizations, governments, and businesses to provide resources for older adults
	National Resource Center on LGBTQ+ Aging (https://lgbtagingcenter.org/)	Provides training, technical assistance, and educational resources to providers, organizations, and LGBTQ+ older adults
	Program of All-Inclusive Care for the Elderly (https://www.npaonline.org/)	Provides comprehensive medical and social services to those who are 55 or older, are eligible for nursing home care, and could live safely in the community. These criteria may change as PACE is being tested with new populations.
	The Center for Prolonged Grief (http://complicatedgrief.org/)	Provides resources for patients, providers, and family members about managing complicated grief
Mobile application	Medisafe (Google Play store, Android and Apple iOS)	Reminds individuals to take and refill medications; also checks for drug interactions, dosage, and side effects

with appropriate clinics (e.g., neuropsychology). In these cases, as well as in cases in which memory loss does not appear to be related to dementia, we offer to discuss methods that could be used to improve remembering.

Assist

Systematic reviews have suggested that cognitive interventions in healthy older adults and those with mild cognitive impairment improve cognitive functioning (e.g., memory performance, executive functioning, attention; M. Martin et al., 2011; Reijnders et al., 2013); however, these interventions often involve multiple hours of training. Some evidence indicates that leisure cognitive activity can improve cognitive functioning (Iizuka et al., 2019). Similarly, some evidence supports the effect of physical activity on cognitive functioning in those with mild cognitive impairment (Langa & Levine, 2014), but systematic reviews of the impact of aerobic exercise have failed to support the relation between improved cardiorespiratory fitness and cognitive benefit in healthy adults (J. Young et al., 2015). We often recommend using memory cues and devices, engaging in cognitively stimulating activities, completing physical exercise, and using relaxation techniques to improve functioning, particularly when one is having difficulty remembering; however, we avoid making unsubstantiated claims about the impact of these exercises and interventions.

Memory Cues and Devices

Developing systems to help patients remember everyday tasks or objects may help reduce some of the stress associated with memory difficulties. These memory cues and devices might include identifying common areas where things are placed, using reminder notes or a calendar to plan tasks and appointments, or learning skills to remember information more efficiently. Pill reminder systems (e.g., pill boxes, mobile applications) can be helpful for managing medication use. A BHC might say the following:

> It can be helpful to incorporate the use of reminders and devices to help you remember. Establish a place to put important objects, such as a hook by the door for keys and a bin on your dresser for your wallet and cell phone. You can use daily to-do lists to help you remember what you need to do each day. Memory strategies, such as remembering things together in groups, can help you remember. For example, rather than trying to remember the individual numbers in a phone number, try putting the numbers together. So instead of 5-5-5-7-3-0-9, remember the number as five hundred and fifty-five and seven thousand, three hundred and nine.

Cognitive Exercises

Engaging in tasks and games that are stimulating and require sustained concentration and planning may help to engage the patient's memory. For example, a BHC could say the following:

> Engaging your memory by participating in activities that require careful thinking may also help your memory. Some examples of these activities are learning a new skill, learning to play an instrument, and playing games or completing puzzles that require complex thinking, such as chess, crossword puzzles, or Sudoku. Some older adults enjoy writing or orally sharing their life stories as a way to exercise their memory. Is there anything that you used to do or would like to do to engage your memory?

Physical Activity

We often talk with PCPs about a patient's physical limitations and make appropriate recommendations about increasing physical activity. It may be necessary to have a physical therapist develop an appropriate program for physical activity; however, if the PCP recommends increased physical activity, we help the patient get started by saying the following:

> Physical activity may improve your ability to think and remember. Would it be reasonable for you to start a walking program? Because you haven't been walking for physical activity, perhaps we could start out by just walking for 10 minutes a day. What days and times could you plan to do that walk?

Relaxation

When someone has difficulty remembering something, it is common for that person to become increasingly frustrated or distressed. Teaching a relaxation technique, such as relaxed breathing, which patients could use when they become distressed about remembering, may help reduce unnecessary sympathetic arousal and distress. The techniques we discussed in Chapter 3 may be useful to consider when introducing relaxation strategies. A BHC could say the following:

> When you are having difficulty remembering something, it is important to try to remain calm. If you get upset, your stress response makes it even harder for you to remember. Taking a couple of deep breaths can help to reduce the stress response that sometimes interferes with remembering.

Arrange

If a BHC is seeing many older adults, it is helpful to have relationships with neuropsychologists or other medical professionals who can assist with more extensive testing for dementia when necessary. In addition, relationships with social workers and hospice staff can help the PCP manage the care of older adults more efficiently. Because of the progressive nature of many dementias (e.g., Alzheimer's disease), it can be helpful to the PCP for a BHC to schedule follow-up appointments with the patient and family member to help monitor changes in functioning. Setting follow-up appointments (e.g., 6 months to 1 year) for individuals with memory complaints who do not screen positive for a cognitive disorder can also be helpful to monitor for any significant changes. In addition, knowing local resources for older adults can help patients and their families get more immediate support for difficulties that they may be encountering.

INCONTINENCE

Among noninstitutionalized older adults in the United States, 55% of women and 30% of men reported experiencing urinary leakage, and 15.9% of men and 19% of women reported accidental bowel leakage (Gorina et al., 2014). Incontinence can have a profound impact on an individual, as it can affect employment and leisure activities, can lead to avoidance of sexual activities, and is a primary reason older adults move into a residential or nursing care facility (National Institute for Health and Care Excellence [NICE], 2019).

If incontinence results from physical exertion (e.g., sneezing, climbing stairs, running), it is called *stress incontinence*, whereas if the incontinence occurs when the individual needs to void, it is called *urge incontinence*. The combination of stress and urge incontinence is termed *mixed incontinence*. Two other forms of incontinence are *overflow* and *functional incontinence*. Frequent urination, increased urgency, or constant dripping of urine are symptoms of overflow incontinence, which occurs because the bladder is overdistended. Functional incontinence refers to individuals who can normally control their urine; however, because of some impairment (e.g., mobility limitations, dementia) the patient is not able to get to the bathroom in time to urinate.

Behavioral interventions for urinary incontinence have often been used in primary care clinics as well as in other medical settings (e.g., urology, obstetrics, and gynecology clinics). A systematic review of the literature revealed that pelvic floor muscle training (PFMT), also known as Kegel exercises, significantly reduces incontinence for women (Dumoulin et al., 2014; NICE, 2019), and some evidence shows that PFMT is effective for men as well (MacDonald et al., 2007). PFMT using at least eight contractions three times per day for a period of at least 3 months is recommended as a first-line treatment for women with stress or mixed urinary incontinence (NICE, 2019). In addition, adjunctive biofeedback, which is performed by some specially trained behavioral health professionals, may be a useful treatment for urinary incontinence in women who struggle with PFMT (Kopańska et al., 2020; NICE, 2019).

Assess

A BHC will not make the diagnosis of incontinence, but they may spend time assessing its effect on functioning. As with any functional assessment, it is important to gain an understanding of frequency, duration, intensity, what is associated with it or triggers it, and consequences of the symptoms. The following are some helpful questions:

- How long has incontinence been a problem? How much urine do you lose?

- How many times a day do you lose urine? Do you lose urine when you're physically active?

- What situations seem to make the incontinence worse? Better?

- When do you have an urge to urinate? Do you avoid situations or activities because you are concerned that you may lose control? If so, what situations or activities?

Increased caffeine use (e.g., greater than 100 mg per day), obesity, and excessive fluid intake may also increase the risk of urinary incontinence (NICE, 2019), so these should also be assessed as potential contributing factors. Other conditions such as abdominal masses, congestive heart failure, cerebral vascular accident, and some medications (e.g., antihypertensives, pain relievers, antidepressants, sedatives, hypnotics) may also contribute to incontinence.

Advise

We discuss behavioral methods of managing stress or mixed urinary incontinence, which may supplement or substitute for pharmacological interventions (e.g., oxybutynin) that may be used to treat incontinence, as follows:

> One method for improving your ability to control your urine flow is to strengthen the muscles that you use to control your urine. Strengthening these muscles is just like strengthening other muscles in your body; by repeatedly contracting these muscles they will increase in strength over time, and your ability to control your urine will likely improve.

We inform patients that these exercises are considered the first line of intervention for stress or mixed incontinence and can be an effective intervention that will allow them to engage in activities that they may be avoiding.

Agree

The behavioral interventions for incontinence require regular practice to be effective. Before we teach the behavioral interventions, we determine patients' motivation to change, as we discussed in Chapter 4, by assessing the importance of the change, their confidence in change, and their willingness to practice these skills. We emphasize that the muscle training may not have an immediate effect on their ability to control their urine, but with time and practice, those skills will gradually improve. Once we have some acceptance from the patient, we move to the assist phase.

Assist

When we teach PFMT, we spend time educating patients about urinary incontinence and how PFMT can help improve control of their incontinence:

> Sometimes we develop incontinence because the muscles that we use to control our urine get weaker as we age. Just like other muscles in our body, if we exercise those muscles, we can make the muscles stronger. If the muscles are stronger, we can control our urine flow more easily. Therefore, we're going to discuss an exercise routine to help you strengthen those muscles. As you are sitting here, see whether you can squeeze the muscles that you use to control your urine flow. The squeezing should not cause you any pain and you shouldn't need to move your body, just gently squeeze those muscles. Are you able to do that? To practice, squeeze the muscles that you use to stop the flow of urine and hold that squeeze for 10 seconds, then let the muscles relax for 10 seconds. Repeat the squeezing and relaxing 10 times at least three times a day.

If patients have difficulty identifying which muscles to contract, encourage them to practice stopping their urine midflow or, for women, to place a finger into the vagina (this will likely require the use of a water-based lubricant) and practice squeezing their finger. Individuals should practice this technique for at least 3 months before determining whether the technique is effective (NICE, 2019).

In addition to PFMT, bladder training should also be considered as a first-line treatment for women with urge or mixed urinary incontinence (Hersh & Salzman, 2013; NICE, 2019). Bladder training requires the patient to wait for increasingly longer periods between voiding. The amount of time is determined by starting out with the current amount of time between voiding and increasing the amount of time by a length that is accepted by the patient (e.g., "Wait an additional 5 minutes after you have the urge to go, then see if you can wait 7 minutes, then 10 minutes, and so on").

If the patient is drinking caffeine or appears to be consuming an excessive amount of liquids, we will discuss ways to reduce consumption, such as gradually tapering by one daily glass or cup per week. If the person is obese, we may offer to use the interventions we discuss in Chapter 6 for targeting weight.

Arrange

We like to have patients return in 2 to 3 weeks to assess whether they are continuing to practice the skills. They also come back after 3 months of practice to determine the effectiveness of the intervention. Should the PFMT and bladder training not work, an anticholinergic medicine (e.g., oxybutynin [Ditropan], tolterodine [Detrol]) may be added as a treatment (NICE, 2019); however, this medication is not recommended for patients with dementia. Complementary interventions, such as acupuncture, hypnosis, and herbal medications, have not been found to have significant therapeutic benefits (NICE, 2019). If the more conservative treatments for urinary incontinence fail, other interventions such as bladder wall injection with botulinum toxin A, percutaneous sacral nerve stimulation, and surgery may be considered (Hersh & Salzman, 2013; NICE, 2019).

CAREGIVER BURDEN

When working with older adults in primary care, it is important to assess whether the patient is a caregiver for another adult (e.g., an ill or disabled spouse, sibling, or friend). Caring for another adult, although potentially rewarding and contributing to meaning in life, can be a chronic stressor for caregivers and may contribute to increased risk of physical and behavioral health problems in the caregiver (Swartz & Collins, 2019). In addition, the caregiver may be incurring additional financial burden and not have the preparation, knowledge, and skills necessary for caregiving, which contributes to additional strain (Swartz & Collins, 2019). If a caregiver's physical or behavioral health is significantly impaired, the person who is being cared for may be at risk as well. For this reason, it also is helpful to assess factors related to caregiver burden for any person who is caring for the patient. The assessment of caregiver burden should include questions related to the context of care (e.g., relationship between caregiver and care recipient), perception of the health of the care recipient (e.g., cognitive functioning, physical health), values (e.g., cultural norms), the caregiver's health (e.g., physical and behavioral health), knowledge and skills (e.g., confidence, competence), and resources (Adelman et al., 2014). Multiple measures are available to help screen for caregiver burden; however, the Zarit Burden Interview (ZBI; Zarit et al., 1985) has been described as the most useful (Van Durme et al., 2012). Brief versions (e.g., ZBI-12, ZBI-7, ZBI-6) of the original 22-item ZBI have been developed and found to be valid and reliable for those with advanced conditions (Higginson et al., 2010), including the one-item ZBI-1 (i.e., "Overall, how burdened do you feel in caring for your relative?" with possible responses "not at all," "a little," "moderately," "quite a bit," or "extremely"; Higginson et al., 2010).

To decrease burden among caregivers it is important to

- promote self-care (e.g., encourage taking care of own health needs, physical activities, and other value-based activities);

- encourage respite care;

- provide education and information (e.g., about the recipient's illness and signs of progression, information about caregiver stress, techniques for appropriately lifting patients, support groups);

- encourage use of technology support (e.g., automatic medication dispensers, webcam monitoring, lift systems); and

- encourage use of community assistance (e.g., Family Caregiver Alliance [https://www.caregiver.org/]) and other supportive services, such as housecleaning, cooking, and visiting nurses. Note: BHCs should assess the family's financial resources before recommending hiring these services so as not to lose credibility and trust with the patient and their caregiver.

Psychoeducational interventions, psychotherapy, support groups, and multicomponent therapy (e.g., individual and family therapy) are useful for reducing caregiver distress (Adelman et al., 2014; Gallagher-Thompson & Coon, 2007; Swartz & Collins, 2019). Interventions based on cognitive behavioral therapy, acceptance and commitment therapy, mindfulness-based stress reduction, and internet-based interventions (i.e., interventions that are provided virtually or by phone) that are tailored to the individual have all shown benefits for caregivers (Cheng et al., 2019). It can also be important for the BHC to give caregivers "permission" to take care of themselves and/or to take a break from assistance for a few hours per week. For example, a BHC might say the following:

> It sounds like almost all of your time is devoted to taking care of your spouse. I wonder what toll that is taking on you. It can be helpful to take some time for yourself to do something you might enjoy or just to take a break. By taking those little breaks, caregivers can find more energy to take care of their loved ones. Is that something you could consider doing?

It is common for caregivers to believe they would be doing something wrong by taking time for themselves. Telling them it is important to take care of themselves as well can help them to be more willing to engage in other activities. Websites for caregivers are included in Figure 13.1.

DEPRESSION AND ANXIETY

The prevalence of major depressive disorder ranges from 5% to 13% among older adults seen in primary care, and an additional 10% demonstrate subthreshold depressive symptoms (O'Connor et al., 2009). The U.S. Preventive Services Task Force recommends screening for depression among older adults (Siu et al., 2016). Integrating behavioral health providers into the primary care setting to enhance the assessment and treatment of older adults demonstrating depressive symptoms has been "strongly recommended" (Steinman et al., 2007). The Geriatric Depression Scale (GDS; Yesavage et al., 1982–1983) was developed specifically for use with older adults. The original scale may be too lengthy for regular use in primary care settings; however, the GDS-5 and the GDS-15 (see Figure 13.2) are valid, shorter versions that take less than 5 minutes to administer (Karlin & Fuller, 2007). Other measures of depressive symptoms such as the Patient Health Questionnaire-9 (Kroenke et al., 2001) and the Beck Depression Inventory-II (Beck et al., 1996) may not be appropriate for patients with limited physical functioning. When assessing depressive symptoms, it is particularly important to ask about suicidal thoughts, as older adults have the highest suicide rate in the United States among all age groups (CDC, 2022c). Although depression is an important risk factor for older adults attempting or dying by suicide, other factors, including a history of serious suicidal ideation, functional impairment, stressful life events, substance abuse, and physical illness, are also associated with significant increased risk (Raue et al., 2014). Cognitive and behaviorally based treatments, such as the ones that we discussed in Chapter 4, have been shown to be just as effective with older adults as with younger adults (Haigh et al., 2018).

Assessment and treatment of anxiety in older adults has not been widely studied, and most studies are not conducted in primary care settings (Balsamo et al., 2018; Wetherell et al., 2005). The prevalence of anxiety disorders among older adults ranges between 3.2% and 14.2% (Wolitzky-Taylor et al., 2010). Meta-analyses show that PCPs identify 30.5% of individuals experiencing anxiety (Olariu et al., 2015), suggesting that most older adults who experience anxiety are not being identified. To screen for anxiety disorders in older adults, the Generalized Anxiety Disorder-7 (Spitzer et al., 2006) and the Beck Anxiety Index for primary care (Beck & Steer, 1993) have been examined in a broad age range of patients, but it is unclear how useful these measures are for older adults (Karlin & Fuller, 2007). The Geriatric Anxiety Inventory, which is comprised of 20 dichotomous questions; the Geriatric Anxiety Inventory-Short Form, which has five items; the Geriatric Anxiety Scale, a 30-item, 4-point Likert scale; and the shorter Geriatric Anxiety Scale-10, which has 10 items,

FIGURE 13.2. Geriatric Depression Scale 5/15

	Section I		
1.	Are you basically satisfied with your life?	YES	**NO**
2.	Do you often get bored?	**YES**	NO
3.	Do you often feel helpless?	**YES**	NO
4.	Do you prefer to stay home rather than going out and doing new things?	**YES**	NO
5.	Do you feel pretty worthless the way you are now?	**YES**	NO

*Calculate score in the box below. Answers in **bold** are worth 1 point.*

Score from first five questions = _____

If a score of 2 or more above, please continue with remaining 10 questions, otherwise depression may not be a problem.

	Section II		
6.	Have you dropped many of your activities and interests?	**YES**	NO
7.	Do you feel that your life is empty?	**YES**	NO
8.	Are you in good spirits most of the time?	YES	**NO**
9.	Are you afraid that something bad is going to happen to you?	**YES**	NO
10	Do you feel happy most of the time?	YES	**NO**
11.	Do you feel you have more problems with memory than most?	**YES**	NO
12.	Do you think it is wonderful to be alive now?	YES	**NO**
13.	Do you feel full of energy?	YES	**NO**
14.	Do you feel your situation is hopeless?	**YES**	NO
15.	Do you think that most people are better off than you are?	**YES**	NO

*Calculate score in the box below. Answers in **bold** are worth 1 point.*

Score from all 15 questions = _____

For clinical purposes a score above 5 points is suggestive of depression and should warrant a follow-up interview. Scores above 10 are almost always depression.

Note. Adapted from original scale in "Development and Validation of a Geriatric Depression Screening Scale: A Preliminary Report," by J. A. Yesavage, T. L. Brink, T. L. Rose, O. Lum, V. Huang, M. B. Adey, and V. O. Leirer, 1982–1983, *Journal of Psychiatric Research, 17*(1), p. 41 (https://doi.org/10.1016/0022-3956(82)90033-4). Copyright 1983 by Pergamon Press Ltd.; scoring method in "Comparing Various Short-Form Geriatric Depression Scales Leads to the GDS-5/15," by S. K. Weeks, P. E. McGann, T. K. Michaels, and B. W. Penninx, 2003, *Journal of Nursing Scholarship, 35*(2), p. 136 (https://doi.org/10.1111/j.1547-5069.2003.00133.x). Copyright 2003 by Sigma Theta Tau International. Adapted with permission.

have been developed to screen for anxiety among older adults and may be appropriate for use in primary care settings (Balsamo et al., 2018).

Overall, we have found techniques such as those presented in Chapter 4 to be clinically useful for targeting anxiety symptoms among older adults. There is an obvious need for more empirical studies that examine depression and anxiety treatment of older adults in primary care settings.

FALL RISK

Among adults 65 years and older, falls are the leading cause of nonfatal and fatal injuries (Moncada & Mire, 2017). When screening for anxiety among older adults, it is important to assess the patient's fear of falling. Among U.S. older adults, 36% report being "moderately" or "very" afraid of falling, which is related to a decline in functioning (R. Boyd & Stevens, 2009). A fear of falling and impact on functioning can be assessed by asking the following questions:

- Have you fallen or had near misses or unsteadiness when you were afraid that you might fall?

- Do you worry about falling or losing your balance when you walk inside? What about outside?

- Do you avoid or limit activities because of your concerns about falling?

To help reduce the risk of falling and the fear of falling, BHCs should encourage the development of an appropriate physical activity regimen. Medical evaluations and interventions regarding orthostatic blood pressure changes, vision impairments, foot care, ADLs, medications, cognitive functioning, and environmental hazards should also be encouraged. Assessment and interventions across these areas have been shown to reduce the risk of falling (Moncada & Mire, 2017).

SEXUALITY

The majority of older women and men up to age 85 are engaged in regular sexual activity, particularly if they consider their health to be at least "good" (Lindau et al., 2007). Chapter 12 discusses the sexual problems most commonly reported by older adults, including, for men, erectile dysfunction and premature ejaculation and, for women, orgasmic disorder, vaginal dryness, and pain (Lindau et al., 2007). Often older adults do not discuss their sexual functioning problems with their medical providers (Lindau et al., 2007). Therefore, it is important for the BHC to integrate questions about sexual functioning and health into their assessments and be prepared to provide recommendations for targeting these problem areas. Nusbaum and Hamilton (2002) provided some practical advice for assessing sexual history in primary care patients. It is perhaps most important to ask about sexual health in a matter-of-fact and sensitive manner, such as in the following example:

> Sexual functioning is often an important part of an individual's life that isn't always discussed in medical appointments. Would it be okay for me to ask a few questions about your functioning in this area? [If yes, then ask the following.] Do you have any concerns about your sexual functioning, including concerns about a lack of interest in sex or problems during sex, such as pain, difficulty with lubrication, or having an orgasm [women] or maintaining an erection or premature ejaculation [men]?

If the patient answers affirmatively, then asking the questions presented in Chapter 12 may provide important information the BHC can use to design interventions that would be appropriate. As part of the primary care team, BHCs must be comfortable with discussing all aspects of functioning, no matter what the person's age.

It is also important for the BHC to consider the sexual preferences of older adults. Historically, more than 20% of lesbian, gay, bisexual, transgender, and questioning or queer (LGBTQ) older adults do not disclose their sexual or gender identity to their physicians (CDC, 2013b). LGBTQ older adults are at greater risk of illness, disability, and premature death (CDC, 2013b). It is important to consider these patients' history of discrimination, concern about discrimination from health care providers, and possible lack of support from family members (Preston, 2022). Resources specifically for LGBTQ older adults are available at https://lgbtagingcenter.org.

SOCIAL ROLE AND SOCIAL SUPPORT CHANGES

Older adults often struggle with significant changes in their social roles (e.g., retirement) and social support structure. As we age, our social support networks often get smaller, but the relative importance of the individuals within that support network significantly increases (Lang & Carstensen, 1994). Therefore, the loss of individuals within a close network of support may be particularly difficult for the older adult. In extraordinary circumstances, such as the social restrictions associated with COVID-19 response, the impacts on older adults may be amplified. In primary care, BHCs can help PCPs screen for whether a particular symptom presentation is more consistent with depression, bereavement, loneliness, or another presenting problem.

Following a significant loss, most individuals experience acute grief symptoms that naturally reduce over time and are usually at a low level after 6 months; however, there may be surges in grief symptoms around holidays or other special occasions (Shear et al., 2011). Some individuals demonstrate symptoms of *complicated grief*, also referred to as prolonged grief disorder. Prolonged grief disorder was added to the fifth edition of the *Diagnostic and Statistical Manual of Mental Disorders, Text Revision* as a formal diagnosis. It is estimated that 2% to 3% of the population experiences complicated grief, and 10% to 20% of those who lose a romantic partner experience complicated grief; the complicated grief prevalence is highest among women older than 60 years (Shear, 2015). Compared with acute grief, complicated grief is unusually severe and prolonged; impairs functioning; and is associated with intense yearning, longing, or emotional pain; preoccupation with the deceased person; an inability to accept the loss; and difficulty imagining a meaningful future (Shear, 2015).

When seeing someone who is bereaved, the first step is to evaluate whether the patient's grief response is an acute grief response or a complicated grief response and to differentiate these responses from other possible clinical diagnoses, such as depression or posttraumatic stress disorder. One of the most important indicators of healthy functioning is whether the patient is beginning to engage or reengage with activities, friends, and family members after the loss. If patients report staying at home and avoiding activities, we recommend that BHCs establish a behavioral activation plan to help the patient reengage with activities and other people. We use a handout, such as the one in Figure 13.3, to educate patients and describe possible methods of coping with their distress. In addition, BHCs may use the strategies we presented in Chapters 4 and 5 to help patients decrease the depressive and anxiety symptoms they may demonstrate. Some evidence suggests that those who experience complicated grief are helped by antidepressants (Shear, 2015). Consider following up with these patients in 2 to 4 weeks to reassess their functioning.

PRACTICAL CONSIDERATIONS

Irrespective of disease processes, as people age, physical functioning, including vision, hearing, and mobility, decreases. If BHCs commonly have older adults as patients, some practical considerations include the following:

- Write down all recommendations for the patient with the specific plan for how to implement those recommendations.

- Use font sizes of 14 to 16 points on handouts to increase readability and should not be printed on high-gloss paper that may increase glare. Consider having magnifying glasses available for use when reviewing handouts with patients.

- Remember that the current cohort of older adults has a lower literacy rate than other cohorts of adults. Determine whether the patient has difficulty reading when interpreting testing or using handouts to guide interventions.

- Consider keeping a pocket amplifier available to assist those older adults who may have difficulty hearing or who have forgotten to bring their hearing aids.

- Maximize lighting in the room and ensure that there is good light on the BHC's face. Look toward patients when talking, as older adults may use the movement of lips to supplement their hearing.

- Have room in the office space for a wheelchair or a plan for how to accommodate someone who relies on a wheelchair for mobility.

- Have enough seating available for the patient and caregivers.

- Consider slowing the rate of speech and avoiding multiple, complex questions.

FIGURE 13.3. Bereavement, Grief, and Mourning Handout

Bereavement, Grief, and Mourning

Bereavement is the state of having lost a significant other to death. *Grief* is the personal response to the loss. *Mourning* is the public expression of that loss.

What Is "Normal" Grief?

Grief reactions vary depending on who we are, whom we lost, our relationship with that person, the circumstances around their passing, and how much their loss affects our day-to-day functioning. Different people may express grief differently, and you may even have different grief responses between one loss and another. Reactions to grief and loss include not just emotional symptoms but also behavioral and physical symptoms. These reactions often change over time. All are normal for a short period of time.

- **Emotional:** shock, denial, numbness, sadness, anxiety, guilt, fear, anger, irritability
- **Behavioral:** crying unexpectedly, sleep changes, not eating, withdrawing from others, restlessness, trouble making decisions
- **Physical:** concentration problems, exhaustion/fatigue, decreased energy, memory problems, upset stomach, pain and headaches

Symptoms that are not normal and may signal the need to talk to a professional include use of drugs, alcohol, violence, and thoughts of killing oneself.

The *duration* of grief varies from person to person. Research shows that the average recovery time is 18 to 24 months. Grief reactions can be stronger around significant dates, like the anniversary of the person's death, birthdays, and holidays.

Give yourself time to grieve. It is normal and important to express your grief and to work through the concerns that arise for you at this time. "Stuffing" your feelings may not be helpful and may delay or prolong your grief.

- **Find supportive people to reach out to during your grief.** This is the time when the support of others may be the most helpful. Don't be afraid to tell them how they can best help, even if it means just listening. It is often very helpful to talk about your loss with people who will allow you to express your emotions.
- **Take care of your health.** Often after a loss, we stop doing the things we need to for health care, such as exercising, eating correctly, or taking prescribed medications. If you are on a health care regimen, it is important to continue to follow that plan.
- **Postpone major life changes.** Give yourself time to adjust to your loss before making plans, for example, to change jobs, move or sell your home, or remarry. Grief can sometimes cloud your judgment and ability to make decisions.
- **Consider keeping a journal.** It is often helpful to write or tell the story of your loss and what it means to you as a way to work through your feelings.
- **Participate in activities.** Staying active through exercise, enjoyable activities, outings with supportive others, and the start of new hobbies can help us get through tough times while providing opportunities for constructive development and use of energy.
- **Find a way to memorialize your loved one.** Planting a tree or garden in the name of your loved one, dedicating a work to their memory, contributing to a charity in their name, and other such activities can be helpful.

Consider joining grief-support groups or contacting a grief counselor for additional support and help. Depressive symptoms (feeling sad) are a normal part of bereavement. Staying active and finding support from others can help you through the grief process.

Note. Adapted from *Bereavement, Grief, and Mourning* [Unpublished handout], by R. A. Nicholas, 2016. In the public domain.

- Make goals for change and interventions concise and specific. Consider asking the patient to repeat back the plan for change.

- Consider the impact of medication side effects on functioning. Although this is true for any patient, older adults are more likely to be taking multiple medications. The complex interactions of medications may affect functioning. It may be helpful to evaluate when patients take their medications and what impact those medications have on the patient's functioning.

- Consider that among older adults, physical activity is an important recommendation for a variety of health reasons, including disease management, memory improvement, and emotional regulation. However, the types of physical activities that are recommended should be considered in close coordination with the medical provider. Consideration should be given to avoiding falls and managing fear of falling.

SUMMARY

Older adults are a diverse population who are often living active lifestyles. Adapting health care to the needs of this growing population will help them to live their later years with a higher quality of life. When working with older adults, it is important to become familiar with some of the common problems that older adults experience and strategies for adapting care to their needs. The information in this chapter can be used as a foundation on which to build assessment and intervention skills.

14

Obstetrics and Gynecology

omen have unique health care needs and concerns. In addition to
being knowledgeable about common physiological problems among
women, such as gynecological and premenstrual disorders, individuals providing health care to women must be prepared to address issues such as infer-
tility, family planning and pregnancy, termination of pregnancy or pregnancy
loss, partner relationship discord, and domestic violence. Although these latter issues do not exclusively affect women, they are prevalent among women,
and health care providers must understand the unique ways in which they
affect women and be skilled in addressing their effects and implications.
Women's health clinics have become an increasingly popular model for
addressing the specific needs of women, including delivering gynecological
care as well as general primary care.

The primary care behavioral health model of service delivery we have advo-
cated throughout this book is applicable to behavioral health providers working
in women's health clinics, and they can apply the clinical guidance as one
would in a general primary care practice. This chapter, however, provides special guidance for behavioral health consultants (BHCs) working in women's
health clinics on three clinical areas that are specifically relevant in that environment: peripartum depression, chronic pelvic pain (CPP), and menopause.

https://doi.org/10.1037/0000380-015
*Integrated Behavioral Health in Primary Care: Step-by-Step Guidance for Assessment and
Intervention, Third Edition*, by C. L. Hunter, J. L. Goodie, M. S. Oordt, and
A. C. Dobmeyer

PERIPARTUM DEPRESSION

Peripartum refers to the time during pregnancy and for a period of time after the birth of a child. This period is often broken up into the perinatal (i.e., during pregnancy), antenatal (i.e., during the birth), and postnatal (i.e., for a time after pregnancy) periods. Throughout the peripartum period, women may receive care in a specialty obstetrics and gynecology (OB/GYN) clinic, a women's health clinic, or a family medicine clinic. When peripartum care is offered in a specialty clinic (i.e., OB/GYN), that clinic typically becomes the woman's primary care clinic throughout the peripartum period. At some point following the completion of the pregnancy, care is transitioned back to a general medical practice. This transition can create problems for continuity of care as well as for screening and intervention for postpregnancy complications such as postpartum depression. When working in an OB/GYN clinic, it is important to consider these factors and develop a plan that optimizes the transition of care back to the primary care provider (PCP). Likewise, if one is working in a primary care or women's health clinic, carefully consider when and how peripartum depression screening should take place and the most effective modes of intervention within one's primary care setting. Screening for peripartum depression is essential because of its high prevalence. Perinatal depression prevalence in the United States is 13.2% on average, ranging from 9.7% to 23.5% depending on geographic region (Bauman et al., 2020). Prevalence is higher for those who smoked cigarettes during the last 3 months of pregnancy or postpartum, breastfed for less than 8 weeks, experienced intimate partner violence before or during pregnancy, had their child die since birth, or had self-reported depression (greatest risk factor) before or during pregnancy (Bauman et al., 2020; Langan & Goodbred, 2016). Although no specific causative factor for postpartum depression has been identified, meta-analytic findings consistently show the importance of psychosocial variables like stressful life events, marital conflict, and lack of social support on postpartum depression (Dennis & Dowswell, 2013).

Peripartum depression (i.e., postpartum depression) is associated with significant neonatal morbidity, such as attachment disorder, failure to thrive, and developmental delay at 1 year of age (Langan & Goodbred, 2016). It is also associated with significant maternal morbidity, including sleep disturbances, poor concentration, disruption of maternal–infant bonding and healthy family dynamics, poor concentration and decreased energy, and mortality, with maternal suicide a more common cause of death during peripartum than mortality from postpartum hemorrhage or hypertensive disorders (Langan & Goodbred, 2016).

Cultural and Diversity Considerations

In their review, O'Hara and McCabe (2013) noted that although some studies have found support for race/ethnicity (African American and Latinx), younger age, and lower education as risk factors for postpartum depression, other studies have found the association is better accounted for by socioeconomic status.

This suggests poverty may be the common factor among demographic correlates. Additional research by Ceballos et al. (2017) showed that the risk for postpartum depression in African American and Latina mothers living in small cities, towns, and rural communities is 80% and 40% greater, respectively, compared with White mothers in those same communities. Bauman et al. (2020) found higher peripartum depression prevalence in women who were 24 years old or younger; were non-Hispanic Asian/Pacific Islander, non-Hispanic Black, or non-Hispanic American Indian/Alaska Native; were not married (includes living with partner); and had 12 or fewer years of completed education, in comparison with those who were 25 years old or older, were Hispanic or non-Hispanic White, had completed greater than 12 years of education, and were married.

Specialty Mental Health

Treatments and outcomes for postpartum depression are similar to those of depressed women who are not pregnant or postpartum (Dennis & Hodnett, 2007; Sockol et al., 2011). Although psychological and pharmacological interventions for postpartum depression are effective (Molyneaux et al., 2015; O'Connor et al., 2016; Siu et al., 2016), medication concerns may be greater because of pregnancy and breastfeeding, leading to a patient preference for nonpharmacological treatment.

Primary Care Adaptation

Consistent screening is an important part of identifying women who might benefit from BHC services. The following highlights important screening and assessment strategies in primary care.

Assess

The U.S. Preventive Services Task Force (USPSTF; Siu et al., 2016) recommends screening patients for depression, including peripartum women, in primary care settings when a system is in place to confirm an accurate diagnosis and provide effective treatment and follow-up. There is convincing evidence that screening increases the accurate identification of adult patients with depressed mood in primary care and treatment of those who are identified decreases clinical morbidity (Siu et al., 2016). Depending on U.S. geographic location, rate of screening for depression may have substantial room for improvement. Bauman et al. (2020) reported that on average 79.1% of women indicate being asked about depression during pregnancy, with a range of 51.3% to 90.7%, and on average 87.4% indicate being asked postpartum, with a range of 50.7% to 96.2%. The USPSTF (Siu et al., 2016) also found that cognitive behavioral therapy (CBT) improves clinical outcomes in peripartum women with depression. BHCs in primary care or women's health clinics have a significant opportunity to educate and support an active screening program for pregnant and postpartum women. In our experience, PCPs are much more likely to implement a standard screening practice if they know they have support to effectively further assess and treat patients who screen positive.

Edinburgh Postnatal Depression Scale. A number of screening instruments can be used throughout the peripartum period (for reviews, see R. C. Boyd et al., 2005; Gaynes et al., 2005; and O'Connor et al., 2016). The best measure to use will depend on the setting and resources available; however, we recommend using the Edinburgh Postnatal Depression Scale (EPDS) as a primary screening tool (to download, see https://www.apa.org/pubs/books/integrated-behavioral-health-primary-care-third-edition). This instrument measures cognitive and emotional symptoms of depression and excludes somatic symptoms, except for sleep problems, that are more likely to occur during these times, which would increase the number of false positives (R. C. Boyd et al., 2005). It is the most widely researched and used screening measure for pregnant and postpartum women, demonstrating moderate to good reliability, sensitivity, and specificity with women from different countries and languages (R. C. Boyd et al., 2005; Gaynes et al., 2005; O'Connor et al., 2016). The positive predictive value for depression at a score of 13 or more ranges from 70% to 90% (Buist et al., 2002). It can be easily administered by a variety of primary care personnel and typically takes less than 5 minutes to complete (O'Connor et al., 2016). In one large study (Buist et al., 2006), 90% of the women found it easy to complete. In addition to the EPDS, we recommend routinely screening this population for suicidal risk. See Chapter 17 for further guidance on suicide risk assessment and intervention.

Times for screening. The current literature is unclear as to the best peripartum times to screen for depressive symptoms (Siu et al., 2016). We believe optimum screening would take place at every visit during pregnancy and every visit for a year postpartum. However, money, time demands, and personnel make this difficult in many clinics. Results from one study implementing screening in 20 departmental obstetric practices found screening accomplished between 28 and 32 weeks of gestation and at a 6-week postpartum visit was feasible if practices had access to mental health staff who would assist with at-risk patients (Gordon et al., 2006). Another model we have found feasible in women's health clinics involves screening women at the time of pregnancy diagnosis, during all visits between 28 and 32 weeks of pregnancy, and again at 6 weeks postpartum.

Once a positive screen exists, conducting a further assessment to clarify the diagnosis and functional impact of symptoms is likely a role the BHC will fulfill. See Chapter 5 for suggestions on depression assessment. Tailoring the assessment to address unique issues with peripartum depression might include the following:

- exploring the patient's view of the pregnancy (e.g., wanted/unwanted, fears/concerns about having this child, concerns about miscarriage);

- presence and quality of social support (and practical support) during and after pregnancy;

- any fears or anxieties regarding the pregnancy or childbirth; and

- any prior episodes of peripartum or postpartum depression and, if so, any psychotic features (as risk is higher for recurrence of psychotic features).

Advise

Results from research on effective treatments for pregnant and postpartum women are consistent with those for others who are depressed. Treatments include medication; cognitive and behavioral therapies; and group treatment, education, and support (Bledsoe & Grote, 2006; Shaw et al., 2006; Siu et al., 2016). See Chapter 5 of this volume for suggestions for treatment of depression within a primary care setting. Patients with depression may prefer nonpharmacological treatments given potential risks and side effects of medication (Gartlehner et al., 2017). Between 58% and roughly 66% of depressed individuals in primary care prefer a nonpharmacological treatment for their symptoms (Dorow et al., 2018; van Schaik et al., 2004). It is likely that a higher percentage of pregnant and breastfeeding women will not consider medication treatment as a first option because of concerns about how it might affect the fetus or child. The U.S. Department of Veterans Affairs and Department of Defense (2022) *Clinical Practice Guideline for the Management of Major Depressive Disorder* suggested that women with mild to moderate major depressive disorder who are pregnant or breastfeeding be offered evidence-based psychotherapy as a first-line treatment. For those with a major depressive disorder history prior to pregnancy who responded to antidepressant medication treatment and are currently stable on pharmacotherapy, consider the benefit/risk balance to mother and fetus in treatment decisions. Medications can be effective and should be included as an option, weighing the pros and cons of risk to mother and fetus or child. Although empirical data are limited, there is general support and extensive use of antidepressant medication as a first-line treatment for peripartum depression (Molyneaux et al., 2015; Ross et al., 2013). Research on the safety and effectiveness of antidepressant medication for peripartum depression will continue to evolve, and it is important that BHCs stay up to date in order to assist medical staff in balancing the benefits and risks for each individual patient.

Another option to consider for this population is educational classes and group treatments within the primary care setting. This might include new parent education support classes or psychoeducational depression treatment groups. We suggest homogenous group treatments that specifically target pregnant or postpartum women, allowing the patients to get valuable information from each other on how they are managing common challenges, which goes beyond what they might get through individual treatment. In their review of group treatments for postpartum depression, J. H. Goodman and Santangelo (2011) found that of the 11 studies meeting inclusion criteria, all but one showed statistically significant improvement from pretreatment to posttreatment on depression scores, suggesting that group treatment is effective in reducing depression symptoms. Interventions included unstructured approaches, interpersonal psychotherapy, CBT, education, workshops, and social support. Classes allow intervention to occur for a large number of patients (e.g., 10) in a relatively short period. Interacting in a group setting may also increase motivation to continue with a treatment strategy that has yet to produce results because other patients may be having similar difficulties and are continuing the treatment. A baby stroller walking group might be another valuable group intervention. In these walking groups, mothers walk together with their infants in a stroller. Evidence suggests that a stroller walking group can be an effective adjunctive treatment for depression (for a review, see Daley et al., 2007). Walking for as little as 40 minutes two times a week with a group of mothers and their infants in strollers and one time a week alone at a moderate intensity (i.e., 60%–75% of maximum heart rate) has been shown to significantly lower EPDS scale scores in 12 weeks when compared with a social support control group. Stroller walking groups could be scheduled after a psychoeducational class, or a person from the clinic could meet with the group and lead the patients through muscle stretches before and after walking. Where and how this group meets will depend on the weather, location, and resources available at each clinic. Alternatively, BHCs can assist new mothers in finding stroller walking groups near their homes (i.e., through internet or social media searches) and provide support and problem-solving interventions to facilitate regular participation.

Agree

In our experience, most women are willing to agree to try the changes a BHC suggests because they are motivated to improve their functioning so they can take better care of their child. If the patient agrees to make multiple changes, it may be beneficial to start on one change to avoid having them feel overwhelmed and to create the best chances for successful change. Initiating the easiest change (e.g., increasing frequency of exercise by walking with the baby in the stroller three times a week for 10 minutes) might be the best place to start.

Assist

There are several standard depression interventions one might start:

- behavioral activation (i.e., increasing exercise, like pushing the stroller on scheduled days for increasing time duration or via other fun, valuable, enjoyable activities that are just for the patient or involve the patient and their partner only),

- cognitive disputation (i.e., developing more accurate ways to view the situation, such as "Even though I feel overwhelmed and exhausted, I am dealing with many things well, I have support, and I don't have to do everything on my own"),

- problem-solving and/or communication skills training focused on obtaining needed social support or practical support (i.e., engage partner or others to assist with specific caregiving activities, allowing patient to have a break), and

- sleep strategies to help improve quality or quantity of sleep that may be disrupted due to depression but also the realities of a newborn in the home (i.e., the typical prohibition on naps may need to be modified for mothers up at night nursing a baby).

See Chapter 5 for more specific guidance on behavioral activation and cognitive disputation. Additional information on goal setting, cognitive disputation, and problem solving can be found in Chapter 4.

Patients might be interested in websites or self-help books to assist in managing their peripartum or postpartum depression. Some of these resources are summarized in Figure 14.1.

Arrange

At a minimum, we recommend at least one follow-up consultation after the initial appointment to help determine whether the patient was able to follow the plan and whether symptoms and functioning are improving. If they did not follow through, then problem solve barriers, reinitiate, or change the plan and suggest an additional follow-up visit with the BHC. If symptoms are improving, then a follow-up might be arranged with the BHC or the PCP in 2 weeks to reassess symptoms and functioning. Follow-up appointments can vary between individuals because of their life circumstances and the severity of their depressive symptoms. In our experience, it is usual for patients to return after the initial consultation appointment and report that they have successfully implemented the plan and are functioning more effectively; depressed mood has usually decreased; and other symptoms, such as energy level, are improving. In pregnant patients with improving symptoms, it may be warranted to schedule a follow-up appointment within 4 to 6 weeks after delivery to reassess symptoms and provide relapse prevention strategies. Some individuals may return for two or three appointments and report that they have not changed their thinking or behaviors and that their symptoms remain unchanged. Consider recommending these patients for specialty mental health treatment if obvious barriers cannot be overcome. Furthermore, BHCs should keep in mind that postpartum depression, though common, can become severe in some cases and pose serious risk to the well-being of the child. Assessment and treatment should always include monitoring, to the degree possible, the impact of the depressive symptoms on the child, especially when the mother is not responding to treatment. When necessary, appropriate actions must be taken to ensure the infant's well-being, including engaging with other family members and/or mandated reporting to local child protective services, when applicable.

CHRONIC PELVIC PAIN

Chronic pelvic pain is defined as "pain perceived to originate from the pelvis, typically lasting more than 6 months, and is often associated with negative cognitive, behavioral, sexual, and emotional consequences and symptoms suggestive of lower urinary tract, sexual, bowel, myofascial, or gynecologic dysfunction"

FIGURE 14.1. Resources for Patients Demonstrating Peripartum Depression: Websites and Books

Type	Location	Description
Websites	National Institute of Mental Health (https://www.nimh.nih.gov/health/publications/postpartum-depression-facts/index.shtml)	Provides patient materials defining peripartum and postpartum symptoms as well as information on treatment and how family and friends can help
	U.S. National Library of Medicine (Medline Plus; https://www.nlm.nih.gov/medlineplus/postpartumdepression.html)	Provides patient information on peripartum and postpartum symptoms and treatment
	Mayo Clinic (https://www.mayoclinic.org/diseases-conditions/postpartum-depression/basics/definition/con-20029130)	Provides information on symptoms, causes, risk factors, complications, treatments, coping, and support
Book	*The Postpartum Depression Workbook: Strategies to Overcome Negative Thoughts, Calm Stress, and Improve Your Mood* (Burd, 2020)	"This depression workbook is here to guide you on your journey, providing supportive strategies and tools grounded in cognitive behavioral therapy (CBT) proven to help you understand, cope with, and reduce your PPD symptoms. Discover common signs of PPD, what it is, and what you can do about it. Explore your thoughts, feelings, and relationships, plus self-care practices through a variety of practical and insightful exercises in this depression workbook. This depression workbook includes: • Primer on PPD—Discover if you might have PPD, take a look at common causes and risk factors, and see how PPD can impact your partner. • Lasting relief—The CBT-based postpartum strategies in this depression workbook will help you adopt a positive mindset, improve your mood, deepen your relationships, and find time to recharge. • Parents like you—Find kinship in real-life scenarios from other parents, paired with practical advice, simple tips, and interactive exercises. This depression workbook provides the strategies, tools, and support you'll need for a healthy and happy transition into parenthood." (Simon & Schuster, 2020, paras. 3–8)

Note. PPD = postpartum depression.

(Lamvu et al., 2021, p. 1). Although prevalence estimates of CPP related to any given etiology is variable, it is estimated to affect 26% of the world's female population (Lamvu et al., 2021), with the most recent study of overall CPP in the United States estimating prevalence at 14.7% for women 18 to 50 years old (Mathias et al., 1996).

CPP symptoms and pathology can be related to a variety of conditions such as endometriosis, pelvic floor abnormalities, dyspareunia, dysmenorrhea, ovulation pain, chronic pelvic inflammatory disease, pelvic venous congestion, fibroids, interstitial cystitis, myofascial pain with trigger points, and pelvic pain of unknown etiology or pathology (Grinberg et al., 2020; Lamvu et al., 2021; Vincent & Moore, 2010). It is a challenging syndrome to diagnose and manage due to the wide range of possible causes; the lack of an identifiable etiology in many patients (Bruckenthal, 2011; Grinberg et al., 2020; Lamvu et al., 2021); and potential complicated interactions between visceral, neurological, musculoskeletal, and psychological symptoms (Grinberg et al., 2020; Lamvu et al., 2021). CPP, like other chronic pain conditions, is often associated with negative emotional, behavioral, cognitive, functional, sexual, and quality of life consequences (Baranowski, 2013; Grinberg et al., 2020; Lamvu et al., 2021). Despite the impact, less than 1% of these individuals seek care from a pain specialist (Brookoff, 2009), likely seeking care instead from PCPs, urologists, and gynecologists.

Although there may be overlap, it is important not to confuse causal, predisposing factors and maintaining factors of CPP (Baranowski, 2013). A variety of causes (e.g., physical trauma [including surgery], infection, cancer and other medical conditions) can produce similar symptoms. In any one person, multiple factors (e.g., neurological factors; neuroendocrine factors; immunological factors; nervous system dysfunction; adverse childhood experiences, abuse, trauma, and psychological distress; mental health disorders; dysfunctional response to stress) may predispose that individual to develop chronic pain in response to those causes (Baranowski, 2013; Grinberg et al., 2020; Lamvu et al., 2021). If the cause is ongoing, focus should be on symptomatic treatment of the cause. If the cause is no longer ongoing, focus should shift to the impact of current mechanisms (e.g., stress, anxiety, depression, posttraumatic stress disorder, partner relationships, fear avoidance) as well as effective chronic pain management skills (Grinberg et al., 2020; Lamvu et al., 2021).

Women often undergo many exams and procedures and see multiple specialists with no definitive diagnosis or treatment, leaving providers and patients frustrated with unrelieved suffering during this time (Levesque et al., 2018). Furthermore, when a referral is made to a behavioral health pain specialist, it is often made as a last resort, and the individual may feel abandoned by the medical system or believe that others think the pain is purely psychological. It has been suggested that once a diagnosis of CPP is made, surgical procedures that offer no pain relief or an exacerbation of the condition should be minimized. Instead, treatment should be multidisciplinary and focused on symptomatic pain management and optimizing function and quality of life, with the same general multidisciplinary approach as any pain syndrome (American College of Obstetricians and Gynecologists [ACOG], 2020; Grinberg et al., 2020; Lamvu et al., 2021). Working in primary care gives behavioral health providers a ripe opportunity to create processes for care within the clinic whereby every woman who has a CPP diagnosis receives a focused biopsychosocial assessment and treatment as part of comprehensive pain management regardless of whether there is evidence of pathology.

Cultural and Diversity Considerations

Mathias et al.'s (1996) study of CPP in the United States found no difference in age, race/ethnicity, or education for women with CPP in comparison to women with no CPP.

Specialty Mental Health

Mental health treatments are generally not designed exclusively for CPP. The studies examining mental health treatments for CPP have been done outside of the primary care setting and include management strategies effective for other chronic pain conditions. A variety of interventions may lead to decreased frequency and/or intensity of pain, improved functioning, and decreased psychological sequelae. Strategies with some empirical support include stress management techniques, such as diaphragmatic breathing, progressive muscle relaxation, and mindfulness; interpersonal psychotherapy for depression; sex therapy and education; cognitive therapy for beliefs, thoughts, feelings, stress, and pacing; and acceptance and commitment therapy (Brooks et al., 2021; Poleshuck et al., 2014; Twiddy et al., 2015).

Primary Care Adaptation

Assessing and treating women with CPP will require asking questions about areas that can be uncomfortable or elicit strong emotional responses. The 5As approach is likely to help the BHC assess and interview efficiently and effectively while helping to minimize patient discomfort.

Assess

Assessing CPP is similar to assessing other chronic pain conditions. Main areas of assessment might include (a) variability in pain and factors associated with increased or decreased pain, (b) effect of pain on daily activities, (c) adaptive coping responses to pain, and (d) social and environmental influences on pain perception. Guidance on specific questions for a pain assessment is found in Chapter 10. In addition to these foundational assessment areas, there are several additional important areas to assess.

Sexual and physical abuse. Because physical, sexual, or psychological trauma can be associated with CPP, it is important to use screening questions to assess this history and its current effect. The provider should carefully balance eliciting detail with minimizing distress during this focused assessment to avoid retraumatizing the patient. Furthermore, we suggest that questions about sexual and physical abuse be asked toward the end of the functional assessment to avoid having the patient believe that the BHC thinks their pain is psychological in nature. Focused questions for sexual and physical abuse in primary care might include the following:

- Have you experienced any physical or sexual abuse or traumas as a child or adult?
  If yes, then ask the following:

- Was it physical, sexual, or both? Was it as a child, adult, or both?

- Have those incidents been affecting you in any way over the last 6 months?
  If yes, then ask the following:

- How have those incidents been affecting you?

The symptoms and impairments a patient may be experiencing as a result of abuse might include anxiety, depression, posttraumatic stress disorder (PTSD), partner intimacy problems, and/or intense anxiety or fear during gynecological exams. All of these conditions have the propensity to make CPP worse and significantly interfere with effective CPP management (ACOG, 2020; Grinberg et al., 2020; Lamvu et al., 2021). If physical or sexual abuse is endorsed, one may want to consider a brief screen using the Primary Care PTSD Screen (Bovin et al., 2021) found in Chapter 5.

Sexual dysfunction. As might be expected, given the anatomical location of pain in individuals with CPP, patients often have sexual dysfunction, including female orgasmic disorder, dyspareunia, postcoital pain, dissatisfaction with sexual frequency, and decrease in sexual desire. In addition to lubrication problems, increased pain during thrusting and in different sexual positions can be common (Howard, 2012; Levesque et al., 2018). Furthermore, sexual dysfunction may inhibit intimate relationships in a manner that starts or increases a stress response, anxious and/or depressed mood, anger, and resentment and thus can interfere with effective pain management, functioning, and quality of life (Howard, 2012). The assessment and management of sexual dysfunction is important with any pain condition; however, it may be especially relevant for CPP. The following questions will allow one to assess sexual dysfunction and use the information obtained to make recommendations for treatment as indicated (for additional questions, see Chapter 12):

- On a scale of 0 to 10, with 0 being not satisfied at all with your current sexual activities and 10 being the most satisfied you can imagine being with your sexual activities, how satisfied are you with your current sexual activities?

If the answer is below 7, consider asking the following questions:

- Do you have pain before, during, or after sexual activity?
  If yes, ask the following questions:

- When does the pain occur?

- Where is the pain located? [Ask about frequency, duration, and intensity.]

- What makes the pain worse during sex (e.g., your partner thrusting, certain sexual positions)?

- Does your partner know you are in pain? [If yes, ask the following.] How does your partner respond to your pain?

- Is lubrication a problem?

- Do you have orgasms? [If yes, ask the following.] Do you have pain during orgasm?

- Do you have distressing or stressful thoughts during sex?

Summary. If a patient is focused exclusively on physiological or disease-based explanations for CPP, they may not be as interested in pursuing nonmedical, nonsurgical pain management strategies. Therefore, it is important to strike a balance in communicating one's understanding of their symptoms and functional impairments and summarizing psychosocial and behavioral factors that may be contributing to CPP. Suggest that ongoing medical evaluations, if still needed, should be pursued, and at the same time, patients may be able to get started on managing their current pain differently, in a way that decreases pain and suffering. Highlight how thoughts, emotions, and physical symptoms are interconnected. The summary might sound like the following:

> For the last 6 months, you have had recurring pelvic pain. You've had multiple tests that have not shown a specific diagnosable condition that your doctor can treat. That doesn't mean your pain is in your head. There are a host of reasons, including tests not being sensitive enough to identify the problem, past injuries, activities, and genetic vulnerabilities, that could be interacting to produce your pain. Even if there was a definitive diagnosis, it doesn't necessarily mean there would be a medical or surgical treatment that could eliminate your pain. Being frustrated or stressed seems to increase your pain. On good days, you go full force, then end up paying the price over the next 2 days with increased pain and decreased activity. You are more irritable than you would like to be, you've decreased sexual activity in response to the pain, and you feel like you are not being the kind of partner you would like to be. The thought of continuing like this leads you to feel more desperate and depressed. You're not sleeping well, and you are feeling hopeless regarding your future.

Advise

The results of your assessment will guide what a BHC advises for treatment or self-management. Common areas for intervention might include negative emotions (e.g., anxiety, depressed mood), negative or catastrophic thinking, improving communication, increasing activities, pacing, and physiological arousal management. A primary goal of pain management is to reduce exacerbation of pain and improve functioning with pain. It is important to explain what the advised management strategies are designed to accomplish so that the patient does not get the false hope that their pain is going to be eliminated. See Chapter 10 for additional recommendations on the advise process for pain management and how different interventions may help to improve pain management.

If sexual or physical abuse is affecting current functioning to the extent that the patient may be experiencing PTSD, address symptoms and functioning with PTSD intervention strategies appropriate for primary care (for PTSD assessment and intervention guidance, see Chapter 5). Primary care behavioral health services might be appropriate for addressing some issues of sexual or physical abuse in primary care regardless of whether the patient meets PTSD criteria. We recommend discussing the potential primary care interventions that might be useful and benefits and drawbacks of primary care versus specialty care treatment.

If sexual dysfunction is a concern, then also advise on how treatment of sexual dysfunction may be helpful. Advice might focus on improving lubrication, decreasing muscle tension or bracing, altering the focus of sexual activity to nonintercourse interactions, changing intercourse positions and movement, and improving communication. Goals of these changes would be to decrease pain and to improve the frequency and enjoyment of sexual activity. See Chapter 12 for additional recommendations on the advise process for female orgasmic disorder.

Agree, Assist, and Arrange

Chapter 10 elaborates on strategies to use in the agree, assist, and arrange phases for chronic pain management, and in Chapter 12, we discuss strategies to use in the agree, assist, and arrange phases for female orgasmic disorder. For sexual or physical abuse and/or PTSD, one may want to have a list of mental health professionals within their system or local community that one knows and works with on a regular basis who have expertise in evidence-based treatment for these problems for referral if primary care treatment for sexual or physical abuse and/or PTSD is not effective or seems unwarranted given a patient's unique presentation or if the patient prefers specialty services. A BHC might offer this list to the patient or help their PCP to initiate a consult.

Patients might be interested in websites, mobile device applications, or self-help books to assist in managing their CPP. Some of these resources are summarized in Figure 14.2.

MENOPAUSE

Natural *menopause* is the term used to mark the permanent cessation of menstruation for 12 months (Minkin, 2019). *Perimenopause* is defined as the entire

FIGURE 14.2. Resources for Patients Demonstrating Chronic Pelvic Pain: Websites, Mobile Applications, and Books (*continues*)

Type	Location	Description
Websites	UpToDate (https://www.uptodate.com/contents/chronic-pelvic-pain-in-women-beyond-the-basics)	Includes links to information on causes, diagnosis, treatment, and coping by disease
	WebMD (https://www.webmd.com/women/tc/chronic-female-pelvic-pain-topic-overview)	Includes information on cause, symptoms, risks, exams and tests, prevention, medication, and treatment
Mobile application	Branch Health (Google Play store, Android and Apple iOS)	"Branch Health is a mobile companion for chronic pain management. An app for pain patients available on iOS and Android, and offered as a reimbursable service by Medicare and many commercial insurance providers, Branch Health has been named the official patient engagement app of the U.S. Pain Foundation and has been used by more than 30,000 patients in both private practice and at some of the nation's leading health systems. Branch offers evidence-backed tools to help engage people who live with chronic pain: • pain and medication tracking • mindfulness and physical therapy • community support • educational resources • clinical integration" (Upside Health, n.d., paras. 1–8)
Books	*Managing Pain Before It Manages You*, 4th ed. (Caudill, 2016)	Details 10 steps that can change the way pain sufferers feel, both physically and emotionally. It includes treatments for coping with flareups, solving everyday problems, and using power of relaxation techniques; content on mindfulness; a "Quick Skill" section in each chapter with simple exercises, supplementary reading, and resources (including smartphone apps); and more. Practical tools include MP3 audio downloads and easy-to-use worksheets that purchasers can download and print.

FIGURE 14.2. Resources for Patients Demonstrating Chronic Pelvic Pain: Websites, Mobile Applications, and Books (*continued*)

Type	Location	Description
Books (continued)	*Breaking Through Chronic Pelvic Pain: A Holistic Approach for Relief* (Weiss, 2019)	"Do you suffer from chronic pelvic pain your practitioner is unable to treat effectively? Or are you a practitioner who has struggled to identify the cause and treat your patients' pelvic pain? Having developed his ground-breaking holistic approach over 20 years ago, Dr. Weiss has become a world-renowned authority in this oft-overlooked field. *Breaking Through Chronic Pelvic Pain* will empower you to discover the true source of debilitating pelvic pain and finally alleviate it." (Weiss, 2019, back cover)
	The Pain Management Workbook: Powerful CBT and Mindfulness Skills to Take Control of Pain and Reclaim Your Life (Zoffness, 2020)	"In this groundbreaking workbook, you'll find a comprehensive outline of this effective biopsychosocial approach, as well as scientifically supported interventions rooted in cognitive-behavioral therapy (CBT), mindfulness, and neuroscience to help you take control of your pain—and your life! You'll learn strategies for creating a pain plan for home and work, reducing reliance on medications, and breaking the pain cycle. Also included are tips for improving sleep, nutrition for pain, methods for resuming valued activities, and more." (New Harbinger Publications, 2020, para. 3)

menopausal transition phase, up to 3 years before final menstrual period and including the first 2 years after the final period (Minkin, 2019). Throughout this chapter, we use the term "menopause" to refer to the perimenopause phase when menstruation is still occurring and "postmenopause" to refer to the 24-month span when menstruation has first stopped.

As a result of fluctuating hormone levels during menopause, a variety of problematic symptoms can occur, the most common being vasomotor symptoms such as hot flashes or flushes and night sweats, which are reported by approximately 75% of women (Monteleone et al., 2018). Of women reporting hot flashes, 87% report having them daily, with 33% experiencing more than 10 per day (ACOG, 2014). Vasomotor symptoms like hot flashes are also the most common menopausal sequelae for which women seek medical assistance

(ACOG, 2014). Vaginal dryness is reported by 42%, and prevalence of sleep disturbances ranges from 40% to 60%, believed to be primarily triggered by vasomotor symptoms (Monteleone et al., 2018; Santoro et al., 2021). Data suggest that women in postmenopause are more likely to report depressive symptoms in comparison to premenopausal women (Monteleone et al., 2018). Women with high levels of anxiety premenopause continue to experience those levels of anxiety during menopause and postmenopause, and those with low anxiety premenopause are at increased risk of developing high levels of anxiety during menopause and postmenopause (Monteleone et al., 2018).

It is hypothesized that vasomotor symptoms are related to hormonal changes affecting the hypothalamus, which is responsible for temperature regulation in the body. The exact mechanism of action is unclear; however, fluctuating estrogen levels may cause the hypothalamus to perceive the body to be hot and therefore respond by trying to dissipate heat, which produces the hot flash (Minkin, 2019; Santoro et al., 2021). Increased frequency of vasomotor symptoms has been associated with increased stress, anxiety, and depression; lower perceived control (E. W. Freeman et al., 2005; Pimenta et al., 2011); alcohol use; hot beverages or food; caffeine; smoking; physical exercise; and a higher body mass index (Koo et al., 2017; Minkin, 2019; Pimenta et al., 2011).

Hormone replacement therapy is one of the most effective treatments available to relieve menopausal symptoms (Flores et al., 2021). Beyond the benefits of controlling vasomotor symptoms and genitourinary syndrome of menopause symptoms (i.e., vaginal dryness, vaginal burning, vaginal discharge, genital itching, burning with urination, urgency with urination, frequent urination, recurrent urinary tract infections), there is reduction in risk for fracture and Type 2 diabetes (Flores et al., 2021). In the absence of comorbid risk factors, such as poorly controlled diabetes, hypertension, cardiovascular disease, risk factors for stroke, morbid obesity, and clotting disorders, healthy postmenopausal women with postmenopausal symptoms younger than 60 years of age and/or within 10 years since menopause onset without contraindications are excellent candidates for hormone replacement therapy (Flores et al., 2021). Some women with one or more comorbid risk factors may be at increased risk for morbidity and mortality with hormone replacement therapy. However, that risk will vary from patient to patient. The patient and PCP should discuss those risks and benefits so the patient can make an informed decision on whether hormone replacement therapy is right for them. Despite the accrued data over the last 20 years, hormone replacement therapy uptake has remained low (Flores et al., 2021). Given the potential benefit minus risk factors and low uptake, we recommend that BHCs read the Flores et al. (2021) article to be fully informed and share that article with the staff in their clinic.

Cultural and Diversity Considerations

Data from the multiethnic, multiracial, multisite study of middle-aged women called the Study of Women's Health Across the Nation found, when comparing

Caucasian, African American, Chinese, Japanese, and Hispanic women, that Caucasian women reported significantly more psychosomatic symptoms than other racial/ethnic groups and African American women reported significantly more vasomotor symptoms (Avis et al., 2001). When followed longitudinally, data showed the odds of high depressive symptoms increased significantly during the first 8 years in Hispanic and Japanese women compared with Caucasian women; the odds for African American and Chinese women were not significantly different than those for the Caucasian women (Bromberger & Kravitz, 2011). For sexual functioning, Chinese and Japanese women reported less importance, desire, and arousal and more pain, whereas African American women reported greater importance, frequency, and pain but less arousal, emotional satisfaction, and physical pleasure than Caucasian women (Avis et al., 2009).

Specialty Mental Health

Most specialty mental health studies examining interventions to reduce menopause symptoms used a CBT intervention package that included education and skill development on physiological, cognitive, behavioral, and emotional components of hot flashes and night sweats; cognitive (e.g., questioning alarming thoughts) and behavioral strategies (e.g., relaxed breathing) to reduce the impact of hot flashes and night sweats; education on mechanisms of sleep; and cognitive and behavioral strategies for dealing with night sweats and nighttime waking. M. Hunter's (2021) review of CBT studies for menopausal symptoms concluded that CBT is acceptable for patients and effective in reducing the impact of vasomotor symptoms; improves quality of life and sleep; and can be delivered effectively via self-help books, online platforms with and without support, and in-person groups.

Primary Care Adaptation

Adapting specialty mental health treatments for menopause can be done smoothly using the 5As approach. Education and cognitive and behavior management strategies are likely to be primary BHC intervention strategies.

Assess

The primary care functional assessment that we present in Chapter 3 is an appropriate generic assessment for women with menopause symptom complaints. Assessment and treatment of vasomotor symptoms related to stress, sleep problems related to night sweats, and sexual difficulties are appropriate primary areas of focus. See Figure 14.3 for recommendations of questions to ask in these areas.

The following is an example of how a summary might sound at the end of the assessment phase:

> You've had symptoms for the last 6 months that include hot flashes one to three times a day, each lasting for about 5 minutes, in which you are

sweating and have a flushed face. Sometimes these seem to happen for no reason at all; at other times, they seem to happen when you're feeling stressed. You have night sweats that wake you two to three times a night; you have trouble falling back to sleep and lie awake in bed for about 45 minutes worrying about falling back to sleep and how that will affect your ability to perform at work the next day. You don't feel rested in the morning, and you have increased your coffee intake from 16 to 48 ounces a day so that you can concentrate better at work. You've noticed that you don't have as much lubrication during intercourse, but that isn't a problem as you and your partner use lubricants. Over the last 3 months, your symptoms have gotten worse; this seems to be related to increased job stress given the extra responsibility in your new position. You feel embarrassed at work because people see your face flush and they ask what is going on. You don't like people at

FIGURE 14.3. Additional Functional Assessment Questions for Women Going Through Menopause

Women experiencing menopause may have a variety of problem symptoms. Some of the most common are hot flashes, sleep problems, and vaginal dryness. Do you have any of these or other bothersome symptoms?

Hot Flashes
Inquire about stressful environments and other triggers.

- Over the last month, have you found you are stressed, worried, anxious, frustrated, or agitated? If yes, then:
- What times and situations do you feel this way?
- What are the physical symptoms you notice?
- What thoughts do you have in these situations?
- How do others respond to you?
- What do you do to manage these symptoms?
- Is there anything that makes the symptoms better or worse?
- Were there other times in your life when you felt this way?

If not specifically identified, assess caffeine and alcohol use, hot drinks, and hot environments as triggers.

Sleep Problems/Night Sweats

- Use the standard sleep behavior assessment from Chapter 5.
- When do night sweats wake you?
- Once awake, what do you do to manage?
- What thoughts typically go through your mind when you cannot sleep?
- Is there anything that makes your night sweats better or worse?
- Does room temperature seem to have an impact on the number of night sweats?

Sexual Difficulties Related to Decreased Lubrication

- Do you have problems with vaginal lubrication (too dry during sex)? If yes, then inquire specifically about the problem(s), then ask:
- Have you done anything to help improve vaginal lubrication?

Expectations/Interpretations

- On a 0 to 10 scale with 0 = worst coping ever and 10 = best coping ever, how would you rate your ability to cope with your symptoms?
- Sometimes women feel embarrassed about their symptoms. Do you feel that way?
- Do you worry about not being in control of your symptoms?
- What do you know about menopause?

work knowing your personal health business, and you are becoming increasingly worried about when hot flashes will occur in the future. Do I have it right, or is there something I've missed?

Advise

On the basis of the unique symptoms and behavioral and functional impairments of the patient, BHCs should provide advice on treatment options that might best address the problems, explaining what the intervention is and how it might help. Common areas of advice might include the following.

General education about menopause. One might say, "Most people don't know a lot about menopause, so it might be helpful to go over what is typical, what to expect, and other specific information on the topic." The following websites contain free educational material that can be downloaded for an interactive discussion, as needed:

- https://www.mayoclinic.org/diseases-conditions/menopause/basics/definition/con-20019726,

- https://www.medicinenet.com/search/mni/menopause, and

- https://www.nlm.nih.gov/medlineplus/menopause.html.

Monitoring symptoms. One might say, "You have some idea of what triggers the hot flashes, but at other times they seem to come out of the blue. It might be helpful to track your symptoms to see whether we can identify other triggers that you could avoid or modify" (see Figure 14.4).

Questioning thoughts. One might say the following:

> At work and in bed at night, your mind gets you stressed or anxious. We know that the more stressed or anxious you get, the more difficult it is to fall back to sleep, and that increased stress response is associated with increased number and intensity of hot flashes. We can't stop your mind from initially telling you things that are stressful, but we can help you get better at noticing those thoughts, not reacting to them, and generating more helpful reassuring thoughts that can decrease your stress response and help you fall back to sleep more easily and perhaps decrease the number of hot flashes at work.

See Figure 14.5 for identifying unhelpful thinking about hot flashes and how one might develop more helpful thought responses to reduce stress.

Relaxation. One might say the following:

> By helping you to decrease your body's physiological stress response, we can likely help you improve your sleep and decrease your hot flashes. One of the ways we can do that is to teach you how to do relaxed breathing so you can turn the volume down on your stress response. We can also make a plan for physical relaxation to be a habit throughout the day.

See Chapter 4 for relaxation training guidance.

FIGURE 14.4. Hot Flash Symptom Diary

Date	Time	Severity (0–10)	Length	Situation/ triggers	Action taken

Please use this form to record all hot flashes. Severity scale ranges from 0 (no symptoms) to 10 (the most extreme hot flash symptoms you can imagine). "Situation/triggers" could include stressors, activities, thoughts, alcohol, or other factors you believe may trigger or worsen your hot flashes. "Action taken" refers to what you did when the hot flash occurred (e.g., left the room, removed clothing, took some deep breaths, told yourself calming thoughts).

FIGURE 14.5. Managing Menopausal Hot Flashes With Reassuring Thinking (*continues*)

Stressful, alarming thoughts may increase the severity of menopausal hot flashes. Alarming thoughts about the hot flashes may also lead to more difficulty coping effectively with the symptoms. One tool to help better manage menopausal symptoms is to change or disrupt a pattern of alarming or unhelpful thoughts by replacing them with more reassuring or supportive statements consistent with your values and how you want to live your life.

1.   Identify Your Negative Self-Talk
The first step in changing unhelpful thinking is to identify your negative, alarming self-talk related to menopausal symptoms. Here are some examples of common thoughts women may have about these symptoms. *Place a check mark next to any thoughts that seem relevant to you.*

❑ Oh no—here it comes.

❑ Everyone is noticing how much I'm sweating right now.

❑ I can't deal with this right now.

❑ People will think I'm strange/anxious/old/etc.

❑ Something is physically wrong with me.

❑ I can't stand this.

❑ This sweating is so embarrassing.

What other alarming or negative self-talk might you notice when you experience hot flashes? Please list them below:

_____

_____

FIGURE 14.5. Managing Menopausal Hot Flashes With Reassuring Thinking (*continued*)

2. Develop Reassuring Coping Statements

The second step in changing alarming thinking is to accept what's happening by making reassuring, calming, and helpful statements to yourself. This may help to keep your initial symptoms from escalating to higher levels and can give you a greater sense of control over the situation.

Some people find it helpful to write or record several coping statements on their phone or on a 3 × 5 index card. When hot flash symptoms begin, refer to those coping statements and repeat them to yourself to help manage the symptoms and your reaction in a healthier manner.

Here are some examples of positive coping statements that people have found helpful when they first feel the symptoms of hot flashes coming on. *Place a check mark next to the coping statements you believe could be most helpful for you.*

- ❏ I don't *like* feeling this way, but I can *accept* it.
- ❏ I can feel like this and still be okay.
- ❏ I can handle these symptoms or sensations.
- ❏ These symptoms are natural—I'm perfectly healthy.
- ❏ I'm going to go on with what I'm doing and wait for my symptoms to decrease.
- ❏ I'll just let my body do its thing. This will pass.
- ❏ I can do my coping strategies (e.g., relaxation) and allow this to pass.
- ❏ Fighting and resisting isn't going to help—so I'll just let it flow.
- ❏ My symptoms are not very noticeable—they feel stronger than they look to others.
- ❏ So what?

What additional coping statements do you believe would be helpful for you to combat your own alarming self-talk? _____
_____
_____
_____

Altering sleep behaviors. See Chapter 5 for a discussion on improving sleep. It may be important to help the patient have realistic expectations about sleep improvements by commenting that although hot flashes at night will likely not be eliminated, it is realistic to expect that changing her response to the awakenings may help her return to sleep more rapidly.

Altering environment and avoiding triggers. One might say the following:

> By avoiding or decreasing things such as caffeine and alcohol that seem to trigger your hot flashes, you can probably decrease the number of hot flashes you have each day. Also, by making your room cooler at night, we can probably decrease night sweats.

Agree

After describing the options, ask what the patient would like to do. If there are several areas they would like to target, ask what is the most important and/or easiest for the patient to initiate and start there.

Assist

There are a variety of treatment options appropriate to target symptoms and improve functioning. What one does should be tailored to the individual. Common areas of intervention are as follows:

- Educate by reviewing fact-related information about menopause.

- Have the patient monitor symptoms for further assessment of problem areas and as a way to assess symptom change (for additional details on self-monitoring, see Chapter 4).

- Teach strategies for questioning and challenging stressful or anxiety-provoking thoughts (for additional details, see Chapter 4).

- Teach deep breathing and cue-controlled relaxation (for additional details, see Chapter 4).

- If deep breathing and cue-controlled relaxation do not produce maximal effect, use passive or progressive muscle relaxation as an additional relaxation strategy (for additional details, see Chapter 4).

- Establish a sleep behavior change plan (for additional details, see Chapter 5).

- Have the patient alter their substance use associated with symptoms (e.g., caffeine, alcohol, tobacco use).

- Have the patient lower the temperature in her bedroom to 64 degrees to decrease night sweats. Freedman and Roehrs (2006) showed a significant reduction in the number of night sweats at this temperature.

Patients might be interested in websites, mobile device applications, or self-help books to assist in managing their menopause symptoms. Some of these resources are summarized in Figure 14.6.

Arrange

We suggest starting an intervention on the first appointment. If one is unable to start anything, the patient should return to establish the planned changes, learn new skills, and implement the plan. One might suggest having one or more return appointments to ensure the plan is working, to solve problems, or to add additional skills, as needed.

SUMMARY

Undetected or ineffectively treated depression during and after pregnancy, CPP, and menopausal symptoms such as hot flashes can lead to unnecessary suffering. In addition to the patient's personal functional impairments stemming from these conditions, other important individuals in women's lives can be affected as well. Effective behavioral health treatment for women with these problems is certainly possible and likely preferable in the primary care setting using a behavioral health consultation model.

An active screening program for depression during and after pregnancy is vital. If one does not know depression is present, they cannot treat it. Additionally, behavioral health assessment and intervention early in the course of CPP is consistent with a multidisciplinary model believed to offer the best management approach and has the possibility of reducing suffering and disability, regardless of whether an organic explanation for the pain is identified. We strongly recommend BHCs discuss with their medical team the possibility of developing a standard process of care within the clinic to include giving most women with CPP an initial behavioral health assessment to determine whether effective behavioral health interventions for managing symptoms are indicated. Finally, women going through menopause can vary greatly in the physiological changes they experience, and hormone replacement therapy works well for many women in managing these symptoms. For other women who cannot or choose not to engage in hormone replacement therapy, consider implementing a standard process of care whereby these women receive an initial behavioral health assessment to determine what, if any, management strategies might help.

FIGURE 14.6. Resources for Patients With Menopause: Websites, Mobile Applications, and Books (*continues*)

Type	Location	Description
Website	The North American Menopause Society (https://www.menopause.org/for-women)	Provides information on symptoms, treatment, and coping
Mobile applications	MenoPro (Apple iOS and Android)	Free mobile application helps patients work with their provider to personalize treatment decisions (e.g., hormone vs. nonhormone options). It includes links to education materials, including a downloadable *MenoNote* on behavioral and lifestyle modifications to reduce hot flashes, information pages on the pros and cons of hormone versus nonhormone therapy options, a discussion of pill versus patch therapy, and information on treatment options for vaginal dryness and pain with sexual activities, with links to tables with information about different medications.
	balance - Menopause Support (Apple iOS and Android)	"Understand more about your menopause with the help of expert medically approved content that's tailored around you. Keep an eye on your symptoms and health with the help of the balance journal. Understand your treatment options in the review section, where others have shared their honest experiences of both HRT and alternatives. Prepare for any healthcare appointments you may have by downloading your own personalised Health Report®. Our 'at-glance' summary allows your healthcare professional to diagnose your peri/menopause more quickly and discuss treatment options with you.

FIGURE 14.6. Resources for Patients With Menopause: Websites, Mobile Applications, and Books (*continued*)

Type	Location	Description
Mobile applications (*continued*)	balance - Menopause Support (Apple iOS and Android) (*continued*)	Track any changes to, or patterns in, your symptoms and health over time with the help of graphs to show you how things are going. Join experiments that have each been specifically designed to help relieve certain symptoms of the menopause. Share your stories and read others', balance is a safe place to talk about this time in your life with people who understand. Here you can feel supported whilst also helping others." (Paused for Thought, n.d., paras. 12–18)
Books	*Managing Hot Flushes and Night Sweats: A Cognitive Behavioural Self-Help Guide to the Menopause*, 2nd ed. (M. Hunter & Smith, 2020)	"Offers up-to-date and evidence-based information about the menopause and about hot flushes and night sweats, which are the main reason that women seek medical help. The four-week self-help guide uses cognitive behavioral therapy, providing information and strategies for managing hot flushes and night sweats, as well as stress and sleep. The guide is interactive with exercises and homework tailored to women's individual circumstances and lifestyles. It challenges myths about menopause and aging and provides better understanding of flushes which in turn reduces stress and improves post-menopausal well-being. The various chapters discuss processes of identification and modification of triggers of hot flushes and offers tips to women on dealing with hot flushes in social and work situations. The guide can be as effective as eight hours of group CBT and will help women who want to try a non-medical treatment that is brief and effective without side effects, or just want to be better informed." (Taylor & Francis Group, 2020, paras. 1–3)
	The Menopause Book (Kantrowitz & Wingert, 2018)	"Incorporates the latest medical findings, cutting-edge research, and best-practices advice. Expertly separating fact from fiction in the latest 'breakthrough' medical studies, it shows you what to pay attention to, and what you can ignore. Learn about the role of hormones and the latest advances in hormone therapy. The truth about hot flashes and how to deal with getting one at work. The impact of menopause on sexuality and how to manage an up-and-down libido. There are chapters on heart health (how to protect it), moods (how to ride them out), and exercise (how to stretch without strain). And finally, why this period of life can be a natural springboard to staying healthy, feeling great, and looking beautiful for the next act of your life." (Workman, 2018, para. 1)

15

Children, Adolescents, and Parenting

By the time they are 16 years old, 37% to 39% of children will have been diagnosed with a behavioral or emotional disorder at some point in their lives (Weitzman et al., 2015). Identifying and targeting these problems in primary care can be essential for promoting optimal development (Weitzman et al., 2015). Broadly defined, integrated medical–behavioral care has been found to improve behavioral health outcomes in primary care among children and adolescents (Asarnow et al., 2015). In this chapter, we focus on three common presenting concerns in primary care among children and adolescents that afford behavioral health consultants (BHCs) opportunities to provide assistance: (a) child and adolescent behavior management, (b) bedwetting, and (c) attention-deficit/hyperactivity disorder (ADHD). Concerns such as anxiety, depression, and obesity are also very common within these populations, and we encourage BHCs to become familiar with the specific guidance for these problems in the child and adolescent populations (e.g., Hampl et al., 2023; Selph & McDonagh, 2019; Styne et al., 2017; Wehry et al., 2015); often cognitive and behavioral or interpersonal therapy interventions are recommended as evidence-based treatments. The American Academy of Pediatrics and the American Academy of Family Physicians have online resources for targeting a broad range of behavioral health concerns (see Figure 15.1). Similarly, as we mention in Chapter 6, the American Academy of Pediatrics published guidelines for treating obesity in children and adolescents (Hampl et al., 2023). Summary guidance on interventions for other

https://doi.org/10.1037/0000380-016

Integrated Behavioral Health in Primary Care: Step-by-Step Guidance for Assessment and Intervention, Third Edition, by C. L. Hunter, J. L. Goodie, M. S. Oordt, and A. C. Dobmeyer

FIGURE 15.1. Resources for Patients With Behavior Management Problems: Websites, Mobile Applications, and Books

Type	Location	Description
Websites	American Academy of Pediatrics (https://www.aap.org/en-us/advocacy-and-policy/aap-health-initiatives/Mental-Health/Pages/default.aspx)	Provides a broad selection of tools and resources for addressing behavioral and emotional challenges in children and adolescents with screening measures and evidence-based behavioral interventions for a broad set of problems
	American Academy of Family Physicians (https://familydoctor.org/familydoctor/en/kids/parenting.html)	Provides a section devoted to parenting resources
	Alan Kazdin and the Yale Parenting Center (https://alankazdin.com/)	Provides resources for parents and providers regarding effective behavior management strategies, including an online Coursera course
	PCIT International (https://www.pcit.org/)	Provides information and resources for parents and providers for PCIT
	Triple P Parenting Program (https://www.triplep.net/; https://www.triplep-parenting.net/)	Resources, primarily for parents, related to the Triple P program
Mobile application	Privilege Points Chore Tracker (https://www.privilegepoints.com/)	Allows parents to track tasks and chores and assigns point values
Books	*The Everyday Parenting Toolkit: The Kazdin Method for Easy, Step-by-Step, Lasting Change for You and Your Child* (Kazdin & Rotella, 2013)	Provides practical, evidence-based parenting guidance for all children
	The Kazdin Method for Parenting the Defiant Child: With No Pills, No Therapy, No Contest of Wills (Kazdin, 2009)	Provides practical, evidence-based parenting guidance for children who are "out of control," including a DVD demonstrating parenting methods

Note. PCIT = parent–child interaction therapy.

specific childhood concerns that BHCs may assist with, including sleep issues, thumb-sucking, picky eating, school readiness, and oral health, were discussed by Nasir and Nasir (2015).

CHILD AND ADOLESCENT BEHAVIOR MANAGEMENT

Parents and caregivers frequently will ask their primary care providers (PCPs) about effective parenting methods or describe difficulties with their children, concerned that an underlying condition (e.g., developmental or affective disorder) is the cause. The BHC can assist the PCP in assessing these concerns and developing methods for targeting behavioral problems.

Cultural and Diversity Considerations

There is a wide breadth of parenting practices across cultures, and cultural influences on parenting shape parental thinking even before children are born. Some cultures will value promoting individual autonomy versus interdependence in their children. Individuals in some cultures will prefer direct commands and will seek to promote assertiveness, whereas others will promote passiveness and self-control (Bornstein, 2012). Before recommending behavior management changes, it is important to determine whether changes are consistent with cultural norms and consider the likelihood that changes might not be implemented if they are inconsistent with those norms. Therefore, BHCs should discuss cultural norms with the individuals engaging in the parenting practices (i.e., parents, guardians), recognizing that there may be disagreements about what is acceptable, particularly if individuals have different expectations based on diverse cultural backgrounds. BHCs may need to consider ways of adapting evidence-informed interventions to increase the likelihood that changes will be implemented.

Specialty Mental Health

Meta-analyses have found that parenting programs are effective for changing parenting behaviors and improving child behavior problems (Kaminski et al., 2008). Although multiple programs have been found to be effective, we discuss four programs here that are prominent throughout the literature and have a breadth of evidence supporting their use.

Parent–child interaction therapy (PCIT) was developed for caregivers of children 4 to 7 years old. PCIT uses child-directed interaction and parent-directed interaction phases to coach parents and teach effective strategies for managing behaviors (McNeil & Hembree-Kigin, 2010). PCIT establishes an authoritative parenting style in the context of a nurturing relationship and clear parent–child communication (Berkovits et al., 2010). In PCIT, child-directed interaction is used to develop parent–child attachment and positive parenting, whereas parent-directed interactions are used to develop clear parental directives, consistency, and follow-through with directives (Berkovits et al., 2010). In specialty behavioral health care settings, therapists often use bug-in-the-ear technology or other forms of coaching to provide guidance to parents while they are interacting with their children. PCIT is effective for decreasing disruptive, hyperactive, negative, and externalizing problems (Thomas et al., 2017; Valero-Aguayo et al., 2021).

The Triple P (Positive Parenting Program) uses five intervention levels on a tiered continuum of interventions to target parenting skills and behavior management strategies (Sanders, 2012; Sanders & Murphey-Brennan, 2010; Thomas & Zimmer-Gembeck, 2007). The levels of the Triple P are as follows (Sanders, 2012):

- Level 1: media communication regarding positive parenting (e.g., public advertising),

- Level 2: brief parenting interventions (e.g., large group parenting seminars),

- Level 3: narrow focused parenting programs (e.g., three to four individual face-to-face or telephone appointments),

- Level 4: broad focused parenting programs (e.g., ten 60-minute individual appointments, eight online modules), and

- Level 5: intensive family interventions (e.g., eight individual appointments that may include home visits).

The level and intensity of the intervention is dependent on the behavior problems and situation of the family (e.g., general population vs. family going through divorce). Triple P is considered effective for improving child, parent, and family well-being (Sanders et al., 2014).

Kazdin and colleagues developed problem-solving skills training and parent management training (PMT) to treat children between 5 and 12 years old who meet diagnostic criteria for oppositional defiant disorder or conduct disorder (Kazdin, 2010). Problem-solving skills training teaches children to use problem-solving steps (e.g., identifying the problem and possible solutions, considering possible outcomes), and PMT teaches parents to use techniques such as positive reinforcement, prompting, shaping, and time-out to manage unwanted behaviors.

Behavioral Health in Primary Care

A small number of studies have evaluated teaching behavior management strategies in primary care settings. Berkovits et al. (2010) compared the use of four weekly, 1.5-hour group appointments in primary care to implement PCIT, which included parent coaching by a therapist, with a group that received PCIT self-guided materials. Both groups resulted in improved child behavior management that was sustained at a 6-month follow-up assessment, and there were no differences in outcomes between the groups at any point in time (Berkovits et al., 2010). McCormick et al. (2014) trained pediatric residents in Triple P skills and found that the residents' parenting consultation skills and the parents' disciplinary practices improved.

Gomez et al. (2014) provided preliminary evidence that BHCs could implement PMT within the context of the primary care behavioral health model. Caregivers reported reductions in distress and high levels of satisfaction.

Together, these findings provide some evidence that brief interventions, based on well-established approaches and provided in primary care, may improve parenting skills and behavior problems, particularly among young children. A systematic review of parenting interventions provided in primary care found that these interventions could improve the functioning of children and parents (J. D. Smith et al., 2020). In addition to the evidence associated with PCIT, the implementation of the Triple P program and PMT have been evaluated in a variety of settings outside of specialty behavioral health care settings and have been shown to be effective (Michelson et al., 2013; Sanders, 2012).

Primary Care Adaptation

Research from specialty mental health and behavioral health in primary care provides a foundation for implementing the 5As in primary care settings.

Assess

When parents and caregivers present with concerns about child or adolescent behavior problems, it is important to consider whether behavior problems may be due to other behavioral health or developmental disorders (e.g., anxiety, autism spectrum disorder, ADHD, depression, substance use) or medical disorders (e.g., headaches, other pain, sleep disorder). This assessment may not be possible without an evaluation of the child; however, knowing whether there are behavior problems in other settings (e.g., at school, when spending time with friends) can help guide decisions about whether additional evaluations are necessary. When assessing behavior management strategies, it is also important to consider whether there is evidence of maltreatment. Caregiver factors (e.g., criminal history, inappropriate expectations of the child and child development, substance abuse), child factors (e.g., behavior problems, medical fragility, special needs), and family and environmental factors (e.g., high local unemployment, intimate partner violence, poverty, social isolation) are related to higher levels of child maltreatment (McDonald, 2007). The following questions help to screen for current behavior management practices and problems:

- How often do you need to discipline your child?

- Where does your child experience behavior problems? At home? At school? With friends?

- What do you do when your child does not do what you ask?

- How do you respond to tantrums?

- What types of discipline do you use most often? What types of discipline have you used less often or perhaps when your typical discipline is not working? What types of discipline do you believe should always be avoided?

- Are you and your significant other typically on the same page when you discipline your child? Do you support each other's disciplining decisions?

- In situations when you don't agree on disciplining decisions, how do you manage those disagreements?

- Are there relationship dynamics between individuals who are involved in disciplining the child that may be affecting/sabotaging effective behavior management?

In addition, several screening measures may help BHCs and PCPs systematically screen for child behavior problems. The Strengths and Difficulties Questionnaire (https://www.sdqinfo.org/) has parent, teacher, and self-report versions in multiple languages and includes 25 items for assessing a broad range of emotional symptoms, conduct problems, hyperactivity and inattention, peer relationship problems, and prosocial behaviors (R. Goodman, 1997, 2001). The Pediatric Symptom Checklist (PSC) is completed by the parent or caregiver and has 35- and 17-item versions (Massachusetts General Hospital, n.d.). Overall scores above 28 on the PSC-35 and above 15 on the PSC-17 (Gardner et al., 2007) are suggestive of psychosocial dysfunction (Jellinek et al., 1988); there are three subscales (attention problems, internalizing problems, and externalizing problems) that can also be used to specify problem areas. There are versions for self-report by adolescents and in multiple languages. The PSC has one of the strongest evidence bases among brief psychosocial screening tools (Becker-Haimes et al., 2020; Jellinek & Murphy, 2021).

Advise

If there are signs of child maltreatment, it is critical for the BHC to coordinate with the PCP about the next steps for keeping the child safe, which may require contacting local child protective services. The BHC will need to advise the parent or caregiver about the steps that need to be taken. If there are no significant concerns about maltreatment or other behavioral health or medical concerns, it is important to discuss with the parent or caregiver their role in managing the behaviors of the child. It can be helpful to frame the changes in terms of the parent or caregiver needing special skills to manage some of these behaviors. You might say the following:

> It sounds like your daughter can be very difficult to manage at times, and it is completely understandable how that could be frustrating. Sometimes parents can benefit from learning special skills to specifically help to manage some of these behaviors. Some of these skills you may have heard of before, like time-out, but we often find that parents can learn how to apply these skills in slightly different ways so that they are more effective.

When advising parents and caregivers, it is important to anticipate potential resistance or skepticism about the effectiveness of these interventions. Interventions, such as time-out, are often discussed in the lay press and media, but unless the skills are implemented in a manner that has been shown to work, the interventions are less likely to be effective.

Agree

During the agree phase it is critical to consider personal or cultural beliefs and concerns regarding behavior management of children and adolescents. Some interventions, such as reinforcing positive behaviors, may be viewed by some individuals as spoiling the child. Similarly, there may be a belief that corporal punishment is the most effective strategy for managing behaviors. Additionally, it will be important to ensure that, if multiple caregivers are involved in discipline, consistency will be maintained between the caregivers in how to approach behavior management. If there are concerns that the caregivers will not be consistent, it may be worth scheduling appointments when all of the caregivers can be present.

Assist

As described by Banks (2002), there are important principles of discipline that should be followed. If two parents are involved, it is important for both to be unified in their approach to discipline. Rules and consequences should be clear and appropriate for the child or adolescent's age. As children get older, it can be helpful to engage them in decision making regarding appropriate consequences, although parents should remain the final decision makers.

Basic behavioral concepts, including positive and negative reinforcement and positive and negative punishment, are key when discussing discipline techniques. Banks (2002) provided a useful table for summarizing age-appropriate techniques for childhood discipline, which we have reprinted in Figure 15.2. The following are key points to discuss with patients when discussing behavior management.

Maintain consistency between parents and caregivers. Children will quickly learn if one parent or caregiver is more lenient than another. Parents and caregivers must agree to support each other in front of the child and discuss differences privately. Ideally, parents and caregivers should discuss how they plan to implement behavior change strategies before a situation develops.

Consequences should immediately follow the behavior. Regardless of whether the parents or caregivers are working to increase or decrease a behavior, the

FIGURE 15.2. Age-Appropriate Techniques for Childhood Discipline

Intervention	Infant	Toddler	School-age	Adolescent
Positive reinforcement	+	+	+	+
Redirecting	+	+	+	0
Verbal instruction/explanation	0	Ltd	+	+
Time-out	0	+	+	0
Establishment of rules	0	0	+	+
Grounding	0	0	+	+
Withholding privileges	0	0	+	+

Note. 0 = little or no effectiveness; + = effective/recommended; Ltd = limited, may work in certain situations or with more mature toddlers. From "Childhood Discipline: Challenges for Clinicians and Parents," by J. B. Banks, 2002, *American Family Physician, 66*(8), p. 1448 (https://www.aafp.org/content/dam/brand/aafp/pubs/afp/issues/2002/1015/p1447.pdf). Copyright 2002 by the American Academy of Family Physicians. Reprinted with permission.

consequence (e.g., the praise, the time-out) should occur as soon after the behavior as possible.

Catch the child engaging in desired behaviors. Often parents are quick to pay attention to unwanted behaviors and are less likely to pay attention to a child when they are engaged in wanted behaviors. Some have estimated that children receive 4 times more attention for unwanted behaviors than for wanted behaviors. One goal is to reverse that ratio so that children are receiving 4 times more positive attention than negative attention or at least receiving just as much praise as corrective feedback. For behavior change interventions to be effective, it is critical for the majority of interactions to be positive.

Use labeled praise. In PCIT interventions, the use of labeled praise is emphasized. Parents and caregivers are encouraged to be specific about what they like about the child's behaviors. For example, rather than saying "good job" a parent might say, "I like how you are sitting quietly at the table."

Work to shape and practice the desired behavior. Often it will be unrealistic to expect a child or adolescent to engage precisely in the desired behavior (e.g., sitting in a seat throughout a meal). Therefore, it is important to gradually shape the behavior by reinforcing approximations of the desired behavior and developing the behavior over time. For example, at first praise sitting at the table for 3 minutes, then 5 minutes, then 8 minutes, and so on, until the child is sitting throughout the meal.

Anticipate and plan for situations that are high risk for unwanted behaviors. Parents and caregivers should work to identify situations that are more likely to elicit unwanted behaviors and develop a plan for how those behaviors will be managed. For example, if a child is known to act out in restaurants, planning could include telling the child what the consequences will be if they engage in unwanted behaviors, which includes providing examples of the unwanted behaviors (e.g., getting out of the chair, throwing food, screaming or yelling), deciding what those consequences will be (e.g., going to a time-out spot away from others), and identifying who will deliver the consequence.

Use time-out effectively. The primary purpose of time-out is to remove a child from things that may increase the likelihood of unwanted behavior, including attention. Time-out should be administered immediately after the unwanted behaviors. A child should be taught to go or be gently led to a chair or place (e.g., the corner of a wall) away from attention from others and things that would be distracting (e.g., a television). Zisser and Eyberg (2010) provided instructions for how to implement time-out in PCIT, which can be adapted to primary care environments. Time-out may be initiated by saying, "You have a choice: You can either sit quietly in your chair or get a time-out." After 5 seconds, if the child has not engaged in the desired behavior, then the parent should say, "You chose not to sit quietly; therefore, you have to go to the time-out chair. Stay on the chair until I tell you to get off." It is not necessary to leave a child in time-out for extended periods of time; approximately 3 minutes is typically enough time. However, it may be useful to start with shorter times if the child is younger and when time-out is first being introduced. While the child is in time-out, parents should actively ignore the child and avoid engaging in conversation or rebutting anything that the child says. If there is a concern about safety, parents may stay in the room but turn away from the child. Once the time is up, it is important to wait for 5 seconds of quiet before removing the child from the time-out location. Otherwise, the child may learn to engage in yelling or other behaviors to get out of time-out. At the end of the time-out period, parents should ask, "Are you ready to sit in your chair at the dining table (i.e., the desired behavior)?" If the child says no, then the child is left in the time-out chair for another 3 minutes. Once the child is engaging in the desired activity, parents should look for other behaviors that can be reinforced through praise.

Monitor progress. It is valuable to provide feedback to both the child and parents about how often the child is engaging in desirable behavior. Using a simple chart to track days without a time-out or days when a particular desired behavior is observed will help track changes in behavior.

Avoid administering consequences when emotions are high. When parents are experiencing frustration or anger, they may be more likely to say things that they do not mean or use unintended force. Consequences should be delivered in a calm, systematic manner. If a parent is having difficulty managing emotions, it may be necessary for the parent to remove themselves from the situation until they are calmer.

Avoid saying things that you do not mean. Sometimes parents and caregivers will make threats that they are unlikely to enforce beyond the situation. Parents and caregivers should say what they mean when describing behavior consequences. For example, a parent might say, "If you don't clean up your room now, you are never going to be allowed to go outside again." Such a statement is likely an empty threat, and it undermines the effectiveness of the consequences. An alternative would be to say, "If you don't put your clothes in your hamper within the next 2 hours, you will lose your phone for the rest of today."

Avoid aversive consequences. Yelling, threatening, and hitting are examples of aversive consequences. These are reactions that are intended to invoke negative emotions in the child or inflict pain. These actions may result in an immediate reduction in an unwanted behavior, but they are not associated with long-term improvements in behavior. Severe and frequent spanking has been shown to have negative consequences on childhood development; the data are less clear regarding the long-term impact of mild or occasional spanking

(Avezum et al., 2022; Benjet & Kazdin, 2003). Beliefs about spanking vary across cultures, regions of the country, and socioeconomic status (Avezum et al., 2022). It is important to work with the individuals involved in spanking to be clear on the limits of mild and occasional spanking if they are not willing to avoid all spanking. Resources, such as the Play Nicely program (Monroe Carell Jr. Children's Hospital, n.d.), may help to change attitudes about using spanking (Burkhart et al., 2018; Richardson & Damashek, 2022). No aversive consequence will be effective, no matter how mild, if the focus is on unwanted behaviors the majority of time.

Overall, adherence to these guidelines will likely enhance behavior management. Additional resources, including websites, mobile device applications, and self-help books, that might be used in conjunction with BHC appointments or by patients who will be following up with their PCP are summarized in Figure 15.1. *The Everyday Parenting Toolkit* (Kazdin & Rotella, 2013) introduces evidence-based interventions in an easy-to-read format and is a particularly useful book for parents to read for managing unwanted behaviors in children. Additional useful parenting strategies for managing child behaviors in primary care settings are discussed by Kavan et al. (2018).

Arrange

In many cases, it will be valuable to have the parent or caregiver return for at least one additional appointment to assess what worked and what did not work. Based on the responses received, BHCs may want to schedule an additional appointment to further or maintain progress or collaborate with the PCP to refer the patient to specialty mental health if there have been no changes with the problem behaviors. If BHCs consider specialty mental health, it will be valuable to identify community mental health providers who can provide the evidence-based interventions we discuss in the specialty mental health section. Given the successes of teaching parenting skills in group settings, it is also valuable to consider whether a BHC could develop a class that is offered regularly in the primary care clinic to specifically target teaching behavior management skills.

BED-WETTING

Bed-wetting, formally described as nocturnal enuresis, is common among young children. As many as 10% to 15% of children 6 years of age will experience bed-wetting, but most individuals will outgrow it by adulthood so that only 1% to 2% of adults demonstrate bed-wetting (Bayne & Skoog, 2014). Strong evidence suggests that there is a genetic component to bed-wetting (Butler, 2004). Nocturnal enuresis is defined in the fifth edition of the *Diagnostic and Statistical Manual of Mental Disorders, Text Revision* (*DSM-5-TR*; American Psychiatric Association, 2022, pp. 399–402) as voluntary or involuntary voiding of urine in bed, at least twice a week for 3 months or causing clinically significant distress or impairment, in children 5 years of age or older. Bed-wetting is associated with social isolation, humiliation, and fear of detection in children, and parents often express concern about the social and emotional impact on the child, while some report intolerance and react to bed-wetting with punishment (Butler, 2004). Bed-wetting is associated with other behavioral health problems; 20% to 30% of children who demonstrate bed-wetting meet criteria for another behavioral health problem (Van Herzeele et al., 2015).

Cultural and Diversity Considerations

Sociocultural factors may affect the degree to which bed-wetting is viewed as a problem and the reactions of children and parents; however, the data have been unclear. Some have found that Asian countries have higher prevalence rates, but others have found that those in a Chinese population had low prevalence rates when compared with European countries (Butler, 2004).

Specialty Mental Health

Several behavioral interventions have been evaluated in specialty care, including fluid restriction, lifting (i.e., carrying a child, while still asleep, to the bathroom), scheduled wakening (i.e., waking the child during the night to encourage urination), rewarding (e.g., using stars on a chart to reinforce dry nights), and bladder training and retention control training (e.g., delaying urination when there is an urge, interrupting the stream of urination). All of these interventions have been found to be better than no intervention (Caldwell et al., 2013). The most effective intervention is a bed-wetting alarm; the other behavioral interventions are not as effective (Caldwell et al., 2020). The bed-wetting alarm uses sensors embedded in a pad, sheets, or nightclothes. When the sensor becomes wet, an auditory alarm and/or vibration are triggered, which causes the child to wake and to cease voiding; this alarm prompts the child to get up and go to the bathroom. Parents often need to ensure that the child has gotten out of bed rather than fallen back asleep (Vande Walle et al., 2012).

Behavioral Health in Primary Care

The use of the bed-wetting alarm is considered a first-line treatment in primary care settings (Bayne & Skoog, 2014). In addition to the bed-wetting alarm, desmopressin (DDAVP), a synthetic form of vasopressin, reduces urine production and has been shown to be effective for helping to manage bed-wetting (Bayne & Skoog, 2014).

Primary Care Adaptation

In the case of bed-wetting, there is a fair amount of overlap between what is being done in specialty care and primary care settings as a first step toward targeting bed-wetting. The 5As helps to organize the appointment and strategies used in primary care.

Assess

During the assessment phase, it is important to conduct a functional analysis of the bed-wetting, including the frequency of the problem and other possible causes of the bed-wetting. The following questions help guide bed-wetting assessment (Vande Walle et al., 2012):

- How often does your child wet the bed?

- How much does your child drink during the day? In the evening, does your child drink more than one glass? Does your child drink anything at night?

- When do you find out that your child wet the bed? As soon as it happens? In the morning?

- What happens when the bed-wetting is discovered? What do you do? What does the child do?

- How does bed-wetting affect your child's life? Are there situations your child avoids (e.g., sleepovers)? How does bed-wetting affect your life?

- Is there evidence of leakage throughout the day? How often? How much?

- How often does your child urinate during the day?

- Does your child demonstrate a sudden urge to urinate? How often?

- Do you notice your child trying to hold urine, such as by crossing legs or standing on tiptoes?

- Is your child constipated, for example, having three or fewer bowel movements per week? Is there any poop in your child's underpants? Does your child experience pain when pooping?

Children who demonstrate frequent urination throughout the day, signs of difficulty controlling urination, or signs of fecal incontinence may have other problems (e.g., overactive bladder, dysfunctional voiding, diabetes), which would interfere with the effectiveness of bed-wetting interventions. Given the increased likelihood of other behavioral health problems, it is also helpful to screen for depressive, anxiety, ADHD, and other posttraumatic stress disorder symptoms. Van Hoecke et al. (2007) developed and tested the Short Screening Instrument for Psychological Problems in Enuresis. This instrument screens for emotional problems and symptoms of ADHD in children and is provided in Figure 15.3. It may be helpful to have parents or caregivers monitor bed-wetting after the initial appointment if there is not time to discuss interventions. Figure 15.4 is an example of a monitoring chart that could be used to assess bed-wetting before and after the initiation of an intervention.

FIGURE 15.3. Short Screening Instrument for Psychological Problems in Enuresis

Short Screening Instrument for Psychological Problems in Enuresis (SSIPPE)

Name: _____ Date of birth: _____

	Emotional symptoms: If more than two positive items, full screening required		
1.	Has your child **sometimes** felt that others are reacting negatively?	YES	NO
2.	Does your child **sometimes** feel worthless or less confident?	YES	NO
3.	Does your child **sometimes** have headaches?	YES	NO
4.	Does your child **sometimes** feel sick?	YES	NO
5.	Does your child **sometimes** have abdominal pain?	YES	NO
6.	Is your child **sometimes** less active or lacking energy?	YES	NO
7.	Does your child **sometimes** feel unhappy, sad, or depressive?	YES	NO
	Inattention symptoms: If more than two positive items, full screening required		
1.	Does your child **frequently** pay insufficient attention to details or make careless defaults in schoolwork?	YES	NO
2.	Does your child **frequently** have difficulties with organizing tasks and activities?	YES	NO
3.	Does your child **frequently** forget in daily practice?	YES	NO
	Hyperactivity/impulsivity symptoms: If more than two positive items, full screening required		
1.	Does your child **frequently** talk continuously?	YES	NO
2.	Is your child **frequently** busy?	YES	NO
3.	Does your child **frequently** run or climb in situations in which this is inappropriate?	YES	NO

Note. From "Early Detection of Psychological Problems in a Population of Children With Enuresis: Construction and Validation of the Short Screening Instrument for Psychological Problems in Enuresis," by E. Van Hoecke, D. Baeyens, H. Vanden Bossche, P. Hoebeke, and J. Vande Walle, 2007, *The Journal of Urology*, *178*(6), p. 2614 (https://doi.org/10.1016/j.juro.2007.08.025). Copyright 2007 by American Urological Association. Reprinted with permission.

Advise

If a BHC identifies other problems that may be contributing to the bed-wetting, take time to discuss these with the PCP to determine the next steps in the patient's care. When BHCs are advising parents, caregivers, and children about bed-wetting, it is valuable to provide education about how common it is for children to experience bed-wetting and to provide reassurance that bed-wetting can be treated. The following is an example of what a BHC could say:

> It is understandable why bed-wetting would be a frustrating experience for everyone. It sounds like this has interfered with your sleep and with your willingness to engage in potentially enjoyable activities. In fact, bed-wetting among children 5 and older is common; approximately 10% to 15% of children in this age group may demonstrate bed-wetting. The good news is that we have several treatments that are effective and can help reduce bed-wetting frequency.

FIGURE 15.4. Bed-wetting Monitoring Chart

		Example	Monday	Tuesday	Wednesday	Thursday	Friday	Saturday	Sunday
Complete Before Bedtime	Number of glasses of liquid within 2 hours of bedtime	1 glass of water							
	Bedtime	8:30 p.m.							
Complete After Waking	Number of times woke up to pee or alarm went off	1							
	Number of times peed in bed	2							
	Wakeup time	7:00 a.m.							

Approximately 66% of children stop bed-wetting during treatment using a bed-wetting alarm, and 50% sustain improvements following treatment (Glazener et al., 2005). Most children who use DDAVP demonstrate immediate improvement but relapse when the medication is discontinued (Glazener et al., 2005).

Agree

Regardless of whether the family will be pursuing behavioral and/or medication interventions for bed-wetting, adherence to the plan will be critical for success. Therefore, getting buy-in from everyone will be important. BHCs could say the following to help get everyone on the same page:

> We have a few treatments that have been found to be most effective. One involves focusing on changing behaviors at night and using a system to alert Tommy when he is about to pee. You can also consider the use of medications to help reduce peeing or a combination of both techniques. Whatever you decide, the interventions will involve the whole family and it will be important to use the intervention consistently. Is that something that you would be willing to do? Let me take a little time to describe these interventions.

Encouraging family involvement can help to ensure that everyone is committed to following through with the planned changes. If there is evidence that the family members or the child are reluctant to engage in the behavior changes, consider whether there are any cultural or individual barriers and consider the use of motivational interviewing techniques described in Chapter 4.

Assist

One of the most important interventions will be the implementation of the bed-wetting alarm. A bed-wetting alarm can be purchased from a variety of vendors; examples of websites are provided in Figure 15.5. If the PCP recommends the alarm, it may be covered by insurance. To assist children and families, there are several important points to discuss:

- It is important that there are no efforts to shame the child and that expressions of frustration or anger are avoided.

- Children should understand that the purpose of the alarm is to wake them up as soon as they start to pee and that they need to wake up and go directly to the bathroom. Ultimately, we want the child to wake before the alarm is activated.

- At first, parents and caregivers should be prepared to wake and help the child get to the bathroom, as children often will fall back asleep after the alarm.

- Fluids should not be restricted during the day. During the 2 hours before bedtime the child may drink fluids if they are thirsty, but they should avoid fluids that contain caffeine, which serves as a diuretic.

- The pathway to the bathroom should be lit (e.g., nightlights) and clear of obstructions.

FIGURE 15.5. Resources for Patients Who Wet the Bed: Websites and Books

Type	Location	Description
Websites	Vendors for bed-wetting alarms (https://www.sleepdryalarm.com/; https://bedwettingstore.com/; https://wetstop.com/)	A variety of vendors sell bed-wetting alarms. These sites may make claims that are not supported by evidence (e.g., cures bed-wetting).
	U.S. National Library of Medicine (https://www.nlm.nih.gov/medlineplus/bedwetting.html)	Consolidates information regarding bed-wetting resources for parents and providers
	American Academy of Pediatrics (https://www.healthychildren.org/English/ages-stages/toddler/toilet-training/Pages/Bedwetting.aspx)	Provides additional information for parents about bed-wetting causes and treatments
Books	*Bedwetting and Accidents Aren't Your Fault: How Potty Accidents Happen and How to Make Them Stop* (Hodges & Schlosberg, 2017)	Children's book discusses bed-wetting; written by a pediatric urologist
	Waking Up Dry: A Guide to Help Children Overcome Bedwetting (H. J. Bennett, 2015)	Describes evidence-based approaches to reducing bed-wetting; written by a practicing pediatrician

- Reward the child for nights without bed-wetting.

- The rate of response will vary and may take multiple weeks or months. This intervention should be tried for at least 2 to 3 months (Bayne & Skoog, 2014).

In situations where the bed-wetting alarm is not effective or when it would be inconvenient to use the alarm (e.g., during a sleepover), it may be valuable to discuss with the family and the PCP whether DDAVP should be considered as a supplemental or alternative method for helping to manage bed-wetting.

Arrange

It may be helpful to have the patients return one to two times to assess whether the intervention is effective and then to follow up after 2 to 3 months if treatment is successful to ensure that the child did not relapse. In situations where neither the bed-wetting alarm nor other behavioral interventions are effective, consider referring to specialty behavioral health. Also consider whether other factors may be contributing to the bed-wetting and whether those factors can be addressed in primary care. Additional resources, including websites and self-help books, that might be used in conjunction with BHC appointments or by patients who will be following up with their PCP are summarized in Figure 15.5.

ATTENTION-DEFICIT/HYPERACTIVITY DISORDER

Among children, ADHD is the most common behavioral disorder (Wolraich et al., 2019). To meet criteria for ADHD as defined in the *DSM-5-TR* (American Psychiatric Association, 2022, pp. 68–76), children must demonstrate six or more inattentive symptoms (e.g., failure to give close attention to details, difficulty sustaining attention in tasks, forgetfulness in daily activities) and/or six or more hyperactivity and impulsive symptoms (e.g., fidgeting with hands or feet, talking excessively, difficulty waiting for their turn) before the age of 12; in previous versions of the *DSM*, the age cutoff was 6 years old. These symptoms must occur in at least two settings and interfere with functioning. ADHD may be specified as predominately inattentive presentation, hyperactive/impulsive presentation, or a combined presentation. ADHD is a chronic condition that can affect academic achievement, socialization, and overall health (Wolraich et al., 2019). ADHD is associated with worse health-related behaviors and physical outcomes, including smoking, illicit substance use disorders, accidental injuries, obesity, and suicide (Nigg, 2013). Adolescents with ADHD are at higher risk for substance abuse and risky driving behaviors (Sibley et al., 2014).

An estimated 9.8% of children between the ages of 3 and 17 years have been diagnosed with ADHD; boys are twice as likely as girls to be diagnosed with ADHD (Bitsko et al., 2022). Among children and adolescents diagnosed with ADHD, 69% were taking a medication for ADHD, 51% received treatment or counseling from a mental health professional, and 82.5% were receiving either medication or mental health treatment (Visser et al., 2014).

Cultural and Diversity Considerations

Although the reported prevalence of ADHD varies widely throughout the world, this variance is hypothesized to be related to methodological limitations of studies rather than actual differences (Polanczyk et al., 2015). Parents and teachers rate Black children and adolescents as having more ADHD symptoms compared with their White counterparts, but Black youth are diagnosed with ADHD at two thirds the rate of White youth; the reasons for the discrepancies are unclear (T. W. Miller et al., 2009; Slobodin & Masalha, 2020). As we discuss later, stimulant medication is considered a first-line treatment for ADHD; however, Latinx, Black, and Asian adolescents are less likely to be prescribed and use stimulant medication compared with their White peers (Johansen et al., 2015; Slobodin & Masalha, 2020). Although the reasons for these discrepancies are unclear, some have suggested that they may be related to differences in cultural norms, attitudes toward mental health, and limited access to care (Johansen et al., 2015; Slobodin & Masalha, 2020). Research specifically investigating interventions for ADHD that reduce these discrepancies across ethnic and cultural groups is needed (Pfiffner & Haack, 2015).

Specialty Mental Health

Stimulant medications, such as methylphenidate (e.g., Concerta, Ritalin) and amphetamines (e.g., Adderall XR, Vyvanse), are considered first-line treatments for ADHD in children and adolescents 6 years old and older. However, there may be concerns with the abuse of stimulant medication, and some patients may experience insomnia, appetite loss, and/or irritability. Second-line medications, which are not stimulants, include atomoxetine (Strattera) and alpha-2 receptor agonists (Tenex, Catapres) and may be preferred by some family members and patients or in situations when providers are concerned about stimulant misuse or side effects. Other medications that have not been approved by the Food and Drug Administration for ADHD but are used off-label include bupropion (Wellbutrin), risperidone (Risperdal), aripiprazole (Abilify), and carbamazepine (Tegretol; Felt et al., 2014).

Behavioral treatments for ADHD usually include behavioral parent training, behavioral classroom management/interventions, child skills training, or a combination of these interventions (Pfiffner & Haack, 2015). These treatments are considered first-line therapy for those 4 to 6 years old and should be included with medication treatment for older children and adolescents (Wolraich et al., 2019). Similar to the behavioral interventions described in this chapter regarding behavior management of children and adolescents, behavioral parent training focuses on educating parents about ADHD and targeting the antecedents and consequences associated with behaviors (e.g., increasing positive parental attention, using effective praise, using time-outs; Antshel, 2015). Employing similar strategies for classroom management (e.g., increasing attention for appropriate behaviors, using time-out for inappropriate behaviors) has also been found to be effective (Antshel, 2015). Child and adolescent skills training focuses on teaching strategies for organization, time management, and effective planning, which have also been found to be helpful for improving functioning (Antshel, 2015). The Homework, Organization, and Planning Skills program is one example of skills training that has been found to be effective in adolescents (Langberg et al., 2012).

Studies have examined the impact of electroencephalogram (EEG) neurofeedback to improve symptoms of ADHD. Most children diagnosed with ADHD show increased slow-wave and decreased fast-wave EEG activity. It is hypothesized that, by providing feedback to focus on these waves, patients can learn to change this activity and decrease ADHD symptoms. There is mixed evidence regarding the effectiveness of EEG-neurofeedback. Some studies have found positive benefits; however, when compared with placebo or sham feedback, EEG-neurofeedback has minimal or no impact (Holtmann et al., 2014; Vollebregt et al., 2014). Overall, the most effective strategy for targeting ADHD is the use of psychostimulant medication, combined with behavioral interventions in educational and specialty behavioral health settings (Watson et al., 2015).

Behavioral Health in Primary Care

The current American Academy of Pediatrics clinical practice guidelines for ADHD (Wolraich et al., 2019) recommend that preschool-aged children (i.e., 4–6 years of age) who demonstrate ADHD receive evidence-based parent- and/ or teacher-administered behavior therapy. Elementary-school-aged children (i.e., 6–12 years of age) should receive approved medications for ADHD in conjunction with behavior therapy (Wolraich et al., 2019). Adolescents between 12 and 18 years of age should receive approved ADHD medications; behavior therapy may be recommended, but the evidence for the effectiveness of behavior therapy in this age group is not as strong as the evidence for preschool- and elementary-school-aged children (Wolraich et al., 2019). Some experts disagree with this conclusion (e.g., Sibley et al., 2014) and suggest that behavior therapy interventions have substantial impact on measures of impairment, which were not used in pharmacotherapy trials, and that 80% to 90% of teens are nonadherent with medication use (Sibley et al., 2014).

A care management model has been found to improve the effectiveness of ADHD treatment in a primary care setting (Silverstein et al., 2015). No published studies have specifically examined the use of BHCs to target ADHD in primary care, and it is unknown whether brief behavioral interventions provided in primary care would have a meaningful impact on functioning in those with ADHD.

Primary Care Adaptation

In primary care settings, BHCs can play an important role in helping clinics develop systematic assessment approaches for ADHD symptoms and then developing approaches to target those problem behaviors. Planning a clear stepped-care approach within the clinic can help patients and families receive the care they need at that moment.

Assess

When assessing for ADHD, consider whether the observed difficulties may be better described by an emotional or behavioral condition (e.g., conduct disorder, mood or anxiety disorder, oppositional defiant disorder, posttraumatic stress disorder), developmental condition (e.g., learning disorder, intellectual disability), or physical condition (e.g., sleep-related problems, insufficient sleep; Felt et al., 2014; Wolraich et al., 2019). The first edition of the Vanderbilt Assessment Scale, along with scoring instructions for the *DSM-5-TR* criteria, is available for free from the National Institute for Children's Health Quality (n.d.). Parent and teacher forms are also available that can be completed and scored. The Centers for Disease Control and Prevention provides a simple checklist on its website, which is also presented in Figure 15.6.

It can be particularly important to consider ADHD in situations when children are described as not living up to their potential, described as being

FIGURE 15.6. Resources for Patients With Attention-Deficit/Hyperactivity Disorder: Websites and Books

Type	Location	Description
Websites	American Academy of Child and Adolescent Psychiatry (https://www.aacap.org/AACAP/Families_and_Youth/Resource_Centers/ADHD_Resource_Center/Home.aspx)	Provides a broad range of resources for patients, parents, providers, and students
	American Academy of Pediatrics (https://www.healthychildren.org/english/health-issues/conditions/adhd/Pages/default.aspx)	Provides information for parents, primarily through a series of brief articles and handouts about ADHD
	Centers for Disease Control and Prevention (https://www.cdc.gov/ncbddd/adhd)	Provides information for providers and parents about ADHD, including summaries of research, educational materials, and data
	Children and Adults With ADHD (https://www.chadd.org; http://www.help4adhd.org)	Nonprofit organization provides education, advocacy, and support for ADHD. Their website has a wide breadth of ADHD materials for parents, children, and providers.
Book	*Taking Charge of ADHD: The Complete, Authoritative Guide for Parents*, 4th ed. (Barkley, 2020)	Written by one of the leading national researchers on ADHD, book provides a breadth of information for parents and caregivers about ADHD and evidence-based methods for managing ADHD

Note. ADHD = attention-deficit/hyperactivity disorder.

daydreamers, failing to complete homework, or demonstrating difficulty with reading. Although this behavior certainly does not mean that child meets criteria for ADHD, children who are acting out or are disruptive (i.e., those demonstrating hyperactivity or impulsivity difficulties) may be more likely to be identified with ADHD compared with those who are demonstrating difficulty with attention and concentration. Additionally, it is important to consider whether there are health conditions that might affect treatment and medication recommendations (e.g., tic disorders). To assist with screening for other concerns, some clinics may find it helpful to use the Child Behavior Checklist (CBCL; Achenbach & Rescorla, 2001). The CBCL is completed by the parents, and there are forms for teachers (i.e., the Teacher's Report Form) and a measure for children 11 and older (i.e., the Youth Self-Report). The CBCL and related forms are purchased from https://store.aseba.org/. Given the time and cost involved with completing the CBCL, BHCs should consider whether it is best to complete the assessments within primary care or whether the patient should be referred to specialty care.

Advise

BHCs may play an important role in describing the benefits and limitations of available treatments for children and adolescents. Given the strong evidence supporting medication use to treat ADHD, an important role for the BHC can be to reinforce the value of medication treatment in those cases when medication is being considered.

Agree
The BHC should work with the parents or caregivers and child or adolescent (in collaboration with the PCP) to agree on the course of treatment and the importance of adherence to behavioral and/or medication interventions. Lack of adherence to treatment recommendations can significantly affect the effectiveness of interventions for ADHD; therefore, using motivational interviewing skills, such as those described in Chapter 4, is important when agreeing on the course of treatment for ADHD.

Assist
School-aged children with ADHD may be eligible for accommodations in school per Section 504 of the Rehabilitation Act or under the Individuals With Disabilities Education Act (Felt et al., 2014). The BHC can help the PCP and family begin to advocate for a formal evaluation that can inform an individualized education plan in the school. It is critical to provide children who are struggling in the classroom with the appropriate school interventions to help manage their behaviors. The behavior management strategies discussed in this chapter are one of the first places to start when intervening with the behavioral challenges associated with ADHD symptoms. Good behavior management skills that focus on identifying the antecedents, behaviors, and consequences that can be targeted can help parents more effectively manage ADHD behaviors.

In addition to behavior management strategies, focusing on developing social skills can also be helpful, particularly among children demonstrating social withdrawal or comorbid anxiety problems (Mikami et al., 2014). Children with ADHD symptoms may have difficulty engaging appropriately with other children. Parents can be encouraged to set up controlled playdates. Often it works best if only one friend is invited over and siblings are kept away. The parent can work with the child to practice common social skills, such as cleaning and preparing for the arrival of the guest, establishing rules of the house (e.g., not going into the parent's bedroom), introducing the guest to other family members, engaging in a structured activity (e.g., craft, baking), and appropriately saying goodbye. It is important for the parent to avoid scolding or punishing the child during the playdate.

BHCs may also help the PCP by monitoring for signs of medication adherence or misuse. Asking children and parents about concerns about the medication use, concerns about side effects, and whether there are significant changes in functioning may provide useful information about medication use.

Arrange
In situations where symptoms of ADHD are not improving with primary-care-based interventions, consider referring to a specialty behavioral health provider that offers evidence-based care for ADHD. Given the prevalence of ADHD, it

may be helpful to identify the local resources and providers offering these services. It may be particularly useful to consider a psychoeducational group or shared medical appointment, as we discuss in Chapter 18, for the children and/or parents to address the child's adaptive behaviors and parenting skills. We provide additional resources for children, parents, and providers in Figure 15.6. As adolescents are managing ADHD transition into adulthood, it could be helpful to discuss additional management strategies (e.g., National Institute of Mental Health, 2021b).

SUMMARY

Behavior problems, bed-wetting, and ADHD, in addition to depressive and anxiety symptoms, are some of the most common problems that will be referred to a BHC in the primary care context. In most cases, we do not have clear evidence that the interventions offered by BHCs will result in long-term effectiveness. However, these interventions are informed by the existing evidence and are an important part of a stepped-care model. It is important for BHCs to understand the limits of their scope of practice and to ensure they have the knowledge and skills to provide a full range of services to the PCPs. Even if the majority of training that a BHC received focused on adult-related problems, it is critical for BHCs to become familiar with the problems that are most common in primary care settings. Offering these assessments and interventions represents an important addition to primary care services.

16

Couple Distress

Intimate partner relationships and health are intertwined. Although significant relationships can come in many forms, much of the research literature focuses on the physical and mental health effects associated with heterosexual marriage. Although marriage itself may confer protective health benefits, the quality of the relationship matters. Individuals who are in distressed marriages are at risk for negative health consequences, whereas those in happier marriages are more likely to have better physical and mental health (Robles, 2014; Robles et al., 2014). In fact, individuals in unhappy marriages have health outcomes similar to or worse than those who are divorced, separated, widowed, or never married (Lawrence et al., 2019). In sum, couples may mutually influence each other's mental and physical health status, in both positive and negative trajectories (Kiecolt-Glaser & Wilson, 2017).

These well-documented links between relationship distress and a myriad of health problems suggest the importance of addressing partner relationship concerns in primary care. Primary care settings also present a front-line opportunity to identify and assist individuals experiencing intimate partner violence (IPV) who may not present to their primary care provider (PCP) with an IPV injury as their primary reason for visit (Vicard-Olagne et al., 2022).

PCPs and behavioral health consultants (BHCs) have an important role in identifying and assisting couples experiencing relationship distress. PCPs often provide guidance and brief counseling regarding relationship troubles, and BHCs have the opportunity to develop and implement more nuanced interventions for

https://doi.org/10.1037/0000380-017

Integrated Behavioral Health in Primary Care: Step-by-Step Guidance for Assessment and Intervention, Third Edition, by C. L. Hunter, J. L. Goodie, M. S. Oordt, and A. C. Dobmeyer

patients and targeted recommendations for PCPs to better assist patients experiencing distress in their primary intimate relationship.

KEY BIOPSYCHOSOCIAL FACTORS

A host of biopsychosocial factors may influence the development and maintenance of problems in intimate relationships, and likewise, intimate relation problems can affect physical and emotional health. Physical, emotional, cognitive, behavioral, social/environmental, and diversity factors present in each member of the couple form a complex set of interrelated influences on relationship functioning and satisfaction. Although a thorough review of this literature is beyond the scope of this chapter, key biopsychosocial factors related to intimate relationship functioning are highlighted next.

Physical Factors

The relationships among health and marital status and relationship quality, as described previously, are well established. Medical conditions may impair daily life functioning and affect the responsibilities, roles, work, and leisure activities of both members in a relationship. Physical changes related to aging or comorbid medical conditions may affect sexual functioning, altering patterns of intimacy. The presence of IPV is associated with both acute and long-term health problems (summarized by the U.S. Preventive Services Task Force [USPSTF]; Curry, Krist, Owens, Barry, Caughey, Davidson, Doubeni, Epling, Grossman, Kemper, Kubik, Kurth, et al., 2018).

Emotional and Cognitive Factors

Mental health problems can have a profound effect on relationship functioning and satisfaction, and relationship distress can negatively affect mental health (Bodenmann & Randall, 2013; Braithwaite & Holt-Lunstad, 2017). For example, alcohol use disorders have a bidirectional relationship with marital distress (Rodriguez et al., 2014). Even in couples without a diagnosed mental illness, emotional and cognitive factors can clearly affect the relationship. For example, core beliefs about intimacy, trust, and self-worth may affect patterns of communication, conflict resolution, fidelity, and intimacy. Violence in intimate relationships is associated with a host of negative mental health outcomes (Curry, Krist, Owens, Barry, Caughey, Davidson, Doubeni, Epling, Grossman, Kemper, Kubik, Kurth, et al., 2018).

Behavioral Factors

Learned patterns of behavior, whether protective or detrimental, also may affect multiple domains of relationship functioning. Individuals bring into their intimate relationship a learning history regarding how to address problems; respond to conflict; communicate needs; and express emotion, appreciation, and affection. Behavioral patterns, whether adaptive or not, may be intentionally or inadvertently reinforced by partners' responses.

Environmental Factors

A host of environmental, economic, and social factors may affect the nature and quality of intimate relationships. For example, transition to parenthood affects communication, marital functioning, and relationship satisfaction (Delicate et al., 2018). The presence of other family members in the home (e.g., children, adult parents, stepchildren) and the nature of those relationships may affect couples' relationship functioning and satisfaction. Connections to the community and a network of social support may serve as protective factors for intimate relationships. Economic hardships may increase family stress and contribute to increased couple conflict (Neppl et al., 2016). Finally, a history of childhood abuse may negatively affect current relationship functioning and satisfaction (Nguyen et al., 2017).

Cultural and Diversity Considerations

Aspects of diversity, such as spiritual beliefs and religious practices, culture, ethnicity, age, sex, gender identity, and sexual orientation crosscut all the biopsychosocial domains discussed previously, with potential to influence physical, emotional, cognitive, behavioral, and environmental variables. Thus, any formulation of couples' functioning should carefully consider the potential impact of diversity variables on the relationship. This could range from the emotional or economic impact of discrimination, to communication patterns shaped by cultural beliefs or gender norms, to the impact of microaggressions on a sexual minority couple. Philosophies and beliefs regarding marriage, separation, and divorce in different cultures and religions can influence decisions regarding maintaining or ending the relationship. Cultural background may also affect gender norms and expectations and hence relationship functioning. These may manifest as conflicts between the couple (e.g., a woman desiring more independence in the context of a partner strongly adhering to a male-dominant hierarchy) or as a stressor between the couple and a cultural environment holding different norms (e.g., the couple may not have internal disagreements regarding gender role expectations, but external cultural pressures may cause distress). The presence of similar cultural values and religious beliefs and practices within both members may serve as protective factors within the relationship. Close attention to diversity variables and their impact on both the individual and couple remains an essential element of care, whether it is provided in specialty behavioral health or primary care settings.

SPECIALTY MENTAL HEALTH INTERVENTION

Behavioral marital therapy (BMT) is an established, evidence-based treatment for relationship problems in couples. A classic meta-analysis of 30 randomized controlled trials comparing levels of distress in couples who received BMT versus those who received no treatment found significantly lower levels of distress in the BMT groups (Shadish & Baldwin, 2005). The core evidence-based components in BMT protocols included "communication training, problem-solving training, contingency contracting, behavior exchanges, desensitization, cognitive restructuring, [and] emotional expressiveness training" (Shadish & Baldwin, 2005, p. 6). Of these, communication training and problem-solving interventions were associated with the largest effect sizes.

Cognitive behavioral couple therapy (CBCT) represents another established approach to working with distressed couples. This treatment focuses on the influence of cognitions, behavioral interactions, and emotions both within each member and between the members of the couple. Intervention strategies may focus on changing unhelpful thought patterns, decreasing problematic behavioral interactions, enhancing communication and problem-solving skills, and improving ability to experience and regulate emotions (Baucom et al., 2020; Dattilio & Epstein, 2021; N. B. Epstein & Zheng, 2017). A summary of the outcome literature concluded that there is significant empirical support for the efficacy of CBCT, particularly the behavioral components, which have received more attention in the literature than the cognitive restructuring components (Dattilio & Epstein, 2021).

Integrative behavioral couple therapy (IBCT), a third wave cognitive behavioral approach, contains increased emphasis on mindfulness and emotional acceptance, as well as renewed focus on functional analysis of behavior. A summary of the IBCT outcome literature reported that 70% of couples receiving IBCT demonstrated significant improvements in relationship satisfaction during treatment (Lebow et al., 2012). Gains were maintained over a 5-year follow-up interval for 50% of couples. The results at the follow-up assessment were similar to those who received traditional BMT.

Overall, a recent meta-analytic review of couple therapy (Roddy et al., 2020) found significant positive impacts of couple therapy on global relationship satisfaction, communication, relationship cognitions, and emotional intimacy. The review included studies of various modalities (e.g., BCT, CBCT, IBCT, emotionally focused couple therapy) and found no significant differences between therapy approaches. Of note, the studies included only male/female couples, the majority of whom were married.

Treatment approaches to address relationship problems in sexual and gender minority couples are also being developed. Sexual and gender minority populations include individuals who identify as gay, lesbian, bisexual, transgender, gender nonbinary, intersex, and/or asexual, among others. Pentel and Baucom (2022) provided a clinical framework for working with sexual minority couples designed to aid therapists in tailoring existing evidence-based couple therapy. The framework emphasizes attention to universal factors (relevant to the relationship functioning of all couples), sexual minority-specific factors, and within-group diversity. Sexual minority-specific environmental factors affecting the couple may include discrimination, problems with family of origin and social support systems, stressors surrounding "outness" and relationship disclosure, and the presence of few sexual minority relationship role models for navigating relationship roles and responsibilities. The authors illustrate how this framework could be used within a CBCT approach and describe a small pilot study with cisgender same-sex female couples that yielded improvements in relationship functioning, decreases in relationship distress, and satisfaction with the intervention.

BEHAVIORAL HEALTH IN PRIMARY CARE

Empirical data on effectiveness of couples interventions in primary care by either PCPs or integrated BHCs is scant. One of the few published studies on couples interventions in primary care settings evaluated a version of Cordova et al.'s (2014) marriage checkup prevention and early intervention program. In this longitudinal randomized controlled trial, the marriage checkup intervention was adapted for BHCs in military primary care clinics (Cigrang et al., 2022). The intervention consisted of three 30-minute appointments focused on identifying partner strengths, addressing each partner's primary relationship concern (using IBCT approaches), providing feedback, and exploring ways for continued relationship growth (drawing from motivational interviewing approaches). The results showed improved outcomes in a number of domains, including communication skills, relationship satisfaction, intimacy, and depressive symptoms in intervention couples at 1- and 6-months postintervention compared with control group couples.

Effective primary care screening and intervention for IPV have been described in the literature. A USPSTF report (Curry, Krist, Owens, Barry, Caughey, Davidson, Doubeni, Epling, Grossman, Kemper, Kubik, Kurth, et al., 2018) advised routine screening for IPV in women of reproductive age and recommended that women experiencing IPV be provided ongoing supportive intervention components. These components may include counseling, parenting support for new mothers, and home visits. Of note, merely giving information on referrals or providing brief (rather than ongoing) intervention was not effective. No studies on screening or intervention for IPV in men were found. Couples counseling is not indicated when IPV is suspected. Although no evaluations of interventions targeting IPV using BHCs have been published, BHCs may certainly assist their primary care teams in providing supportive and skill-based interventions over time as a core member of the care team.

PRIMARY CARE ADAPTATION

Many of the key components of evidence-based treatments for couple distress can be readily adapted for implementation by BHCs. Cognitive behavioral approaches to couple treatment may appeal to many patients due to their pragmatic, skill-building, action-oriented approach. For these same reasons, adaptations of evidence-based interventions such as problem solving, communication training, and behavior exchange, among others, represent a good fit with primary care culture, norms, and expectations of both patients and primary care providers.

Adapting the existing evidence-based interventions for improving relationship functioning and satisfaction can be enhanced through following the 5As approach to primary care management of behavioral health conditions. The following sections provide specific recommendations on putting such interventions into practice.

Assess

Assessment of couples' distress may begin with screening at PCP appointments and be followed by additional evaluation by the BHC.

Screening at PCP Appointments

The first step in assisting couples experiencing relationship distress is to identify the presence of a problem. Failure to identify individuals experiencing significant relationship distress certainly may occur in primary care clinics, given the complexity and number of problem areas that PCPs address in a brief appointment. Unless the patient spontaneously discloses difficulties or the PCP directly asks, such problems may remain undetected. Brief screening for relationship distress can be used effectively at PCP appointments to identify patients who might benefit from intervention. A one-item primary care screening measure, "On a score of 1 to 10, rate your overall satisfaction with your marriage, with 1 being very unsatisfied and 10 being extremely satisfied" (Bailey et al., 2012, p. 106) has a positive correlation with the widely used and validated 32-item Dyadic Adjustment Scale (Spanier, 1976). A cut point of 7 on the one-item screener (rating of 7 or less indicating relationship dissatisfaction) was found to best maximize sensitivity (86%) and specificity (86%) in the primary care population (Bailey et al., 2012). Although reliability of assessment instruments may decrease when standard administration is not followed, it may be useful to incorporate more inclusive language (e.g., substituting "intimate relationship" for "marriage").

Clinics following USPSTF guidance (Curry, Krist, Owens, Barry, Caughey, Davidson, Doubeni, Epling, Grossman, Kemper, Kubik, Kurth, et al., 2018) regarding IPV screening in women of childbearing age have several options for primary care screening measures with adequate psychometric properties: the four-item Hurt, Insult, Threaten, Scream measure (Sherin, n.d.; Sherin et al.,

1998) available in English and Spanish; the eight-item Woman Abuse Screening Tool (J. B. Brown et al., 2000); and the four-item Humiliation, Afraid, Rape, Kick measure (Sohal, n.d.; Sohal et al., 2007).

Assessment at BHC Appointments

Once the PCP has identified and referred the patient (or couple) to the BHC, the BHC conducts further assessment, drawing from multiple sources of information. As with individual patients, the BHC will obtain relevant information about the current concern and relevant history from the PCP as well as a review of the patient's electronic health record. The BHC may also make use of a brief self-report assessment measure, such as the Revised Dyadic Adjustment Scale (Busby et al., 1995). This questionnaire, a shorter but highly correlated version of the Dyadic Adjustment Scale (14 vs. 32 items), shows strong ability to differentiate between distressed and nondistressed couples and can be quickly administered, scored, and interpreted within a primary care environment.

In some cases, it is useful for the BHC to have an individual initial appointment with each member of the couple separately prior to a joint appointment. This separate initial appointment serves several functions. First, it provides a confidential environment for screening and assessment of IPV, which should not be assessed with both partners present. If the PCP has not directly screened for IPV, having a separate initial BHC appointment with each member is recommended. Second, it provides a forum for the BHC to assess each partner's perceptions of the challenges and strengths in the relationship, as well as the impact of the relationship problems on key areas of psychosocial functioning. Questions regarding infidelity in the marriage may be answered more honestly in an individual appointment. Third, in situations in which motivation to change or to attend joint appointments may be questionable, an individual appointment provides an environment for the BHC to implement motivational enhancement interventions. Of note, the BHC should clarify the level of confidentiality that will be maintained regarding information shared in individual appointments.

Assessment questions designed to obtain information useful in guiding problem solving and other behavioral interventions can be employed. Such questions could include the following:

- What problem is most distressing to each of you?

- What factors make each of these problems worse? Better?

- What strategies to address these problems have you tried?

- What does each of you see as the biggest strength of the other?

- What does each of you see as the biggest strength in the relationship?

- What problem would each of you like to address first?

Figure 16.1 provides additional examples of specific assessment questions that the BHC might ask when working with couples.

FIGURE 16.1. Relationship Problems Sample Assessment Questions

Appointment type	Sample assessment questions
Individual	Do you feel safe in your relationship?
	Have you been physically hurt or threatened by your partner?
	Has your partner forced you to have sex?
	Do you feel controlled or frightened by your partner?
	Has there been any infidelity in your relationship?
Joint	Describe your main concerns with the relationship.
	What affects your relationship problems the most?
	What problem occurs most frequently? How often?
	What problem has the most negative effect on your relationship?
	Describe a recent disagreement and how you resolved it.
	What seems to improve the closeness you feel?
	How often do you spend time in leisure activities together?
	What have you tried so far to improve the relationship problems?
	Have you ever participated in any couples therapy?
	Have you read any self-help relationship materials?
	What problem would you like to target first?
	What do you think would help improve the relationship?

Advise

The results of the assessment and functional analysis guide the recommendations provided to the patient. Given the clinical complexity that often occurs when working with a dyad, there may be more than one identified problem area that could be targeted for intervention. The task at this point is to discuss with the couple their options for care, provide recommendations, and guide them toward making a joint decision regarding how to proceed.

This might involve working together over the course of several BHC appointments to learn and implement one or two evidence-based strategies for improving communication, increasing intimacy, or jointly solving problems. It could involve an approach using self-help materials and books rather than follow-up with a professional. Alternately, with couples who have significant relationship dysfunction, it could involve seeking more intensive forms of specialty behavioral health treatment, particularly if initial interventions within primary care do not lead to improvements in relationship functioning. For others, the BHC might recommend a specialty behavioral health referral for one (or both) members to address a significant mental health comorbidity in one or both partners that precludes effective primary care intervention for relationship distress.

The following is an example of how a BHC might begin a discussion with a couple about the recommended or desired level of care:

> Based on the assessment, it sounds like the two of you have a number of problem areas you could work on to improve your relationship. Some of the major

ones are disagreements about discipline for the kids, distribution of work around the house, relationships with extended family, and how money is spent. Here in the primary care clinic setting, we can do some focused training on communication and problem-solving skills that are likely to be helpful for you in working on these problems. In fact, research shows that this type of focused skill training alone increases relationship satisfaction for many couples. However, some couples benefit more from extended help to work through each of these issues with a therapist. If that is the case, it may be more beneficial to refer you to a specialty relationship counselor because that type of therapy is more than we can do here. Would you like to start with skills training and assess how that is working for you, or would you prefer I make the referral now?

Presentations that might warrant a higher level of care include the presence of IPV (discussed earlier), intermediate or high acute risk for suicide (for more information on assessing suicide risk, see Chapter 17), or severe mental health disorders (e.g., psychotic disorders, severe depression, significant personality disorder). For these patients, the advise phase of the appointment should include a frank discussion about the BHC's recommendation that the patient (or couple) initiate care through the specialty behavioral health system, as well as the rationale for this recommendation and the potential negative outcomes of attempting to solely manage the problem in the primary care environment or on their own. When indicated, BHCs can continue to see the couple or the individual to bridge any gaps in care prior to engagement with specialty behavioral health.

Regardless of the level of severity, the goal in this phase of the appointment is to clearly describe the options for care as well as to share the BHC's professional opinion regarding which ones are most recommended and why. This process gives the couple the opportunity to make an informed, joint decision regarding how to proceed during the next phase of the appointment.

Agree

Reaching agreement regarding the direction of care during the agree phase of the appointment often poses a greater challenge when working with couples, compared with working with an individual, as all three parties (the BHC and both patients) need to reach consensus regarding the direction for intervention. The goal is to agree on both a broad and a specific approach to managing the problem. Initially, agreement needs to be reached on broad setting of care (i.e., appointments with BHC, follow-up with PCP only, referral for specialty couples counseling, or no follow-up care).

If the couple opts to engage in additional consultation with the BHC, agreement then should be reached on one or more specific intervention approaches (e.g., communication training, increasing shared positive experiences, joint problem solving). Socratic questioning and motivational interviewing with one or both partners can assist in increasing willingness to try an approach. The following is an example of lines of discussion and questioning a BHC might use when working with a couple who does not initially agree on an approach:

We've discussed several options available to you. I've shared my recommendation that we work together for several appointments to improve how the two of
you communicate, particularly during conflicts. Mark, it sounds like you are in
favor of this approach and would like to try it out. But Sarah, you're leaning
more toward the self-help option and are interested in working through a book
with Mark on ideas for improving your marriage. Is that right? [Both nod in
agreement.] The choice is certainly up to you. The most important thing is that
whichever option you select, both of you commit to giving it your best effort.
And there is nothing wrong with choosing one approach, trying it out for a
couple of months, and then evaluating how it's going and whether you'd like to
try something else. Maybe to help make a decision you can both agree upon, we
could discuss what each of you see as the pros and cons of both options and
what you'd be willing to try over the next 2 months.

Assist

Once agreement is reached with the couple regarding the direction of care, the
BHC shifts to the assist phase of the appointment, providing education or teaching specific self-management skills. In initial appointments, this phase typically
lasts 5 to 10 minutes due to the length of time needed for assessment and building agreement. In follow-up appointments, more time (often 15 to 20 minutes
of a 30-minute appointment) is available for intervention. The following sections provide details on a number of evidence-based interventions for relationship distress, adapted for the primary care environment: communication
training, problem-solving training, motivational enhancement approaches,
behavioral strategies for increasing desired behavior, behavior exchange, and
addressing safety.

Communication Training

Improving a couple's ability to communicate effectively is often a primary
focus of intervention with distressed couples in primary care, as many couples experience difficulty discussing problematic topics without engaging in
behaviors that impair effective problem resolution (e.g., arguing, accusing,
withdrawing). Communication training forms a core component of many
specialty behavioral health approaches to couple distress. In primary care,
communication training tailored to the needs of the couple may be as brief as
one appointment followed by home practice or may include several appointments incorporating modeling by the BHC and role play by the couple. Skill
development focuses on both listener and speaker strategies. Many effective
speaker strategies rely on assertive communication approaches as a cornerstone. Methods to improve assertive communication are described in detail in
Chapter 4. Key components to teach patients include differentiating between
aggressive, passive, and assertive communication styles; using appropriate
nonverbal communication; improving ability to use "I" statements; and effectively expressing feelings or thoughts in response to their partner's behavior
(e.g., use of the "XYZ formula"). Figure 4.10 can be used with couples to assist
with developing speaker communication skills. BHCs can further assist

patients in improving expressive communication skills by teaching and modeling strategies such as keeping expressions brief, mentioning positives when discussing a problem in the partner, and using specific (rather than global) language (Dattilio & Epstein, 2021).

Effective communication requires both partners to have good skills in not just assertive communication but, perhaps even more importantly, listening. BHCs can assist couples in improving nonverbal communication while listening (e.g., appropriate eye contact and posture), as well as developing skills in minimizing interruptions and summarizing and reflecting the speaker's content and/or emotion prior to sharing their own thoughts and feelings on the topic. Figure 16.2 summarizes these key points.

While listening, some patients continue to inappropriately interrupt their partner, particularly when an emotionally charged topic is discussed. This can be related to a belief or fear that they will not later have the opportunity (or remember) to bring up their point or side of the argument. Introducing the pad-and-pencil technique (Dattilio, 2010) can teach partners to listen without interrupting. In this approach, patients are asked to briefly jot down their thoughts or feelings on a notepad (rather than interrupt their partner) during conversation. Partners agree that each will have the opportunity to discuss the content later. This approach can effectively reduce interruptions and increase each partner's sense that they have been heard.

An additional method is the speaker–listener technique (Markman et al., 2010), used to decrease interruptions during conflict, ensure that each partner has an opportunity to speak, and increase likelihood that partners are heard. Partners take turns as speaker and listener, with the speaker "having the floor"

FIGURE 16.2. Effective Listening Handout

Improving Communication Through Effective Listening

Good Communication = Speaking + Listening

Sometimes when people try to improve communication with their partner, they focus only on how to better express their thoughts or get their own point across. While being a good *speaker* is important, effective communication also requires that partners be good *listeners*. The following strategies can help you improve your ability to listen effectively. Practice these components of good listening and ask for feedback on how you are doing.

Key Strategies for Effective Listening

- **Nonverbal behavior:** Face the speaker and maintain good eye contact. Nodding at appropriate times can also show you continue to listen.
- **Avoid interrupting:** Interruptions communicate a lack of respect for the speaker. If you have trouble with this, briefly jot down your thoughts and ideas on a pad of paper while your partner is speaking. This allows your partner to express their thoughts uninterrupted and provides you the opportunity to remember and discuss your ideas later.
- **Summarize:** When your partner has finished speaking, summarize what you heard. Ask questions if you don't understand something they said.
- **Reflect:** Reflect the key thoughts and emotions you heard. This tells your partner you accurately understood what they were trying to communicate (whether or not you agree with the point or perspective).

and holding an agreed-upon object (e.g., a pen) to designate them as the speaker. Speakers are encouraged to use "I" statements, keep their statements brief, and stop to let the partner paraphrase. Listeners are encouraged to wait their turn, paraphrase their partner's comments, and avoid rebuttal. Listeners will have the opportunity to share their point of view when it is their turn as the speaker.

Structuring an intervention to improve communication will vary based on the unique needs of the couple and, depending on the rate of a couple's progress, may span two or more appointments. However, a general intervention framework could include the following:

- educating the couple about speaker and listener skills (supplemented by written handouts summarizing key points);

- modeling effective speaker skills and/or listener skills, with each member of the couple taking turns engaging in the role play;

- having patients practice (during appointment) the speaker and listener skills when discussing a relatively neutral topic, with feedback from each other and the BHC; and

- developing a home communication practice plan, including information on number of days per week, time of day, and a list of topics of increasing difficulty for the couple. In some cases, patients benefit from the BHC assisting them with developing a gradual series of topics to be discussed in these at-home communication practice sessions. A sample home communication practice plan is included in Figure 16.3.

FIGURE 16.3. Communication Practice Plan Handout

Home Practice Plan for Improving Communication

1. We will review the handouts on assertive communication and effective listening at least _____ time(s) in the upcoming week.
2. We will practice effective communication (good speaking and good listening skills) _____ times per week for at least _____ minutes each time.
3. Time of day that we will set aside for practice: _____
4. We will practice communication skills using the following topics (in order from least to most difficult to discuss):
   a) _____
   b) _____
   c) _____
   d) _____
   e) _____
   f) _____
   g) _____

We will remember that the goal of these communication practice times is not necessarily to solve a problem or resolve a conflict. The goal is to improve our ability to discuss difficult issues in healthier ways through effective speaking and listening.

Problem-Solving Training

Improving a couple's ability to effectively solve problems typically requires that both members have adequate prerequisite skills in effective communication. If couples remain stuck in arguing about a problem, effective problem solving cannot occur. However, effective communication does not automatically lead to good problem resolution, and many couples benefit from explicit intervention to improve their ability to resolve specific problems.

Training in problem solving or decision making typically involves multiple phases. One basic method of delineating the steps involves a three-phase approach: problem definition, problem solution, and evaluation. All phases need to involve joint input from each partner in a context free from argument or escalating emotion. Steps in problem definition include the following:

- Both members agree on a time and place to discuss a specific problem.

- One partner states the problem in specific behavioral terms. Only one problem area should be introduced. The partner can express how the problem affects them or why the problem is important.

- The other partner summarizes the content shared by their partner and then shares their own understanding of the issues. The partners should attempt to remain nondefensive and avoid justifying or defending their actions. Solutions should not yet be proposed.

- The couple jointly develops a concise written statement of the problem that they both agree on and are willing to address.

Once both partners have agreed on a common definition of the problem, they proceed to the second phase, problem solution, consisting of the following steps:

- The couple brainstorms potential solutions together, writing down or verbalizing all possible solutions without regard to evaluation or judgment.

- The couple identifies pros and cons of each possible solution. Couples should focus on identifying solutions that take the needs of both people into consideration. Through this process, couples eliminate unacceptable solutions and identify the solution(s) that appear acceptable to both and may comprise the final plan.

- If the couple is unable to find a solution that meets the needs of both people, a compromise plan can be developed. If the couple is unable to develop a compromise plan, then they should agree to a solution that meets the preferences of one person.

- The couple puts the final solution into writing. The change plan should be specific, including details regarding who will do what actions, when, and in what context.

The final phase of problem solving involves evaluation of how well the solution is working during an initial trial period. Steps include the following:

- The couple agrees on the length of the trial period and implements the solution to the best of their ability during this time.

- At the conclusion of the trial period, the couple evaluates how well the solution worked.

- The couple modifies their original solution as needed, using the problem-solving steps again.

BHCs may find the handout included in Figure 16.4 useful for couples who are working on improving their ability to jointly make decisions and solve problems.

The following example illustrates use of a problem-solving approach with a couple, Steven and Joseph, who felt they were "growing apart," bickering more frequently about small issues, and isolating themselves in the evenings. They engaged in a joint problem-solving process and developed the following problem statement: "We do not spend enough time doing fun activities together anymore." After a process of brainstorming and evaluation of potential solutions, they developed the following plan: "On 2 nights each week, Tuesday and Friday, we will spend 1 hour in a fun activity together (e.g., playing chess, preparing a meal together, going for a walk)." They agreed to take turns selecting and planning the activity and to give it a trial period of 2 weeks before evaluating the plan.

Motivational Enhancement Strategies

In relationships, as in other areas of life, plans to change behavior may not successfully translate to sustained behavior change. Even after appropriate communication and joint problem solving, it can remain a challenge for couples to actually translate their intentions for change into new habits of behavior. Through motivational interviewing strategies, as well as behavioral interventions to increase desired behaviors, BHCs can assist couples who have identified problematic behaviors influencing their relationship but have had trouble making the change. This section will focus on the first intervention: enhancing motivation for change in patients who have ambivalence regarding making a specific change to behavior.

Chapter 4 contains information on applying motivational interviewing strategies in primary care settings. Methods such as using a readiness-to-change ruler, followed by discussion of strengths and barriers, or conducting a cost–benefit analysis to assist the patient in identifying and resolving ambivalence can be adapted for use with couples. For example, a BHC might conduct a cost–benefit analysis (i.e., pros and cons) around a proposed behavior change by one member by asking both partners to independently write down the perceived benefits and drawbacks of the individual making the proposed change. The BHC asks the couple to discuss their perceptions with each other. This

FIGURE 16.4. Problem-Solving Guidelines for Couples Handout

Couples Guidelines for Problem Solving

Effectively solving problems or making difficult decisions as a couple can prove difficult. Many couples find that following a specific set of guidelines when resolving an important issue helps them arrive at a solution that is acceptable to both individuals and minimizes arguing or defensiveness. The following guidelines summarize a three-step approach to solving problems together.

1. Define the problem.
   a) Agree on a time and place to discuss the problem.
   b) Partner A describes the problem in specific behavioral terms and shares how the problem has impacted them. Partners should focus on one problem at a time and avoid accusations, arguing, or proposing solutions.
   c) Partner B summarizes what was shared by Partner A, and then describes their own understanding of the issue. Partners should avoid arguing, becoming defensive, or proposing solutions.
   d) Together, the couple develops a brief written statement of the problem that they both agree on and are willing to address.

2. Identify a solution.
   a) The couple brainstorms potential solutions.
   b) The couple identifies pros and cons of each possible solution, eliminating unacceptable ones and identifying those that appear acceptable to both.
   c) If unable to find a solution that meets the needs of both, the couple develops a compromise plan.
   d) The couple writes down the final solution, including specific details on who will do what actions, when, and in which situations.

3. Evaluate the solution.
   a) The couple agrees upon a trial period to implement the solution.
   b) At the end of the trial period, the couple evaluates how well the solution worked.
   c) If needed, the couple modifies their original solution using the problem-solving steps again.

Problem-Solving Worksheet for Couples

1. Statement of the problem (developed jointly):
   _____
   _____

2. List of possible solutions (brainstorming):
   _____
   _____
   _____
   _____
   _____

3. Best options: Discuss the pros and cons of each possible solution. Considering the preferences of both individuals, place an X by options that are unacceptable. Of those remaining, select the best one and circle it.

4. Statement of solution (include who will do what, when, and in which situations):
   _____
   _____

5. Length of trial period: _____

6. Evaluation of solution: Did the solution work well enough? If yes, continue the plan developed above. If changes are needed, set aside time for joint problem solving to modify or improve the solution.

allows the patient to verbalize their own reasons for change (as well as costs or barriers) but also hear the potential impact that making such a change may have on their partner. Having a fuller understanding of the costs and benefits to the couple (not just the individual) may assist with resolving ambivalence and increasing readiness to change.

Consider again the example of Steven and Joseph. During the trial period for their new planned behavior change (spending 1 hour in joint enjoyable activity, 2 evenings per week), Joseph had particular trouble with "disconnecting" from reading online news to spend time with Steven. He checked his smartphone frequently and sent and responded to texts during the times they had set aside for each other. He also did not follow through on his responsibility for planning one of the activities each week. The BHC used a motivational enhancement strategy by asking the couple to independently write down what they saw as the benefits and the drawbacks of following the plan (planning and engaging in joint activities twice per week). The BHC then asked the couple to discuss these together. Steven had the opportunity to express the specific reasons why it was important to him to spend time connecting with Joseph in the evenings. Joseph identified a barrier to making the change that they were able to problem solve together. Joseph's willingness and intention to make the change increased.

Behavioral Interventions for Increasing Desired Behavior
Behavior change interventions are founded in behavioral learning principles. Strategies such as rewarding desired behavior or selectively ignoring (nonreinforcing) certain behaviors can successfully be used with couples with minimal adaptation. To implement, BHCs should discuss with the couple the rationale for the intervention, assist the couple in identifying the specific behavior to be targeted, collaboratively develop a monitoring plan and schedule of reinforcement, and identify the reward(s) to be used. For example, a BHC might initiate the intervention by saying the following:

> It sounds like Sarah feels very frustrated when you, Luis, come home from the gym and leave your gym bag and towel on the kitchen table. Sarah, you've responded by repeated reminders and sometimes yelling, but it doesn't seem to change his behavior. Luis, you have shared that you often "forget" and don't understand why this is such a "big deal." You also don't like it when Sarah continually reminds you to clean up. Sarah, you said Luis "occasionally" remembers to put his gym items in the laundry room but acknowledged that when he does so, you typically make sarcastic comments. I'm wondering if the two of you might be willing to try an experiment. Luis, your role would be to set a goal of putting your gym clothes in the laundry room each time. Perhaps you can attach something to your bag or place a note on the table to remind you. Sarah, your role is to "catch" Luis when he's following through on the plan and reward him, right then and there. It could be a smile and a thank you, a kiss, or whatever else you think would work. What do you both think about trying this approach for the next 2 weeks? Let's talk a little more to flesh out the specifics of this plan.

Assisting couples with problematic behavior patterns may involve substituting alternate behavior patterns during the problematic interaction. The BHC can assist the couple with identifying a more appropriate behavior, if needed. Strategies to increase success with behavior change, such as behavioral rehearsal, monitoring of behavior over time, and rewarding success, should be considered. When possible, incorporate both members of the couple in these behavioral strategies. For example, rather than asking an individual to self-monitor the frequency that the new/alternate behavior is used, the couple could be encouraged to track this change together (joint monitoring). Couples can be asked to role play desired interactions or behaviors together, both during the appointment and at home, to rehearse the desired behavior change. Lists of short- and long-term rewards for meeting goals for behavior change could include couples-based rewards, such as going out to eat together or giving and receiving massages.

Behavior Exchange

One core component of traditional cognitive behavioral therapy for distressed couples that is quite amenable to the primary care setting is *behavior exchange*, a process aimed to increase positive interactions (which may be infrequent in distressed relationships) and relationship satisfaction (Dattilio & Epstein, 2021). BHCs could introduce the idea of behavior exchange with the following description:

> Often when couples are having difficulty in their relationship, they focus a lot on the negatives or the problems that come up. Less and less time is spent in positive interactions that actually build up relationship strength and satisfaction. It sounds like this may be occurring in your relationship. As you've had more conflicts about money and friends, and you've become busier with work and kids, you've put less emphasis on showing each other you care in your everyday interactions. Many couples find that by intentionally planning and doing positive interactions, their satisfaction in the relationship increases. For example, each person might intentionally do something that demonstrates caring for the other several times each week and then discuss its impact. Would you be interested in learning more about this strategy?

One method of implementing a behavior exchange strategy is to have each partner independently generate a list of actions they could do for their partner that might make their partner feel appreciated or cared for. The BHC can guide the patients to list a range of activities, both large and small, that are inexpensive and easily implemented. For example, a list could include greeting the partner with a smile, a hug, and a kiss when they arrive home at the end of the day; making a partner's favorite food; filling the partner's car with gas; taking care of a task that typically falls to the partner (e.g., making the bed, brewing the coffee, shoveling the walk); or planning a special evening out. Some couples prefer to review the lists together to ensure that items would truly be reinforcing or desired; others opt to keep the lists private to retain a sense of surprise or spontaneity. The BHC can then assist the couple in determining how frequently they would like to engage in the positive exchanges (e.g., daily vs. several per week) as well as a developing a plan for reviewing their progress. This review should include a discussion about what they did, whether they felt appreciated, how difficult it was to accomplish, and what they might consider differently for the future. Some couples may plan to review their actions together at the end of the week; others may benefit from reviewing with the BHC in a future appointment. Figure 16.5 may be useful in working with patients on implementing this strategy.

Addressing Safety

A primary intervention for patients experiencing IPV involves addressing personal safety. If a patient discloses IPV or is afraid for their safety, the BHC should prioritize assisting with developing a safety plan, discussing options, identifying additional resources, and linking to specialty care. Couples counseling is not indicated when IPV is present. A safety plan can be developed collaboratively during the individual appointment. Safety plans should include information about steps the patient will take to prepare in advance of future episodes of IPV (e.g., money and cell phone on hand, neighbor or friend alerted, weapons inaccessible); steps to take if IPV escalates (e.g., escape plan); and resources for assistance, including information on crisis lines, local IPV shelters, and 911 for emergencies. An example of a safety plan is included in Figure 16.6. Referral to

FIGURE 16.5. Behavior Exchange Handout

Taking Action to Show Your Partner You Care

Often when couples are having difficulties in their relationship, they do not spend as much time in positive interactions showing each other they care. Making a point to do something for your partner on a regular basis that shows you care for them, appreciate them, or are simply thinking of them can increase intimacy and relationship satisfaction.

Step 1
Make a list of actions you could do for your partner that would show them you care for and appreciate them. These should be easy to implement and not cost much money. Examples could include making a favorite food, giving a back rub, doing a chore that normally falls to the other partner, or giving a smile and a hug when returning home.

_____	_____
_____	_____
_____	_____
_____	_____

Step 2
Decide with your partner whether you will share your lists or keep them private.

Step 3
Decide with your partner how frequently you will each do an activity from your list (e.g., number of times per day or week): _____ per _____

Step 4
Plan a date with your partner when you will review progress, discuss what seemed to work well, and make changes and future plans: _____

FIGURE 16.6. Sample Intimate Partner Violence Safety Plan

My Safety Plan

❑ I will go to a safe area of the home if I am in danger. A safe area is an area of the home where there are no weapons and where there is a way to escape. My safe area is:

_____

❑ I will have a cell phone with me at all times, if possible. Numbers to call for help include:

- 911 (call if life or safety are in danger)
- Local violence shelter: _____
- Friend/family: _____
- National Domestic Violence Hotline: 1-800-799-SAFE (7233)

❑ I will tell a trusted neighbor, friend, or family member of my situation. I will develop a safety plan and a signal to use with them when I need help:

_____

_____

_____

❑ I will keep weapons (like knives or guns) locked away or as difficult to access as possible. This location is: _____

❑ Other: _____

_____

_____

specialty behavioral health services is recommended; however, if patients are unwilling or unable to access these services, then continued ongoing support from the primary care team, including the PCP, the BHC, and case managers, if available, should be provided.

BHCs can provide information on several ways to access information and immediate support from the National Domestic Violence Hotline:

- 24/7 phone hotline: 1-800-799-SAFE (7233), TTY 1-800-787-3224

- Website: https://www.thehotline.org/

- Text support: text "START" to 88788

Hotline operators are trained to provide support, guidance, and information on resources to victims of IPV. The website contains information on IPV, strategies for safety, a variety of tips on healthy relationships, additional resources for those affected by IPV, downloadable safety plan handouts, and a link for accessing live chat support.

Arrange

Follow-up appointments with the BHC, if indicated, ideally should be arranged prior to the patient departing the clinic. In some cases, it is advisable to time these visits to coincide with future PCP appointments, particularly in situations in which the patient(s) perceives a burden of multiple medical appointments. For others, it can be more helpful to stagger appointments with the PCP and BHC, in order to allow reinforcement of the plan from the PCP during the interval between BHC appointments. For couples who intend to initiate care through specialty behavioral health, the BHC can assist the PCP with placing a referral and ensuring patients are aware of the steps required to follow through on the referral. If the BHC questions whether a couple will be successful in linking with a specialty behavioral health provider, proactive telephone follow-up from the BHC is recommended, with the BHC calling the couple after a reasonable interval (e.g., 2 weeks) to determine whether they need additional assistance in finding a provider and getting scheduled for an intake. BHCs may continue to meet with the couple to bridge any gaps in care as they work to get linked with a specialty provider.

The BHC can also provide the couple with a variety of additional resources that might be used in conjunction with BHC appointments or be used by patients who opt to follow up with their PCP only. Many couples may be interested in websites, mobile device applications, and self-help books to improve their relationships. These resources may be used by the couple alone, without professional assistance, or as resources for guided self-help in conjunction with BHC appointments. Ideally, both members of the couple will read and discuss the material together. A number of these resources are summarized in Figure 16.7. Of note, the mobile application listed was developed out of an existing evidence base regarding components of healthy relationships; however, there is not a solid research base demonstrating the effectiveness of use of mobile applications to improve relationships at this time.

SUMMARY

Primary care BHCs can play a key role in assisting PCPs with assessing patients' satisfaction with their intimate relationship functioning and in implementing focused, evidence-based interventions for improving partner relationships and decreasing relationship distress. BHCs can also assist the PCP in identifying which patients are not benefiting from intervention at the primary care level and recommend referrals to specialty behavioral health providers when indicated.

A number of specialty behavioral health care treatments have been proven effective for improving couples' relationship functioning. The challenge for BHCs is to appropriately select and implement discrete components of these larger treatment packages, modified to fit within a primary care behavioral health model of service delivery. This chapter provided recommendations for how BHCs might approach this task, with a particular focus on evidence-based treatment components that appear most amenable to a primary care environment: strategies for improving communication and joint problem-solving skills, enhancing patient motivation for change, increasing desired behavior through behavioral approaches, increasing positive exchanges demonstrating appreciation or caring, and addressing safety issues in relationships affected by IPV.

FIGURE 16.7. Resources for Couples: Websites, Mobile Applications, and Books (*continues*)

Type	Location	Description
Websites	National Domestic Violence Hotline Website (https://www.thehotline.org/)	Contains information on IPV, strategies for safety, a variety of tips on healthy relationships, additional resources for those affected by IPV, and downloadable safety plan handouts
	The American Association for Marriage and Family Therapy (https://www.aamft.org/)	Contains a locator service for marriage and family therapists, as well as information about a variety of topics related to family and relationship functioning
	Help Guide (https://www.helpguide.org/)	Offers a section on relationships, including advice for strengthening relationships, improving communication skills, increasing emotional intelligence, setting healthy boundaries, and resolving conflicts
	University of Minnesota: Taking Charge of Your Health and Well-Being (https://www.takingcharge.csh.umn.edu/relationships)	Contains information on healthy relationships; offers a number of strategies for couples in distress; and describes ways to nurture relationships, improve communication, practice forgiveness, and resolve conflict
	The Gottman Institute (https://www.gottman.com/)	Contains evidence-based information and resources for couples and professionals and provides links to additional resources and information on workshops for couples and trainings for professionals
Mobile application	The Gottman Institute Card Decks (https://www.gottman.com/couples/apps/)	Contains more than 1,000 virtual flashcards to help couples improve their relationship. It includes questions, statements, and ideas for relationship enhancement.
Books	*Fighting for Your Marriage: A Deluxe Revised Edition of the Classic Best-Seller for Enhancing Marriage and Preventing Divorce* (Markman et al., 2010)	Offers various enhancement skills for relationships including communication, teamwork, and conflict resolution. It also emphasizes the importance of fun and friendship between couples and shows how these can lead to a healthy and happy relationship.
	The Seven Principles for Making Marriage Work (Gottman & Silver, 2015)	Book based on the research and clinical experience of Dr. John Gottman, who studied couples for years and turned his research and experience into a pathway for couples to succeed in their relationship. The authors offer principles of living to help couples stay together.

FIGURE 16.7. Resources for Couples: Websites, Mobile Applications, and Books (*continued*)

Type	Location	Description
Books (*continued*)	*What Makes Love Last? How to Build Trust and Avoid Betrayal* (Gottman & Silver, 2012)	Another book by noted relationship researcher Dr. John Gottman, provides strategies and tools for repairing and healing relationships that have been affected by betrayal
	The 5 Love Languages: The Secret to Love That Lasts (Chapman, 2015)	Bestselling relationship book focuses on strategies to express love in a manner that is meaningful to one's partner (i.e., using their preferred "emotional love language"). Although the book is not evidence-based, many couples have responded positively.
	Working It Out: A Lesbian Relationship Primer (Fuchs, 2009)	Interactive workbook focuses on improving lesbian relationships. It contains exercises to improve communication skills, manage conflicts, and address challenges related to coming out.
	Ten Smart Things Gay Men Can Do to Improve Their Lives, 2nd ed. (Kort, 2016)	Identifies the struggles gay men may go through in life and recommends different strategies that can enhance their life and relationships and help them address the challenges of being gay in modern society

Note. IPV = intimate partner violence.

SPECIAL ISSUES

17

Managing Suicide Risk in the Primary Care Setting

In response to alarming rates of suicidality in recent years, professional associations, government organizations, and health care systems have increasingly released guidance to clinicians for effectively assessing and managing risk in primary care and other medical settings. This is a welcome and much-needed development. As recently as 20 to 30 years ago, little standardized training or practice guidelines existed to help professionals respond to suicidal ideation or behavior, even among mental health specialists (Oordt et al., 2009). Many primary care providers (PCPs) were not well trained to inquire about or recognize risk factors for self-harm. In recent years, much more guidance has become available as well as strong evidence that training PCPs to recognize and treat suicide risk factors, such as depression, is effective for preventing suicide (Mann et al., 2021).

The growth in training and guidance on recognizing and managing suicide risk is essential because rates of suicidal behavior and completed suicides have skyrocketed. In 2020, suicide was among the top four causes of death in the United States for people ages 10 to 14, 15 to 24, 25 to 34, and 35 to 44 (Centers for Disease Control and Prevention, 2022c). It was in the top 10 causes of death for every age group except infant to age 4 and ages 65+. Studies indicate 4.9% of adults report experiencing thoughts of suicide in the past year, and this percentage increases to 11.3% among young adults ages 18 to 25 (Substance Abuse and Mental Health Services Administration [SAMHSA], 2021a). In 2020, there were 1.2 million suicide attempts in the United States (SAMHSA,

https://doi.org/10.1037/0000380-018

Integrated Behavioral Health in Primary Care: Step-by-Step Guidance for Assessment and Intervention, Third Edition, by C. L. Hunter, J. L. Goodie, M. S. Oordt, and A. C. Dobmeyer

2021a). Data from the Centers for Disease Control and Prevention (2022c) show that between 2000 and 2018, the U.S. suicide rate increased from 10.4 to 14.2 per 100,000, a 36.5% increase. Among male individuals, the rate increased from 17.7 per 100,000 in 2000 to a high of 22.8 per 100,000 in 2018. Slight decreases occurred in 2019 and 2020 for both male individuals and the total population.

PCPs are on the front lines for addressing suicide risk. Over 60% of individuals who complete suicide had a medical visit within a year of their death, with 20% seeing a PCP in the 4 weeks preceding their death (Ahmedani et al., 2014). As many as 73% of older adults who die by suicide see a PCP in the month prior (Juurlink, 2004). Since many people who attempt or complete suicide are not under the care of a mental health clinician, it is far more likely for a suicidal individual to have contact with a PCP than a specialty mental health provider (Ahmedani et al., 2014). Statistics such as these suggest that PCPs and behavioral health professionals working in a primary care setting must be prepared to screen, assess, manage, and intervene to address suicidal risk.

Bryan and Rudd (2010) provided the only full-length book to date on addressing suicidal risk in primary care. Although much research has been done since its publication, it still serves as a valuable resource. They outlined four principles that guide care for suicidal patients in the primary care setting that are foundational to our discussion in this chapter. First, clinical approaches must be consistent with the context of primary care. Providers should not apply the techniques, structures, and expectations appropriate for specialty mental health settings when working in primary care. To do so intensifies risk for the patient, decreases likelihood for a positive outcome, and increases provider liability. Second, approaches to suicide risk assessment and management must be consistent with the consultative model. The consultative relationship between the PCP and the behavioral health provider is key to successful and comprehensive care for the patient. Care for suicidal patients can increase vulnerability for malpractice liability when an adverse outcome occurs, and this is one reason PCPs tend to be quick in referring patients with suicidal ideation to specialty mental health care. Nevertheless, some levels of suicidal risk can be appropriately managed in primary care. The outcome for some patients may be better in primary care, particularly in situations in which the patient and provider have established rapport and when the patient is unlikely to follow through on a specialty care referral. Furthermore, malpractice liability can be reduced in the primary care setting when the primary care medical provider maintains primary decision-making authority. Third, clinical approaches must be informed by empirical data. The needs for efficiency inherent in the primary care model of care require that the highest commitment to evidence-based care be maintained. Finally, clinical approaches must be based in competency. Behavioral health providers in primary care must have mastery over a defined clinical skill set that directly contributes to best practices in care to address suicide risk.

KEY BIOPSYCHOSOCIAL FACTORS
Physical Factors

Physical illness and disability are often contributing factors when primary care patients are struggling with thoughts of suicide. Chronic medical illnesses that have been associated with suicide include asthma, back pain, brain injury, cancer, congestive heart failure, chronic obstructive pulmonary disorder, diabetes, epilepsy, HIV/AIDS, heart disease, hypertension, migraine, Parkinson's disease, psychogenic pain, renal disorder, sleep disorders, stroke, and osteoporosis (Ahmedani et al., 2017; Webb et al., 2012). Patients with chronic pain are also at elevated risk of suicide (Racine, 2018), particularly related to feelings of perceived burdensomeness on others (Kanzler et al., 2012).

Emotional Factors

Emotional distress is also a strong factor in suicidal risk. Feelings of loss, depression, despair, anxiety, and hopelessness are common correlates. The emotional consequences of experienced trauma can also contribute (Ásgeirsdóttir et al., 2018; Bahk et al., 2017). Examples include sexual assault, childhood trauma, domestic violence, and exposure to death and severe violence. Meta-analyses of studies on anxiety and suicide have shown a weak but statistically significant association with suicidality, although not with completed suicides, with post-traumatic stress disorder (PTSD) having the strongest associations (Bentley et al., 2016; Krysinska & Lester, 2010). A recent population study of 3.1 million people in Sweden found that women with PTSD were at 6.74 times higher risk for suicide than those without PTSD, and risk for men with PTSD was 3.96 times higher than for those without PTSD (Fox et al., 2021).

Cognitive Factors

Cognitions related to suicide and death are a central part of suicide symptoms. Early factor analytic work by Joiner et al. (1997) was seminal in understanding the role of cognitions in suicidal risk. They concluded that suicide symptoms fall into two factors, each of which is primarily related to cognitions. The first factor is *suicidal desire and ideation* and includes the following:

- limited reasons for living,
- wish to die,
- frequency of ideation,
- wish not to live,
- passive attempt,
- desire for attempt,
- expectancy of attempt,

- lack of deterrents to attempt, and

- talk of death and/or suicide.

The second factor is *resolved plans and preparation*. This includes the following:

- sense of courage to make an attempt,

- sense of competence to make an attempt,

- availability of means for an attempt,

- opportunity to make an attempt,

- specificity of plans for an attempt,

- preparations for an attempt,

- duration of suicidal ideation, and

- intensity of suicidal ideation.

Although suicidal symptoms from both factors are important, those in the resolved plans and preparation category are indicative of greater risk of making a suicide attempt.

Two additional cognitive states that also have strong links to suicide involve perceptions of one's relation to other people. These cognitive states are integral to Joiner's (2005) interpersonal theory of suicide. These are perceived burdensomeness and a sense of low belongingness or social alienation. *Perceived burdensomeness* is the perception that one's life is an extreme burden to family and friends and one's death would be worth more to others than one's life. A *sense of low belongingness* relates to the perception one is not integral to one's circle of friends and family. Research over 20 years on the interpersonal theory of suicide has supported the theory that a low sense of belongingness and perceived burdensomeness are significantly associated with suicidal ideation. The interaction between a low sense of belongingness, perceived burdensomeness, and a capability for suicide is significantly related to a greater number of prior suicide attempts, although effect sizes are somewhat modest (C. Chu et al., 2017).

Behavioral Factors

A history of past suicide attempts is one of the most robust risk factors for suicidal behavior (G. K. Brown et al., 2000; Miranda et al., 2008). Furthermore, multiple attempters appear to be a unique group compared with those who experience suicidal ideation and those who have attempted suicide only once. Multiple attempters present a more severe clinical picture and should be viewed as having a greater baseline risk (Nichter et al., 2021; Rudd et al., 1996; L. Smith et al., 2021). They tend to have more severe psychopathology; more severe suicidality; and more problems such as interpersonal stress and conflicts, social isolation, lower personal achievement, lower ability to control emotions, and more social welfare problems (Choi et al., 2013; L. Smith et al., 2021). Multiple attempt status should be carefully assessed and incorporated into treatment planning.

Environmental Factors

Access to one or more practical means for suicide is a significant environmental risk factor. For example, availability of firearms has been documented to be associated with increased risk for suicide (Swanson et al., 2021). Methods for suicide are numerous, and many are always available. The primary concerns, however, are the methods the patient is considering and whether they have access to those means. Limiting access to lethal means is an important step for maximizing safety, and evidence suggests it can be effective in lowering risk, particularly in contexts where substitution of one means for another is less likely to occur (Florentine & Crane, 2010).

Cultural and Diversity Factors

Individuals from any demographic category can experience suicidal symptoms, engage in suicidal behavior, and complete suicide. However, significant differences in risk exist between demographic groups and within diversity categories. This is relevant for understanding *static risk*, which is risk that is fixed and not modifiable. The rates reported in the following sections are 2019 data reported by the American Association of Suicidology (Drapeau & McIntosh, 2020) expressed in number per 100,000 in the U.S. population.

Gender
Female individuals attempt suicide 3 times more often than males; however, male individuals complete suicide at a rate 3.6 times greater than their female counterparts. The 2019 rate of completed suicide for male individuals was 23, whereas the rate for female individuals was 6.2.

Age
The highest rate of suicide is among individuals aged 45 to 54. In 2019, the rate for this age group was 19.6. For comparison, the 2019 U.S. suicide rate for all ages was 14.5. Suicide by adults ages 55 to 64 occurred at a rate of 19.4—the second highest age category. Among adults ages 65 and older, the suicide rate was 17. Notably, in 2019 the 65+ age group made up 16.5% of the population and 19.3% of suicides. Suicide is the second leading cause of death for teens and young adults; nevertheless, the rate is significantly lower than other age categories with a rate of 13.

Race
In the U.S. population, White individuals have the highest suicide rate at 16.4. In 2019, 88.3% of all U.S. suicides were completed by White individuals. In the

same reporting period, the rate was 7.4 for Asian/Pacific Islander, 7.1 for African American, and 7.2 for Latinx individuals.

Lesbian, Gay, Bisexual, Transgender, and Queer or Questioning

Studies have repeatedly shown higher rates of suicidal ideation and behavior for lesbian, gay, bisexual, transgender, and queer or questioning (LGBTQ) individuals compared with others (di Giacomo et al., 2018). The Trevor Project's 2022 National Survey on LGBTQ Youth's Mental Health found that 45% of LGBTQ youths seriously considered suicide in the previous year and 14% reported attempting suicide in the previous year (Trevor Project, 2022). The percentage of LGBTQ young people ages 13 to 17 who contemplated suicide (50%) and who attempted suicide (18%) were higher than those in the 18 to 24 age group (37% and 8%, respectively). Most studies on LGBTQ suicide risk address the youth and young adult populations, and there are limited data on other age groups. Government statistics on suicide do not include sexual minority status as a variable.

SPECIALTY MENTAL HEALTH APPROACHES

Outpatient specialty care for suicidal individuals typically involves four components: (a) assessment of the risk for suicide, (b) initial safety planning prior to being released from acute care, (c) treatment using empirically supported approaches in the least restrictive setting that is appropriate to level of risk, and (d) follow-up monitoring. Treatment should address both suicidality itself as well as underlying mental health conditions that may be contributing to the individual's suicide risk. Several clinical practice guidelines for specialty behavioral health providers have been developed, the most recent update being the *U.S. Department of Veterans Affairs and Department of Defense Clinical Practice Guideline for Assessment and Management of Patients at Risk for Suicide* (VA/DoD, 2019a). Treatment modalities may involve psychotherapy, pharmacotherapy, or a combination of both. Patients whose safety cannot be managed adequately on an outpatient basis should be referred for inpatient care. Careful monitoring and management are essential during transition from a higher level of care to a lower level (i.e., inpatient to outpatient), as this can be a particularly high-risk period.

PRIMARY CARE ADAPTATION

The 5As format can be readily applied to addressing suicide risk in primary care.

Assess

The assess phase includes two components: screening and assessment. As a low-base-rate event, suicidal behavior cannot be predicted accurately; therefore, the goal should be to assess risk in a manner that is reasonable and consistent in order to guide interventions. Behavioral health consultants (BHCs) can play an essential role in helping PCPs integrate appropriate screening and assessment into their practices, as well as assisting clinics with establishing standardized protocols for identifying and managing suicide risk.

The U.S. Preventive Services Task Force's most recent review concluded there is insufficient evidence to either recommend or not recommend routine screening of the general population for suicidal ideation (LeFevre, 2014). This is true only when screening patients who would not otherwise be identified based on mental health diagnosis, emotional distress, or a previous suicide attempt. When a known risk factor is present, screening is essential. This includes patients with psychiatric disorders, medical disorders (e.g., those listed in the section on physical risk factors), or conditions such as sleep difficulties or who are postpartum. Additionally, screening is indicated for patients experiencing psychosocial stressors, such as legal, financial, or relationship issues, or who have experienced a significant loss (e.g., death of family member or friend, job loss). Figure 17.1 contains a list of risk factors and protective factors for suicide that can be used as a handout to educate patients and members of their support network.

FIGURE 17.1. Protective and Risk Factors for Suicide (*continues*)

Circumstances That Protect Against Suicide Risk

Many factors can reduce risk for suicide. Similar to risk factors, a range of factors at the individual, relationship, community, and societal levels can protect people from suicide. Everyone can help prevent suicide. We can take action in communities and as a society to support people and help protect them from suicidal thoughts and behavior.

Individual Protective Factors
These personal factors protect against suicide risk:

- Effective coping and problem-solving skills
- Reasons for living (e.g., family, friends, pets)
- Strong sense of cultural identity

Relationship Protective Factors
These healthy relationship experiences protect against suicide risk:

- Support from partners, friends, and family
- Feeling connected to others

Community Protective Factors
These supportive community experiences protect against suicide risk:

- Feeling connected to school, community, and other social institutions
- Availability of consistent and high-quality physical and behavioral health care

Societal Protective Factors
These cultural and environmental factors within the larger society protect against suicide risk:

- Reduced access to lethal means of suicide among people at risk
- Cultural, religious, or moral objections to suicide

FIGURE 17.1. Protective and Risk Factors for Suicide (*continued*)

Circumstances That Increase Suicide Risk

Individual Risk Factors

Suicide is rarely caused by a single circumstance or event. Instead, a range of factors—at the individual, relationship, community, and societal levels—can increase risk. These risk factors are situations or problems that can increase the possibility that a person will attempt suicide. These personal factors contribute to risk:

- Previous suicide attempt
- History of depression and other mental illnesses
- Serious illness such as chronic pain
- Criminal/legal problems
- Job/financial problems or loss
- Impulsive or aggressive tendencies
- Substance misuse
- Current or prior history of adverse childhood experiences
- Sense of hopelessness
- Violence victimization and/or perpetration

Relationship Risk Factors

These harmful or hurtful experiences within relationships contribute to risk:

- Bullying
- Family/loved one's history of suicide
- Loss of relationships
- High-conflict or violent relationships
- Social isolation

Community Risk Factors

These challenging issues within a person's community contribute to risk:

- Lack of access to health care
- Suicide cluster in the community
- Stress of acculturation
- Community violence
- Historical trauma
- Discrimination

Societal Risk Factors

These cultural and environmental factors within the larger society contribute to risk:

- Stigma associated with help seeking and mental illness
- Easy access to lethal means of suicide among people at risk
- Unsafe media portrayals of suicide

Note. Adapted from *Risk and Protective Factors*, by the Centers for Disease Control and Prevention, 2022 (https://www.cdc.gov/suicide/factors/index.html). In the public domain.

Clinical Question

Several approaches to screening are available to primary care clinics. One approach is to verbally inquire about suicidal ideation as part of the initial assessment. Typically, vital sign measurements are taken as part of the clinic's routine check-in procedures, and a question can easily be asked during that part of the encounter, such as "Over the past 2 weeks, have you had any thoughts of suicide?"

Patient Health Questionnaire-9

The VA/DoD (2019a) clinical practice guideline referenced previously recommends using a validated screening tool to identify individuals at risk for suicide. Item 9 from the Patient Health Questionnaire-9 is suggested based on their findings of weak but positive evidence supporting use of the tool. The full questionnaire is available at https://www.phqscreeners.com/. Item 9 is "Over the past 2 weeks, how often have you been bothered by thoughts that you would be better off dead or of hurting yourself in some way?" Response options are "not at all," "several days," "more than half the days," or "nearly every day." Louzon et al. (2016) found that a response of "several days" to this question increased risk for suicide by 75%, "more than half the days" increased risk by 115%, and "nearly every day" increased risk by 185%.

Columbia-Suicide Severity Rating Scale

The Columbia-Suicide Severity Rating Scale (Bjureberg et al., 2021; Posner et al., 2011) is a brief screening tool with plain-language questions about suicidal thoughts and behavior that anyone can administer. It contains initial screening questions related to suicidal ideation. If the individual answers yes to having thoughts about killing themselves, three additional questions are asked related to suicidal thoughts, behaviors, and intentions. A sixth question related to suicidal preparation or behaviors is always asked. The protocol indicates high risk when individuals give positive responses to questions regarding intention to act on suicidal thoughts, developing suicidal plans, or suicidal behaviors or preparations. The Columbia-Suicide Severity Rating Scale protocol and information about it can be found on the Columbia Lighthouse Project website (https://cssrs.columbia.edu).

Ask Suicide Screening Questions

The National Institute of Mental Health recommends using the Ask Suicide-Screening Questions (ASQ), which is provided as part of an ASQ Toolkit (National Institute of Mental Health, 2021a). The ASQ is a brief set of four screening questions that can be administered in less than half a minute. It is in the public domain and is reprinted in Figure 17.2. Studies found an answer of yes to one or more of the four questions accurately identified both young people and adults at risk for suicide with high specificity in primary care and emergency room settings (Aguinaldo et al., 2021; Horowitz et al., 2012, 2020).

P4 Screener

Another useful primary care screening tool for suicide risk is the P4 (Dube et al., 2010). The P4 screener contains four items that cover the "4 P's": past suicide attempts, suicide plan, probability of completing suicide, and preventive factors. Based on responses to these items, patients are classified as minimal, lower, and higher risk. The P4 questions and scoring procedures are available in the article by Dube et al. (2010). Whichever approach is used, the BHC can

FIGURE 17.2. ASQ Suicide Risk Screening Tool

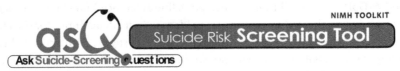

NIMH TOOLKIT

asQ Suicide Risk **Screening Tool**

Ask Suicide-Screening Questions

Ask the patient:

1. In the past few weeks, have you wished you were dead? ○ Yes   ○ No

2. In the past few weeks, have you felt that you or your family would be better off if you were dead? ○ Yes   ○ No

3. In the past week, have you been having thoughts about killing yourself? ○ Yes   ○ No

4. Have you ever tried to kill yourself? ○ Yes   ○ No

   If yes, how? _____

   _____

   _____

   When? _____

   _____

If the patient answers Yes to any of the above, ask the following acuity question:

5. Are you having thoughts of killing yourself right now? ○ Yes   ○ No

   If yes, please describe: _____

Next steps:

- If patient answers "No" to all questions 1 through 4, screening is complete (not necessary to ask question #5). No intervention is necessary (*Note: Clinical judgment can always override a negative screen*).

- If patient answers "Yes" to any of questions 1 through 4, or refuses to answer, they are considered a positive screen. **Ask question #5 to asses acuity:**

  ☐ "Yes" to question #5 = **acute positive screen** (imminent risk identified)
    - **Patient requires a STAT safety/full mental health evaluation.** Patient cannot leave until evaluated for safety.
    - Keep patient in sight. Remove all dangerous objects from room. Alert physician or clinician responsible for patient's care.

  ☐ "No" to question #5 = **non-acute positive screen** (potential risk identified)
    - **Patient requires a brief suicide safety assessment to determine if a full mental health evaluation is needed.** Patient cannot leave until evaluated for safety.
    - Alert physician or clinician responsible for patient's care.

Provide resources to all patients

- 24/7 National Suicide Prevention Lifeline 1-800-273-TALK (8255) En Español: 1-888-628-9454
- 24/7 Crisis Text Line: Text "HOME" to 741-741

asQ Suicide Risk Screening Toolkit   **NATIONAL INSTITUTE OF MENTAL HEALTH (NIMH)**   NIH 7/1/2020

Note. Reprinted from *Ask Suicide-Screening Questions (ASQ) Toolkit*, by National Institute of Mental Health, 2021 (https://www.nimh.nih.gov/research/research-conducted-at-nimh/asq-toolkit-materials). In the public domain.

assist with establishing a usual and customary practice that is applied consistently in clinical care.

Suicide risk is not static; therefore, clinics conducting universal screening may benefit from administering a tool at every visit, and the BHC can facilitate this screening. Some patients will be reluctant to admit suicidal thoughts during a screening interview; therefore, it may be prudent to ask again later in the interview after rapport has been established. Any positive response to a screening question should be followed up by the PCP or the BHC with a full assessment of suicidal risk. The goal of the assessment is to understand the level of risk and factors contributing to the patient's suicidality and to formulate an intervention plan to reduce risk for self-harm or death. Figure 17.3 contains the components to cover in a comprehensive assessment of suicide risk.

FIGURE 17.3. Suicide Risk Assessment Components

Ideation	Frequency of suicidal thoughts
	Duration of suicidal thoughts
	Intensity of suicidal thoughts
	Intent to act on suicidal thoughts
	Desire/plan to act on suicidal thoughts
	Meaning of suicidal thoughts—particular focus should be given to thoughts of perceived "burdensomeness" on others and sense of hopelessness
	Plans for attempting suicide
Environment	Means and access to means they have considered
Behavior	Overt presuicidal behavior • Talking about suicide • Rehearsal behaviors • Visiting places to attempt suicide • Writing a suicide note
	Substance use and abuse
History	Past suicide attempts (history of multiple suicide attempts elevates risk significantly)
	History of impulsivity
	History of family suicide
	History of physical, emotional, or sexual abuse
	History of other trauma
Psychosocial factors	Psychosocial stressors • Financial problems • Legal issues • Relationship difficulties • Job difficulties
	Recent loss • Death of a friend/family member • Job loss • Divorce/relationship breakup
Static risk factors	Age: Risk escalates with age, particularly after age 45
	Sex: Risk greater for male individuals
	Previous psychiatric diagnosis
Protective factors	Social support
	Evidence of past problem solving
	Higher level of investment in current treatment

Advise

BHCs should assist clinics in establishing standardized protocols for managing potential suicide risk dispositions in primary care, including involuntary hospitalization when necessary. Based on the results of assessment, the BHC should advise the PCP regarding the patient's level of risk and recommended intervention and assist implementing the appropriate protocol. Patients who are considering suicide often feel desperate and hopeless and may resist engaging in care for fear of losing freedom to choose suicide as an option to escape pain and despair. In discussing interventions with the patient, be clear about the benefits of help seeking and communicate that problems and accompanying distress can improve. Patients at imminent risk for harm require hospitalization, whether voluntarily or involuntarily. Helping them to understand the benefits of inpatient care and the goal of returning to independent life as soon as possible is essential. An adversarial confrontation should be used only as a last resort when there is no other way to secure the patient's safety. Maintaining trust and a collaborative patient–provider relationship will be beneficial for facilitating a commitment to treatment. When patients are not at imminent risk, it can be helpful to discuss the full scope of resources that can be used to manage suicidal thoughts, feelings, and impulses. These range from personal support systems (e.g., friends, family), use of individual coping resources (e.g., exercise, music, meditation, faith/religion, hobbies), support from primary care at the lower end of the risk spectrum, and specialty mental health care and inpatient care at the higher end. The BHC should include in the discussion the patient's perspective as well as their own perspective on what level of care is needed.

Agree

Identify a mutually agreeable plan to recommend to the PCP to keep the patient safe, reduce distress, maintain the highest level of autonomy possible, and support commitment to staying engaged in treatment. Include a short-term plan for dealing with crisis, which includes increasing levels of intervention as needed. Also include a longer term plan for addressing underlying issues. The agreed-upon plan should address both suicidal symptoms and risk specifically, as well as any underlying mental health disorder.

Assist

The characteristics of primary care settings will often not provide the treatment intensity to adequately manage higher levels of suicide risk. However, lower levels of risk can be effectively monitored and managed in primary care and, when appropriate, may be preferable for patients who may feel stigma or who otherwise might resist a referral to an outside mental health care provider. Figure 17.4 provides a helpful rubric for categorizing risk and interventions to consider at each risk level from the VA/DoD (2019a) clinical practice guidelines. This guidance is specifically directed to providers in

FIGURE 17.4. Recommended Actions for Primary Care Providers for Levels of Suicide Risk (*continues*)

Risk of suicide attempt	Essential features	Action
High acute risk	• Suicidal ideation with intent to die by suicide • Inability to maintain safety, independent of external support or help Common warning signs: • A plan for suicide • Recent attempt and/or ongoing preparatory behaviors • Acute major mental illness (e.g., major depressive episode, acute mania, acute psychosis, recent/current drug relapse) • Exacerbation of personality disorder (e.g., increased borderline symptomatology)	• This typically requires psychiatric hospitalization to maintain safety and aggressively target modifiable factors. • These individuals may need to be directly observed until they are transferred to a secure unit and kept in an environment with limited access to lethal means (e.g., keep away from sharps, cords or tubing, toxic substances). • During hospitalization co-occurring conditions should also be addressed.
Intermediate acute risk	• Suicidal ideation to die by suicide • Ability to maintain safety, independent of external support/help These individuals may present similarly to those at high acute risk, sharing many of the features. The only difference may be lack of intent, based upon an identified reason for living (e.g., children), and ability to abide by a safety plan and maintain their own safety. Preparatory behaviors are likely to be absent.	• Consider psychiatric hospitalization, if related factors driving risk are responsive to inpatient treatment (e.g., acute psychosis). • Outpatient management of suicidal thoughts and/or behaviors should be intensive and include frequent contact, regular reassessment of risk, and a well-articulated safety plan. • Mental health treatment should also address co-occurring conditions.
Low acute risk	• No current suicidal intent AND • No specific and current suicidal plan AND • No recent preparatory behaviors AND • Collective high confidence (e.g., patient, care provider, family member) in the ability of the patient to independently maintain safety Individuals may have suicidal ideation, but it will be with little or no intent or specific current plan. If a plan is present, the plan is general and/or vague and without any associated preparatory behaviors (e.g., "I'd shoot myself if things got bad enough, but I don't have a gun"). These patients will be capable of engaging appropriate coping strategies and are willing and able to utilize a safety plan in a crisis situation.	• This can be managed in primary care. • Outpatient mental health treatment may also be indicated, particularly if suicidal ideation and co-occurring conditions exist.

FIGURE 17.4. Recommended Actions for Primary Care Providers for Levels of Suicide Risk (*continued*)

Risk of suicide attempt	Essential features	Action
High chronic risk	Common warning sign: • Chronic suicidal ideation Common risk factors: • Chronic major mental illness and/or personality disorder • History of prior suicide attempt(s) • History of substance use disorders • Chronic pain • Chronic medical condition • Limited coping skills • Unstable or turbulent psychosocial status (e.g., unstable housing, erratic relationships, marginal employment) • Limited ability to identify reasons for living	These individuals are considered to be at chronic risk for becoming acutely suicidal, often in the context of unpredictable situational contingencies (e.g., job loss, loss of relationships, and relapse on drugs). These individuals typically require: • Routine mental health follow-up • A well-articulated safety plan, including lethal means safety (e.g., no access to guns, limited medication supply) • Routine suicide risk screening • Coping skills building • Management of co-occurring conditions
Intermediate chronic risk	• These individuals may feature similar chronicity as those at high chronic risk with respect to psychiatric, substance use, and medical and pain disorders. • Protective factors, coping skills, reasons for living, and relative psychosocial stability suggest enhanced ability to endure future crisis without engaging in self-directed violence.	These individuals typically require: • Routine mental health care to optimize psychiatric conditions and maintain/enhance coping skills and protective factors • A well-articulated safety plan, including lethal means safety (e.g., safe storage of lethal means, medication disposal, blister packaging) • Management of co-occurring conditions
Low chronic risk	• These individuals may range from persons with no or little in the way of mental health or substance use problems, to persons with significant mental illness that is associated with relatively abundant strengths/resources. • Stressors historically have typically been endured absent of suicidal ideation. The following factors will generally be missing: • History of self-directed violence • Chronic suicidal ideation • Tendency towards being highly impulsive • Risky behaviors • Marginal psychosocial functioning	• This is appropriate for mental health care on an as-needed basis, some may be managed in primary care. • Others may require mental health follow-up to continue successful treatments.

Note. From *VA/DoD Clinical Practice Guideline for the Assessment and Management of Patients at Risk for Suicide* (pp. 23–24), by U.S. Department of Veterans Affairs and Department of Defense, 2019 (https://www.healthquality.va.gov/guidelines/MH/srb/VADoDSuicideRiskFullCPGFinal5088212019.pdf). In the public domain.

the primary care setting; however, it does not take into consideration the presence of a behavioral health specialist in the clinic. The presence of an integrated BHC will allow some of the recommended actions to occur within the primary care setting rather than referring to a specialty behavioral health setting.

Regardless of whether treatment will be provided in the primary care setting or a referral will be made to a specialty behavioral health provider, a safety plan should be discussed. Behavioral health providers can assist the primary care manager by developing a safety plan in collaboration with the patient. The plan should be detailed and tailored specifically to the patient.

BHCs should understand that a safety plan is not the same as a no-suicide contract. Although a contract with the patient to not harm themselves is still commonly used by some clinicians, it is inadequate and there is no empirical support for using no-suicide contracts. In contrast, a safety plan is a tangible set of steps the patient agrees to take when certain triggers occur. A safety plan should include the following:

- Identification of signs and symptoms that warrant an immediate reevaluation by a health care provider. Examples include thoughts or feelings of intent to act on suicidal thoughts, suicide preparation acts, or suicide rehearsal behaviors.

- Contact information for suicide help lines and the location of nearby emergency departments that will be used if these high-risk signs and symptoms occur.

- Identification of early warning signs (events, thoughts, feelings, behaviors) that may trigger high levels of distress and escalate into suicidal thoughts and behaviors.

- Steps that can be taken to help regulate emotions when these warning signs occur, such as calling a friend, exercising, or using relaxation techniques.

- Actions the patient should take to limit access to means of self-harm. This may include having a friend or family member take possession of a firearm or disposing of a stockpile of medications.

Once the plan is formulated, the BHC should ensure that the PCP is aware of the details of the safety plan so they can inquire about adherence to the plan and reinforce its use during future PCP appointments.

An essential component to the safety plan is a crisis response plan (Bryan & Rudd, 2010) that collaboratively identifies steps the patient will take when feeling in crisis or when thinking about harming themselves, instead of engaging in suicidal behaviors. A worksheet for developing a crisis response plan is provided in Figure 17.5. An example of a completed crisis response plan is presented in Figure 17.6.

- The plan should define when it is to be used, for example, when suicidal thoughts occur.

FIGURE 17.5. Crisis Response Planning Worksheet

In the past, what events, thoughts, and feelings have precipitated suicidal thoughts and behaviors?
     Events:
     Thoughts:
     Feelings:

In the past, what activities have been helpful in reducing negative thoughts and feelings? What has been the result of engaging in these activities? Activity: Result:
What are some thoughts that have been helpful in reducing distress?
Who is the best source of emotional support?
What behaviors should be avoided?
What lethal means are available?
What steps should be taken to limit access to these means?

What are the best resources to use in case of emergency (i.e., strong suicidal thoughts and intent)?
     Daytime contact number?
     Suicide hotline number?
     Location of emergency department?
     Who can be called for help getting to the emergency department?

FIGURE 17.6. Sample Crisis Response Plan

Crisis Response Plan

When I have suicidal thoughts of any kind or any intensity, I will proceed through the following steps until I no longer feel suicidal:

1.   Listen to classical music on my cell phone.
2.   Take a walk.
3.   Take a shower.
4.   Call my friend Joe and talk about sports to distract myself.
5.   Call the suicide hotline at 988.
6.   Go to the emergency room at General Hospital on 57th Street.

- The plan should provide specific actions the patient will use to enhance safety and decrease the intensity and frequency of suicidal thoughts.

- In developing the plan, have the patient identify behaviors that have helped with coping in the past.

- The plan can be written on a card or completed electronically and carried by the patient on a smartphone or tablet.

- The plan should be individually developed with the patient to ensure it contains steps the patient is willing and able to take. A generic, preprinted plan is less likely to be used.

Numerous studies have empirically evaluated treatment modalities for patients at risk for suicide. Readers are referred to the VA/DoD (2019a) clinical practice guidelines for a review. A recommendation to the PCP to evaluate the patient for medication may be indicated if there appears to be an underlying mental disorder involved. Time-limited cognitive behavioral treatment addressing distortions in thinking and teaching adaptive coping skills has been shown to be effective in reducing suicidal ideation and behavior compared with control groups receiving treatment as usual (Gøtzsche & Gøtzsche, 2017; Riblet et al., 2017). The VA/DoD clinical practice guidelines rate the quality of evidence for these interventions as strong and in favor of cognitive behavioral therapy. Studies have evaluated other treatment modalities for suicidality, such as dialectical behavior therapy for borderline personality disorder (McMain et al., 2017) and problem-solving therapy (Hatcher et al., 2011), with positive results. The VA/DoD guideline found evidence in favor of these approaches, although concludes the evidence is weak.

Bryan and Rudd (2010) identified six brief interventions that apply to primary care and can help the PCP and BHC manage suicide risk for appropriate patients. These interventions include the following:

- use of coping cards to address distorted beliefs and self-perceptions,

- creation of a "survival kit" or "hope box" to target suicidal emotional states,

- developing a "reasons for living list,"

- behavioral activation,

- relaxation exercises, and

- mindfulness exercises.

Figure 17.7 briefly reviews the application of these techniques to patients with suicidal symptoms. Further details on some of these interventions can be found in Chapter 4.

Finally, research has shown various brief contact interventions to be effective for managing suicide risk (Milner et al., 2016). These interventions involve reaching out to patients periodically to check on how they are doing, remind them of available resources, and probably most importantly, let them know

FIGURE 17.7. Brief Suicide Management Interventions Applicable to Primary Care

Intervention	Description	Target
Coping cards	The patient writes suicidal beliefs on a 3 × 5 card using their exact words. On the reverse side, the patient writes more adaptive responses. The patient carries the cards to read when the patient notices thoughts that are in a suicidal mode.	Helps patients distance themselves from the suicidal belief systems and change their response to typical triggers of suicidal beliefs and thoughts.
Survival kit/ hope box	A container is filled with tangible objects that have positive associations for the patient. Examples include photographs of happy events, souvenirs, inspirational quotes, letters from loved ones, and photos of loved ones. The patient discusses their rationale for including each item in the kit with the provider at a follow-up appointment.	Helps patients strengthen positive memories and heighten emotional associations with the objects. The intervention also aims to strengthen a sense of mastery of the suicidal state by showing patients that they can generate positive emotions.
Reasons for living list	The patient generates a list of reasons to live and writes them on a 3 × 5 card. These might include people, goals, values, and anticipated positive events. The patient is instructed to read the list at a given time daily or as needed when experiencing triggers to the suicidal mode.	Helps patients expand awareness of the meaningful and positive aspects of their life and distracts them from focusing on negative aspects.
Behavioral activation	The provider conducts a functional analysis to identify dysfunctional behavior patterns. The provider and patient collaboratively identify desired behavioral alternatives and then set realistic goals to achieve the desired behaviors.	Helps patients overcome avoidance behaviors that disrupt daily activities. Engaging in inherently rewarding behaviors reduces emotional distress in the short term and disrupts patterns of avoidance and withdrawal that can result in a downward spiral of emotional and cognitive dysfunction.
Relaxation exercises	The provider teaches relaxation exercises and instructs the patient to practice them daily and as needed to manage emotional arousal and distress.	Helps the patient gain mastery over physiological arousal contributing to distress.
Mindfulness exercises	The provider teaches skills for focusing on the present moment without judgment and to observe rather than react to thoughts and emotions.	Helps the patient respond to thoughts and emotions with less reactivity to reduce distress.

someone is thinking of them and cares about them. Examples include actions such as a health care professional making postdischarge telephone calls; sending a text message; and making contact by email, postcards, or letters. Milner et al.'s (2016) review of 16 studies suggested the most likely mechanisms underpinning brief contact interventions are social support and improved suicide prevention literacy. Although brief intervention contacts generally are not the first line of intervention for at-risk patients, they provide a means of intervention when patients decline to engage in further care, when patients are discharged from care, or as adjunctive to other treatment modalities.

Arrange

Patients who present with suicidal risk factors but are assessed to be at minimal risk should be monitored for indications of increasing risk. Follow-up visits at weekly intervals are recommended during which the screening tool can be readministered and any life stressors that have occurred can be discussed. This is also a good opportunity to review the crisis response plan and talk through successes and/or difficulties in using it. If low levels of suicide risk are maintained and no additional treatment for an underlying mental health disorder is indicated, monitoring visits can be spaced further apart. However, because suicidal risk factors have been present, the patient should be directed to schedule a same-day appointment if a significant life stressor occurs or if emotional symptoms such as depression or anxiety worsen. To maintain a collaborative therapeutic alliance and to encourage return visits during a potential suicidal crisis, regular check-in visits with the BHC are beneficial even when suicidal risk remains low. These visits might occur with decreasing frequency such as monthly, then every other month, and then quarterly, and then biannually. Patients needing more frequent appointments for monitoring, emotional support, or psychological interventions (i.e., weekly visits) over an extended period may need to be referred to a specialty mental health provider.

When an underlying mental health disorder is present, an evaluation for medications may be indicated. Additionally, a referral for specialty behavioral health services may be helpful. Following up with patients to ensure they have followed through with the referral is recommended. Because of the potential life-threatening risk of not receiving treatment, patients who do not follow through with referrals may need more assistance.

Inpatient Treatment
If a patient is judged to be at significant risk for self-harm, inpatient treatment should be considered to keep the patient safe. As previously discussed, it is best if a patient collaboratively agrees to participate in inpatient care. However, if an imminently suicidal patient is unwilling to consent to inpatient treatment, they may need to be involuntarily hospitalized. This may require a court order or an evaluation by the mental health assessment team of a local law enforcement agency. Clinicians should become familiar with local laws and procedures for involuntary hospitalization.

When a patient who is at significant risk for suicide does not qualify for involuntary hospitalization yet also is refusing a referral for more intensive services outside of primary care, the BHC will need to work with the patient to reduce resistance to referral. This can be time intensive but is necessary to maximize safety. Explore the patient's concerns about more intensive care with empathy and a genuine desire to understand their perspective. Sometimes the patient will have distorted or mistaken ideas about what psychiatric hospitalization will be like, often derived from movies or television. Gently correcting these distortions may reduce fear or anxiety about more intensive care. A patient also may have had negative personal experiences in the past with hospitalization, which are underlying their resistance. The BHC can use motivational enhancement techniques (discussed in Chapter 4) to empathetically discuss these experiences, specifically drawing on ambivalence the patient may have about dying and helping the patient weigh the potential benefits of intensive levels of care against their fears and anxieties. Focusing on the patient's use of coping skills to get through past negative experiences with inpatient care and their ultimate survival during past suicidal episodes may be helpful. Furthermore, patients may view suicide as the only way to escape their pain and suffering if it becomes unbearable and may resist hospitalization out of fear that they will lose this option. The reality is that individuals never completely lose the option to commit suicide even when in a more controlled environment or following discharge from inpatient care. BHCs may hesitate to bring this truth to a patient's attention due to concerns it will elevate the person's risk. However, to the degree that the patient will be more accepting of potentially lifesaving care and accept hospitalization, discussing the patient's continuing ability to make choices about suicide can be a helpful and ethical approach. When a patient continues to refuse more intensive care despite the behavioral health provider's interventions to reduce resistance, every effort must be made to maximize safety without hospitalization. Steps include working with the patient to identify a family member or friend to be with them at all times, discussing ways to remove means of harm, and scheduling a follow-up appointment with the BHC the following day.

Mobile Applications, Helplines, and Websites

For many people, computers, tablets, and smartphones are the first source they use for finding information, resources, and assistance related to health care. Accordingly, an increasing number of websites and mobile applications are available to provide both clinicians and patients with information and tools relevant to management of suicide risk. Websites and applications, as well as suicide hotlines, have the advantage of being available 24 hours per day, which can be essential for people in crisis. Application and website users can access suicide hotline links and phone numbers as well as coping tools such as relaxation exercises, reminders of positive relationships and pleasant events, positive activity planning, and distraction tools. Electronic resources can also provide depression and suicide risk self-assessment and advise when symptoms and risk factors should be evaluated by a clinician.

In the United States, the 988 Suicide Crisis Hotline was implemented in 2022 to replace the 10-digit 1-800-SUICIDE National Suicide Hotline. Modeled after the 911 emergency number, it is an easy-to-remember number that will connect a person at risk for suicide with a trained mental health professional. As 988 becomes more widely known, the 10-digit number will continue to be operational, but the call will be automatically routed to the 988 service.

Web-based resources and mobile applications are not regulated, and information available is of varying quality. Unfortunately, patients may have difficulty discerning which resources and mobile applications provide valid and reliable information (Luxton et al., 2011). Figure 17.8 contains a selection of resources that may be helpful for at-risk patients.

SUMMARY

Vigilance regarding suicide risk is an essential component to primary health care. In the fast-paced structure of primary care practices, it is essential that potentially lethal signs and symptoms of suicidality are not overlooked or minimized. Behavioral health providers working in primary care can ensure appropriate screening, assessment, and safety planning. Furthermore, a skilled behavioral health provider in primary care can deliver evidence-based care to patients with lower acuity suicidality and, in doing so, can help prevent escalation of risk to the patient and potentially avoid the need for referral to higher levels of care.

FIGURE 17.8. Resources for Patients With Suicidal Ideation: Telephone, Websites, and Mobile Applications (*continues*)

Type	Location	Description
Telephone	Dial 988	988 is the national Suicide and Crisis Lifeline in the United States. It is available in English and Spanish and operates 24 hours per day.
	Dial 988, then press 1	Pressing 1 after dialing 988 accesses the Veteran's Crisis Line in the United States.
Websites	The 988 Suicide and Crisis Lifeline (https://988lifeline.org)	988 Suicide and Crisis Lifeline provides free and confidential emotional support to people in suicidal crisis or emotional distress.
	The American Association of Suicidology (AAS; https://suicidology.org/)	AAS leads the advancement of suicide prevention through research, education, training, development of standards, and resources for professionals and the public, as well as survivor support services.
	Substance Abuse and Mental Health Services Administration (SAMHSA; https://www.samhsa.gov/)	SAMHSA provides numerous publications and resources for understanding and managing suicidal risk and behavior.

FIGURE 17.8. Resources for Patients With Suicidal Ideation: Telephone, Websites, and Mobile Applications (*continued*)

Type	Location	Description
Mobile applications	The Virtual Hope Box (Google Play store, Android and Apple iOS)	The Virtual Hope Box is a free mobile application for smartphones or tablets developed by the National Center for Telehealth and Technology, a U.S. Department of Defense Center of Excellence for Psychological Health and Traumatic Brain Injury. It helps patients use healthy coping skills and facilitate emotional regulation. It is best used with guidance from providers. Patients can add individually tailored content into various sections of the app, such as family photos, videos and recorded messages from friends and family, inspirational quotations, soothing music, reminders of previous successes and positive life experiences, future goals, and statements about their worth. The app also contains areas for positive activity planning, distraction tools, and relaxation exercises.
	notOK (Google Play store, Android and Apple iOS)	Free application intended for teenagers features a large, red button that can be clicked to let designated friends or family in their support network know help is needed. Their current GPS location is sent to their contacts with a message that reads: "Hey, I'm not OK! Please call, text, or come find me." A green button can be pressed to let contacts know they are feeling better.
	Suicide Safe (Google Play store, Android and Apple iOS)	Suicide prevention learning tool for primary care and behavioral health providers by SAMHSA based on Suicide Assessment Five-Step Evaluation and Triage practice guidelines. It helps providers feel confident in assisting patients who present suicidal ideation. The app offers suggestions on how to communicate effectively with patients and their support networks, make helpful decisions, and make referrals.

18

Developing Clinical Pathways and Implementing Shared Medical Appointments

The U.S. medical system has historically been geared to treat acute illness and, as such, is poorly matched for today's health care needs. With 129 million American adults (51.8%) managing at least one of 10 chronic conditions (hypertension, coronary heart disease, stroke, diabetes, cancer, arthritis, hepatitis, weak or failing kidneys, asthma, and chronic obstructive pulmonary disease; Boersma et al., 2020), the system is inadequate to address the population's health concerns. However, with an increased focus on delivering primary medical care in patient-centered medical homes, systems are producing innovations in health care that lead to improved access, outcomes, cost management, and patient satisfaction with care (John et al., 2020; National Committee for Quality Assurance, 2019; Nielsen et al., 2015). This shift in health care service delivery has coincided with innovations in electronic health records, telemedicine, messaging, and patient health data gathering/tracking (Atasoy et al., 2019; H. M. Young & Nesbitt, 2017) to facilitate high-quality patient-centered care in a timely manner. Along those lines, methods to deliver primary care services using clinical pathways that include a behavioral health consultant (BHC) and the use of a BHC in a group format through shared medical appointments (SMAs) are increasingly incorporated as a standard primary care practice to help deliver easily accessible and efficient evidence-based care.

https://doi.org/10.1037/0000380-019

Integrated Behavioral Health in Primary Care: Step-by-Step Guidance for Assessment and Intervention, Third Edition, by C. L. Hunter, J. L. Goodie, M. S. Oordt, and A. C. Dobmeyer

CLINICAL PATHWAYS

We introduced the concept of clinical pathways and the rationale behind their use in the Introduction and Chapter 1 and conclude with additional practical detail on how one might develop and implement them effectively in their own clinic. In sum, clinical pathways can be used as a team-based approach to deliver evidence-based care to a given population of interest (e.g., everyone with a new chronic pain diagnosis, patients with a hemoglobin A1C of 8% or greater, those with a body mass index equal to or greater than 30, everyone with a Patient Health Questionnaire-9 score of 10 or more).

Sometimes people confuse clinical practice guidelines and clinical pathways. To avoid confusion, it is important to understand that clinical practice guidelines are "statements that include recommendations, intended to optimize patient care, that are informed by a systematic review of evidence and an assessment of the benefits and harms of alternative care options" (Institute of Medicine Committee on Standards for Developing Trustworthy Clinical Practice Guideline, 2011, p. 4). In other words, clinical practice guidelines tell providers *what* to do based on the current evidence (e.g., screening, assessment, intervention).

Clinical pathways, on the other hand, have been described as "a documented sequence of clinical interventions, placed in an appropriate timeframe, written and agreed to by a multidisciplinary team. They help a patient with a specific condition or diagnosis move progressively through a clinical experience to a desired outcome" (National Assembly for Wales, 1999, p. 10). There is no agreed-upon definition of a clinical pathway (also referred to as a care map, integrated clinical pathway, critical pathway, or care pathway). However, Lawal et al. (2016) outlined the following as an operational definition of what constitutes a clinical pathway:

- The intervention is a structured multidisciplinary plan of care.

- The intervention is used to translate guidelines or evidence into local structures.

- The intervention details the steps in a course of treatment or care in a plan, pathway, algorithm, guideline, protocol, or other inventory of actions (i.e., the intervention has timeframes or criteria-based progression).

- The intervention aims to standardize care for a specific population.

In their review of care pathway literature in the United States, Chawla et al. (2016) concluded that care pathways appear to provide a good way to incorporate evidence-based care into real-world clinical practice, offering flexibility in implementation while using high-quality evidence in pathway development. We believe implementing clinical pathways can be an effective way to leverage standard operating procedures to make sure those who might benefit from team-based care that includes the BHC are consistently identified and have access to these services. We have included pathway materials on the companion website to this book (https://www.apa.org/pubs/books/integrated-behavioral-health-primary-care-third-edition) that can be used to discuss with one's team how they might tailor and launch a standard clinical pathway for alcohol misuse, anxiety, chronic pain, depression, diabetes, insomnia, obesity, and tobacco use. These resources also provide base pathways that one can tailor to their specific needs to address the following:

- identifying those who could benefit,

- connecting the patient with the BHC,

- delivering the intervention, and

- outcomes.

In addition, we recommend *Integrated Care Pathways: A Guide to Good Practice* (N. Davis, 2005) for additional guidance on pathway development.

SHARED MEDICAL APPOINTMENTS

Although it may seem counterintuitive that patients would appreciate receiving services in a group setting, clinical experience and data show high patient and provider satisfaction with group-based care, as well as improved health care outcomes with the use of SMAs (S. D. Cunningham et al., 2021; Jaber et al., 2006; Noffsinger, 2013). Wadsworth et al. (2019), in their examination of 20 high-quality primary research articles, concluded that there are nine mechanisms to explain how SMAs work:

1. Group exposure in SMAs combats isolation, which in turn helps to remove doubts about one's ability to manage illness.

2. Patients learn about disease self-management vicariously by witnessing others' illness experiences.

3. Patients feel inspired by seeing others who are coping well.

4. Group dynamics lead patients and providers to develop more equitable relationships.

5. Providers feel increased appreciation and rapport toward colleagues, leading to increased efficiency.

6. Providers learn from the patients how better to meet their patients' needs.

7. Adequate time allotment of the SMA leads patients to feel supported.

8. Patients receive professional expertise from the provider in combination with first-hand information from peers, resulting in more robust health knowledge.

9. Patients have the opportunity to see how the medical provider interacts with fellow patients, which allows them to get to know the physician and better determine their level of trust.

Group appointments allow a primary care provider (PCP) to see more patients in a given amount of time without sacrificing care quality. One critical way group appointments save time is that they allow a provider and BHC to have conversations with an entire group that often happen on a one-on-one basis. For example, many health conditions treated in primary care would be improved or managed more effectively if patients engaged in more physical activity. In a group appointment, the BHC can discuss methods for increasing physical activity with group patients at one time, rather than having a similar conversation with each patient individually. In addition to the guidance provided by the BHC, the group patients hear ideas from other patients. This chapter describes the three main SMA models of service delivery and the BHC's role within these models.

DROP-IN GROUP MEDICAL APPOINTMENT

The drop-in group medical appointment (DIGMA) is a provider-focused group that always includes the PCP and a BHC and focuses on the patients enrolled to an individual PCP's practice (Agency for Healthcare Research and Quality, 2017; Jaber et al., 2006; Liebhaber et al., 2011; Noffsinger, 2013; Noffsinger & Scott, 2000b). This model was designed to help providers see more patients in a given amount of time, improve access to care, attend to psychosocial factors, improve provider and patient satisfaction with care, and increase quality of care through more frequent follow-up (Noffsinger & Scott, 2000b).

These groups can be viewed as consecutive individual office visits with other patients in the room (Pennachio, 2003). Each patient can have their individual needs attended to while being supported by group members, learning as others are examined, and asking additional questions throughout the time the group is together (Pennachio, 2003).

DIGMAs are typically run weekly for 60, 90, or 120 minutes, but most are 90 minutes and consist of 10 to 22 patients with three to six family members (Christianson & Warrick, 2003; Noffsinger & Scott, 2000b). An ideal size for most clinics is 10 to 16 patients (Noffsinger, 2013). Although a DIGMA might be offered weekly, individual patients only attend at the frequency recommended by their PCP (e.g., monthly, quarterly) or when they feel a need to drop in for additional, unscheduled care. Patients are recruited to a DIGMA through physician invitation, a scheduler call, or attendance on a drop-in or unscheduled basis when they have a medical question or need (Christianson & Warrick, 2003).

There are three DIGMA subtypes: homogenous, heterogeneous, and mixed (Christianson & Warrick, 2003; Noffsinger 2013). The homogenous type consists of patients grouped by diagnosis (e.g., hypertension, diabetes). The heterogeneous type includes patients with different diagnoses or conditions; utilization behavior; and personal characteristics like age, sex, or socioeconomic level. A third type uses a mixed model in which, for example, weekly visits could be focused on one of four diagnoses or problem areas like cardiopulmonary, chronic pain, weight management, diabetes, or gastrointestinal problems, but patients could also be seen in a group visit at any time.

BHC Roles in DIGMAs

DIGMAs are designed for follow-up visits with established patients and are particularly well suited for patients who require more time and may have more psychosocial needs to address than a typical individual appointment would allow (Noffsinger, 2013; Pennachio, 2003). Patients not appropriate for a DIGMA include new or one-time evaluations and those who speak a different language, have a cognitive impairment, have an infectious disease, have emergencies, or require complex procedures.

The BHC is active throughout each DIGMA, including introducing the group concept and procedures for the day. The BHC is also responsible for helping the PCP stay on time and address psychosocial issues as they arise through interactive group discussions. This allows the PCP the freedom to focus on delivering high-quality individual care within a supportive group setting (Noffsinger, 1999). The BHC is also able to address individual behavioral health concerns outside of the group through individual appointments as needed. A growing body of literature shows that DIGMAs, like other SMAs, result in improved satisfaction with and access to care (e.g., Heyworth et al., 2014), improved health management knowledge (e.g., Jhagroo et al., 2013), improvements in health behaviors like physical activity (e.g., Dickman et al., 2012), better quality of life (e.g., Seesing et al., 2014), and better physical health measures like hemoglobin A1C and systolic blood pressure (e.g., Edelman et al., 2015).

Critical Success Factors

A number of pregroup planning activities have been cited as important for a successful DIGMA start-up (Christianson & Warrick 2003; Noffsinger, 2013):

• Designate an administrative champion responsible for the DIGMA program to include development and deployment throughout the facility and ensure adequate administrative support.

• Include only those PCPs who want to do DIGMAs and who have panel enrollment large enough to start using this model.

• Secure patient buy-in through marketing with professional materials (e.g., wall posters, letters to patients) and PCP intervention, such as taking 15 to 30 seconds during every office visit to explain the benefits of a DIGMA to patients and hand them a flyer.

• Assign a scheduler with dedicated time for DIGMA support to invite and book patients and a medical assistant to take vital signs, review and order tests, and review forms.

- Choose a BHC who has a skill and practice set that is appropriately matched to the physician and the group. This person will introduce the group and manage time so the group runs smoothly. The BHC may need to help the PCP interact with the group and limit time spent with each individual in order to keep the group running smoothly. The BHC will assess and address psychosocial concerns with each patient and include other group members with similar concerns. Also, helping to resolve patient anger or other negative emotions when the PCP is absent from the room may be required in this model (Noffsinger, 1999). This person must have compassion for the chronically ill, be skilled in running groups, and have a solid knowledge base regarding psychosocial needs of medical patients (Noffsinger, 1999). Clinical health psychologists and medical social workers are ideal for these types of groups. Other specialists can also effectively serve in this role, especially with homogeneous groups (e.g., diabetes), by developing the knowledge and skills needed through educational readings, workshops, and consultation or training with behavioral health providers knowledgeable in health psychology or behavioral medicine.

- Have a budget dedicated to the development and production of attractive professional promotional material.

- Provide adequate preparation and training for the PCP and staff on how to run a DIGMA.

- Provide adequate space for the group.

Typical DIGMA Session Profile

- Patients arriving early for the DIGMA immediately have their vitals taken by a nurse or other medical assistant and complete additional paperwork. Those who arrive as the group starts or show up late are pulled out of the group by the nurse or medical assistant to perform these tasks.

- Patients sit in a circular arrangement if the room configuration allows, and the PCP and BHC sit together.

- The BHC starts the group by introducing medical team members, making introductory comments about the group and what will occur, and explaining how patients can get the most from the group appointment (for an introduction guide, see Figure 18.1). Patients complete confidentiality forms prior to or during the introduction. Next, the BHC asks each person to introduce themselves one at a time in whatever manner they would like, starting with those who have to leave early. Patients are asked to state what their medical condition is and what assistance or information they are seeking. An alternative could include having a nurse or medical technician get this information during vitals or having the patient write it out on a sheet before the visit. This cuts down on the time away from patient care. This process takes 10 to 15 minutes.

FIGURE 18.1. DIGMA Appointment Introduction

Introduce the team: discuss the roles of each person present

- BHC paces and manages the group.
- Discuss types of medical care the physician will provide.
- Explain what is expected of patients during the group appointment.
- Complete confidentiality forms and paperwork.

Describe the DIGMA: extended medical appointment, meets weekly, 90 minutes

Benefits of DIGMA: more time, faster access, physical and behavioral aspects, closer follow-up care, more social support

Explain that medical services are provided during the DIGMA: medical questions will be answered, prescriptions can be changed or refilled, procedures (e.g., foot check if diabetic) and referrals will be ordered, test results may be discussed

DIGMAs are voluntary:

> *It is your choice to be here today, and we are happy you made it. You can attend this group today or see Dr. Franzos individually as before. Many people will have times when they want to meet with Dr. Franzos individually, but most things can be handled well in this setting. Please let us know if you do become uncomfortable at any time.*

Confidentiality and sensitivity in group: confidentiality form must be signed, brief private time with physician can be available at end of group per physician's discretion or patient request

Reminders:

- Groups are held every week, but the physician may be gone during some weeks.
- Active participation is always welcome.
- Beverages are provided if available, and there are bathrooms.
- Ask patients to bring a list of questions and any medications they want the physician to review.
- Ask patients to keep questions or issues for the physician to two main concerns. If time is available later on, additional questions can be asked, or patients are welcome to attend the next convenient group to get their questions answered.
- Patients can ask about their medical, emotional, or behavioral concerns.
- Patients may briefly break away from the group so a nurse or medical technician can take and record their vital signs if needed.
- After patients have seen the physician, they should stay until they get their patient instruction sheet from the technician. This sheet will have all the information about follow-up scheduling, lab work, or medication adjustments.
- Patients may need to get up and stretch or walk around. Ask if there is anyone who needs to leave early.

Note. DIGMA = drop-in group medical appointment; BHC = behavioral health consultant.

- Starting with patients who must leave early, the PCP begins the history taking and medical decision making one patient at a time while other patients watch and listen. Problem presentation is typically limited to no more than two areas of concern. Average individual patient time will depend on the number of patients and their concerns or needs (e.g., 15 patients would allow an average of 4 minutes with each patient). Although only a few minutes is spent with each individual, patients often perceive that they have spent more time with the provider than they would have in an individual appointment because they have been learning from the group for 90 minutes. The PCP and BHC can interact with other individuals in the group as each person is being seen so group learning can occur. For example, a patient who started on blood pressure medication may report feeling fatigued or lethargic as a side effect of the medication. The question can then be asked,

How many of you are taking blood pressure medication and have felt this way?

This can open a discussion of why patients get this response, what can be done about it, and how individual patients have coped effectively with this symptom in the past.

- Medical record documentation happens with each patient as the exam is done. How this occurs will vary depending on paper or electronic records and available support staff. The goal is to have the PCP finished with all documentation by the end of the 90-minute period.

- The final 15 minutes of the group can be used for individual, brief private exams outside of the room by the PCP if needed. However, these are not needed regularly and should be limited as much as possible. Most of the care takes place within the group setting. The BHC continues to run the group while the PCP is away. Patients are free to leave at this point, or they may stay if they have additional questions or need to be seen privately.

Specific Skills to Develop for BHC

In DIGMAs, the BHC will need to be assertive and organized and have broad health and general psychology knowledge. For example, BHCs are responsible for providing the structure for the group appointment by explaining confidentiality, what topics will be discussed, how brief examinations will be conducted by the PCP, and the length of the entire group. To keep the appointment running smoothly, a BHC may need to tell a PCP who has spent enough time with a patient that there is a need to move on by saying,

Dr. Smith, would it be okay if we moved on to the next person? I think we will have time at the end of the appointment to finish this discussion, or we can schedule more time if needed.

Such a statement brings to the attention of the PCP that moving along with the appointment is imperative, yet they have the choice about how to use the time. Another example is a case in which an obvious referral is in order (e.g., a tobacco user). One might interject into the PCP's assessment and ask the patient,

Have you ever thought of quitting? Would you like to try again?

If the answer is yes, then one might say,

Dr. Smith, do you believe Mr. Jones will benefit from a referral for help with tobacco cessation? A lot of your other patients have certainly benefited from the various methods of help available at the hospital's Wellness Center, such as in-person support groups, virtual and texting support, and nicotine replacement therapy.

A quick educational comment like this from the BHC will go beyond addressing the needs of this individual patient and will educate all group members on the available resources. And if the answer from the PCP is yes, the BHC can say,

> I will go ahead and put that referral in for you if you would like. Mr. Jones, at your appointment with the Wellness Center they will work with you to determine what will be the best approach for your success.

In this way the BHC provides some structure, sticks to the behavioral agenda, and assists the PCP in identifying and making appropriate referrals. Remember, BHCs are the primary facilitator for the appointment, but the PCP and group members are the stars.

One must have the ability to process what is being said and not said, anticipating where it will go and how those subject areas might be leveraged for group education. For instance, when the PCP finishes an encounter for blood pressure with an individual and is completing the documentation, one might ask,

> Who else in the appointment today has been told they have high blood pressure?

In a typical group of primary care patients, many will have a hypertension diagnosis, so one can expect to see raised hands. In response, one can now ask if people would like to hear more information about the behavioral management of hypertension. The answer from the group should be yes, which opens the door for one to discuss a topic of choice, such as behavioral techniques for weight management, exercise, and nutrition.

The BHC may need to foster the PCP's interactions with the rest of the group while interacting with an individual. Most PCPs are not accustomed to dealing with patients in a group setting, so they tend to focus on one individual, lowering their voice and neglecting the group process. For example, while the PCP is interacting with a diabetes patient, the BHC might say,

> Dr. Smith, I wonder if anyone else in the group would be interested in hearing more about diabetes and the average hemoglobin A1C that is typically recommended by the American Diabetes Association?

A question like this will draw the PCP back into engaging the entire group as they spend a moment teaching before returning to the specifics of the individual patient and finishing that appointment. In this way individual needs are met, the group process is attended to, and many individuals gain prevention and educational information.

PHYSICAL SHARED MEDICAL APPOINTMENT

As detailed by Noffsinger (2013), the physical shared medical appointment (PSMA) model is viable for any patient in a practice that will need a physical examination conducted in private while they are disrobed (e.g., prenatal exam). PSMAs can be used when a new patient is entering a medical system or to address any chronic illness that requires a private physical examination, if ease of access to an examination is important (Noffsinger, 2013).

PSMAs have three components:

- a patient packet with a detailed history questionnaire that is sent to the participant to complete in advance of the PSMA, as well as completed previsit labs;

- a private physical exam during the first half of the PSMA; and

- an interactive group time run by the BHC during the last half of the PSMA that looks much as it would in a DIGMA.

PSMAs are usually held weekly for 90 minutes but could be longer or shorter based on a unique clinic need. PSMAs may be divided by sex or age group and consist of six to nine patients and, like DIGMAs, can be homogeneous, heterogeneous, or mixed.

PCPs efficiently conduct the physical examinations during the first half of the PSMA with the help of two medical assistants or nurses and two to four properly equipped exam rooms. A documenter is also present during the private exam and the group room activities to ensure that the PCP never has to wait but goes from room to room where the patient is ready for the physical examination. The PCP can defer most discussions, including questions patients have during the physical exam, for the group setting by saying,

> That is a great question others will want to hear the answer to. Please ask that again when we go back to the group room.

As the PCP conducts physical exams, the BHC interacts with the group of unroomed rotating patients in the following steps:

1. Arrive 5 to 10 minutes early in the group room and welcome the group.

2. Discuss confidentiality twice to ensure those who are getting physical exams first also get this information.

3. Write down patient questions on a whiteboard to discuss with the PCP during the second half of the appointment.

4. Productively interact with patients to include the integration of support of other patients into each individual's unique situation, deliver patient education, and attend to relevant biopsychosocial issues.

5. As time allows, also start reviewing the patient packet and perform any additional duties requested by the physician (e.g., reviewing educational handouts).

The PCP returns to the group room after physical exams are completed and can immediately see whiteboards with patient concerns and previsit lab results listed prior to the appointment by a nurse or medical assistant, with abnormal results circled in red. During the second half of the appointment, the PCP answers questions from the whiteboard and determines a course of action for any abnormal labs.

COOPERATIVE HEALTH CARE CLINIC

The cooperative health care clinic (CHCC) model targets those who have medical contact two or more times a month and/or those in specific high-risk groups, such as frail patients over the age of 65 or those with conditions like hypertension, diabetes, hyperlipidemia, cardiovascular disease, asthma, and depression (Jaber et al., 2006; Junling et al., 2015; Noffsinger, 2013; Noffsinger & Scott, 2000b). Optimal group size is 15 to 20 patients that meet once a month at the same time and place. Total time set aside for the group is 2.5 hours to include 90 minutes of group time followed by 1 hour for one-on-one provider appointments as needed, which typically covers six or seven patients (Noffsinger, 2013; Noffsinger & Scott, 2000b). The BHC will play different roles and may be involved significantly less or not at all in the CHCC compared with the DIGMA and PSMA models. Depending on one's setting, a BHC might be on a rotating schedule with other specialists to target specific educational topics or serve as an additional support that attends monthly to help answer or address psychosocial topics as they arise (e.g., Jaber et al., 2006; Noffsinger & Scott, 2000a, 2000b).

CHCC group visits are designed to work in conjunction with the typical office visit and not to replace such visits. These groups

- allow more time for self-management education, provider–patient interaction, skill building, social and emotional support, problem solving, modeling, and increased self-efficacy (Jaber et al., 2006);

- include components of a typical individual visit such as private one-on-one exams and typically have the same individuals from visit to visit;

- include education focused on self-management with topics like physical activity, nutrition, medication management, and psychosocial factors related to good health (Jaber et al., 2006; Noffsinger & Scott, 2000b); and

- include guest speakers (e.g., pharmacist, psychologist) who are part of the team and are brought in on a periodic or rotating basis to address specific specialty content areas.

In reviews of the group visit literature, Jaber et al. (2006) and Wadsworth et al. (2019) found sufficient data to support the effectiveness of CHCC group visits in decreasing emergency room and specialist visits and improving quality of care, quality of life, biophysical outcomes, and physician and patient satisfaction.

Each CHCC group visit has five components, including socialization time, education time, a working break, time for questions and answers, and planning for the next CHCC appointment (Noffsinger, 2013). Limits of confidentiality must be addressed, which can be done verbally at the beginning of the group. Clinics or providers requiring a more formal documentation of this process can use informed consent regarding confidentiality or Health Insurance Portability and Accountability Act release documents. A 90-minute CHCC group session typically moves through the following stages:

1. Socialization time (10–15 minutes): This spontaneous or organized time includes introduction of team members, patients, and sharing of personal information to build group cohesion.

2. Education time (30 minutes): During the 1st year, core topics like advance directives, emergency care, and health maintenance requirements may be areas of focus. As the group continues, topics selected by the group are introduced. Education can be interactive, didactic, or a combination of both approaches.

3. Working break time (20–30 minutes): The primary PCP and a nurse start on opposite sides of a U-shaped seating arrangement and address various concerns of the group. Activities like blood pressure measurement and medication refills are accomplished, and each member has one-on-one contact. Patients not engaged with the provider or nurse can interact with other group members and may partake of snacks brought by group members designated to bring items for that appointment.

4. Question and answer time (10–15 minutes): This interactive and varied time can range from topics or problems covered that day to other complex medical issues.

5. Planning time (5–10 minutes): This encompasses deciding on a topic for the following month and specifying the time and day of the group visit.

A 60-minute individual care segment follows the group appointment. Patients that require an individual encounter with the provider are seen within this hour. Situations that may require an individual encounter include exacerbation of a chronic condition or the need for health maintenance (e.g., physical exams) that could not be conducted within the group setting.

ADAPTATION

Regardless of what SMA model one uses or if one chooses to blend them, we think it is important to take into consideration the context of one's clinic, patients, and any alterations you may need to make in SMA service delivery in order to provide the most effective care. For example, Noya et al. (2019)

culturally adapted an SMA intervention for Latinx patients with diabetes referred to as ALDEA (Latinxs con Diabetes en Acción). Adaptations included the following:

- consideration of social determinants (low socioeconomic status/insurance status and low health literacy), with a low-cost pharmacy, low-cost/free diabetes supplies, screening for low health literacy at intake, and food distribution established on-site; and

- cultural considerations, including a bilingual team, cultural humility training for the team, an invitation of family members to participate, consideration of family in planning and execution of SMART (specific, measurable, achievable, relevant, time-bound) goals, provision of a flexible schedule, normalization of late arrival, and integration of assessment of herbal medicine into the intake form.

The adapted SMA intervention participants had a significantly greater number of individuals (58%) achieve target hemoglobin A1C 6 months into the program in comparison with individuals (31%) receiving usual primary care services (Noya et al., 2019).

In addition to the information in this chapter, several resources on the internet can provide additional guidance and user-friendly forms that one might find useful. See Figure 18.2 for links and descriptions.

SUMMARY

In this chapter, we expanded on the use of clinical pathways introduced in Chapter 1. We have provided specific clinical pathway materials on the companion website to this book that one can readily adapt to their setting. We believe that implementing clinical pathways can lead to consistent identification and care engagement of patients who could benefit from BHC services.

We have also outlined the three primary SMAs, their delivery format and goals, and the BHC's role in each. If one is in a clinic that may be interested in starting an SMA program, we encourage BHCs to help their team prepare for success through readings (e.g., Noffsinger, 2009, 2013; Noffsinger & Scott, 2000a, 2000b) and in-person training from SMA experts who have experience effectively running these groups and teaching others how to effectively run them.

In our experience, successful clinical pathway implementation and SMAs have been rewarding for patients and providers. They can produce good outcomes, increase patient satisfaction with health care, and help the team function at their peak scope of practice. BHCs can be important advocates for examining the clinic population, assessing provider interest, and determining whether a clinical pathway or SMA is appropriate for initiation to serve the clinic's patient population more efficiently and effectively.

FIGURE 18.2. Provider Resources

Type	Location	Description
Resources	University of Massachusetts Chan Medical School MGV Training (https://www. umassmed.edu/cipc/ continuing-education/ MGVTraining/)	This link will take you to a webpage where you access MGV course curriculum and training and 11 MGV guides developed by different health systems.
	American Diabetes Association Starter Kit (https://www.sfhp. org/wp-content/files/ Diabetes_Medical_Group_ Visit_Toolkit.pdf)	This 41-page group medical visit starter kit is designed for health care teams who want to begin offering group medical visits for their patients. It contains information on (a) what are group medical visits, (b) why they are useful, (c) how to plan and implement the visits, (d) a task list and timeline, (e) who does what, (f) a sample letter for patients, (g) sample agendas, (h) information on a "Patient Workbook" for the participants, (i) group medical visit norms, (j) a vitals record for patients, (k) a clinic information sheet, (l) a list of resources to help you get started, (m) sources for patient education materials, and (n) tips on facilitating groups.

Note. MGV = medical group visit.

REFERENCES

Achenbach, T. M., & Rescorla, L. A. (2001). *Manual for the ASEBA school-age forms & profiles*. University of Vermont, Research Center for Children, Youth, & Families.

Adelman, R. D., Tmanova, L. L., Delgado, D., Dion, S., & Lachs, M. S. (2014). Caregiver burden: A clinical review. *The Journal of the American Medical Association, 311*(10), 1052–1059.

Administration on Aging. (2021). *2020 profile of older Americans*. U.S. Department of Health and Human Services. https://acl.gov/sites/default/files/aging%20and%20Disability%20In%20America/2020Profileolderamericans.final_.pdf

Agency for Healthcare Research and Quality. (2017). *The CAHPS ambulatory care improvement guide: Practical strategies for improving patient experience: Section 6: Strategies for improving patient experience with ambulatory care*. https://www.ahrq.gov/sites/default/files/wysiwyg/cahps/quality-improvement/improvement-guide/6-strategies-for-improving/access/cahps-strategy-6m.pdf

Aguinaldo, L. D., Sullivant, S., Lanzillo, E. C., Ross, A., He, J. P., Bradley-Ewing, A., Bridge, J. A., Horowitz, L. M., & Wharff, E. A. (2021). Validation of the Ask Suicide-Screening Questions (ASQ) with youth in outpatient specialty and primary care clinics. *General Hospital Psychiatry, 68*, 52–58. https://doi.org/10.1016/j.genhosppsych.2020.11.006

Agustí, A., Soler, J. J., Molina, J., Muñoz, M. J., García-Losa, M., Roset, M., Jones, P. W., & Badia, X. (2012). Is the CAT questionnaire sensitive to changes in health status in patients with severe COPD exacerbations? *COPD: Journal of Chronic Obstructive Pulmonary Disease, 9*(5), 492–498. https://doi.org/10.3109/15412555.2012.692409

Ahles, T. A., Wasson, J. H., Seville, J. L., Johnson, D. J., Cole, B. F., Hanscom, B., Stukel, T. A., & McKinstry, E. (2006). A controlled trial of methods for managing pain in primary care patients with or without co-occurring psychosocial problems. *Annals of Family Medicine, 4*(4), 341–350. https://doi.org/10.1370/afm.527

Ahmedani, B. K., Peterson, E. L., Hu, Y., Rossom, R. C., Lynch, F., Lu, C. Y., Waitzfelder, B. E., Owen-Smith, A. A., Hubley, S., Prabhakar, D., Williams, L. K., Zeld, N., Mutter, E., Beck, A., Tolsma, D., & Simon, G. E. (2017). Major physical health conditions and risk of suicide. *American Journal of Preventive Medicine, 53*(3), 308–315. https://doi.org/10.1016/j.amepre.2017.04.001

Ahmedani, B. K., Simon, G. E., Stewart, C., Beck, A., Waitzfelder, B. E., Rossom, R., Lynch, F., Owen-Smith, A., Hunkeler, E. M., Whiteside, U., Operskalski, B. H., Coffey, M. J., & Solberg, L. I. (2014). Health care contacts in the year before suicide death. *Journal of General Internal Medicine, 29*(6), 870–877. https://doi.org/10.1007/s11606-014-2767-3

Åkerberg, A., Söderlund, A., & Lindén, M. (2016). Investigation of the validity and reliability of a smartphone pedometer application. *European Journal of Physiotherapy, 18*(3), 185–193. https://doi.org/10.3109/21679169.2016.1174297

Alageel, S., Gulliford, M. C., McDermott, L., & Wright, A. J. (2017). Multiple health behaviour change interventions for primary prevention of cardiovascular disease in primary care: Systematic review and meta-analysis. *BMJ Open, 7*(6), Article e015375. https://doi.org/10.1136/bmjopen-2016-015375

Albee, G. W. (1983). Psychopathology, prevention, and the just society. *The Journal of Primary Prevention, 4*(1), 5–40. https://doi.org/10.1007/BF01359083

Alda, M., Luciano, J. V., Andrés, E., Serrano-Blanco, A., Rodero, B., del Hoyo, Y. L., Roca, M., Moreno, S., Magallón, R., & García-Campayo, J. (2011). Effectiveness of cognitive behaviour therapy for the treatment of catastrophisation in patients with fibromyalgia: A randomised controlled trial. *Arthritis Research & Therapy, 13*(5), Article R173. https://doi.org/10.1186/ar3496

Aldus, C. F., Arthur, A., Dennington-Price, A., Millac, P., Richmond, P., Dening, T., Fox, C., Matthews, F. E., Robinson, L., Stephan, B. C. M., Brayne, C., & Savva, G. M. (2020). Undiagnosed dementia in primary care: A record linkage study. *Health Services and Delivery Research, 8*(20), 1–108. https://doi.org/10.3310/hsdr08200

Alipour, Z., Kazemi, A., Kheirabadi, G., & Eslami, A. A. (2020). Marital communication skills training to promote marital satisfaction and psychological health during pregnancy: A couple focused approach. *Reproductive Health, 17*(1), Article 23. https://doi.org/10.1186/s12978-020-0877-4

Allan, R., & Fisher, J. (Eds.). (2012). *Heart and mind: The practice of cardiac psychology* (2nd ed.). American Psychological Association. https://doi.org/10.1037/13086-000

Allen, M. S., & Walter, E. E. (2019). Erectile dysfunction: An umbrella review of meta-analyses of risk-factors, treatment, and prevalence outcomes. *Journal of Sexual Medicine, 16*(4), 531–541. https://doi.org/10.1016/j.jsxm.2019.01.314

Althof, S. E., McMahon, C. G., Waldinger, M. D., Serefoglu, E. C., Shindel, A. W., Adaikan, P. G., Becher, E., Dean, J., Giuliano, F., Hellstrom, W. J., Giraldi, A., Glina, S., Incrocci, L., Jannini, E., McCabe, M., Parish, S., Rowland, D., Segraves, R. T., Sharlip, I., & Torres, L. O. (2014). An update of the International Society of Sexual Medicine's guidelines for the diagnosis and treatment of premature ejaculation (PE). *Sexual Medicine, 2*(2), 60–90. https://doi.org/10.1002/sm2.28

Alzheimer's Association. (2013, January 4). *Disclosing an Alzheimer's diagnosis* [Video]. YouTube. https://www.youtube.com/watch?v=jBJ6XccZnPg

Amaral, A. S., Afonso, R. M., Simões, M. R., & Freitas, S. (2022). Decision-making capacity in healthcare: Instruments review and reflections about its assessment in the elderly with cognitive impairment and dementia. *Psychiatric Quarterly, 93*(1), 35–53. https://doi.org/10.1007/s11126-020-09867-7

American Academy of Family Physicians. (n.d.). *Primary care.* https://www.aafp.org/about/policies/all/primary-care.html

American Academy of Family Physicians. (2017). *Addressing alcohol use practice manual: An alcohol screening and brief intervention program.* https://www.aafp.org/dam/AAFP/documents/patient_care/alcohol/alcohol-manual.pdf

American Academy of Family Physicians, American Academy of Pediatrics, American College of Physicians, & American Osteopathic Association. (2007). *Joint principles of the patient-centered medical home.* https://www.aafp.org/dam/AAFP/documents/practice_management/pcmh/initiatives/PCMHJoint.pdf

American Bar Association & American Psychological Association. (2008). *Assessment of older adults with diminished capacity: A handbook for psychologists.* https://www.apa.org/pi/aging/programs/assessment/capacity-psychologist-handbook.pdf

American College of Obstetricians and Gynecologists. (2014). Management of menopausal symptoms (Practice Bulletin No. 141). *Obstetrics and Gynecology, 123*(1), 202–216. https://doi.org/10.1097/01.AOG.0000441353.20693.78

American College of Obstetricians and Gynecologists. (2020). Chronic pelvic pain (ACOG Practice Bulletin No. 218). *Obstetrics and Gynecology, 135*(3), e98–e109. https://doi.org/10.1097/AOG.0000000000003716

American College of Preventive Medicine. (2011). *Use, abuse, misuse and disposal of prescription pain medication time tool: A resource from the American College of Preventive Medicine.*

American Diabetes Association. (2020). *The official pocket guide to diabetic food choices* (5th ed.).

American Diabetes Association Professional Practice Committee. (2022a). Classification and diagnosis of diabetes: Standards of medical care in diabetes—2022. *Diabetes Care, 45*(Suppl. 1), S17–S38. https://doi.org/10.2337/dc22-S002

American Diabetes Association Professional Practice Committee. (2022b). Comprehensive medical evaluation and assessment of comorbidities: Standards of medical care in diabetes—2022. *Diabetes Care, 45*(Suppl. 1), S46–S59. https://doi.org/10.2337/dc22-S004

American Diabetes Association Professional Practice Committee. (2022c). Facilitating behavior change and well-being to improve health outcomes: Standards of medical care in diabetes—2022. *Diabetes Care, 45*(Suppl. 1), S60–S82. https://doi.org/10.2337/dc22-S005

American Diabetes Association Professional Practice Committee. (2022d). Glycemic targets: Standards of medical care in diabetes—2022. *Diabetes Care, 45*(Suppl. 1), S83–S96. https://doi.org/10.2337/dc22-S006

American Diabetes Association Professional Practice Committee. (2022e). Improving care and promoting health in populations: Standards of medical care in diabetes—2022. *Diabetes Care, 45*(Suppl. 1), S8–S16. https://doi.org/10.2337/dc22-S001

American Diabetes Association Professional Practice Committee. (2022f). Management of diabetes in pregnancy: Standards of medical care in diabetes—2022. *Diabetes Care, 45*(Suppl. 1), S232–S243. https://doi.org/10.2337/dc22-S015

American Diabetes Association Professional Practice Committee. (2022g). Pharmacologic approaches to glycemic treatment: Standards of medical care in diabetes—2022. *Diabetes Care, 45*(Suppl. 1), S125–S143. https://doi.org/10.2337/dc22-S009

American Diabetes Association Professional Practice Committee. (2022h). Prevention or delay of Type 2 diabetes and associated comorbidities: Standards of medical care in diabetes—2022. *Diabetes Care, 45*(Suppl. 1), S39–S45. https://doi.org/10.2337/dc22-S003

American Lung Association. (2023, May 30). *Join Freedom From Smoking®.* https://www.lung.org/quit-smoking/join-freedom-from-smoking

American Psychiatric Association. (2022). *Diagnostic and statistical manual of mental disorders* (5th ed., text rev.). https://doi.org/10.1176/appi.books.9780890425787

American Psychological Association. (2014). Guidelines for psychological practice with older adults. *American Psychologist, 69*(1), 34–65. https://doi.org/10.1037/a0035063

American Psychological Association. (2017). *Clinical practice guideline for the treatment of posttraumatic stress disorder (PTSD).* https://www.apa.org/ptsd-guideline/ptsd.pdf

American Psychological Association. (2019). *Clinical practice guideline for the treatment of depression across three age cohorts.* https://www.apa.org/depression-guideline

American Psychological Association. (2022). *Behavioral health integration fact sheet.* https://www.apa.org/health/behavioral-integration-fact-sheet

Anderson, K. (2010). *How to change your drinking: A harm reduction guide to alcohol* (2nd ed.). HAMS Harm Reduction Network.

Andrews, A. R., III, Gomez, D., Larey, A., Pacl, H., Burchette, D., Hernandez Rodriguez, J., Pastrana, F. A., & Bridges, A. J. (2016). Comparison of integrated behavioral health treatment for internalizing psychiatric disorders in patients with and without Type 2 diabetes. *Families, Systems, & Health, 34*(4), 367–377. https://doi.org/10.1037/fsh0000224

Antshel, K. M. (2015). Psychosocial interventions in attention-deficit/hyperactivity disorder: Update. *Child and Adolescent Psychiatric Clinics of North America, 24*(1), 79–97. https://doi.org/10.1016/j.chc.2014.08.002

Apter, A. J., Wan, F., Reisine, S., Bender, B., Rand, C., Bogen, D. K., Bennett, I. M., Bryant-Stephens, T., Roy, J., Gonzalez, R., Priolo, C., Have, T. T., & Morales, K. H. (2013). The association of health literacy with adherence and outcomes in moderate-severe asthma. *The Journal of Allergy and Clinical Immunology, 132*(2), 321–327. https://doi.org/10.1016/j.jaci.2013.02.014

Archer, J., Bower, P., Gilbody, S., Lovell, K., Richards, D., Gask, L., Dickens, C., & Coventry, P. (2012). Collaborative care for depression and anxiety problems. *Cochrane Database of Systematic Reviews, 10*, Article CD006525. https://doi.org/10.1002/14651858.CD006525.pub2

Arnett, D. K., Blumenthal, R. S., Albert, M. A., Buroker, A. B., Goldberger, Z. D., Hahn, E. J., Himmelfarb, C. D., Khera, A., Lloyd-Jones, D., McEvoy, J. W., Michos, E. D., Miedema, M. D., Muñoz, D., Smith, S. C., Jr., Virani, S. S., Williams, K. A., Sr., Yeboah, J., & Ziaeian, B. (2019). 2019 ACC/AHA guideline on the primary prevention of cardiovascular disease: A report of the American College of Cardiology/American Heart Association Task Force on Clinical Practice Guidelines. *Circulation, 140*(11), e596–e646. https://doi.org/10.1161/CIR.0000000000000678

Asarnow, J. R., Rozenman, M., Wiblin, J., & Zeltzer, L. (2015). Integrated medical-behavioral care compared with usual primary care for child and adolescent behavioral health: A meta-analysis. *JAMA Pediatrics, 169*(10), 929–937. https://doi.org/10.1001/jamapediatrics.2015.1141

Ásgeirsdóttir, H. G., Valdimarsdóttir, U. A., Þorsteinsdóttir, Þ. K., Lund, S. H., Tomasson, G., Nyberg, U., Ásgeirsdóttir, T. L., & Hauksdóttir, A. (2018). The association between different traumatic life events and suicidality. *European Journal of Psychotraumatology, 9*(1), Article 1510279. https://doi.org/10.1080/20008198.2018.1510279

Atasoy, H., Greenwood, B. N., & McCullough, J. S. (2019). The digitization of patient care: A review of the effects of electronic health records on health care quality and utilization. *Annual Review of Public Health, 40*(1), 487–500. https://doi.org/10.1146/annurev-publhealth-040218-044206

A-Tjak, J. G., Davis, M. L., Morina, N., Powers, M. B., Smits, J. A., & Emmelkamp, P. M. (2015). A meta-analysis of the efficacy of acceptance and commitment therapy for clinically relevant mental and physical health problems. *Psychotherapy and Psychosomatics, 84*(1), 30–36. https://doi.org/10.1159/000365764

Avery-Clark, C., Weiner, L., & Adams-Clark, A. A. (2019). Sensate focus for sexual concerns: An updated, critical literature review. *Current Sexual Health Reports, 11*(2), 84–94. https://doi.org/10.1007/s11930-019-00197-9

Avezum, M. D. M. D. M., Altafim, E. R. P., & Linhares, M. B. M. (2022). Spanking and corporal punishment parenting practices and child development: A systematic review. *Trauma, Violence, & Abuse.* Advance online publication. https://doi.org/10.1177/15248380221124243

Avis, N. E., Brockwell, S., Randolph, J. F., Jr., Shen, S., Cain, V. S., Ory, M., & Greendale, G. A. (2009). Longitudinal changes in sexual functioning as women transition through menopause: Results from the Study of Women's Health Across the Nation. *Menopause, 16*(3), 442–452. https://doi.org/10.1097/gme.0b013e3181948dd0

Avis, N. E., Stellato, R., Crawford, S., Bromberger, J., Ganz, P., Cain, V., & Kagawa-Singer, M. (2001). Is there a menopausal syndrome? Menopausal status and symptoms across racial/ethnic groups. *Social Science & Medicine, 52*(3), 345–356. https://doi.org/10.1016/S0277-9536(00)00147-7

Babb, S., Malarcher, A., Schauer, G., Asman, K., & Jamal, A. (2017). Quitting smoking among adults—United States, 2000–2015. *Morbidity and Mortality Weekly Report, 65*(52), 1457–1464. https://doi.org/10.15585/mmwr.mm6552a1

Bahk, Y. C., Jang, S. K., Choi, K. H., & Lee, S. H. (2017). The relationship between childhood trauma and suicidal ideation: Role of maltreatment and potential mediators. *Psychiatry Investigation, 14*(1), 37–43. https://doi.org/10.4306/pi.2017.14.1.37

Bai, Z., Luo, S., Zhang, L., Wu, S., & Chi, I. (2020). Acceptance and commitment therapy (ACT) to reduce depression: A systematic review and meta-analysis. *Journal of Affective Disorders, 260*, 728–737. https://doi.org/10.1016/j.jad.2019.09.040

Bailey, J., Kerley, S., & Kibelstis, T. (2012). A brief marital satisfaction screening tool for use in primary care medicine. *Family Medicine, 44*(2), 105–109. https://www.stfm.org/familymedicine/vol44issue2/Bailey105

Bair, M. J., Richardson, K. M., Dobscha, S. K., Yi, E., Gerrity, M., & Kroenke, K. (2005). Chronic pain management guidelines: A systematic review of content and strength of evidence. *Journal of General Internal Medicine, 20*(Suppl. 1), 62.

Baird, M., Blount, A., Brungardt, S., Dickinson, P., Dietrich, A., Epperly, T., Green, L., Henley, D., Kessler, R., Korsen, N., McDaniel, S., Miller, B., Pugno, P., Roberts, R., Schirmer, J., Seymour, D., & deGruy, F. (2014). Joint principles: Integrating behavioral health care into the patient-centered medical home. *Annals of Family Medicine, 12*(2), 183–185. https://doi.org/10.1370/afm.1634

Ball, J., Kearney, B., Wilhelm, K., Dewhurst-Savellis, J., & Barton, B. (2000). Cognitive behaviour therapy and assertion training groups for patients with depression and comorbid personality disorders. *Behavioural and Cognitive Psychotherapy, 28*(1), 71–85. https://doi.org/10.1017/S1352465800000072

Balsamo, M., Cataldi, F., Carlucci, L., & Fairfield, B. (2018). Assessment of anxiety in older adults: A review of self-report measures. *Clinical Interventions in Aging, 13*, 573–593. https://doi.org/10.2147/CIA.S114100

Banks, J. B. (2002). Childhood discipline: Challenges for clinicians and parents. *American Family Physician, 66*(8), 1447–1452. https://www.aafp.org/content/dam/brand/aafp/pubs/afp/issues/2002/1015/p1447.pdf

Baranowski, A. (2013). Chronic pelvic pain of uncertain origin. In M. Chin, R. Fillingim, & T. Ness (Eds.), *Pain in women* (pp. 273–283). Oxford University Press.

Barkley, R. A. (2020). *Taking charge of ADHD: The complete, authoritative guide for parents* (4th ed.). Guilford Press.

Barnes, P. J. (2016). Sex differences in chronic obstructive pulmonary disease mechanisms. *American Journal of Respiratory and Critical Care Medicine, 193*(8), 813–814. https://doi.org/10.1164/rccm.201512-2379ED

Barnes, R. D., & Ivezaj, V. (2015). A systematic review of motivational interviewing for weight loss among adults in primary care. *Obesity Reviews, 16*(4), 304–318. https://doi.org/10.1111/obr.12264

Barstow, C., Shahan, B., & Roberts, M. (2018). Evaluating medical decision-making capacity in practice. *American Family Physician, 98*(1), 40–46. https://www.aafp.org/content/dam/brand/aafp/pubs/afp/issues/2018/0701/p40.pdf

Bartels, S. J., Coakley, E. H., Zubritsky, C., Ware, J. H., Miles, K. M., Areán, P. A., Chen, H., Oslin, D. W., Llorente, M. D., Costantino, G., Quijano, L., McIntyre, J. S., Linkins, K. W., Oxman, T. E., Maxwell, J., Levkoff, S. E., & the PRISM-E Investigators. (2004). Improving access to geriatric mental health services: A randomized trial comparing treatment engagement with integrated versus enhanced referral care for depression, anxiety, and at-risk alcohol use. *The American Journal of Psychiatry, 161*(8), 1455–1462. https://doi.org/10.1176/appi.ajp.161.8.1455

Bastien, C. H., Vallières, A., & Morin, C. M. (2001). Validation of the Insomnia Severity Index as an outcome measure for insomnia research. *Sleep Medicine, 2*(4), 297–307. https://doi.org/10.1016/S1389-9457(00)00065-4

Batelaan, N. M., Seldenrijk, A., Bot, M., van Balkom, A. J., & Penninx, B. W. (2016). Anxiety and new onset of cardiovascular disease: Critical review and meta-analysis.

The British Journal of Psychiatry, 208(3), 223–231. https://doi.org/10.1192/bjp.bp.114.
156554

Baucom, D. H., Fisher, M. S., Corrie, S., Worrell, M., & Boeding, S. E. (2020). *Treating relationship distress and psychopathology in couples: A cognitive-behavioural approach.* Routledge.

Bauman, B. L., Ko, J. Y., Cox, S., D'Angelo, D. V., Warner, L., Folger, S., Tevendale, H. D., Coy, K. C., Harrison, L., & Barfield, W. D. (2020). Vital signs: Postpartum depressive symptoms and provider discussions about perinatal depression—United States, 2018. *Morbidity and Mortality Weekly Report, 69*(19), 575–581. https://doi.org/10.15585/mmwr.mm6919a2

Bayne, A. P., & Skoog, S. J. (2014). Nocturnal enuresis: An approach to assessment and treatment. *Pediatrics in Review, 35*(8), 327–335. https://doi.org/10.1542/pir.35.8.327

Bazzano, L. A., Green, T., Harrison, T. N., & Reynolds, K. (2013). Dietary approaches to prevent hypertension. *Current Hypertension Reports, 15*(6), 694–702. https://doi.org/10.1007/s11906-013-0390-z

Beck, A. T., & Steer, R. A. (1993). *Beck Anxiety Inventory manual.* Psychological Corporation.

Beck, A. T., Steer, R. A., & Brown, G. K. (1996). *Manual for Beck Depression Inventory II (BDI-II).* APA PsycTests. https://doi.org/10.1037/t00742-000

Becker-Haimes, E. M., Tabachnick, A. R., Last, B. S., Stewart, R. E., Hasan-Granier, A., & Beidas, R. S. (2020). Evidence base update for brief, free, and accessible youth mental health measures. *Journal of Clinical Child and Adolescent Psychology, 49*(1), 1–17. https://doi.org/10.1080/15374416.2019.1689824

Beehler, G. P., Dobmeyer, A. C., Hunter, C. L., & Funderburk, J. S. (2018). *Brief cognitive behavioral therapy for chronic pain: IBHC manual.* Defense Health Agency.

Beehler, G. P., Funderburk, J. S., King, P. R., Possemato, K., Maddoux, J. A., Goldstein, W. R., & Wade, M. (2020). Validation of an expanded measure of integrated care provider fidelity: PPAQ-2. *Journal of Clinical Psychology in Medical Settings, 27*(1), 158–172. https://doi.org/10.1007/s10880-019-09628-0

Beehler, G. P., Murphy, J. L., King, P. R., & Dollar, K. M. (2021). *Brief cognitive behavioral therapy for chronic pain: Therapist manual, version 2.0.* U.S. Department of Veterans Affairs.

Beehler, G. P., Murphy, J. L., King, P. R., Dollar, K. M., Kearney, L. K., Haslam, A., Wade, M., & Goldstein, W. R. (2019). Brief cognitive behavioral therapy for chronic pain: Results from a clinical demonstration project in primary care behavioral health. *The Clinical Journal of Pain, 35*(10), 809–817. https://doi.org/10.1097/AJP.0000000000000747

Bell, A. C., & D'Zurilla, T. J. (2009). Problem-solving therapy for depression: A meta-analysis. *Clinical Psychology Review, 29*(4), 348–353. https://doi.org/10.1016/j.cpr.2009.02.003

Benjet, C., & Kazdin, A. E. (2003). Spanking children: The controversies, findings, and new directions. *Clinical Psychology Review, 23*(2), 197–224. https://doi.org/10.1016/S0272-7358(02)00206-4

Bennett, H. J. (2015). *Waking up dry: A guide to help children overcome bedwetting* (2nd ed.). American Academy of Pediatrics.

Bennett, S., & Thomas, A. J. (2014). Depression and dementia: Cause, consequence or coincidence? *Maturitas, 79*(2), 184–190. https://doi.org/10.1016/j.maturitas.2014.05.009

Benson, L. A., McGinn, M. M., & Christensen, A. (2012). Common principles of couple therapy. *Behavior Therapy, 43*(1), 25–35. https://doi.org/10.1016/j.beth.2010.12.009

Bentley, K. H., Franklin, J. C., Ribeiro, J. D., Kleiman, E. M., Fox, K. R., & Nock, M. K. (2016). Anxiety and its disorders as risk factors for suicidal thoughts and behaviors: A meta-analytic review. *Clinical Psychology Review, 43*, 30–46. https://doi.org/10.1016/j.cpr.2015.11.008

Benuto, L. T., Gonzalez, F. R., & Singer, J. (Eds.). (2020). *Handbook of cultural factors in behavioral health: Guide for the helping professional.* Springer. https://doi.org/10.1007/978-3-030-32229-8

Berger, W. E. (2010). *Asthma for dummies, pocket edition.* Wiley.

Berkovits, M. D., O'Brien, K. A., Carter, C. G., & Eyberg, S. M. (2010). Early identification and intervention for behavior problems in primary care: A comparison of two abbreviated versions of parent-child interaction therapy. *Behavior Therapy, 41*(3), 375–387. https://doi.org/10.1016/j.beth.2009.11.002

Bernal, G., & Domenech Rodríguez, M. M. (Eds.). (2012). *Cultural adaptations: Tools for evidence-based practice with diverse populations.* American Psychological Association. https://doi.org/10.1037/13752-000

Bernal, G., Jiménez-Chafey, M. I., & Domenech Rodríguez, M. M. (2009). Cultural adaptation of treatments: A resource for considering culture in evidence-based practice. *Professional Psychology: Research and Practice, 40*(4), 361–368. https://doi.org/10.1037/a0016401

Bernardy, K., Klose, P., Welsch, P., & Häuser, W. (2018). Efficacy, acceptability and safety of cognitive behavioural therapies in fibromyalgia syndrome—A systematic review and meta-analysis of randomized controlled trials. *European Journal of Pain, 22*(2), 242–260. https://doi.org/10.1002/ejp.1121

Berner, M., & Günzler, C. (2012). Efficacy of psychosocial interventions in men and women with sexual dysfunctions—A systematic review of controlled clinical trials. *Journal of Sexual Medicine, 9*(12), 3089–3107. https://doi.org/10.1111/j.1743-6109.2012.02970.x

Berwick, D. M., Nolan, T. W., & Whittington, J. (2008). The triple aim: Care, health, and cost. *Health Affairs, 27*(3), 759–769. https://doi.org/10.1377/hlthaff.27.3.759

Bholat, M. A., Ray, L., Brensilver, M., Ling, K., & Shoptaw, S. (2012). Integration of behavioral medicine in primary care. *Primary Care, 39*(4), 605–614. https://doi.org/10.1016/j.pop.2012.08.003

Biener, A. I., Decker, S. L., & Rohde, F. (2019). Prevalence and treatment of chronic obstructive pulmonary disease (COPD) in the United States. *JAMA, 322*(7), 602. https://doi.org/10.1001/jama.2019.10241

Bitsko, R. H., Claussen, A. H., Lichstein, J., Black, L. I., Jones, S. E., Danielson, M. L., Hoenig, J. M., Davis Jack, S. P., Brody, D. J., Gyawali, S., Maenner, M. J., Warner, M., Holland, K. M., Perou, R., Crosby, A. E., Blumberg, S. J., Avenevoli, S., Kaminski, J. W., & Ghandour, R. M. (2022). Mental health surveillance among children—United States, 2013–2019. *MMWR Supplements, 71*(2), 1–42. https://doi.org/10.15585/mmwr.su7102a1

Bjureberg, J., Dahlin, M., Carlborg, A., Edberg, H., Haglund, A., & Runeson, B. (2021). Columbia–Suicide Severity Rating Scale Screen Version: Initial screening for suicide risk in a psychiatric emergency department. *Psychological Medicine, 52*(16), 1–9. https://doi.org/10.1017/S0033291721000751

Bledsoe, S. E., & Grote, N. K. (2006). Treating depression during pregnancy and the postpartum: A preliminary meta-analysis. *Research on Social Work Practice, 16*(2), 109–120. https://doi.org/10.1177/1049731505282202

Bleich, S. N., Pickett-Blakely, O., & Cooper, L. A. (2011). Physician practice patterns of obesity diagnosis and weight-related counseling. *Patient Education and Counseling, 82*(1), 123–129. https://doi.org/10.1016/j.pec.2010.02.018

Blumenthal, J. A., Hinderliter, A. L., Smith, P. J., Mabe, S., Watkins, L. L., Craighead, L., Ingle, K., Tyson, C., Lin, P. H., Kraus, W. E., Liao, L., & Sherwood, A. (2021). Effects of lifestyle modification on patients with resistant hypertension: Results of the TRIUMPH randomized clinical trial. *Circulation, 144*(15), 1212–1226. https://doi.org/10.1161/CIRCULATIONAHA.121.055329

Bodenheimer, T., & Sinsky, C. (2014). From triple to quadruple aim: Care of the patient requires care of the provider. *Annals of Family Medicine, 12*(6), 573–576. https://doi.org/10.1370/afm.1713

Bodenmann, G., & Randall, A. K. (2013). Close relationships in psychiatric disorders. *Current Opinion in Psychiatry*, *26*(5), 464–467. https://doi.org/10.1097/YCO.0b013e3283642de7

Boersma, P., Black, L. I., & Ward, B. W. (2020). Prevalence of multiple chronic conditions among U.S. adults: Preventing chronic disease. *Preventing Chronic Disease*, *17*, Article E106. https://doi.org/10.5888/pcd17.200130

Bogner, H. R., Morales, K. H., de Vries, H. F., & Cappola, A. R. (2012). Integrated management of Type 2 diabetes mellitus and depression treatment to improve medication adherence: A randomized controlled trial. *Annals of Family Medicine*, *10*(1), 15–22. https://doi.org/10.1370/afm.1344

Bogner, H. R., Morales, K. H., Post, E. P., & Bruce, M. L. (2007). Diabetes, depression, and death: A randomized controlled trial of a depression treatment program for older adults based in primary care (PROSPECT). *Diabetes Care*, *30*(12), 3005–3010. https://doi.org/10.2337/dc07-0974

Bogucki, O. E., Craner, J. R., Berg, S. L., Wolsey, M. K., Miller, S. J., Smyth, K. T., Johnson, M. W., Mack, J. D., Sedivy, S. J., Burke, L. M., Glader, M. A., Williams, M. W., Katzelnick, D. J., & Sawchuk, C. N. (2021). Cognitive behavioral therapy for anxiety disorders: Outcomes from a multi-state, multi-site primary care practice. *Journal of Anxiety Disorders*, *78*, Article 102345. https://doi.org/10.1016/j.janxdis.2020.102345

Bohlmeijer, E., ten Klooster, P. M., Fledderus, M., Veehof, M., & Baer, R. (2011). Psychometric properties of the Five Facet Mindfulness Questionnaire in depressed adults and development of a short form. *Assessment*, *18*(3), 308–320. https://doi.org/10.1177/1073191111408231

Bond, F. W., Hayes, S. C., Baer, R. A., Carpenter, K. M., Guenole, N., Orcutt, H. K., Waltz, T., & Zettle, R. D. (2011). Preliminary psychometric properties of the Acceptance and Action Questionnaire–II: A revised measure of psychological inflexibility and experiential avoidance. *Behavior Therapy*, *42*(4), 676–688. https://doi.org/10.1016/j.beth.2011.03.007

Bootzin, R. R., & Epstein, D. R. (2000). Stimulus control. In K. L. Lichstein & C. M. Morin (Eds.), *Treatment of late-life insomnia* (pp. 167–184). Sage Publications. https://doi.org/10.4135/9781452225555.n7

Bornstein, M. H. (2012). Cultural approaches to parenting. *Parenting: Science and Practice*, *12*(2–3), 212–221. https://doi.org/10.1080/15295192.2012.683359

Boulet, L. P., Vervloet, D., Magar, Y., & Foster, J. M. (2012). Adherence: The goal to control asthma. *Clinics in Chest Medicine*, *33*(3), 405–417. https://doi.org/10.1016/j.ccm.2012.06.002

Bourne, E. J. (2020). *The anxiety and phobia workbook* (7th ed.). New Harbinger Publications.

Bovin, M. J., Kimerling, R., Weathers, F. W., Prins, A., Marx, B. P., Post, E. P., & Schnurr, P. P. (2021). Diagnostic accuracy and acceptability of the Primary Care Posttraumatic Stress Disorder Screen for the *Diagnostic and Statistical Manual of Mental Disorders* (fifth edition) among US veterans. *Journal of the American Medical Association Network Open*, *4*(2), Article e2036733. https://doi.org/10.1001/jamanetworkopen.2020.36733

Boyd, R., & Stevens, J. A. (2009). Falls and fear of falling: Burden, beliefs and behaviours. *Age and Ageing*, *38*(4), 423–428. https://doi.org/10.1093/ageing/afp053

Boyd, R. C., Le, H. N., & Somberg, R. (2005). Review of screening instruments for postpartum depression. *Archives of Women's Mental Health*, *8*(3), 141–153. https://doi.org/10.1007/s00737-005-0096-6

Braithwaite, S., & Holt-Lunstad, J. (2017). Romantic relationships and mental health. *Current Opinion in Psychology*, *13*, 120–125. https://doi.org/10.1016/j.copsyc.2016.04.001

Brensilver, M., Tariq, S., & Shoptaw, S. (2012). Optimizing pain management through collaborations with behavioral and addiction medicine in primary care. *Primary Care*, *39*(4), 661–669. https://doi.org/10.1016/j.pop.2012.08.007

Breslau, J., Aguilar-Gaxiola, S., Kendler, K. S., Su, M., Williams, D., & Kessler, R. C. (2006). Specifying race-ethnic differences in risk for psychiatric disorder in a USA national sample. *Psychological Medicine, 36*(1), 57–68. https://doi.org/10.1017/S0033291705006161

Broderick, J. E., Keefe, F. J., Schneider, S., Junghaenel, D. U., Bruckenthal, P., Schwartz, J. E., Kaell, A. T., Caldwell, D. S., McKee, D., & Gould, E. (2016). Cognitive behavioral therapy for chronic pain is effective, but for whom? *Pain, 157*(9), 2115–2123. https://doi.org/10.1097/j.pain.0000000000000626

Bromberger, J. T., & Kravitz, H. M. (2011). Mood and menopause: Findings from the Study of Women's Health Across the Nation (SWAN) over 10 years. *Obstetrics and Gynecology Clinics of North America, 38*(3), 609–625. https://doi.org/10.1016/j.ogc.2011.05.011

Brookoff, D. (2009). Genitourinary pain syndromes: Interstitial cystitis, chronic prostatitis, pelvic floor dysfunction, and related disorders. In H. S. Smith (Ed.), *Current therapy in pain* (pp. 205–215). Saunders-Elsevier. https://doi.org/10.1016/B978-1-4160-4836-7.00028-6

Brooks, T., Sharp, R., Evans, S., Baranoff, J., & Esterman, A. (2021). Psychological interventions for women with persistent pelvic pain: A survey of mental health clinicians. *Journal of Multidisciplinary Healthcare, 14*, 1725–1740. https://doi.org/10.2147/JMDH.S313109

Brown, G. K., Beck, A. T., Steer, R. A., & Grisham, J. R. (2000). Risk factors for suicide in psychiatric outpatients: A 20-year prospective study. *Journal of Consulting and Clinical Psychology, 68*(3), 371–377. https://doi.org/10.1037/0022-006X.68.3.371

Brown, J. B., Lent, B., Schmidt, G., & Sas, G. (2000). Application of the Woman Abuse Screening Tool (WAST) and WAST-Short in the family practice setting. *The Journal of Family Practice, 49*(10), 896–903. https://www.researchgate.net/publication/12274837

Bruckenthal, P. (2011). Chronic pelvic pain: Approaches to diagnosis and treatment. *Pain Management Nursing, 12*(1), S4–S10. https://doi.org/10.1016/j.pmn.2010.11.004

Bryan, C. J., & Rudd, M. D. (2010). *Managing suicide risk in primary care.* Springer.

Bu, F., Zaninotto, P., & Fancourt, D. (2020). Longitudinal associations between loneliness, social isolation and cardiovascular events. *Heart, 106*(18), 1394–1399. https://doi.org/10.1136/heartjnl-2020-316614

Buist, A. E., Barnett, B. E., Milgrom, J., Pope, S., Condon, J. T., Ellwood, D. A., Boyce, P. M., Austin, M. P., & Hayes, B. A. (2002). To screen or not to screen—That is the question in perinatal depression. *The Medical Journal of Australia, 177*(S7), S101–S105. https://doi.org/10.5694/j.1326-5377.2002.tb04866.x

Buist, A. E., Condon, J., Brooks, J., Speelman, C., Milgrom, J., Hayes, B., Ellwood, D., Barnett, B., Kowalenko, N., Matthey, S., Austin, M. P., & Bilszta, J. (2006). Acceptability of routine screening for perinatal depression. *Journal of Affective Disorders, 93*(1–3), 233–237. https://doi.org/10.1016/j.jad.2006.02.019

Burch, R., Rizzoli, P., & Loder, E. (2018). The prevalence and impact of migraine and severe headache in the United States: Figures and trends from government health studies. *Headache: The Journal of Head and Face Pain, 58*(4), 496–505. https://doi.org/10.1111/head.13281

Burd, A. (2020). *The postpartum depression workbook: Strategies to overcome negative thoughts, calm stress, and improve your mood.* Simon & Schuster.

Burkhart, K., Knox, M., Hunter, K., Pennewitt, D., & Schrouder, K. (2018). Decreasing caregivers' positive attitudes toward spanking. *Journal of Pediatric Health Care, 32*(4), 333–339. https://doi.org/10.1016/j.pedhc.2017.11.007

Burnes, D., Hancock, D. W., Eckenrode, J., Lachs, M. S., & Pillemer, K. (2021). Estimated incidence and factors associated with risk of elder mistreatment in New York State. *JAMA Network Open, 4*(8), Article e2117758. https://doi.org/10.1001/jamanetworkopen.2021.17758

Busby, D. M., Christensen, C., Crane, D. R., & Larson, J. H. (1995). A revision of the Dyadic Adjustment Scale for use with distressed and nondistressed couples: Construct hierarchy and multidimensional scales. *Journal of Marital and Family Therapy, 21*(3), 289–308. https://doi.org/10.1111/j.1752-0606.1995.tb00163.x

Butler, R. J. (2004). Childhood nocturnal enuresis: Developing a conceptual framework. *Clinical Psychology Review, 24*(8), 909–931. https://doi.org/10.1016/j.cpr.2004.07.001

Butryn, M. L., Crane, N. T., Lufburrow, E., Hagerman, C. J., Forman, E. M., & Zhang, F. (2022). The role of physical activity in long-term weight loss: 36-month results from a randomized controlled trial. *Annals of Behavioral Medicine, 57*(2), 146–154. https://doi.org/10.1093/abm/kaac028

Buysse, D. J., Germain, A., Moul, D. E., Franzen, P. L., Brar, L. K., Fletcher, M. E., Begley, A., Houck, P. R., Mazumdar, S., Reynolds, C. F., III, & Monk, T. H. (2011). Efficacy of brief behavioral treatment for chronic insomnia in older adults. *Archives of Internal Medicine, 171*(10), 887–895. https://doi.org/10.1001/archinternmed.2010.535

Caldwell, P. H. Y., Codarini, M., Stewart, F., Hahn, D., & Sureshkumar, P. (2020). Alarm interventions for nocturnal enuresis in children. *Cochrane Database of Systematic Reviews, 5*, Article CD002911. https://doi.org/10.1002/14651858.CD002911.pub3

Caldwell, P. H. Y., Nankivell, G., & Sureshkumar, P. (2013). Simple behavioural interventions for nocturnal enuresis in children. *Cochrane Database of Systematic Reviews, 7*, Article CD003637. https://doi.org/10.1002/14651858.CD003637.pub3

Caleyachetty, R., Barber, T. M., Mohammed, N. I., Cappuccio, F. P., Hardy, R., Mathur, R., Banerjee, A., & Gill, P. (2021). Ethnicity-specific BMI cutoffs for obesity based on Type 2 diabetes risk in England: A population-based cohort study. *The Lancet Diabetes & Endocrinology, 9*(7), 419–426. https://doi.org/10.1016/S2213-8587(21)00088-7

Candib, L. M. (2007). Obesity and diabetes in vulnerable populations: Reflection on proximal and distal causes. *Annals of Family Medicine, 5*(6), 547–556. https://doi.org/10.1370/afm.754

Cape, J., Whittington, C., Buszewicz, M., Wallace, P., & Underwood, L. (2010). Brief psychological therapies for anxiety and depression in primary care: Meta-analysis and meta-regression. *BMC Medicine, 8*(1), Article 38. https://doi.org/10.1186/1741-7015-8-38

Caramenico, A. (2014) *Medical home must-dos for population health management.* Fierce Healthcare. https://www.fiercehealthcare.com/payer/medical-home-must-dos-for-population-health-management?page=full

Carbone, S., Del Buono, M. G., Ozemek, C., & Lavie, C. J. (2019). Obesity, risk of diabetes and role of physical activity, exercise training and cardiorespiratory fitness. *Progress in Cardiovascular Diseases, 62*(4), 327–333. https://doi.org/10.1016/j.pcad.2019.08.004

Carpenter, B. D., Gatz, M., & Smyer, M. A. (2022). Mental health and aging in the 2020s. *American Psychologist, 77*(4), 538–550. https://doi.org/10.1037/amp0000873

Carpenter, J. K., Andrews, L. A., Witcraft, S. M., Powers, M. B., Smits, J. A. J., & Hofmann, S. G. (2018). Cognitive behavioral therapy for anxiety and related disorders: A meta-analysis of randomized placebo-controlled trials. *Depression and Anxiety, 35*(6), 502–514. https://doi.org/10.1002/da.22728

Carr, D. B., Gray, S., Baty, J., & Morris, J. C. (2000). The value of informant versus individual's complaints of memory impairment in early dementia. *Neurology, 55*(11), 1724–1727. https://doi.org/10.1212/WNL.55.11.1724

Carr, L. T. B., Bell, C., Alick, C., & Bentley-Edwards, K. L. (2022). Responding to health disparities in behavioral weight loss interventions and COVID-19 in Black adults: Recommendations for health equity. *Journal of Racial and Ethnic Health Disparities, 9*(3), 739–747. https://doi.org/10.1007/s40615-022-01269-8

Cass, V. (2007). *The elusive orgasm: A woman's guide to why she can't and how she can orgasm.* Marlowe & Co.

Castro, M. R. (2022). *Mayo Clinic: The essential diabetes book: How to prevent, manage and live with diabetes* (3rd ed.). Mayo Clinic Press.

Caudill, M. A. (2016). *Managing pain before it manages you* (4th ed.). Guilford Press.

Cavalieri, S., Frankowski, A., Galles, J., Milford, C., & Rios, A. (2016). *A roadmap for population health management.* Institute for Health Technology Transformation. https://www.pcpcc.org/sites/default/files/resources/PHM-IBM_Watson-RR.pdf

Cazzola, M., Calzetta, L., Matera, M. G., Hanania, N. A., & Rogliani, P. (2018). How does race/ethnicity influence pharmacological response to asthma therapies? *Expert Opinion on Drug Metabolism & Toxicology, 14*(4), 435–446. https://doi.org/10.1080/17425255.2018.1449833

Ceballos, M., Wallace, G., & Goodwin, G. (2017). Postpartum depression among African-American and Latina mothers living in small cities, towns, and rural communities. *Journal of Racial and Ethnic Health Disparities, 4*(5), 916–927. https://doi.org/10.1007/s40615-016-0295-z

Center for Integrated Healthcare. (2022, May 13). *The Primary Care Behavioral Health Provider Adherence Questionnaire (PPAQ).* U.S. Department of Veterans Affairs. https://www.mirecc.va.gov/cih-visn2/PPAQ.asp

Centers for Disease Control and Prevention. (2013a). Adult participation in aerobic and muscle-strengthening physical activities—United States, 2011. *Morbidity and Mortality Weekly Report, 62*(17), 326–330. https://www.ncbi.nlm.nih.gov/pmc/articles/PMC4604926/pdf/326-330.pdf

Centers for Disease Control and Prevention. (2013b). *The state of aging and health in America 2013.* https://www.cdc.gov/aging/pdf/state-aging-health-in-america-2013.pdf

Centers for Disease Control and Prevention. (2014). *Planning and implementing screening and brief intervention for risky alcohol use: A step-by-step guide for primary care practices.* National Center on Birth Defects and Developmental Disabilities. https://www.cdc.gov/ncbddd/fasd/documents/alcoholsbiimplementationguide.pdf

Centers for Disease Control and Prevention. (2018). *Asthma surveillance data.* National Center for Environmental Health. https://www.cdc.gov/asthma/national-surveillance-data/default.htm

Centers for Disease Control and Prevention. (2019). *About dementia.* Division of Population Health, National Center for Chronic Disease Prevention and Health Promotion. https://www.cdc.gov/aging/dementia/index.html

Centers for Disease Control and Prevention. (2021a). *Gestational diabetes.* https://www.cdc.gov/diabetes/basics/gestational.html

Centers for Disease Control and Prevention. (2021b). *Mortality in the United States, 2020.* National Center for Health Statistics. https://www.cdc.gov/nchs/products/databriefs/db427.htm

Centers for Disease Control and Prevention. (2021c). *Violence prevention: Elder abuse.* National Center for Injury Prevention and Control, Division of Violence Prevention. https://www.cdc.gov/violenceprevention/elderabuse/index.html

Centers for Disease Control and Prevention. (2022a). *National diabetes statistics report website.* https://www.cdc.gov/diabetes/data/statistics-report/index.html

Centers for Disease Control and Prevention. (2022b). *Risk and protective factors.* https://www.cdc.gov/suicide/factors/index.html

Centers for Disease Control and Prevention. (2022c). *10 leading causes of death, United States.* National Center for Injury Prevention and Control. https://www.cdc.gov/injury/wisqars/index.html

Centers for Disease Control and Prevention, National Center for Chronic Disease Prevention and Health Promotion, & Division of Nutrition and Physical Activity. (1999). *Promoting physical activity: A guide for community action.* Human Kinetics.

Centers for Medicare and Medicaid Innovation. (2019). *The Accountable Health Communities Health-Related Social Needs screening tool.* Centers for Medicare and Medicaid Services. https://innovation.cms.gov/files/worksheets/ahcm-screeningtool.pdf

Chan, P. S., Fang, Y., Wong, M. C., Huang, J., Wang, Z., & Yeoh, E. K. (2021). Using Consolidated Framework for Implementation Research to investigate facilitators and barriers of implementing alcohol screening and brief intervention among primary care health professionals: A systematic review. *Implementation Science, 16*(1), Article 99. https://doi.org/10.1186/s13012-021-01170-8

Chapman, G. D. (2015). *The 5 love languages: The secret to love that lasts.* Northfield Publishing.

Chawla, A., Westrich, K., Matter, S., Kaltenboeck, A., & Dubois, R. (2016). Care pathways in U.S. healthcare settings: Current successes and limitations, and future challenges. *The American Journal of Managed Care, 22*(1), 53–62. https://www.ajmc.com/view/care-pathways-in-us-healthcare-settings-current-successes-and-limitations-and-future-challenges

Cheng, S.-T., Au, A., Losada, A., Thompson, L. W., & Gallagher-Thompson, D. (2019). Psychological interventions for dementia caregivers: What we have achieved, what we have learned. *Current Psychiatry Reports, 21*(7), Article 59. https://doi.org/10.1007/s11920-019-1045-9

Cherkin, D. C., Sherman, K. J., Balderson, B. H., Cook, A. J., Anderson, M. L., Hawkes, R. J., Hansen, K. E., & Turner, J. A. (2016). Effect of mindfulness-based stress reduction vs cognitive behavioral therapy or usual care on back pain and functional limitations in adults with chronic low back pain: A randomized clinical trial. *JAMA, 315*(12), 1240–1249. https://doi.org/10.1001/jama.2016.2323

Chernin, J. N. (2006). *Get closer: A gay men's guide to intimacy and relationships.* Alyson Books.

Choi, K. H., Wang, S. M., Yeon, B., Suh, S. Y., Oh, Y., Lee, H. K., Kweon, Y. S., Lee, C. T., & Lee, K. U. (2013). Risk and protective factors predicting multiple suicide attempts. *Psychiatry Research, 210*(3), 957–961. https://doi.org/10.1016/j.psychres.2013.09.026

Chou, R., Loeser, J. D., Owens, D. K., Rosenquist, R. W., Atlas, S. J., Baisden, J., Carragee, E. J., Grabois, M., Murphy, D. R., Resnick, D. K., Stanos, S. P., Shaffer, W. O., Wall, E. M., & American Pain Society Low Back Pain Guideline Panel. (2009). Interventional therapies, surgery, and interdisciplinary rehabilitation for low back pain: An evidence-based clinical practice guideline from the American Pain Society. *Spine, 34*(10), 1066–1077. https://doi.org/10.1097/BRS.0b013e3181a1390d

Christianson, J. B., & Warrick, L. H. (2003). *The business case for drop-in group medical appointments: A case study of Luther Midelfort Mayo System* (Report No. 611). The Commonwealth Fund. https://www.commonwealthfund.org/sites/default/files/documents/___media_files_publications_fund_report_2003_apr_the_business_case_for_drop_in_group_medical_appointments__a_case_study_of_luther_midelfort_mayo_syst_christianson_bcs_drop_ingroup_611_pdf.pdf

Chu, C., Buchman-Schmitt, J. M., Stanley, I. H., Hom, M. A., Tucker, R. P., Hagan, C. R., Rogers, M. L., Podlogar, M. C., Chiurliza, B., Ringer, F. B., Michaels, M. S., Patros, C. H. G., & Joiner, T. E. (2017). The interpersonal theory of suicide: A systematic review and meta-analysis of a decade of cross-national research. *Psychological Bulletin, 143*(12), 1313–1345. https://doi.org/10.1037/bul0000123

Chu, P., Pandya, A., Salomon, J. A., Goldie, S. J., & Hunink, M. G. (2016). Comparative effectiveness of personalized lifestyle management strategies for cardiovascular disease risk reduction. *Journal of the American Heart Association, 5*(3), Article e002737. https://doi.org/10.1161/JAHA.115.002737

Cigrang, J. A., Cordova, J. V., Gray, T. D., Fedynich, A. L., Maher, E., Diehl, A. N., & Hawrilenko, M. (2022). Marriage checkup in integrated primary care: A randomized controlled trial with active-duty military couples. *Journal of Consulting and Clinical Psychology, 90*(5), 381–391. https://doi.org/10.1037/ccp0000734

Cigrang, J. A., Rauch, S. A. M., Avila, L. L., Bryan, C. J., Goode, J. L., Hryshko-Mullen, A., & Peterson, A. (2011). Treatment of active duty military with PTSD in primary care: Early findings. *Psychological Services, 8*(2), 104–113. https://doi.org/10.1037/a0022740

Cigrang, J. A., Rauch, S. A. M., Mintz, J., Brundige, A., Avila, L. L., Bryan, C. J., Goodie, J. L., Peterson, A. L., & the STRONG STAR Consortium. (2015). Treatment of active duty military with PTSD in primary care: A follow-up report. *Journal of Anxiety Disorders, 36,* 110–114. https://doi.org/10.1016/j.janxdis.2015.10.003

Cimini, M. D., & Martin, J. L. (Eds.). (2020). *Screening, brief intervention, and referral to treatment for substance use: A practitioner's guide.* American Psychological Association. https://doi.org/10.1037/0000199-000

Clayton, C., Motley, C., & Sakakibara, B. (2019). Enhancing social support among people with cardiovascular disease: A systematic scoping review. *Current Cardiology Reports, 21*(10), Article 123. https://doi.org/10.1007/s11886-019-1216-7

Cohen, B. E., Edmondson, D., & Kronish, I. M. (2015). State of the art review: Depression, stress, anxiety, and cardiovascular disease. *American Journal of Hypertension, 28*(11), 1295–1302. https://doi.org/10.1093/ajh/hpv047

Collins, C., Hewson, D. L., Munger, R., & Wade, T. (2010). *Evolving models of behavioral health integration in primary care.* The Milbank Memorial Fund. https://www.milbank. org/wp-content/files/documents/10430EvolvingCare/EvolvingCare.pdf

Collins, L. G., & Swartz, K. (2011). Caregiver care. *American Family Physician, 83*(11), 1309–1317. https://www.aafp.org/content/dam/brand/aafp/pubs/afp/issues/2011/ 0601/p1309.pdf

Combs, H., & Markman, J. (2014). Anxiety disorders in primary care. *The Medical Clinics of North America, 98*(5), 1007–1023. https://doi.org/10.1016/j.mcna.2014.06.003

Community Preventive Services Task Force. (2022). *Guide to community preventive services: CPSTF findings for physical activity.* U.S. Department of Health and Human Services. https://www.thecommunityguide.org/pages/task-force-findings-physical-activity.html

Compendium of Physical Activities. (n.d.). *Activity categories.* Lippincott Williams & Wilkins. https://sites.google.com/site/compendiumofphysicalactivities/

Connors, M. H., Teixeira-Pinto, A., Ames, D., Woodward, M., & Brodaty, H. (2022). Distinguishing apathy and depression in dementia: A longitudinal study. *Australian & New Zealand Journal of Psychiatry, 57*(6), 884–894. https://doi.org/10.1177/ 00048674221114597

Cooper, M., Park-Lee, E., Ren, C., Cornelius, M., Jamal, A., & Cullen, K. A. (2022). Notes from the field: E-cigarette use among middle and high school students—United States, 2022. *Morbidity and Mortality Weekly Report, 71*(40), 1283–1285. https://doi. org/10.15585/mmwr.mm7140a3

Cordova, J. V., Fleming, C. J. E., Morrill, M. I., Hawrilenko, M., Sollenberger, J. W., Harp, A. G., Gray, T. D., Darling, E. V., Blair, J. M., Meade, A. E., & Wachs, K. (2014). The Marriage Checkup: A randomized controlled trial of annual relationship health checkups. *Journal of Consulting and Clinical Psychology, 82*(4), 592–604. https://doi. org/10.1037/a0037097

Cornelius, M. E., Loretan, C. G., Wang, T. W., Jamal, A., & Homa, D. M. (2022). Tobacco product use among adults—United States, 2020. *Morbidity and Mortality Weekly Report, 71*(11), 397–405. https://doi.org/10.15585/mmwr.mm7111a1

Corso, K. A., Bryan, C. J., Morrow, C. E., Appolonio, K. K., Dodendorf, D. M., & Baker, M. T. (2009). Managing posttraumatic stress disorder symptoms in active duty military personnel in primary care settings. *Journal of Mental Health Counseling, 31*(2), 119–136. https://doi.org/10.17744/mehc.31.2.1m2238t85rv38041

Corso, K. A., Hunter, C. L., Dahl, O., Kallenberg, G. A., & Manson, L. (2016). *Integrating behavioral health into the medical home: A rapid implementation guide.* Greenbranch Publishing.

Coyne, J. C., Schwenk, T. L., & Fechner-Bates, S. (1995). Nondetection of depression by primary care physicians reconsidered. *General Hospital Psychiatry, 17*(1), 3–12. https:// doi.org/10.1016/0163-8343(94)00056-J

Crowdis, M., Leslie, S. W., & Nazir, S. (2019). Premature ejaculation. In *StatPearls.* StatPearls Publishing. https://www.ncbi.nlm.nih.gov/books/NBK546701/

Cully, J. A., Stanley, M. A., Deswal, A., Hanania, N. A., Phillips, L. L., & Kunik, M. E. (2010). Cognitive-behavioral therapy for chronic cardiopulmonary conditions:

Preliminary outcomes from an open trial. *Primary Care Companion to the Journal of Clinical Psychiatry, 12*(4), Article 26117. https://doi.org/10.4088/PCC.09m00896blu

Cully, J. A., Stanley, M. A., Petersen, N. J., Hundt, N. E., Kauth, M. R., Naik, A. D., Sorocco, K., Sansgiry, S., Zeno, D., & Kunik, M. E. (2017). Delivery of brief cognitive behavioral therapy for medically ill patients in primary care: A pragmatic randomized clinical trial. *Journal of General Internal Medicine, 32*(9), 1014–1024. https://doi.org/10.1007/s11606-017-4101-3

Cunningham, S. D., Sutherland, R. A., Yee, C. W., Thomas, J. L., Monin, J. K., Ickovics, J. R., & Lewis, J. B. (2021). Group medical care: A systematic review of health service performance. *International Journal of Environmental Research and Public Health, 18*(23), Article 12726. https://doi.org/10.3390/ijerph182312726

Cunningham, T. J., Ford, E. S., Chapman, D. P., Liu, Y., & Croft, J. B. (2015). Independent and joint associations of race/ethnicity and educational attainment with sleep-related symptoms in a population-based US sample. *Preventive Medicine, 77*, 99–105. https://doi.org/10.1016/j.ypmed.2015.05.008

Curry, S. J., Krist, A. H., Owens, D. K., Barry, M. J., Caughey, A. B., Davidson, K. W., Doubeni, C. A., Epling, J. W., Jr., Grossman, D. C., Kemper, A. R., Kubik, M., Kurth, A., Landefeld, C. S., Mangione, C. M., Silverstein, M., Simon, M. A., Tseng, C. W., & Wong, J. B. (2018). Screening for intimate partner violence, elder abuse, and abuse of vulnerable adults: U.S. Preventive Services Task Force final recommendation statement. *JAMA, 320*(16), 1678–1687. https://doi.org/10.1001/jama.2018.14741

Curry, S. J., Krist, A. H., Owens, D. K., Barry, M. J., Caughey, A. B., Davidson, K. W., Doubeni, C. A., Epling, J. W., Jr., Grossman, D. C., Kemper, A. R., Kubik, M., Landefeld, C. S., Mangione, C. M., Phipps, M. G., Silverstein, M., Simon, M. A., Tseng, C. W., & Wong, J. B. (2018). Behavioral weight loss interventions to prevent obesity-related morbidity and mortality in adults: U.S. Preventive Services Task Force recommendation statement. *JAMA, 320*(11), 1163–1171. https://doi.org/10.1001/jama.2018.13022

Dalal, H. M., Doherty, P., & Taylor, R. S. (2015). Cardiac rehabilitation. *BMJ, 351*, Article h5000. https://doi.org/10.1136/bmj.h5000

Daley, A. J., Macarthur, C., & Winter, H. (2007). The role of exercise in treating postpartum depression: A review of the literature. *Journal of Midwifery & Women's Health, 52*(1), 56–62. https://doi.org/10.1016/j.jmwh.2006.08.017

D'Amico, E. J., Parast, L., Shadel, W. G., Meredith, L. S., Seelam, R., & Stein, B. D. (2018). Brief motivational interviewing intervention to reduce alcohol and marijuana use for at-risk adolescents in primary care. *Journal of Consulting and Clinical Psychology, 86*(9), 775–786. https://doi.org/10.1037/ccp0000332

Darker, C. D., Sweeney, B. P., Barry, J. M., Farrell, M. F., & Donnelly-Swift, E. (2015). Psychosocial interventions for benzodiazepine harmful use, abuse or dependence. *Cochrane Database of Systematic Reviews, 5*, Article CD009652. https://doi.org/10.1002/14651858.CD009652.pub2

Dattilio, F. M. (2010). *Cognitive-behavioral therapy with couples and families*. Guilford Press.

Dattilio, F. M., & Epstein, N. B. (2021). Cognitive behavioral couple and family therapy. In A. Wenzel (Ed.), *Handbook of cognitive behavioral therapy: Applications* (pp. 513–548). American Psychological Association. https://doi.org/10.1037/0000219-016

David, L. (2017). *Alcohol and you: 21 ways to control and stop drinking: How to give up your addiction and quit alcohol*. Sober Living Books.

Davies, M. J., Gagliardino, J. J., Gray, L. J., Khunti, K., Mohan, V., & Hughes, R. (2013). Real-world factors affecting adherence to insulin therapy in patients with Type 1 or Type 2 diabetes mellitus: A systematic review. *Diabetic Medicine, 30*(5), 512–524. https://doi.org/10.1111/dme.12128

Davis, D. H., Creavin, S. T., Yip, J. L., Noel-Storr, A. H., Brayne, C., & Cullum, S. (2015). Montreal Cognitive Assessment for the diagnosis of Alzheimer's disease and other dementias. *Cochrane Database of Systematic Reviews, 10*, Article CD010775. https://doi.org/10.1002/14651858.CD010775.pub2

Davis, D. M., & Hayes, J. A. (2011). What are the benefits of mindfulness? A practice review of psychotherapy-related research. *Psychotherapy, 48*(2), 198–208. https://doi.org/10.1037/a0022062

Davis, J., Fischl, A. H., Beck, J., Browning, L., Carter, A., Condon, J. E., Dennison, M., Francis, T., Hughes, P. J., Jaime, S., Lau, K. H. K., McArthur, T., McAvoy, K., Magee, M., Newby, O., Ponder, S. W., Quraishi, U., Rawlings, K., Socke, J., . . . Villalobos, S. (2022). 2022 national standards for diabetes self-management education and support. *The Science of Diabetes Self-Management and Care, 48*(1), 44–59. https://doi.org/10.1177/26350106211072203

Davis, N. (2005). *Integrated care pathways: A guide to good practice.* National Leadership and Innovation Agency for Healthcare.

Dawson, D. A., Grant, B. F., Stinson, F. S., & Zhou, Y. (2005). Effectiveness of the derived Alcohol Use Disorders Identification Test (AUDIT-C) in screening for alcohol use disorders and risk drinking in the U.S. general population. *Alcohol: Clinical and Experimental Research, 29*(5), 844–854. https://doi.org/10.1097/01.ALC.0000164374.32229.A2

Deacon, B., Lickel, J., & Abramowitz, J. S. (2008). Medical utilization across the anxiety disorders. *Journal of Anxiety Disorders, 22*(2), 344–350. https://doi.org/10.1016/j.janxdis.2007.03.004

DeGeorge, K. C., Grover, M., & Streeter, G. S. (2022). Generalized anxiety disorder and panic disorder in adults. *American Family Physician, 106*(2), 157–164. https://www.aafp.org/pubs/afp/issues/2022/0800/generalized-anxiety-disorder-panic-disorder.html

de Lannoy, L., Cowan, T., Fernandez, A., & Ross, R. (2021). Physical activity, diet, and weight loss in patients recruited from primary care settings: An update on obesity management interventions. *Obesity Science & Practice, 7*(5), 619–628. https://doi.org/10.1002/osp4.514

Delgado-Lista, J., Alcala-Diaz, J. F., Torres-Peña, J. D., Quintana-Navarro, G. M., Fuentes, F., Garcia-Rios, A., Ortiz-Morales, A. M., Gonzalez-Requero, A. I., Perez-Caballero, A. I., Yubero-Serrano, E. M., Rangel-Zuñiga, O. A., Camargo, A., Rodriguez-Cantalejo, F., Lopez-Segura, F., Badimon, L., Ordovas, J. M., Perez-Jimenez, F., Perez-Martinez, P., Lopez-Miranda, J., & Yubero-Serrano, E. M. (2022). Long-term secondary prevention of cardiovascular disease with a Mediterranean diet and a low-fat diet (CORDIOPREV): A randomised controlled trial. *The Lancet, 399*(10338), 1876–1885. https://doi.org/10.1016/S0140-6736(22)00122-2

Delicate, A., Ayers, S., & McMullen, S. (2018). A systematic review and meta-synthesis of the impact of becoming parents on the couple relationship. *Midwifery, 61*, 88–96. https://doi.org/10.1016/j.midw.2018.02.022

Denford, S., Taylor, R. S., Campbell, J. L., & Greaves, C. J. (2014). Effective behavior change techniques in asthma self-care interventions: Systematic review and meta-regression. *Health Psychology, 33*(7), 577–587. https://doi.org/10.1037/a0033080

Dennis, C. L., & Dowswell, T. (2013). Psychosocial and psychological interventions for preventing postpartum depression. *Cochrane Database of Systematic Reviews, 2*, Article CD001134. https://doi.org/10.1002/14651858.CD001134.pub3

Dennis, C. L., & Hodnett, E. D. (2007). Psychosocial and psychological interventions for treating postpartum depression. *Cochrane Database of Systematic Reviews, 4*, Article CD006116. https://doi.org/10.1002/14651858.CD006116.pub2

Dewitte, M., Bettocchi, C., Carvalho, J., Corona, G., Flink, I., Limoncin, E., Pascoal, P., Reisman, Y., & Van Lankveld, J. (2021). A psychosocial approach to erectile dysfunction: Position statements from the European Society of Sexual Medicine (ESSM). *Sexual Medicine, 9*(6), Article 100434. https://doi.org/10.1016/j.esxm.2021.100434

Dibben, G., Faulkner, J., Oldridge, N., Rees, K., Thompson, D. R., Zwisler, A. D., & Taylor, R. S. (2021). Exercise-based cardiac rehabilitation for coronary heart disease. *Cochrane Database of Systematic Reviews, 11*, Article CD001800. https://doi.org/10.1002/14651858.CD001800.pub4

Dickman, K., Pintz, C., Gold, K., & Kivlahan, C. (2012). Behavior changes in patients with diabetes and hypertension after experiencing shared medical appointments. *Journal of the American Academy of Nurse Practitioners, 24*(1), 43–51. https://doi.org/10.1111/j.1745-7599.2011.00660.x

Dietz, W. H., Douglas, C. E., & Brownson, R. C. (2016). Chronic disease prevention: Tobacco avoidance, physical activity, and nutrition for a healthy start. *JAMA, 316*(16), 1645–1646. https://doi.org/10.1001/jama.2016.14370

di Giacomo, E., Krausz, M., Colmegna, F., Aspesi, F., & Clerici, M. (2018). Estimating the risk of attempted suicide among sexual minority youths: A systematic review and meta-analysis. *JAMA Pediatrics, 172*(12), 1145–1152. https://doi.org/10.1001/jamapediatrics.2018.2731

DiLillo, V., Siegfried, N. J., & West, D. S. (2003). Incorporating motivational interviewing into behavioral obesity treatment. *Cognitive and Behavioral Practice, 10*(2), 120–130. https://doi.org/10.1016/S1077-7229(03)80020-2

DiLillo, V., & West, D. S. (2011). Motivational interviewing for weight loss. *The Psychiatric Clinics of North America, 34*(4), 861–869. https://doi.org/10.1016/j.psc.2011.08.003

DiMatteo, M. R., Giordani, P. J., Lepper, H. S., & Croghan, T. W. (2002). Patient adherence and medical treatment outcomes: A meta-analysis. *Medical Care, 40*(9), 794–811. https://doi.org/10.1097/00005650-200209000-00009

Dobkin, P. L., & Boothroyd, L. J. (2008). Organizing health services for patients with chronic pain: When there is a will there is a way. *Pain Medicine, 9*(7), 881–889. https://doi.org/10.1111/j.1526-4637.2007.00326.x

Dobmeyer, A. C., Hunter, C. L., Corso, M. L., Nielsen, M. K., Corso, K. A., Polizzi, N. C., & Earles, J. E. (2016). Primary care behavioral health provider training: Systematic development and implementation in a large medical system. *Journal of Clinical Psychology in Medical Settings, 23*(3), 207–224. https://doi.org/10.1007/s10880-016-9464-9

Dobscha, S. K., Corson, K., Perrin, N. A., Hanson, G. C., Leibowitz, R. Q., Doak, M. N., Dickinson, K. C., Sullivan, M. D., & Gerrity, M. S. (2009). Collaborative care for chronic pain in primary care: A cluster randomized trial. *JAMA, 301*(12), 1242–1252. https://doi.org/10.1001/jama.2009.377

Dollar, K., Dundon, M., & Kusche, A. (2010). *Tobacco use cessation: A brief primary care intervention.* Center for Integrated Healthcare. https://www.mentalhealth.va.gov/coe/cih-visn2/documents/provider_education_handouts/tobacco_use_cessation_brief_intervention_manual_version_3.pdf

Dorow, M., Löbner, M., Pabst, A., Stein, J., & Riedel-Heller, S. G. (2018). Preferences for depression treatment including internet-based interventions: Results from a large sample of primary care patients. *Frontiers in Psychiatry, 9*, Article 181. https://doi.org/10.3389/fpsyt.2018.00181

Dowell, D., Haegerich, T. M., & Chou, R. (2016). CDC guideline for prescribing opioids for chronic pain—United States, 2016. *JAMA, 315*(15), 1624–1645. https://doi.org/10.1001/jama.2016.1464

Drapeau, C. W., & McIntosh, J. L. (2020). *U.S.A. suicide: 2019 official final data.* American Association of Suicidology. https://suicidology.org/wp-content/uploads/2021/01/2019datapgsv2b.pdf

Dube, P., Kurt, K., Bair, M. J., Theobald, D., & Williams, L. S. (2010). The P4 screener: Evaluation of a brief measure for assessing potential suicide risk in 2 randomized effectiveness trials of primary care and oncology patients. *Primary Care Companion to the Journal of Clinical Psychiatry, 12*(6), e1–e8. https://doi.org/10.4088/PCC.10m00978blu

Dumoulin, C., Hay-Smith, E. J., & Mac Habée-Séguin, G. (2014). Pelvic floor muscle training versus no treatment, or inactive control treatments, for urinary incontinence in women. *Cochrane Database of Systematic Reviews, 5*, Article CD005654. https://doi.org/10.1002/14651858.CD005654.pub3

Dunkel, L. D., & Glaros, A. G. (1978). Comparison of self-instructional and stimulus control treatments for obesity. *Cognitive Therapy and Research, 2*(1), 75–78. https://doi.org/10.1007/BF01172517

Dunkley, A. J., Bodicoat, D. H., Greaves, C. J., Russell, C., Yates, T., Davies, M. J., & Khunti, K. (2014). Diabetes prevention in the real world: Effectiveness of pragmatic lifestyle interventions for the prevention of Type 2 diabetes and of the impact of adherence to guideline recommendations: A systematic review and meta-analysis. *Diabetes Care, 37*(4), 922–933. https://doi.org/10.2337/dc13-2195

Dunn, J. A., Chokron Garneau, H., Filipowicz, H., Mahoney, M., Seay-Morrison, T., Dent, K., & McGovern, M. (2021). What are patient preferences for integrated behavioral health in primary care? *Journal of Primary Care & Community Health, 12*, Article 21501327211049053. https://doi.org/10.1177/21501327211049053

Eaton, W. W., Smith, C., Ybarra, M., Muntaner, C., & Tien, A. (2004). Center for Epidemiologic Studies Depression Scale: Review and revision (CESD and CESD-R). In M. E. Maruish (Ed.), *The use of psychological testing for treatment planning and outcomes assessment: Vol. 3. Instruments for adults* (pp. 363–377). Lawrence Erlbaum.

Ebrahim, S., Taylor, F., Ward, K., Beswick, A., Burke, M., & Davey Smith, G. (2011, January 19). Multiple risk factor interventions for primary prevention of coronary heart disease. *Cochrane Database of Systematic Reviews, 1*, Article CD001561. https://doi.org/10.1002/14651858.CD001561.pub3

Edelman, D., Gierisch, J. M., McDuffie, J. R., Oddone, E., & Williams, J. W., Jr. (2015). Shared medical appointments for patients with diabetes mellitus: A systematic review. *Journal of General Internal Medicine, 30*(1), 99–106. https://doi.org/10.1007/s11606-014-2978-7

Edinger, J. D., & Carney, C. E. (2014). *Overcoming insomnia: A cognitive-behavioral therapy approach* (2nd ed.). Oxford University Press.

Ee, C., Lake, J., Firth, J., Hargraves, F., de Manincor, M., Meade, T., Marx, W., & Sarris, J. (2020). An integrative collaborative care model for people with mental illness and physical comorbidities. *International Journal of Mental Health Systems, 14*(1), Article 83. https://doi.org/10.1186/s13033-020-00410-6

Ehde, D. M., Dillworth, T. M., & Turner, J. A. (2014). Cognitive-behavioral therapy for individuals with chronic pain: Efficacy, innovations, and directions for research. *American Psychologist, 69*(2), 153–166. https://doi.org/10.1037/a0035747

El-Den, S., Chen, T. F., Gan, Y. L., Wong, E., & O'Reilly, C. L. (2018). The psychometric properties of depression screening tools in primary healthcare settings: A systematic review. *Journal of Affective Disorders, 225*, 503–522. https://doi.org/10.1016/j.jad.2017.08.060

Elgaddal, N., Kramarow, E. A., & Reuben, C. (2022). *Physical activity among adults aged 18 and over: United States, 2020.* National Center for Health Statistics. https://www.cdc.gov/nchs/products/databriefs/db443.htm

El-Hamd, M. A., Saleh, R., & Majzoub, A. (2019). Premature ejaculation: An update on definition and pathophysiology. *Asian Journal of Andrology, 21*(5), 425–432. https://doi.org/10.4103/aja.aja_122_18

Emerson, M. A., Moore, R. S., & Caetano, R. (2017). Association between lifetime post-traumatic stress disorder and past year alcohol use disorder among American Indians/Alaska Natives and Non-Hispanic Whites. *Alcoholism, Clinical and Experimental Research, 41*(3), 576–584. https://doi.org/10.1111/acer.13322

Engel, G. L. (1977). The need for a new medical model: A challenge for biomedicine. *Science, 196*(4286), 129–136. https://doi.org/10.1126/science.847460

Epstein, L. H., Paluch, R. A., Kilanowski, C. K., & Raynor, H. A. (2004). The effect of reinforcement or stimulus control to reduce sedentary behavior in the treatment of pediatric obesity. *Health Psychology, 23*(4), 371–380. https://doi.org/10.1037/0278-6133.23.4.371

Epstein, N. B., & Zheng, L. (2017). Cognitive-behavioral couple therapy. *Current Opinion in Psychology, 13,* 142–147. https://doi.org/10.1016/j.copsyc.2016.09.004

Epton, T., Currie, S., & Armitage, C. J. (2017). Unique effects of setting goals on behavior change: Systematic review and meta-analysis. *Journal of Consulting and Clinical Psychology, 85*(12), 1182–1198. https://doi.org/10.1037/ccp0000260

Ernstzen, D. V., Louw, Q. A., & Hillier, S. L. (2017). Clinical practice guidelines for the management of chronic musculoskeletal pain in primary healthcare: A systematic review. *Implementation Science, 12*(1), Article 1. https://doi.org/10.1186/s13012-016-0533-0

Falloon, K., Elley, C. R., Fernando, A., III, Lee, A. C., & Arroll, B. (2015). Simplified sleep restriction for insomnia in general practice: A randomised controlled trial. *The British Journal of General Practice, 65*(637), e508–e515. https://doi.org/10.3399/bjgp15X686137

Farquhar, J. M., Stonerock, G. L., & Blumenthal, J. A. (2018). Treatment of anxiety in patients with coronary heart disease: A systematic review. *Psychosomatics, 59*(4), 318–332. https://doi.org/10.1016/j.psym.2018.03.008

Felt, B. T., Biermann, B., Christner, J. G., Kochhar, P., & Van Harrison, R. (2014). Diagnosis and management of ADHD in children. *American Family Physician, 90*(7), 456–464.

Fernandes, N., Prada, L., Rosa, M. M., Ferreira, J. J., Costa, J., Pinto, F. J., & Caldeira, D. (2021). The impact of SSRIs on mortality and cardiovascular events in patients with coronary artery disease and depression: Systematic review and meta-analysis. *Clinical Research in Cardiology, 110*(2), 183–193. https://doi.org/10.1007/s00392-020-01697-8

Fernando, A., III, Arroll, B., & Falloon, K. (2013). A double-blind randomised controlled study of a brief intervention of bedtime restriction for adult patients with primary insomnia. *Journal of Primary Health Care, 5*(1), 5–10.

Ferrante, T., Manzoni, G. C., Russo, M., Camarda, C., Taga, A., Veronesi, L., Pasquarella, C., Sansebastiano, G., & Torelli, P. (2013). Prevalence of tension-type headache in adult general population: The PACE study and review of the literature. *Neurological Sciences, 34*(S1), 137–138. https://doi.org/10.1007/s10072-013-1370-4

Finger, W. W. (2007). Medications and sexual health. In L. VandeCreek, F. L. Peterson, Jr., & J. W. Bley (Eds.), *Innovations in clinical practice: Focus on sexual health* (pp. 47–61). Professional Resource Press.

Fink, H. A., Hemmy, L. S., Linskens, E. J., Silverman, P. C., MacDonald, R., McCarten, J. R., Talley, K. M. C., Desai, P. J., Forte, M. L., Miller, M. A., Brasure, M., Nelson, V. A., Taylor, B. C., Ng, W. Y., Ouellette, J. M., Greer, N. L., Sheets, K. M., Wilt, T. J., & Butler, M. (2020). *Diagnosis and treatment of clinical Alzheimer's-type dementia: A systematic review: Comparative effectiveness review no. 223* (AHRQ Publication No. 20-EHC003). Agency for Healthcare Research and Quality. https://doi.org/10.23970/AHRQEPCCER223

Fiore, M. C., Jaen, C. R., Baker, T. B., Bailey, W. C., Benowitz, N. L., Curry, S. J., Dorfman, S. F., Froelicher, E. S., Goldstein, M. G., Healton, C. G., Henderson, P. N., Heyman, R. B., Koh, H. K., Kottke, T. E., Lando, H. A., Mecklenburg, R. E., Mermelstein, R. J., Mullen, P. D., Orleans, C. T., . . . Leitzke, C. (2008). *Treating tobacco use and dependence: 2008 update.* U.S. Department of Health and Human Services.

Fisher, L., & Glasgow, R. E. (2007). A call for more effectively integrating behavioral and social science principles into comprehensive diabetes care. *Diabetes Care, 30*(10), 2746–2749. https://doi.org/10.2337/dc07-1166

Fisher, L., Glasgow, R. E., Mullan, J. T., Skaff, M. M., & Polonsky, W. H. (2008). Development of a brief diabetes distress screening instrument. *Annals of Family Medicine, 6*(3), 246–252. https://doi.org/10.1370/afm.842

Fitzpatrick, S. L., Schumann, K. P., & Hill-Briggs, F. (2013). Problem solving interventions for diabetes self-management and control: A systematic review of the literature.

Diabetes Research and Clinical Practice, 100(2), 145–161. https://doi.org/10.1016/j.diabres.2012.12.016

Florentine, J. B., & Crane, C. (2010). Suicide prevention by limiting access to methods: A review of theory and practice. *Social Science & Medicine, 70*(10), 1626–1632. https://doi.org/10.1016/j.socscimed.2010.01.029

Flores, V. A., Pal, L., & Manson, J. E. (2021). Hormone therapy in menopause: Concepts, controversies, and approach to treatment. *Endocrine Reviews, 42*(6), 720–752. https://doi.org/10.1210/endrev/bnab011

Fogelholm, M. (2010). Physical activity, fitness and fatness: Relations to mortality, morbidity and disease risk factors. A systematic review. *Obesity Reviews, 11*(3), 202–221. https://doi.org/10.1111/j.1467-789X.2009.00653.x

Folstein, M. F., Folstein, S. E., & McHugh, P. R. (1975). "Mini-mental state": A practical method for grading the cognitive state of patients for the clinician. *Journal of Psychiatric Research, 12*(3), 189–198. https://doi.org/10.1016/0022-3956(75)90026-6

Ford, E. S., Wheaton, A. G., Cunningham, T. J., Giles, W. H., Chapman, D. P., & Croft, J. B. (2014). Trends in outpatient visits for insomnia, sleep apnea, and prescriptions for sleep medications among U.S. adults: Findings from the National Ambulatory Medical Care survey 1999–2010. *Sleep, 37*(8), 1283–1293. https://doi.org/10.5665/sleep.3914

Forsyth, J. P., & Eifert, G. H. (2016). *The mindfulness and acceptance workbook for anxiety: A guide to breaking free from anxiety, phobias, and worry using acceptance and commitment therapy* (2nd ed.). New Harbinger Publications.

Fox, V., Dalman, C., Dal, H., Hollander, A. C., Kirkbride, J. B., & Pitman, A. (2021). Suicide risk in people with post-traumatic stress disorder: A cohort study of 3.1 million people in Sweden. *Journal of Affective Disorders, 279*, 609–616. https://doi.org/10.1016/j.jad.2020.10.009

Freak-Poli, R., Ryan, J., Neumann, J. T., Tonkin, A., Reid, C. M., Woods, R. L., Nelson, M., Stocks, N., Berk, M., McNeil, J. J., Britt, C., & Owen, A. J. (2021). Social isolation, social support and loneliness as predictors of cardiovascular disease incidence and mortality. *BMC Geriatrics, 21*(1), Article 711. https://doi.org/10.1186/s12877-021-02602-2

Frederick, D. A., John, H. K. S., Garcia, J. R., & Lloyd, E. A. (2018). Differences in orgasm frequency among gay, lesbian, bisexual, and heterosexual men and women in a U.S. national sample. *Archives of Sexual Behavior, 47*(1), 273–288. https://doi.org/10.1007/s10508-017-0939-z

Fredrix, M., McSharry, J., Flannery, C., Dinneen, S., & Byrne, M. (2018). Goal-setting in diabetes self-management: A systematic review and meta-analysis examining content and effectiveness of goal-setting interventions. *Psychology & Health, 33*(8), 955–977. https://doi.org/10.1080/08870446.2018.1432760

Freedman, R. R., & Roehrs, T. A. (2006). Effects of REM sleep and ambient temperature on hot flash-induced sleep disturbance. *Menopause, 13*(4), 576–583. https://doi.org/10.1097/01.gme.0000227398.53192.bc

Freeman, D. S., Manson, L., Howard, J., & Hornberger, J. (2018). Financing the Primary Care Behavioral Health Model. *Journal of Clinical Psychology in Medical Settings, 25*(2), 197–209. https://doi.org/10.1007/s10880-017-9529-4

Freeman, E. W., Sammel, M. D., Lin, H., Gracia, C. R., Kapoor, S., & Ferdousi, T. (2005). The role of anxiety and hormonal changes in menopausal hot flashes. *Menopause, 12*(3), 258–266. https://doi.org/10.1097/01.GME.0000142440.49698.B7

Friedberg, R. D. (2006). A cognitive-behavioral approach to family therapy. *Journal of Contemporary Psychotherapy, 36*(4), 159–165. https://doi.org/10.1007/s10879-006-9020-2

Frost, R., & Donovan, C. (2021). A qualitative exploration of the distress experienced by long-term heterosexual couples when women have low sexual desire. *Sexual and Relationship Therapy, 36*(1), 22–45. https://doi.org/10.1080/14681994.2018.1549360

Fryar, C. D., Carroll, M. D., & Afful, J. (2020). *Prevalence of overweight, obesity, and severe obesity among adults aged 20 and over: United States, 1960–1962 through 2017–2018.* National Center for Health Statistics. https://www.cdc.gov/nchs/data/hestat/obesity-adult-17-18/obesity-adult.htm

Fuchs, F. F. (2009). *Working it out: A lesbian relationship primer.* BookSurge.

Fuller, D., Colwell, E., Low, J., Orychock, K., Tobin, M. A., Simango, B., Buote, R., Van Heerden, D., Luan, H., Cullen, K., Slade, L., & Taylor, N. G. A. (2020). Reliability and validity of commercially available wearable devices for measuring steps, energy expenditure, and heart rate: Systematic review. *Journal of Medical Internet Research mHealth and uHealth, 8*(9), Article e18694. https://doi.org/10.2196/18694

Funderburk, J. S., Dobmeyer, A. C., Hunter, C. L., Walsh, C. O., & Maisto, S. A. (2013). Provider practices in the primary care behavioral health (PCBH) model: An initial examination in the Veterans Health Administration and United States Air Force. *Families, Systems, & Health, 31*(4), 341–353. https://doi.org/10.1037/a0032770

Gagnon, C., Bélanger, L., Ivers, H., & Morin, C. M. (2013). Validation of the Insomnia Severity Index in primary care. *Journal of the American Board of Family Medicine, 26*(6), 701–710. https://doi.org/10.3122/jabfm.2013.06.130064

Galatzer-Levy, I. R., Nickerson, A., Litz, B. T., & Marmar, C. R. (2013). Patterns of lifetime PTSD comorbidity: A latent class analysis. *Depression and Anxiety, 30*(5), 489–496. https://doi.org/10.1002/da.22048

Gallagher-Thompson, D., & Coon, D. W. (2007). Evidence-based psychological treatments for distress in family caregivers of older adults. *Psychology and Aging, 22*(1), 37–51. https://doi.org/10.1037/0882-7974.22.1.37

Gallo, J. J., Zubritsky, C., Maxwell, J., Nazar, M., Bogner, H. R., Quijano, L. M., Syropoulos, H. J., Cheal, K. L., Chen, H., Sanchez, H., Dodson, J., Levkoff, S. E., & the PRISM-E Investigators. (2004). Primary care clinicians evaluate integrated and referral models of behavioral health care for older adults: Results from a multisite effectiveness trial (PRISM-E). *Annals of Family Medicine, 2*(4), 305–309. https://doi.org/10.1370/afm.116

Garcia, J. R., Lloyd, E. A., Wallen, K., & Fisher, H. E. (2014). Variation in orgasm occurrence by sexual orientation in a sample of U.S. singles. *Journal of Sexual Medicine, 11*(11), 2645–2652. https://doi.org/10.1111/jsm.12669

Gardner, W., Lucas, A., Kolko, D. J., & Campo, J. V. (2007). Comparison of the PSC-17 and alternative mental health screens in an at-risk primary care sample. *Journal of the American Academy of Child & Adolescent Psychiatry, 46*(5), 611–618. https://doi.org/10.1097/chi.0b013e318032384b

Garland, E. L., Brintz, C. E., Hanley, A. W., Roseen, E. J., Atchley, R. M., Gaylord, S. A., Faurot, K. R., Yaffe, J., Fiander, M., & Keefe, F. J. (2020). Mind-body therapies for opioid-treated pain: A systematic review and meta-analysis. *JAMA Internal Medicine, 180*(1), 91–105. https://doi.org/10.1001/jamainternmed.2019.4917

Garland, E. L., Hanley, A. W., Nakamura, Y., Barrett, J. W., Baker, A. K., Reese, S. E., Riquino, M. R., Froeliger, B., & Donaldson, G. W. (2022). Mindfulness-oriented recovery enhancement vs. supportive group therapy for co-occurring opioid misuse and chronic pain in primary care: A randomized clinical trial. *JAMA Internal Medicine, 182*(4), 407–417. https://doi.org/10.1001/jamainternmed.2022.0033

Gartlehner, G., Wagner, G., Matyas, N., Titscher, V., Greimel, J., Lux, L., Gaynes, B. N., Viswanathan, M., Patel, S., & Lohr, K. N. (2017). Pharmacological and non-pharmacological treatments for major depressive disorder: Review of systematic reviews. *BMJ Open, 7*(6), Article e014912. https://doi.org/10.1136/bmjopen-2016-014912

Gatchel, R. J., McGeary, D. D., McGeary, C. A., & Lippe, B. (2014). Interdisciplinary chronic pain management: Past, present, and future. *American Psychologist, 69*(2), 119–130. https://doi.org/10.1037/a0035514

Gates, P. J., Sabioni, P., Copeland, J., Le Foll, B., & Gowing, L. (2016). Psychosocial interventions for cannabis use disorder. *Cochrane Database of Systematic Reviews, 5*, Article CD005336. https://doi.org/10.1002/14651858.CD005336.pub4

Gaynes, B. N., Gavin, N. Meltzer-Brody, Lohr, K. N., Swinson, T., Gartlehner, G., Brody, S., & Miller, W. C. (2005). Perinatal depression: Prevalence, screening accuracy, and screening outcomes. *Evidence Report/Technology Assessment*, *119*, 1–8. https://doi.org/10.1037/e439372005-001

Gebauer, S., Salas, J., & Scherrer, J. F. (2017). Neighborhood socioeconomic status and receipt of opioid medication for new back pain diagnosis. *Journal of the American Board of Family Medicine*, *30*(6), 775–783. https://doi.org/10.3122/jabfm.2017.06.170061

Gentzke, A. S., Wang, T. W., Cornelius, M., Park-Lee, E., Ren, C., Sawdey, M. D., Cullen, K. A., Loretan, C., Jamal, A., & Homa, D. M. (2022). Tobacco product use and associated factors among middle and high school students—National Youth Tobacco Survey, United States, 2021. *Morbidity and Mortality Weekly Report Surveillance Summaries*, *71*(5), 1–29. https://doi.org/10.15585/mmwr.ss7105a1

Gentzke, A. S., Wang, T. W., Jamal, A., Park-Lee, E., Ren, C., Cullen, K. A., & Neff, L. (2020). Tobacco product use among middle and high school students—United States, 2020. *Morbidity and Mortality Weekly Report*, *69*(50), 1881–1888. https://doi.org/10.15585/mmwr.mm6950a1

Gewirtz-Meydan, A., & Opuda, E. (2022). The impact of child sexual abuse on men's sexual function: A systematic review. *Trauma, Violence, & Abuse*, *23*(1), 265–277. https://doi.org/10.1177/1524838020939134

Ghazavi, Z., Feshangchi, S., Alavi, M., & Keshvari, M. (2016). Effect of a family-oriented communication skills training program on depression, anxiety, and stress in older adults: A randomized clinical trial. *Nursing and Midwifery Studies*, *5*(1), Article e28550.

Gianfredi, V., Blandi, L., Cacitti, S., Minelli, M., Signorelli, C., Amerio, A., & Odone, A. (2020). Depression and objectively measured physical activity: A systematic review and meta-analysis. *International Journal of Environmental Research and Public Health*, *17*(10), Article 3738. https://doi.org/10.3390/ijerph17103738

Gillies, C. L., Abrams, K. R., Lambert, P. C., Cooper, N. J., Sutton, A. J., Hsu, R. T., & Khunti, K. (2007). Pharmacological and lifestyle interventions to prevent or delay Type 2 diabetes in people with impaired glucose tolerance: Systematic review and meta-analysis. *BMJ*, *334*(7588), 299–307. https://doi.org/10.1136/bmj.39063.689375.55

Gillies, D., Buykx, P., Parker, A. G., & Hetrick, S. E. (2015). Consultation liaison in primary care for people with mental disorders. *Cochrane Database of Systematic Reviews*, *9*, Article CD007193. https://doi.org/10.1002/14651858.CD007193.pub2

Glasgow, R. E., Funnell, M. M., Bonomi, A. E., Davis, C., Beckham, V., & Wagner, E. H. (2002). Self-management aspects of the Improving Chronic Illness Care Breakthrough Series: Implementation with diabetes and heart failure teams. *Annals of Behavioral Medicine*, *24*(2), 80–87. https://doi.org/10.1207/S15324796ABM2402_04

Glasgow, R. E., Nelson, C. C., Strycker, L. A., & King, D. K. (2006). Using RE-AIM metrics to evaluate diabetes self-management support interventions. *American Journal of Preventive Medicine*, *30*(1), 67–73. https://doi.org/10.1016/j.amepre.2005.08.037

Glazener, C. M., Evans, J. H., & Peto, R. E. (2005). Alarm interventions for nocturnal enuresis in children. *Cochrane Database of Systematic Reviews*, *2*, Article CD002911. https://doi.org/10.1002/14651858.CD002911.pub2

Glina, S., Sharlip, I. D., & Hellstrom, W. J. G. (2013). Modifying risk factors to prevent and treat erectile dysfunction. *Journal of Sexual Medicine*, *10*(1), 115–119. https://doi.org/10.1111/j.1743-6109.2012.02816.x

Global Burden of Disease Study 2013 Collaborators. (2015). Global, regional, and national incidence, prevalence, and years lived with disability for 301 acute and chronic diseases and injuries in 188 countries, 1990–2013: A systematic analysis for the Global Burden of Disease Study 2013. *The Lancet*, *386*(9995), 743–800. https://doi.org/10.1016/S0140-6736(15)60692-4

Global Initiative for Asthma. (2022). *Global strategy for asthma management and prevention*. https://ginasthma.org/wp-content/uploads/2022/07/GINA-Main-Report-2022-FINAL-22-07-01-WMS.pdf

Global Initiative for Chronic Obstructive Lung Disease. (2023). *Global strategy for the diagnosis, management, and prevention of chronic obstructive pulmonary disease: 2023 report.* https://goldcopd.org/wp-content/uploads/2023/03/GOLD-2023-ver-1.3-17Feb2023_WMV.pdf

Glover, N. G., Sylvers, P. D., Shearer, E. M., Kane, M. C., Clasen, P. C., Epler, A. J., Plumb-Vilardaga, J. C., Bonow, J. T., & Jakupcak, M. (2016). The efficacy of focused acceptance and commitment therapy in VA primary care. *Psychological Services, 13*(2), 156–161. https://doi.org/10.1037/ser0000062

Golaszewski, N. M., LaCroix, A. Z., Godino, J. G., Allison, M. A., Manson, J. E., King, J. J., Weitlauf, J. C., Bea, J. W., Garcia, L., Kroenke, C. H., Saquib, N., Cannell, B., Nguyen, S., & Bellettiere, J. (2022). Evaluation of social isolation, loneliness, and cardiovascular disease among older women in the US. *JAMA Network Open, 5*(2), Article e2146461. https://doi.org/10.1001/jamanetworkopen.2021.46461

Goldstein, M. G., Whitlock, E. P., DePue, J., & Planning Committee of the Addressing Multiple Behavioral Risk Factors in Primary Care Project. (2004). Multiple behavioral risk factor interventions in primary care: Summary of research evidence. *American Journal of Preventive Medicine, 27*(2), 61–79. https://doi.org/10.1016/j.amepre.2004.04.023

Gomez, D., Bridges, A. J., Andrews, A. R., III, Cavell, T. A., Pastrana, F. A., Gregus, S. J., & Ojeda, C. A. (2014). Delivering parent management training in an integrated primary care setting: Description and preliminary outcome data. *Cognitive and Behavioral Practice, 21*(3), 296–309. https://doi.org/10.1016/j.cbpra.2014.04.003

Gonzalez, J. S., Peyrot, M., McCarl, L. A., Collins, E. M., Serpa, L., Mimiaga, M. J., & Safren, S. A. (2008). Depression and diabetes treatment nonadherence: A meta-analysis. *Diabetes Care, 31*(12), 2398–2403. https://doi.org/10.2337/dc08-1341

Goodie, J. L., Isler, W. C., Hunter, C., & Peterson, A. L. (2009). Using behavioral health consultants to treat insomnia in primary care: A clinical case series. *Journal of Clinical Psychology, 65*(3), 294–304. https://doi.org/10.1002/jclp.20548

Goodie, J. L., Kanzler, K. E., McGeary, C. A., Blankenship, A. E., Young-McCaughan, S., Peterson, A. L., Cobos, B. A., Dobmeyer, A. C., Hunter, C. L., Blue Star, J., Bhagwat, A., & McGeary, D. D. (2020). Targeting chronic pain in primary care settings by using behavioral health consultants: Methods of a randomized pragmatic trial. *Pain Medicine, 21*(Suppl. 2), S83–S90. https://doi.org/10.1093/pm/pnaa346

Goodman, J. H., & Santangelo, G. (2011). Group treatment for postpartum depression: A systematic review. *Archives of Women's Mental Health, 14*(4), 277–293. https://doi.org/10.1007/s00737-011-0225-3

Goodman, R. (1997). The strengths and difficulties questionnaire: A research note. *Journal of Child Psychology and Psychiatry, 38*(5), 581–586. https://doi.org/10.1111/j.1469-7610.1997.tb01545.x

Goodman, R. (2001). Psychometric properties of the strengths and difficulties questionnaire. *Journal of the American Academy of Child & Adolescent Psychiatry, 40*(11), 1337–1345. https://doi.org/10.1097/00004583-200111000-00015

Gordon, T. E. J., Cardone, I. A., Kim, J. J., Gordon, S. M., & Silver, R. K. (2006). Universal perinatal depression screening in an academic medical center. *Obstetrics and Gynecology, 107*(2 Pt. 1), 342–347. https://doi.org/10.1097/01.AOG.0000194080.18261.92

Gorina, Y., Schappert, S., Bercovitz, A., Elgaddal, M. S., & Kramarow, E. (2014). Prevalence of incontinence among older Americans. *Vital and Health Statistics, 3*(36), 1–33. https://www.cdc.gov/nchs/data/series/sr_03/sr03_036.pdf

Gottman, J. M., & Silver, N. (2012). *What makes love last? How to build trust and avoid betrayal.* Simon & Schuster.

Gottman, J. M., & Silver, N. (2015). *The seven principles for making marriage work.* Random House/Crown/Harmony.

Gøtzsche, P. C., & Gøtzsche, P. K. (2017). Cognitive behavioural therapy halves the risk of repeated suicide attempts: Systematic review. *Journal of the Royal Society of Medicine, 110*(10), 404–410. https://doi.org/10.1177/0141076817731904

Graham, G. (2014). Population-based approaches to understanding disparities in cardio-vascular disease risk in the United States. *International Journal of General Medicine, 7*, 393–400. https://doi.org/10.2147/IJGM.S65528

Gray, L. J., Cooper, N., Dunkley, A., Warren, F. C., Ara, R., Abrams, K., Davies, M. J., Khunti, K., & Sutton, A. (2012). A systematic review and mixed treatment comparison of pharmacological interventions for the treatment of obesity. *Obesity Reviews, 13*(6), 483–498. https://doi.org/10.1111/j.1467-789X.2011.00981.x

Greenberg, P. E., Fournier, A. A., Sisitsky, T., Simes, M., Berman, R., Koenigsberg, S. H., & Kessler, R. C. (2021). The economic burden of adults with major depressive disorder in the United States (2010 and 2018). *PharmacoEconomics, 39*(6), 653–665. https://doi.org/10.1007/s40273-021-01019-4

Greenberger, D., & Padesky, C. A. (2015). *Mind over mood: Change how you feel by changing the way you think* (2nd ed.). Guilford Press.

Greenwood, J. L., Joy, E. A., & Stanford, J. B. (2010). The Physical Activity Vital Sign: A primary care tool to guide counseling for obesity. *Journal of Physical Activity & Health, 7*(5), 571–576. https://doi.org/10.1123/jpah.7.5.571

Grinberg, K., Sela, Y., & Nissanholtz-Gannot, R. (2020). New insights about chronic pelvic pain syndrome (CPPS). *International Journal of Environmental Research and Public Health, 17*(9), Article 3005. https://doi.org/10.3390/ijerph17093005

Grundy, S. M., Stone, N. J., Bailey, A. L., Beam, C., Birtcher, K. K., Blumenthal, R. S., Braun, L. T., de Ferranti, S., Faiella-Tommasino, J., Forman, D. E., Goldberg, R., Heidenreich, P. A., Hlatky, M. A., Jones, D. W., Lloyd-Jones, D., Lopez-Pajares, N., Ndumele, C. E., Orringer, C. E., Peralta, C. A., . . . Yeboah, J. (2019). 2018 AHA/ACC/AACVPR/AAPA/ABC/ACPM/ADA/AGS/APhA/ASPC/NLA/PCNA guideline on the management of blood cholesterol: A report of the American College of Cardiology/American Heart Association Task Force on Clinical Practice Guidelines. *Circulation, 139*(25), e1082–e1143. https://doi.org/10.1161/CIR.0000000000000625

Gudzune, K. A., Doshi, R. S., Mehta, A. K., Chaudhry, Z. W., Jacobs, D. K., Vakil, R. M., Lee, C. J., Bleich, S. N., & Clark, J. M. (2015). Efficacy of commercial weight-loss programs: An updated systematic review. *Annals of Internal Medicine, 162*(7), 501–512. https://doi.org/10.7326/M14-2238

Gunn, H. E., Tutek, J., & Buysse, D. J. (2019). Brief behavioral treatment of insomnia. *Sleep Medicine Clinics, 14*(2), 235–243. https://doi.org/10.1016/j.jsmc.2019.02.003

Ha, H., & Gonzalez, A. (2019). Migraine headache prophylaxis. *American Family Physician, 99*(1), 17–24. https://www.aafp.org/content/dam/brand/aafp/pubs/afp/issues/2019/0101/p17.pdf

Haigh, E. A. P., Bogucki, O. E. M. A., Sigmon, S. T. P., & Blazer, D. G. M. D. P. (2018). Depression among older adults: A 20-year update on five common myths and misconceptions. *The American Journal of Geriatric Psychiatry, 26*(1), 107–122. https://doi.org/10.1016/j.jagp.2017.06.011

Hall, K. D., Sacks, G., Chandramohan, D., Chow, C. C., Wang, Y. C., Gortmaker, S. L., & Swinburn, B. A. (2011). Quantification of the effect of energy imbalance on body-weight. *The Lancet, 378*(9793), 826–837. https://doi.org/10.1016/S0140-6736(11)60812-X

Hall, K. S., Hyde, E. T., Bassett, D. R., Carlson, S. A., Carnethon, M. R., Ekelund, U., Evenson, K. R., Galuska, D. A., Kraus, W. E., Lee, I. M., Matthews, C. E., Omura, J. D., Paluch, A. E., Thomas, W. I., & Fulton, J. E. (2020). Systematic review of the prospective association of daily step counts with risk of mortality, cardiovascular disease, and dysglycemia. *The International Journal of Behavioral Nutrition and Physical Activity, 17*(1), Article 78. https://doi.org/10.1186/s12966-020-00978-9

Halm, E. A., Mora, P., & Leventhal, H. (2006). No symptoms, no asthma: The acute episodic disease belief is associated with poor self-management among inner-city adults with persistent asthma. *Chest, 129*(3), 573–580. https://doi.org/10.1378/chest.129.3.573

Hampl, S. E., Hassink, S. G., Skinner, A. C., Armstrong, S. C., Barlow, S. E., Bolling, C. F., Avila Edwards, K. C., Eneli, I., Hamre, R., Joseph, M. M., Lunsford, D., Mendonca, E., Michalsky, M. P., Mirza, N., Ochoa, E. R., Jr., Sharifi, M., Staiano, A. E., Weedn, A. E., Flinn, S. K., . . . Okechukwu, K. (2023). Clinical practice guideline for the evaluation and treatment of children and adolescents with obesity. *Pediatrics, 151*(2), Article e2022060640. https://doi.org/10.1542/peds.2022-060640

Harmon, A. L., Goldstein, E. S. R., Shiner, B., & Watts, B. V. (2014). Preliminary findings for a brief posttraumatic stress intervention in primary mental health care. *Psychological Services, 11*(3), 295–299. https://doi.org/10.1037/a0035846

Harris, P., Loveman, E., Clegg, A., Easton, S., & Berry, N. (2015). Systematic review of cognitive behavioural therapy for the management of headaches and migraines in adults. *British Journal of Pain, 9*(4), 213–224. https://doi.org/10.1177/2049463715578291

Harshfield, E. L., Pennells, L., Schwartz, J. E., Willeit, P., Kaptoge, S., Bell, S., Shaffer, J. A., Bolton, T., Spackman, S., Wassertheil-Smoller, S., Kee, F., Amouyel, P., Shea, S. J., Kuller, L. H., Kauhanen, J., van Zutphen, E. M., Blazer, D. G., Krumholz, H., Nietert, P. J., . . . Davidson, K. W. (2020). Association between depressive symptoms and incident cardiovascular diseases. *JAMA, 324*(23), 2396–2405. https://doi.org/10.1001/jama.2020.23068

Hartmann-Boyce, J., Hong, B., Livingstone-Banks, J., Wheat, H., & Fanshawe, T. R. (2019). Additional behavioural support as an adjunct to pharmacotherapy for smoking cessation. *Cochrane Database of Systematic Reviews, 6*, Article CD009670. https://doi.org/10.1002/14651858.CD009670.pub4

Hartmann-Boyce, J., Livingstone-Banks, J., Ordóñez-Mena, J. M., Fanshawe, T. R., Lindson, N., Freeman, S. C., Sutton, A. J., Theodoulou, A., & Aveyard, P. (2021). Behavioural interventions for smoking cessation: An overview and network meta-analysis. *Cochrane Database of Systematic Reviews, 1*, Article CD013229. https://doi.org/10.1002/14651858.CD013229.pub2

Harvan, J. R., & Cotter, V. (2006). An evaluation of dementia screening in the primary care setting. *Journal of the American Academy of Nurse Practitioners, 18*(8), 351–360. https://doi.org/10.1111/j.1745-7599.2006.00137.x

Harvard Health Publishing. (2020, August 29). *Chest pain: A heart attack or something else?* https://www.health.harvard.edu/heart-health/chest-pain-a-heart-attack-or-something-else

Harvard Health Publishing. (2022, April 5). *Is it dementia or depression?* https://www.health.harvard.edu/mind-and-mood/is-it-dementia-or-depression

Hasin, D. S., Sarvet, A. L., Meyers, J. L., Saha, T. D., Ruan, W. J., Stohl, M., & Grant, B. F. (2018). Epidemiology of adult *DSM-5* major depressive disorder and its specifiers in the United States. *JAMA Psychiatry, 75*(4), 336–346. https://doi.org/10.1001/jamapsychiatry.2017.4602

Hassett, A. L., & Gevirtz, R. N. (2009). Nonpharmacologic treatment for fibromyalgia: Patient education, cognitive-behavioral therapy, relaxation techniques, and complementary and alternative medicine. *Rheumatic Disease Clinics of North America, 35*(2), 393–407.

Hatano, Y. (1993). Use of pedometer for promoting daily walking exercise. *Journal of the International Committee on Health, Physical Education, and Recreation, 29*, 4–8.

Hatcher, S., Sharon, C., Parag, V., & Collins, N. (2011). Problem-solving therapy for people who present to hospital with self-harm: Zelen randomised controlled trial. *The British Journal of Psychiatry, 199*(4), 310–316. https://doi.org/10.1192/bjp.bp.110.090126

Havranek, E. P., Mujahid, M. S., Barr, D. A., Blair, I. V., Cohen, M. S., Cruz-Flores, S., Davey-Smith, G., Dennison-Himmelfarb, C. R., Lauer, M. S., Lockwood, D. W., Rosal, M., & Yancy, C. W. (2015). Social determinants of risk and outcomes for cardiovascular disease: A scientific statement from the American Heart Association. *Circulation, 132*(9), 873–898. https://doi.org/10.1161/CIR.0000000000000228

Hayes, S. C. (2016). Acceptance and commitment therapy, relational frame theory, and the third wave of behavioral and cognitive therapies—Republished article. *Behavior Therapy, 47*(6), 869–885. https://doi.org/10.1016/j.beth.2016.11.006

Hayes, S. C., Strosahl, K. D., & Wilson, K. G. (1999). *Acceptance and commitment therapy: An experiential approach to behavior change.* Guilford Press.

Hayes, S. C., Strosahl, K. D., & Wilson, K. G. (2011). *Acceptance and commitment therapy: The process and practice of mindful change.* Guilford Press.

Health Promotion Research Center. (n.d.). *Rapid Assessment of Physical Activity (RAPA).* University of Washington. https://depts.washington.edu/hprc/programs-tools/tools-guides/rapa/

Heath, B., Wise, R. P., & Reynolds, K. A. (2013). *A standard framework for levels of integrated healthcare.* SAMHSA-HRSA Center for Integrated Health Solutions. https://www.pcpcc.org/sites/default/files/resources/SAMHSA-HRSA%202013%20Framework%20for%20Levels%20of%20Integrated%20Healthcare.pdf

Heron, M. (2021). Deaths: Leading causes for 2019. *National Vital Statistics Reports, 70*(9), 1–114. https://www.cdc.gov/nchs/data/nvsr/nvsr70/nvsr70-09-508.pdf

Herr, N. R., Williams, J. W., Jr., Benjamin, S., & McDuffie, J. (2014). Does this patient have generalized anxiety or panic disorder? The Rational Clinical Examination systematic review. *JAMA, 312*(1), 78–84. https://doi.org/10.1001/jama.2014.5950

Hersh, L., & Salzman, B. (2013). Clinical management of urinary incontinence in women. *American Family Physician, 87*(9), 634–640.

Heyworth, L., Rozenblum, R., Burgess, J. F., Jr., Baker, E., Meterko, M., Prescott, D., Neuwirth, Z., & Simon, S. R. (2014). Influence of shared medical appointments on patient satisfaction: A retrospective 3-year study. *Annals of Family Medicine, 12*(4), 324–330. https://doi.org/10.1370/afm.1660

Hiddinga, L. (2021). *Are you coming? A vagina owner's guide to orgasm.* The Experiment.

Higginson, I. J., Gao, W., Jackson, D., Murray, J., & Harding, R. (2010). Short-form Zarit Caregiver Burden Interviews were valid in advanced conditions. *Journal of Clinical Epidemiology, 63*(5), 535–542. https://doi.org/10.1016/j.jclinepi.2009.06.014

Hilton, L., Hempel, S., Ewing, B. A., Apaydin, E., Xenakis, L., Newberry, S., Colaiaco, B., Maher, A. R., Shanman, R. M., Sorbero, M. E., & Maglione, M. A. (2017). Mindfulness meditation for chronic pain: Systematic review and meta-analysis. *Annals of Behavioral Medicine, 51*(2), 199–213. https://doi.org/10.1007/s12160-016-9844-2

Ho, P. M., Bryson, C. L., & Rumsfeld, J. S. (2009). Medication adherence: Its importance in cardiovascular outcomes. *Circulation, 119*(23), 3028–3035. https://doi.org/10.1161/CIRCULATIONAHA.108.768986

Hodges, S., & Schlosberg, S. (2017). *Bedwetting and accidents aren't your fault: Why potty accidents happen and how to make them stop.* O'Regan Press.

Hoffman, R. S., & Weinhouse, G. L. (2021). Management of moderate and severe alcohol withdrawal syndromes. *UpToDate.* https://www.uptodate.com/contents/management-of-moderate-and-severe-alcohol-withdrawal-syndromes

Hogan, B. E., Linden, W., & Najarian, B. (2002). Social support interventions: Do they work? *Clinical Psychology Review, 22*(3), 381–440. https://doi.org/10.1016/S0272-7358(01)00102-7

Hoge, M. A., Morris, J. A., Laraia, M., Pomernatz, A., & Farley, T. (2014). *Core competencies for integrated behavioral health and primary care.* SAMHSA-HRSA Center for Integrated Health Solutions. https://www.thenationalcouncil.org/wp-content/uploads/2020/01/Integration_Competencies_Final.pdf

Holsinger, T., Deveau, J., Boustani, M., & Williams, J. W., Jr. (2007). Does this patient have dementia? *JAMA, 297*(21), 2391–2404. https://doi.org/10.1001/jama.297.21.2391

Holtmann, M., Sonuga-Barke, E., Cortese, S., & Brandeis, D. (2014). Neurofeedback for ADHD: A review of current evidence. *Child and Adolescent Psychiatric Clinics of North America, 23*(4), 789–806. https://doi.org/10.1016/j.chc.2014.05.006

Holzmeister, L. (2017). *The diabetes carbohydrate & fat gram guide: Quick, easy meal planning using carbohydrate and fat gram counts* (5th ed.). American Diabetes Association.

Hong, J., Tiu, Y. C., Leung, P. Y. B., Wong, M. F., Ng, W. Y., Cheung, D., Mok, H. Y., Lam, W. Y., Li, K. Y., & Wong, C. K. (2022). Interventions that improve adherence to anti-hypertensive medications in coronary heart disease patients: A systematic review. *Postgraduate Medical Journal, 98*(1157), 219–227. https://doi.org/10.1136/postgradmedj-2020-139116

Hooker, S. A., Slattengren, A. H., Boyle, L., & Sherman, M. D. (2020). Values-based behavioral activation for chronic pain in primary care: A pilot study. *Journal of Clinical Psychology in Medical Settings, 27*(4), 633–642. https://doi.org/10.1007/s10880-019-09655-x

Horowitz, L. M., Bridge, J. A., Teach, S. J., Ballard, E., Klima, J., Rosenstein, D. L., Wharff, E. A., Ginnis, K., Cannon, E., Joshi, P., & Pao, M. (2012). Ask Suicide-Screening Questions (ASQ): A brief instrument for the pediatric emergency department. *Archives of Pediatrics & Adolescent Medicine, 166*(12), 1170–1176. https://doi.org/10.1001/archpediatrics.2012.1276

Horowitz, L. M., Snyder, D. J., Boudreaux, E. D., He, J. P., Harrington, C. J., Cai, J., Claassen, C. A., Salhany, J. E., Dao, T., Chaves, J. F., Jobes, D. A., Merikangas, K. R., Bridge, J. A., & Pao, M. (2020). Validation of the Ask Suicide-Screening Questions for adult medical inpatients: A brief tool for all ages. *Psychosomatics, 61*(6), 713–722. https://doi.org/10.1016/j.psym.2020.04.008

Howard, H. S. (2012). Sexual adjustment counseling for women with chronic pelvic pain. *Journal of Obstetric, Gynecologic, and Neonatal Nursing, 41*(5), 692–702. https://doi.org/10.1111/j.1552-6909.2012.01405.x

Howlett, N., Trivedi, D., Troop, N. A., & Chater, A. M. (2019). Are physical activity interventions for healthy inactive adults effective in promoting behavior change and maintenance, and which behavior change techniques are effective? A systematic review and meta-analysis. *Translational Behavioral Medicine, 9*(1), 147–157. https://doi.org/10.1093/tbm/iby010

Huerne, K., & Eisenberg, M. (2023). Vaping cessation interventions in former smokers: A review. *The Canadian Journal of Cardiology.* Advance online publication. https://doi.org/10.1016/j.cjca.2023.04.020

Huey, S. J., Jr., Tilley, J. L., Jones, E. O., & Smith, C. A. (2014). The contribution of cultural competence to evidence-based care for ethnically diverse populations. *Annual Review of Clinical Psychology, 10*(1), 305–338. https://doi.org/10.1146/annurev-clinpsy-032813-153729

Hughes, L. S., Clark, J., Colclough, J. A., Dale, E., & McMillan, D. (2017). Acceptance and commitment therapy (ACT) for chronic pain: A systematic review and meta-analyses. *The Clinical Journal of Pain, 33*(6), 552–568. https://doi.org/10.1097/AJP.0000000000000425

Hui, C. Y., Walton, R., McKinstry, B., Jackson, T., Parker, R., & Pinnock, H. (2017). The use of mobile applications to support self-management for people with asthma: A systematic review of controlled studies to identify features associated with clinical effectiveness and adherence. *Journal of the American Medical Informatics Association, 24*(3), 619–632. https://doi.org/10.1093/jamia/ocw143

Hundt, N. E., Renn, B. N., Sansgiry, S., Petersen, N. J., Stanley, M. A., Kauth, M. R., Naik, A. D., Kunik, M. E., & Cully, J. A. (2018). Predictors of response to brief CBT in patients with cardiopulmonary conditions. *Health Psychology, 37*(9), 866–873. https://doi.org/10.1037/hea0000595

Hungin, A. P., Chang, L., Locke, G. R., Dennis, E. H., & Barghout, V. (2005). Irritable bowel syndrome in the United States: Prevalence, symptom patterns and impact. *Alimentary Pharmacology & Therapeutics, 21*(11), 1365–1375. https://doi.org/10.1111/j.1365-2036.2005.02463.x

Hunter, C. L., Funderburk, J. S., Polaha, J., Bauman, D., Goodie, J. L., & Hunter, C. M. (2018). Primary care behavioral health (PCBH) model research: Current state of the science and a call to action. *Journal of Clinical Psychology in Medical Settings, 25,* 127–156. https://doi.org/10.1007/s10880-017-9512-0

Hunter, C. L., & Goodie, J. L. (2010). Operational and clinical components for integrated-collaborative behavioral healthcare in the patient-centered medical home. *Families, Systems, & Health, 28*(4), 308–321. https://doi.org/10.1037/a0021761

Hunter, M. (2021). Cognitive behavioral therapy for menopausal symptoms. *Climacteric, 24*(1), 51–56. https://doi.org/10.1080/13697137.2020.1777965

Hunter, M., & Smith, M. (2020). *Managing hot flushes and night sweats: A cognitive behavioural self-help guide to the menopause* (2nd ed.). Routledge.

Iestra, J. A., Kromhout, D., van der Schouw, Y. T., Grobbee, D. E., Boshuizen, H. C., & van Staveren, W. A. (2005). Effect size estimates of lifestyle and dietary changes on all-cause mortality in coronary artery disease patients: A systematic review. *Circulation, 112*(6), 924–934. https://doi.org/10.1161/CIRCULATIONAHA.104.503995

Iizuka, A., Suzuki, H., Ogawa, S., Kobayashi-Cuya, K. E., Kobayashi, M., Takebayashi, T., & Fujiwara, Y. (2019). Can cognitive leisure activity prevent cognitive decline in older adults? A systematic review of intervention studies. *Geriatrics & Gerontology International, 19*(6), 469–482. https://doi.org/10.1111/ggi.13671

Institute for Healthcare Improvement. (2009). *Triple aim concept design.* https://www.ihi.org/Engage/Initiatives/TripleAim/Documents/ConceptDesign.pdf

Institute of Medicine. (2011). *Relieving pain in America: A blueprint for transforming prevention, care, education, and research.* The National Academies Press. https://doi.org/10.17226/13172

Institute of Medicine Committee on Standards for Developing Trustworthy Clinical Practice Guidelines. (2011). Introduction. In R. Graham, M. Mancher, D. Miller Wolman, S. Greenfield, & E. Steinberg (Eds.), *Clinical practice guidelines we can trust* (pp. 11–20). National Academies Press. https://www.ncbi.nlm.nih.gov/books/NBK209546/

Jabbarpour, Y., DeMarchis, E., Bazemore, A., & Grundy, P. (2017). *The impact of primary care practice transformation on cost, quality, and utilization: A systematic review of research published in 2016.* https://www.pcpcc.org/sites/default/files/resources/pcmh_evidence_report_08-1-17%20FINAL.pdf

Jaber, R., Braksmajer, A., & Trilling, J. S. (2006). Group visits: A qualitative review of current research. *Journal of the American Board of Family Medicine, 19*(3), 276–290. https://doi.org/10.3122/jabfm.19.3.276

Jacobson, N. S. (1978). A stimulus control model of change in behavioral couples' therapy: Implications for contingency contracting. *Journal of Marital and Family Therapy, 4*(3), 29–35. https://doi.org/10.1111/j.1752-0606.1978.tb00524.x

Jastreboff, A. M., Aronne, L. J., Ahmad, N. N., Wharton, S., Connery, L., Alves, B., Kiyosue, A., Zhang, S., Liu, B., Bunck, M. C., & Stefanski, A. (2022). Tirzepatide once weekly for the treatment of obesity. *The New England Journal of Medicine, 387*(3), 205–216. https://doi.org/10.1056/NEJMoa2206038

Jellinek, M. S., & Murphy, J. M. (2021). Screening for psychosocial functioning as the eighth vital sign. *JAMA Pediatrics, 175*(1), 13–14. https://doi.org/10.1001/jamapediatrics.2020.2005

Jellinek, M. S., Murphy, J. M., Robinson, J., Feins, A., Lamb, S., & Fenton, T. (1988). Pediatric Symptom Checklist: Screening school-age children for psychosocial dysfunction. *The Journal of Pediatrics, 112*(2), 201–209. https://doi.org/10.1016/S0022-3476(88)80056-8

Jenkins, C., Schwartz, E., Onnen, N., Craigmile, P. F., & Roberts, M. E. (2022). Variations in tobacco retailer type across community characteristics: Place matters. *Preventing Chronic Disease, 19,* Article E49. https://doi.org/10.5888/pcd19.210454

Jern, P., Sola, I. M., & Ventus, D. (2020). Do women's relationship satisfaction and sexual functioning vary as a function of their male partners' premature ejaculation symptoms? *Journal of Sex & Marital Therapy, 46*(7), 630–638. https://doi.org/10.1080/0092623X.2020.1766612

Jernelöv, S., Lekander, M., Blom, K., Rydh, S., Ljótsson, B., Axelsson, J., & Kaldo, V. (2012). Efficacy of a behavioral self-help treatment with or without therapist guidance for co-morbid and primary insomnia—A randomized controlled trial. *BMC Psychiatry, 12*(1), Article 5. https://doi.org/10.1186/1471-244X-12-5

Jetty, A., Petterson, S., Westfall, J. M., & Jabbarpour, Y. (2021). Assessing primary care contributions to behavioral health: A cross-sectional study using medical expenditure panel survey. *Journal of Primary Care & Community Health, 12*, 1–6. https://doi.org/10.1177/21501327211023871

Jhagroo, R. A., Nakada, S. Y., & Penniston, K. L. (2013). Shared medical appointments for patients with kidney stones new to medical management decrease appointment wait time and increase patient knowledge. *The Journal of Urology, 190*(5), 1778–1784. https://doi.org/10.1016/j.juro.2013.05.037

Johansen, M. E., Matic, K., & McAlearney, A. S. (2015). Attention deficit hyperactivity disorder medication use among teens and young adults. *The Journal of Adolescent Health, 57*(2), 192–197. https://doi.org/10.1016/j.jadohealth.2015.04.009

John, J. R., Jani, H., Peters, K., Agho, K., & Tannous, W. K. (2020). The effectiveness of patient-centred medical home-based models of care versus standard primary care in chronic disease management: A systematic review and meta-analysis of randomized and non-randomized controlled trials. *International Journal of Environmental Research and Public Health, 17*, Article 6886. https://doi.org/10.3390/ijerph17186886

Johnson, J. A., Lee, A., Vinson, D., & Seale, J. P. (2013). Use of AUDIT-based measures to identify unhealthy alcohol use and alcohol dependence in primary care: A validation study. *Alcoholism, Clinical and Experimental Research, 37*(s1), E253–E259. https://doi.org/10.1111/j.1530-0277.2012.01898.x

Joiner, T. E. (2005). *Why people die by suicide*. Harvard University Press.

Joiner, T. E., Rudd, M. D., & Rajab, M. H. (1997). The Modified Scale for Suicidal Ideation: Factors of suicidality and their relation to clinical and diagnostic variables. *Journal of Abnormal Psychology, 106*(2), 260–265. https://doi.org/10.1037/0021-843x.106.2.260

Jones, P. W., Harding, G., Berry, P., Wiklund, I., Chen, W. H., & Kline Leidy, N. (2009). Development and first validation of the COPD Assessment Test. *The European Respiratory Journal, 34*(3), 648–654. https://doi.org/10.1183/09031936.00102509

Jorm, A. F. (1994). *Short form of the Informant Questionnaire on Cognitive Decline in the Elderly (Short IQCODE)*. Australian National University Center for Mental Health Research. https://www.alz.org/media/documents/short-form-informant-questionnaire-decline.pdf

Jost, B. C., & Grossberg, G. T. (1996). The evolution of psychiatric symptoms in Alzheimer's disease: A natural history study. *Journal of the American Geriatrics Society, 44*(9), 1078–1081. https://doi.org/10.1111/j.1532-5415.1996.tb02942.x

Junling, G., Yang, L., Junming, D., Pinpin, Z., & Hua, F. (2015). Evaluation of group visits for Chinese hypertensives based on primary health care center. *Asia-Pacific Journal of Public Health, 27*(2), NP350–NP360. https://doi.org/10.1177/1010539512442566

Juurlink, D. N., Herrmann, N., Szalai, J. P., Kopp, A., & Redelmeier, D. A. (2004). Medical illness and the risk of suicide in the elderly. *Archives of Internal Medicine, 164*(11), 1179–1184. https://doi.org/10.1001/archinte.164.11.1179

Kahn, E. B., Ramsey, L. T., Brownson, R. C., Heath, G. W., Howze, E. H., Powell, K. E., Stone, E. J., Rajab, M. W., & Corso, P. (2002). The effectiveness of interventions to increase physical activity: A systematic review. *American Journal of Preventive Medicine, 22*(4, Suppl. 1), 73–107. https://doi.org/10.1016/S0749-3797(02)00434-8

Kalogeropoulos, D., & Larouche, J. (2020). An integrative biopsychosocial approach to the conceptualization and treatment of erectile disorder. In K. Hall & Y. Binik (Eds.), *Principles and practice of sex therapy* (6th ed., pp. 87–108). Guilford Press.

Kaminski, J. W., Valle, L. A., Filene, J. H., & Boyle, C. L. (2008). A meta-analytic review of components associated with parent training program effectiveness. *Journal of Abnormal Child Psychology, 36*(4), 567–589. https://doi.org/10.1007/s10802-007-9201-9

Kantrowitz, B., & Wingert, P. (2018). *The menopause book: The complete guide: Hormones, hot flashes, health, moods, sleep, sex.* Workman. https://www.hachettebookgroup.com/titles/barbara-kantrowitz/the-menopause-book/9781523504282/

Kanzler, K. E., Bryan, C. J., McGeary, D. D., & Morrow, C. E. (2012). Suicidal ideation and perceived burdensomeness in patients with chronic pain. *Pain Practice, 12*(8), 602–609. https://doi.org/10.1111/j.1533-2500.2012.00542.x

Kanzler, K. E., Robinson, P. J., McGeary, D. D., Mintz, J., Kilpela, L. S., Finley, E. P., McGeary, C., Lopez, E. J., Velligan, D., Munante, M., Tsevat, J., Houston, B., Mathias, C. W., Potter, J. S., & Pugh, J. (2022). Addressing chronic pain with focused acceptance and commitment therapy in integrated primary care: Findings from a mixed methods pilot randomized controlled trial. *BMC Primary Care, 23*(1), Article 77. https://doi.org/10.1186/s12875-022-01690-2

Kaplun, A., Alperovitch-Najenson, D., & Kalichman, L. (2021). Effect of guided imagery on pain and health-related quality of life in musculoskeletal medicine: A comprehensive narrative review. *Current Pain and Headache Reports, 25*(12), Article 76. https://doi.org/10.1007/s11916-021-00991-y

Karel, M. J., Holley, C. K., Whitbourne, S. K., Segal, D. L., Tazeau, Y. N., Emery, E. E., Molinari, V., Yang, J., & Zweig, R. A. (2012). Preliminary validation of a tool to assess competencies for professional geropsychology practice. *Professional Psychology, Research and Practice, 43*(2), 110–117. https://doi.org/10.1037/a0025788

Karlin, B. E., & Fuller, J. D. (2007). Meeting the mental health needs of older adults. *Geriatrics, 62*(1), 26–35.

Katon, W. J. (2012). Collaborative depression care models: From development to dissemination. *American Journal of Preventive Medicine, 42*(5), 550–552. https://doi.org/10.1016/j.amepre.2012.01.017

Katon, W. J., Lin, E. H., Von Korff, M., Ciechanowski, P., Ludman, E. J., Young, B., Peterson, D., Rutter, C. M., McGregor, M., & McCulloch, D. (2010). Collaborative care for patients with depression and chronic illnesses. *The New England Journal of Medicine, 363*(27), 2611–2620. https://doi.org/10.1056/NEJMoa1003955

Katon, W. J., Russo, J. E., Von Korff, M., Lin, E. H. B., Ludman, E., & Ciechanowski, P. S. (2008). Long-term effects on medical costs of improving depression outcomes in patients with depression and diabetes. *Diabetes Care, 31*(6), 1155–1159. https://doi.org/10.2337/dc08-0032

Katz, S., Ford, A. B., Moskowitz, R. W., Jackson, B. A., & Jaffe, M. W. (1963). Studies of illness in the aged: The index of ADL: A standardized measure of biological and psychosocial function. *JAMA, 185*(12), 914–919. https://doi.org/10.1001/jama.1963.03060120024016

Katzman, R., Brown, T., Fuld, P., Peck, A., Schechter, R., & Schimmel, H. (1983). Validation of a short Orientation-Memory-Concentration Test of cognitive impairment. *The American Journal of Psychiatry, 140*(6), 734–739. https://doi.org/10.1176/ajp.140.6.734

Kavan, M. G., Saxena, S. K., & Rafiq, N. (2018). General parenting strategies: Practical suggestions for common child behavior issues. *American Family Physician, 97*(10), 642–648. https://www.aafp.org/pubs/afp/issues/2018/0515/p642.html

Kazdin, A. E. (2009). *The Kazdin method for parenting the defiant child: With no pills, no therapy, no contest of wills.* Houghton Mifflin.

Kazdin, A. E. (2010). Problem-solving skills training and parent management training for oppositional defiant disorder and conduct disorder. In J. R. Weisz & A. E. Kazdin (Eds.), *Evidence-based psychotherapies for children and adolescents* (2nd ed., pp. 211–226). Guilford Press.

Kazdin, A. E., & Rotella, C. (2013). *The everyday parenting toolkit: The Kazdin method for easy, step-by-step, lasting change for you and your child.* Houghton Mifflin Harcourt.

Kessler, R., Stafford, D., & Messier, R. (2009). The problem of integrating behavioral health in the medical home and the questions it leads to. *Journal of Clinical Psychology in Medical Settings, 16*(1), 4–12. https://doi.org/10.1007/s10880-009-9146-y

Kessler, R. C., Berglund, P. A., Chiu, W. T., Deitz, A. C., Hudson, J. I., Shahly, V., Aguilar-Gaxiola, S., Alonso, J., Angermeyer, M. C., Benjet, C., Bruffaerts, R., de Girolamo, G., de Graaf, R., Maria Haro, J., Kovess-Masfety, V., O'Neill, S., Posada-Villa, J., Sasu, C., Scott, K., . . . Xavier, M. (2013). The prevalence and correlates of binge eating disorder in the World Health Organization World Mental Health Surveys. *Biological Psychiatry, 73*(9), 904–914. https://doi.org/10.1016/j.biopsych.2012.11.020

Kessler, R. C., Chiu, W. T., Jin, R., Ruscio, A. M., Shear, K., & Walters, E. E. (2006). The epidemiology of panic attacks, panic disorder, and agoraphobia in the National Comorbidity Survey Replication. *Archives of General Psychiatry, 63*(4), 415–424. https://doi.org/10.1001/archpsyc.63.4.415

Kessler, R. C., Petukhova, M., Sampson, N. A., Zaslavsky, A. M., & Wittchen, H. U. (2012). Twelve-month and lifetime prevalence and lifetime morbid risk of anxiety and mood disorders in the United States. *International Journal of Methods in Psychiatric Research, 21*(3), 169–184. https://doi.org/10.1002/mpr.1359

Kettle, V. E., Madigan, C. D., Coombe, A., Graham, H., Thomas, J. J. C., Chalkley, A. E., & Daley, A. J. (2022). Effectiveness of physical activity interventions delivered or prompted by health professionals in primary care settings: Systematic review and meta-analysis of randomised controlled trials. *BMJ, 376*, Article e068465. https://doi.org/10.1136/bmj-2021-068465

Kiecolt-Glaser, J. K., & Wilson, S. J. (2017). Lovesick: How couples' relationships influence health. *Annual Review of Clinical Psychology, 13*(1), 421–443. https://doi.org/10.1146/annurev-clinpsy-032816-045111

Kim, H. S., & Kim, E. J. (2018). Effects of relaxation therapy on anxiety disorders: A systematic review and meta-analysis. *Archives of Psychiatric Nursing, 32*(2), 278–284. https://doi.org/10.1016/j.apnu.2017.11.015

Kindig, D. A. (2007). Understanding population health terminology. *The Milbank Quarterly, 85*(1), 139–161. https://doi.org/10.1111/j.1468-0009.2007.00479.x

Kindig, D. A., & Isham, G. (2014). Population health improvement: A community health business model that engages partners in all sectors. *Frontiers of Health Services Management, 30*(4), 3–20. https://doi.org/10.1097/01974520-201404000-00002

King, M., Semlyen, J., Tai, S. S., Killaspy, H., Osborn, D., Popelyuk, D., & Nazareth, I. (2008). A systematic review of mental disorder, suicide, and deliberate self harm in lesbian, gay and bisexual people. *BMC Psychiatry, 8*(1), Article 70. https://doi.org/10.1186/1471-244X-8-70

Kinman, C. R., Gilchrist, E. C., Payne-Murphy, J. C., & Miller, B. F. (2015). *Provider- and practice-level competencies for integrated behavioral health in primary care: A literature review.* Agency for Healthcare Research and Quality. https://integrationacademy.ahrq.gov/sites/default/files/2020-06/AHRQ_AcadLitReview.pdf

Kirk, S. F., Penney, T. L., McHugh, T. L., & Sharma, A. M. (2012). Effective weight management practice: A review of the lifestyle intervention evidence. *International Journal of Obesity, 36*(2), 178–185. https://doi.org/10.1038/ijo.2011.80

Klein, D. A., Sylvester, J. E., & Schvey, N. A. (2021). Eating disorders in primary care: Diagnosis and management. *American Family Physician, 103*(1), 22–32. https://www.aafp.org/pubs/afp/issues/2021/0101/p22.html

Knowler, W. C., Barrett-Connor, E., Fowler, S. E., Hamman, R. F., Lachin, J. M., Walker, E. A., Nathan, D. M., & the Diabetes Prevention Program Research Group. (2002). Reduction in the incidence of Type 2 diabetes with lifestyle intervention or metformin. *The New England Journal of Medicine, 346*(6), 393–403. https://doi.org/10.1056/NEJMoa012512

Koo, S., Ahn, Y., Lim, J. Y., Cho, J., & Park, H. Y. (2017). Obesity associates with vasomotor symptoms in postmenopause but with physical symptoms in perimenopause: A cross-sectional study. *BMC Women's Health, 17*(1), Article 126. https://doi.org/10.1186/s12905-017-0487-7

Koohsari, M. J., Sugiyama, T., Sahlqvist, S., Mavoa, S., Hadgraft, N., & Owen, N. (2015). Neighborhood environmental attributes and adults' sedentary behaviors: Review and research agenda. *Preventive Medicine, 77*, 141–149. https://doi.org/10.1016/j.ypmed.2015.05.027

Kopańska, M., Torices, S., Czech, J., Koziara, W., Toborek, M., & Dobrek, Ł. (2020). Urinary incontinence in women: Biofeedback as an innovative treatment method. *Therapeutic Advances in Urology, 12*, 1–12. https://doi.org/10.1177/1756287220934359

Kopta, S. M., & Lowry, J. L. (2002). Psychometric evaluation of the Behavioral Health Questionnaire-20: A brief instrument for assessing global mental health and the three phases of psychotherapy outcome. *Psychotherapy Research, 12*(4), 413–426. https://doi.org/10.1093/ptr/12.4.413

Kort, J. (2016). *Ten smart things gay men can do to improve their lives* (2nd ed.). Joe Kort.

Krantz, D. S., Shank, L. M., & Goodie, J. L. (2022). Post-traumatic stress disorder (PTSD) as a systemic disorder: Pathways to cardiovascular disease. *Health Psychology, 41*(10), 651–662. https://doi.org/10.1037/hea0001127

Kraus, W. E., Powell, K. E., Haskell, W. L., Janz, K. F., Campbell, W. W., Jakicic, J. M., Troiano, R. P., Sprow, K., Torres, A., Piercy, K. L., & the 2018 Physical Activity Guidelines Advisory Committee. (2019). Physical activity, all-cause and cardiovascular mortality, and cardiovascular disease. *Medicine and Science in Sports and Exercise, 51*(6), 1270–1281. https://doi.org/10.1249/MSS.0000000000001939

Krebs, E. E., Lorenz, K. A., Bair, M. J., Damush, T. M., Wu, J., Sutherland, J. M., Asch, S. M., & Kroenke, K. (2009). Development and initial validation of the PEG, a three-item scale assessing pain intensity and interference. *Journal of General Internal Medicine, 24*(6), 733–738. https://doi.org/10.1007/s11606-009-0981-1

Krist, A. H., Davidson, K. W., Mangione, C. M., Barry, M. J., Cabana, M., Caughey, A. B., Curry, S. J., Donahue, K., Doubeni, C. A., Epling, J. W., Jr., Kubik, M., Ogedegbe, G., Pbert, L., Silverstein, M., Simon, M. A., Tseng, C.-W., Wong, J. B., & the U.S. Preventive Services Task Force. (2020). Screening for unhealthy drug use: U.S. Preventive Services Task Force recommendation statement. *JAMA, 323*(22), 2301–2309. https://doi.org/10.1001/jama.2020.8020

Krist, A. H., Davidson, K. W., Mangione, C. M., Barry, M. J., Cabana, M., Caughey, A. B., Donahue, K., Doubeni, C. A., Epling, J. W., Jr., Kubik, M., Landefeld, S., Ogedegbe, G., Pbert, L., Silverstein, M., Simon, M. A., Tseng, C. W., Wong, J. B., & the U.S. Preventive Services Task Force. (2020). Behavioral counseling interventions to promote a healthy diet and physical activity for cardiovascular disease prevention in adults with cardiovascular risk factors: U.S. Preventive Services Task Force recommendation statement. *JAMA, 324*(20), 2069–2075. https://doi.org/10.1001/jama.2020.21749

Krist, A. H., Davidson, K. W., Mangione, C. M., Barry, M. J., Cabana, M., Caughey, A. B., Donahue, K., Doubeni, C. A., Epling, J. W., Jr., Kubik, M., Ogedegbe, G., Pbert, L., Silverstein, M., Simon, M. A., Tseng, C. W., Wong, J. B., & the U.S. Preventive Services Task Force. (2021). Interventions for tobacco smoking cessation in adults, including pregnant persons: U.S. Preventive Services Task Force recommendation statement. *JAMA, 325*(3), 265–279. https://doi.org/10.1001/jama.2020.25019

Kroenke, K., Spitzer, R. L., & Williams, J. B. (2001). The PHQ-9: Validity of a brief depression severity measure. *Journal of General Internal Medicine, 16*(9), 606–613. https://doi.org/10.1046/j.1525-1497.2001.016009606.x

Kroenke, K., Spitzer, R. L., & Williams, J. B. (2003). The Patient Health Questionnaire-2: Validity of a two-item depression screener. *Medical Care, 41*(11), 1284–1292. https://doi.org/10.1097/01.MLR.0000093487.78664.3C

Kroenke, K., Spitzer, R. L., Williams, J. B. W., Monahan, P. O., & Löwe, B. (2007). Anxiety disorders in primary care: Prevalence, impairment, comorbidity, and detection. *Annals of Internal Medicine, 146*(5), 317–325. https://doi.org/10.7326/0003-4819-146-5-200703060-00004

Krysinska, K., & Lester, D. (2010). Post-traumatic stress disorder and suicide risk: A systematic review. *Archives of Suicide Research, 14*(1), 1–23. https://doi.org/10.1080/13811110903478997

Kubany, E. S., Hill, E. E., Owens, J. A., Iannce-Spencer, C., McCaig, M. A., Tremayne, K. J., & Williams, P. L. (2004). Cognitive trauma therapy for battered women with PTSD (CTT-BW). *Journal of Consulting and Clinical Psychology, 72*(1), 3–18. https://doi.org/10.1037/0022-006X.72.1.3

Laan, E., Rellini, A. H., & Barnes, T. (2013). Standard operating procedures for female orgasmic disorder: Consensus of the International Society for Sexual Medicine. *Journal of Sexual Medicine, 10*(1), 74–82. https://doi.org/10.1111/j.1743-6109.2012.02880.x

Labott, S. M. (2020). *Psychological treatment of patients with chronic respiratory disease.* American Psychological Association. https://doi.org/10.1037/0000189-000

Laliberte, M., McCabe, R. E., & Taylor, V. (2009). *The cognitive behavioral workbook for weight management: A step by step program.* New Harbinger Publications.

Lamb, C. A., Kennedy, N. A., Raine, T., Hendy, P. A., Smith, P. J., Limdi, J. K., Hayee, B., Lomer, M. C. E., Parkes, G. C., Selinger, C., Barrett, K. J., Davies, R. J., Bennett, C., Gittens, S., Dunlop, M. G., Faiz, O., Fraser, A., Garrick, V., Johnston, P. D., . . . Hawthorne, A. B. (2019). British Society of Gastroenterology consensus guidelines on the management of inflammatory bowel disease in adults. *Gut, 68*(Suppl. 3), s1–s106. https://doi.org/10.1136/gutjnl-2019-318484

Lamb, S. E., Hansen, Z., Lall, R., Castelnuovo, E., Withers, E. J., Nichols, V., Potter, R., & Underwood, M. R. (2010). Group cognitive behavioural treatment for low-back pain in primary care: A randomised controlled trial and cost-effectiveness analysis. *The Lancet, 375*(9718), 916–923. https://doi.org/10.1016/S0140-6736(09)62164-4

Lamvu, G., Carrillo, J., Ouyang, C., & Rapkin, A. (2021). Chronic pelvic pain in women: A review. *JAMA, 325*(23), 2381–2391. https://doi.org/10.1001/jama.2021.2631

Lang, F. R., & Carstensen, L. L. (1994). Close emotional relationships in late life: Further support for proactive aging in the social domain. *Psychology and Aging, 9*(2), 315–324. https://doi.org/10.1037/0882-7974.9.2.315

Langa, K. M., & Levine, D. A. (2014). The diagnosis and management of mild cognitive impairment: A clinical review. *JAMA, 312*(23), 2551–2561. https://doi.org/10.1001/jama.2014.13806

Langan, R., & Goodbred, A. J. (2016). Identification and management of peripartum depression. *American Family Physician, 93*(10), 852–858. https://www.aafp.org/content/dam/brand/aafp/pubs/afp/issues/2016/0515/p852.pdf

Langberg, J. M., Epstein, J. N., Becker, S. P., Girio-Herrera, E., & Vaughn, A. J. (2012). Evaluation of the Homework, Organization, and Planning Skills (HOPS) intervention for middle school students with ADHD as implemented by school mental health providers. *School Psychology Review, 41*(3), 342–364. https://doi.org/10.1080/02796015.2012.12087514

Laumann, E. O., Paik, A., & Rosen, R. C. (1999). Sexual dysfunction in the United States: Prevalence and predictors. *JAMA, 281*(6), 537–544. https://doi.org/10.1001/jama.281.6.537

Lawal, A. K., Rotter, T., Kinsman, L., Machotta, A., Ronellenfitsch, U., Scott, S. D., Goodridge, D., Plishka, C., & Groot, G. (2016). What is a clinical pathway? Refinement of an operational definition to identify clinical pathway studies for a Cochrane systematic review. *BioMed Central Medicine, 14*, Article 35. https://doi.org/10.1186/s12916-016-0580-z

Lawrence, E. M., Rogers, R. G., Zajacova, A., & Wadsworth, T. (2019). Marital happiness, marital status, health, and longevity. *Journal of Happiness Studies, 20*(5), 1539–1561. https://doi.org/10.1007/s10902-018-0009-9

Lawton, M. P., & Brody, E. M. (1969). Assessment of older people: Self-maintaining and instrumental activities of daily living. *The Gerontologist, 9*(3, Pt. 1), 179–186. https://doi.org/10.1093/geront/9.3_Part_1.179

Lean, M., Fornells-Ambrojo, M., Milton, A., Lloyd-Evans, B., Harrison-Stewart, B., Yesufu-Udechuku, A., Kendall, T., & Johnson, S. (2019). Self-management interventions for people with severe mental illness: Systematic review and meta-analysis. *The British Journal of Psychiatry, 214*(5), 260–268. https://doi.org/10.1192/bjp.2019.54

LeBlanc, E. S., O'Connor, E., Whitlock, E. P., Patnode, C. D., & Kapka, T. (2011). Effectiveness of primary care-relevant treatments for obesity in adults: A systematic evidence review for the U.S. Preventive Services Task Force. *Annals of Internal Medicine, 155*(7), 434–447. https://doi.org/10.7326/0003-4819-155-7-201110040-00006

Lebow, J. L., Chambers, A. L., Christensen, A., & Johnson, S. M. (2012). Research on the treatment of couple distress. *Journal of Marital and Family Therapy, 38*(1), 145–168. https://doi.org/10.1111/j.1752-0606.2011.00249.x

Lee, H. J., Lee, J. H., Cho, E. Y., Kim, S. M., & Yoon, S. (2019). Efficacy of psychological treatment for headache disorder: A systematic review and meta-analysis. *The Journal of Headache and Pain, 20*(1), Article 17. https://doi.org/10.1186/s10194-019-0965-4

LeFevre, M. L. (2014). Screening for suicide risk in adolescents, adults, and older adults in primary care: U.S. Preventive Services Task Force recommendation statement. *Annals of Internal Medicine, 160*(10), 719–726. https://doi.org/10.7326/M14-0589

Lenferink, A., Brusse-Keizer, M., van der Valk, P. D., Frith, P. A., Zwerink, M., Monninkhof, E. M., van der Palen, J., & Effing, T. W. (2017). Self-management interventions including action plans for exacerbations versus usual care in patients with chronic obstructive pulmonary disease. *Cochrane Database of Systematic Reviews, 8*, Article CD011682. https://doi.org/10.1002/14651858.CD011682.pub2

Lett, H. S., Blumenthal, J. A., Babyak, M. A., Strauman, T. J., Robins, C., & Sherwood, A. (2005). Social support and coronary heart disease: Epidemiologic evidence and implications for treatment. *Psychosomatic Medicine, 67*(6), 869–878. https://doi.org/10.1097/01.psy.0000188393.73571.0a

Levack, W. M., Weatherall, M., Hay-Smith, J. C., Dean, S. G., McPherson, K., & Siegert, R. J. (2016). Goal setting and strategies to enhance goal pursuit in adult rehabilitation: Summary of a Cochrane systematic review and meta-analysis. *European Journal of Physical and Rehabilitation Medicine, 52*(3), 400–416. https://hdl.handle.net/10871/21370

Levesque, A., Riant, T., Ploteau, S., Rigaud, J., Labat, J. J., & the Convergences PP Network. (2018). Clinical criteria of central sensitization in chronic pelvic and perineal pain (Convergences PP Criteria): Elaboration of a clinical evaluation tool based on formal expert consensus. *Pain Medicine, 19*(10), 2009–2015. https://doi.org/10.1093/pm/pny030

Lewington, S., Clarke, R., Qizilbash, N., Peto, R., Collins, R., & the Prospective Studies Collaboration. (2002). Age-specific relevance of usual blood pressure to vascular mortality: A meta-analysis of individual data for one million adults in 61 prospective studies. *The Lancet, 360*(9349), 1903–1913. https://doi.org/10.1016/S0140-6736(02)11911-8

Li, S. Y. H., & Bressington, D. (2019). The effects of mindfulness-based stress reduction on depression, anxiety, and stress in older adults: A systematic review and meta-analysis. *International Journal of Mental Health Nursing, 28*(3), 635–656. https://doi.org/10.1111/inm.12568

Liao, Y., Gao, G., & Peng, Y. (2019). The effect of goal setting in asthma self-management education: A systematic review. *International Journal of Nursing Sciences, 6*(3), 334–342. https://doi.org/10.1016/j.ijnss.2019.04.003

Lichtenstein, A. H., Appel, L. J., Vadiveloo, M., Hu, F. B., Kris-Etherton, P. M., Rebholz, C. M., Sacks, F. M., Thorndike, A. N., Van Horn, L., & Wylie-Rosett, J. (2021). 2021 dietary guidance to improve cardiovascular health: A scientific statement from the American Heart Association. *Circulation, 144*(23), e472–e487. https://doi.org/10.1161/CIR.0000000000001031

Liebhaber, M., Bannister, R., Raffetto, W., & Dyer, Z. (2011). Drop-in group medical appointments for patients with asthma: A four-year outcomes study. *ISRN Allergy, 2011*, Article 178925. https://doi.org/10.5402/2011/178925

Lin, J. S., O'Connor, E., Rossom, R. C., Perdue, L. A., Burda, B. U., Thompson, M., & Eckstrom, E. (2013). *Screening for cognitive impairment in older adults: An evidence update for the U.S. Preventive Services Task Force* (Evidence Report No. 107, AHRQ Publication No. 14-05198-EF-1). Agency for Healthcare Research and Quality. https://www.ncbi.nlm.nih.gov/books/n/es107/pdf/

Lindau, S. T., Schumm, L. P., Laumann, E. O., Levinson, W., O'Muircheartaigh, C. A., & Waite, L. J. (2007). A study of sexuality and health among older adults in the United States. *The New England Journal of Medicine, 357*(8), 762–774. https://doi.org/10.1056/NEJMoa067423

Linde, K., Sigterman, K., Kriston, L., Rücker, G., Jamil, S., Meissner, K., & Schneider, A. (2015). Effectiveness of psychological treatments for depressive disorders in primary care: Systematic review and meta-analysis. *Annals of Family Medicine, 13*(1), 56–68. https://doi.org/10.1370/afm.1719

Lindson, N., Pritchard, G., Hong, B., Fanshawe, T. R., Pipe, A., & Papadakis, S. (2021). Strategies to improve smoking cessation rates in primary care. *Cochrane Database of Systematic Reviews, 9*, Article CD011556. https://doi.org/10.1002/14651858.CD011556.pub2

Lindson, N., Thompson, T. P., Ferrey, A., Lambert, J. D., & Aveyard, P. (2019). Motivational interviewing for smoking cessation. *Cochrane Database of Systematic Reviews, 7*, Article CD006936. https://doi.org/10.1002/14651858.CD006936.pub4

Lindson-Hawley, N., Thompson, T. P., & Begh, R. (2015). Motivational interviewing for smoking cessation. *Cochrane Database of Systematic Reviews, 3*, Article CD006936. https://doi.org/10.1002/14651858.CD006936.pub3

Lippi, G., & Henry, B. M. (2020). Chronic obstructive pulmonary disease is associated with severe coronavirus disease 2019 (COVID-19). *Respiratory Medicine, 167*, Article 105941. https://doi.org/10.1016/j.rmed.2020.105941

Liu, J., Gill, E., & Li, S. (2021). Revisiting cultural competence. *The Clinical Teacher, 18*(2), 191–197. https://doi.org/10.1111/tct.13269

Livingstone-Banks, J., Ordóñez-Mena, J. M., & Hartmann-Boyce, J. (2019). Print-based self-help interventions for smoking cessation. *Cochrane Database of Systematic Reviews, 1*, Article CD001118. https://doi.org/10.1002/14651858.CD001118.pub4

Lobelo, F., Rohm Young, D., Sallis, R., Garber, M. D., Billinger, S. A., Duperly, J., Hutber, A., Pate, R. R., Thomas, R. J., Widlansky, M. E., McConnell, M. V., & Joy, E. A. (2018). Routine assessment and promotion of physical activity in healthcare settings: A scientific statement from the American Heart Association. *Circulation, 137*(18), e495–e522. https://doi.org/10.1161/CIR.0000000000000559

Logan, D. E., Lavoie, A. M., Zwick, W. R., Kunz, K., Bumgardner, M. A., & Molina, Y. (2019). Integrating addiction medicine into rural primary care: Strategies and initial outcomes. *Journal of Consulting and Clinical Psychology, 87*(10), 952–961. https://doi.org/10.1037/ccp0000410

Longstreth, G. F., Thompson, W. G., Chey, W. D., Houghton, L. A., Mearin, F., & Spiller, R. C. (2006). Functional bowel disorders. *Gastroenterology, 130*(5), 1480–1491. https://doi.org/10.1053/j.gastro.2005.11.061

Louzon, S. A., Bossarte, R., McCarthy, J. F., & Katz, I. R. (2016). Does suicidal ideation as measured by the PHQ-9 predict suicide among VA patients? *Psychiatric Services, 67*(5), 517–522. https://doi.org/10.1176/appi.ps.201500149

Lundahl, B., Moleni, T., Burke, B. L., Butters, R., Tollefson, D., Butler, C., & Rollnick, S. (2013). Motivational interviewing in medical care settings: A systematic review and meta-analysis of randomized controlled trials. *Patient Education and Counseling, 93*(2), 157–168. https://doi.org/10.1016/j.pec.2013.07.012

Luoma, J. B., Hayes, S. C., & Walzer, R. D. (2007). *Learning ACT: An acceptance & commitment therapy skills-training manual for therapists.* New Harbinger Publications.

Luxton, D. D., June, J. D., & Kinn, J. T. (2011). Technology-based suicide prevention: Current applications and future directions. *Telemedicine Journal and e-Health, 17*(1), 50–54. https://doi.org/10.1089/tmj.2010.0091

MacDonald, R., Fink, H. A., Huckabay, C., Monga, M., & Wilt, T. J. (2007). Pelvic floor muscle training to improve urinary incontinence after radical prostatectomy: A systematic review of effectiveness. *BJU International, 100*(1), 76–81. https://doi.org/10.1111/j.1464-410X.2007.06913.x

Magill, M., Martino, S., & Wampold, B. E. (2022). Goal setting and monitoring with alcohol and other drug use disorders: Principles and practices. *Journal of Substance Abuse Treatment, 132,* Article 108650. https://doi.org/10.1016/j.jsat.2021.108650

Mahler, D. A. (2022). *COPD: Answers to your most pressing questions about chronic obstructive pulmonary disease.* Johns Hopkins University Press.

Majumdar, S., & Morris, R. (2019). Brief group-based acceptance and commitment therapy for stroke survivors. *British Journal of Clinical Psychology, 58*(1), 70–90. https://doi.org/10.1111/bjc.12198

Manalo, T. A., Biermann, H. D., Patil, D. H., & Mehta, A. (2022). The temporal association of depression and anxiety in young men with erectile dysfunction. *Journal of Sexual Medicine, 19*(2), 201–206. https://doi.org/10.1016/j.jsxm.2021.11.011

Mangione, C. M., Barry, M. J., Nicholson, W. K., Cabana, M., Coker, T. R., Davidson, K. W., Davis, E. M., Donahue, K. E., Jaen, C. R., Kubik, M., Li, L., Ogedegbe, G., Pbert, L., Ruiz, J. M., Stevermer, J., & Wong, J. B. (2022). Behavioral counseling interventions to promote a healthy diet and physical activity for cardiovascular disease prevention in adults without cardiovascular disease risk factors: US Preventive Services Task Force recommendation statement. *JAMA, 328*(4), 367–374. https://doi.org/10.1001/jama.2022.10951

Mann, J. J., Michel, C. A., & Auerbach, R. P. (2021). Improving suicide prevention through evidence-based strategies: A systematic review. *The American Journal of Psychiatry, 178*(7), 611–624. https://doi.org/10.1176/appi.ajp.2020.20060864

Marchand, E. (2021). Psychological and behavioral treatment of female orgasmic disorder. *Sexual Medicine Reviews, 9*(2), 194–211. https://doi.org/10.1016/j.sxmr.2020.07.007

Markman, H. J., Stanley, S. M., & Blumberg, S. L. (2010). *Fighting for your marriage: A deluxe revised edition of the classic best-seller for enhancing marriage and preventing divorce.* John Wiley & Sons.

Martin, J. M. (2020). *Live your life with COPD: 52 weeks of health, happiness, and hope* (2nd ed.). Outskirts Press.

Martin, M., Clare, L., Altgassen, A. M., Cameron, M. H., & Zehnder, F. (2011). Cognition-based interventions for healthy older people and people with mild cognitive impairment. *Cochrane Database of Systematic Reviews, 1,* Article CD006220. https://doi.org/10.1002/14651858.CD006220.pub2

Martin, S. A., Atlantis, E., Lange, K., Taylor, A. W., O'Loughlin, P., & Wittert, G. A. (2014). Predictors of sexual dysfunction incidence and remission in men. *Journal of Sexual Medicine, 11*(5), 1136–1147. https://doi.org/10.1111/jsm.12483

Martinez, M. E., & Clarke, T. C. (2021). QuickStats: Percentage of adults in fair or poor health, by age group and race and ethnicity—National Health Interview Survey, United States, 2019. *Morbidity and Mortality Weekly Report, 70*(9), Article 333. https://doi.org/10.15585/mmwr.mm7009a5

Massachusetts General Hospital. (n.d.). *Pediatric symptom checklist.* https://www.massgeneral.org/psychiatry/treatments-and-services/pediatric-symptom-checklist

Masters, W. H., & Johnson, V. E. (1970). *Human sexual inadequacy*. Little, Brown.

Mathias, S. D., Kuppermann, M., Liberman, R. F., Lipschutz, R. C., & Steege, J. F. (1996). Chronic pelvic pain: Prevalence, health-related quality of life, and economic correlates. *Obstetrics and Gynecology, 87*(3), 321–327. https://doi.org/10.1016/0029-7844(95)00458-0

McCarthy, B., Casey, D., Devane, D., Murphy, K., Murphy, E., & Lacasse, Y. (2015). Pulmonary rehabilitation for chronic obstructive pulmonary disease. *Cochrane Database of Systematic Reviews, 2*, Article CD003793. https://doi.org/10.1002/14651858.CD003793.pub3

McCarthy, B., & McCarthy, E. (2012). *Sexual awareness: Your guide to healthy couple sexuality* (5th ed.). Routledge. https://doi.org/10.4324/9780203123904

McCarthy, B., & McCarthy, E. (2020). *Rekindling desire* (3rd ed.). Routledge.

McCormick, E., Kerns, S. E., McPhillips, H., Wright, J., Christakis, D. A., & Rivara, F. P. (2014). Training pediatric residents to provide parent education: A randomized controlled trial. *Academic Pediatrics, 14*(4), 353–360. https://doi.org/10.1016/j.acap.2014.03.009

McDaniel, S. H., Grus, C. L., Cubic, B. A., Hunter, C. L., Kearney, L. K., Schuman, C. C., Karel, M. J., Kessler, R. S., Larkin, K. T., McCutcheon, S., Miller, B. F., Nash, J., Qualls, S. H., Connolly, K. S., Stancin, T., Stanton, A. L., Sturm, L. A., & Johnson, S. B. (2014). Competencies for psychology practice in primary care. *American Psychologist, 69*(4), 409–429. https://doi.org/10.1037/a0036072

McDonald, K. C. (2007). Child abuse: Approach and management. *American Family Physician, 75*(2), 221–228. https://www.aafp.org/content/dam/brand/aafp/pubs/afp/issues/2007/0115/p221.pdf

McEwan, D., Harden, S. M., Zumbo, B. D., Sylvester, B. D., Kaulius, M., Ruissen, G. R., Dowd, A. J., & Beauchamp, M. R. (2016). The effectiveness of multi-component goal setting interventions for changing physical activity behaviour: A systematic review and meta-analysis. *Health Psychology Review, 10*(1), 67–88. https://doi.org/10.1080/17437199.2015.1104258

McGuire, B. E., Morrison, T. G., Hermanns, N., Skovlund, S., Eldrup, E., Gagliardino, J., Kokoszka, A., Matthews, D., Pibernik-Okanović, M., Rodríguez-Saldaña, J., de Wit, M., & Snoek, F. J. (2010). Short-form measures of diabetes-related emotional distress: The Problem Areas in Diabetes Scale (PAID)-5 and PAID-1. *Diabetologia, 53*, 66–69. https://doi.org/10.1007/s00125-009-1559-5

McKnight, T. L. (2006). *Obesity management in family practice*. Springer.

McMain, S. F., Guimond, T., Barnhart, R., Habinski, L., & Streiner, D. L. (2017). A randomized trial of brief dialectical behaviour therapy skills training in suicidal patients suffering from borderline disorder. *Acta Psychiatrica Scandinavica, 135*(2), 138–148. https://doi.org/10.1111/acps.12664

McNally, R. J. (2003). *Remembering trauma*. Harvard University Press.

McNaughton, J. L. (2009). Brief interventions for depression in primary care: A systematic review. *Canadian Family Physician, 55*(8), 789–796. https://www.ncbi.nlm.nih.gov/pubmed/19675262

McNeil, C., & Hembree-Kigin, T. L. (2010). *Parent-child interaction therapy*. Springer. https://doi.org/10.1007/978-0-387-88639-8

Mechanick, J. I., Youdim, A., Jones, D. B., Garvey, W. T., Hurley, D. L., McMahon, M. M., Heinberg, L. J., Kushner, R., Adams, T. D., Shikora, S., Dixon, J. B., & Brethauer, S. (2013). Clinical practice guidelines for the perioperative nutritional, metabolic, and nonsurgical support of the bariatric surgery patient—2013 update: Cosponsored by American Association of Clinical Endocrinologists, The Obesity Society, and American Society for Metabolic & Bariatric Surgery. *Obesity, 21*(S1), S1–S27. https://doi.org/10.1002/oby.20461

Meinhausen, C., Prather, A. A., & Sumner, J. A. (2022). Posttraumatic stress disorder (PTSD), sleep, and cardiovascular disease risk: A mechanism-focused narrative review. *Health Psychology, 41*(10), 663–673. https://doi.org/10.1037/hea0001143

Meiris, D. C., & Nash, D. B. (2008). More than just a name. *Population Health Management, 11*(4), 181. https://doi.org/10.1089/pop.2008.114801

Melzack, R. (1999). Pain—An overview. *Acta Anaesthesiologica Scandinavica, 43*(9), 880–884. https://doi.org/10.1034/j.1399-6576.1999.430903.x

Melzack, R., & Wall, P. D. (1965, November 19). Pain mechanisms: A new theory. *Science, 150*(3699), 971–979. https://doi.org/10.1126/science.150.3699.971

Merlijn, V. P. B. M., Hunfeld, J. A. M., van der Wouden, J. C., Hazebroek-Kampschreur, A. A. J. M., van Suijlekom-Smit, L. W. A., Koes, B. W., & Passchier, J. (2005). A cognitive-behavioural program for adolescents with chronic pain—A pilot study. *Patient Education and Counseling, 59*(2), 126–134. https://doi.org/10.1016/j.pec.2004.10.010

Metz, M. E., & McCarthy, B. W. (2003). *Coping with premature ejaculation: Overcome PE, please your partner, and have great sex.* New Harbinger.

Metz, M. E., & McCarthy, B. W. (2004). *Coping with erectile dysfunction: How to regain confidence and enjoy great sex.* New Harbinger.

Michelson, D., Davenport, C., Dretzke, J., Barlow, J., & Day, C. (2013). Do evidence-based interventions work when tested in the "real world?" A systematic review and meta-analysis of parent management training for the treatment of child disruptive behavior. *Clinical Child and Family Psychology Review, 16*(1), 18–34. https://doi.org/10.1007/s10567-013-0128-0

Mikami, A. Y., Jia, M., & Na, J. J. (2014). Social skills training. *Child and Adolescent Psychiatric Clinics, 23*(4), 775–788. https://doi.org/10.1016/j.chc.2014.05.007

Mikocka-Walus, A., Bampton, P., Hetzel, D., Hughes, P., Esterman, A., & Andrews, J. M. (2017). Cognitive-behavioural therapy for inflammatory bowel disease: 24-month data from a randomised controlled trial. *International Journal of Behavioral Medicine, 24*(1), 127–135. https://doi.org/10.1007/s12529-016-9580-9

Miller, T. W., Nigg, J. T., & Miller, R. L. (2009). Attention deficit hyperactivity disorder in African American children: What can be concluded from the past ten years? *Clinical Psychology Review, 29*(1), 77–86. https://doi.org/10.1016/j.cpr.2008.10.001

Miller, W. R., & Muñoz, R. F. (2013). *Controlling your drinking: Tools to make moderation work for you* (2nd ed.). Guilford Press.

Miller, W. R., & Rollnick, S. (2013). *Motivational interviewing: Helping people change* (3rd ed.). Guilford Press.

Miller, W. R., Zweben, J., & Johnson, W. R. (2005). Evidence-based treatment: Why, what, where, when, and how? *Journal of Substance Abuse Treatment, 29*(4), 267–276. https://doi.org/10.1016/j.jsat.2005.08.003

Mills, S., Torrance, N., & Smith, B. H. (2016). Identification and management of chronic pain in primary care: A review. *Current Psychiatry Reports, 18*(2), Article 22. https://doi.org/10.1007/s11920-015-0659-9

Milner, A., Spittal, M. J., Kapur, N., Witt, K., Pirkis, J., & Carter, G. (2016). Mechanisms of brief contact interventions in clinical populations: A systematic review. *BMC Psychiatry, 16*(1), Article 194. https://doi.org/10.1186/s12888-016-0896-4

Milton, K., Bull, F. C., & Bauman, A. (2011). Reliability and validity testing of a single-item physical activity measure. *British Journal of Sports Medicine, 45*(3), 203–208. https://doi.org/10.1136/bjsm.2009.068395

Milton, K., Clemes, S., & Bull, F. (2013). Can a single question provide an accurate measure of physical activity? *British Journal of Sports Medicine, 47*(1), 44–48. https://doi.org/10.1136/bjsports-2011-090899

Minen, M. T., Adhikari, S., Padikkala, J., Tasneem, S., Bagheri, A., Goldberg, E., Powers, S., & Lipton, R. B. (2020). Smartphone-delivered progressive muscle relaxation for the treatment of migraine in primary care: A randomized controlled trial. *Headache, 60*(10), 2232–2246. https://doi.org/10.1111/head.14010

Minkin, M. J. (2019). Menopause: Hormones, lifestyle, and optimizing aging. *Obstetrics and Gynecology Clinics of North America, 46*(3), 501–514. https://doi.org/10.1016/j.ogc.2019.04.008

Miranda, R., Scott, M., Hicks, R., Wilcox, H. C., Harris Munfakh, J. L., & Shaffer, D. (2008). Suicide attempt characteristics, diagnoses, and future attempts: Comparing multiple attempters to single attempters and ideators. *Journal of the American Academy of Child & Adolescent Psychiatry*, 47(1), 32–40. https://doi.org/10.1097/chi.0b013e31815a56cb

Mitchell, A. J., Meader, N., Bird, V., & Rizzo, M. (2012). Clinical recognition and recording of alcohol disorders by clinicians in primary and secondary care: Meta-analysis. *The British Journal of Psychiatry*, 201(2), 93–100. https://doi.org/10.1192/bjp.bp.110.091199

Mitchell, A. J., Rao, S., & Vaze, A. (2011). International comparison of clinicians' ability to identify depression in primary care: Meta-analysis and meta-regression of predictors. *The British Journal of General Practice*, 61(583), e72–e80. https://doi.org/10.3399/bjgp11X556227

Modave, F., Bian, J., Leavitt, T., Bromwell, J., Harris, C., III, & Vincent, H. (2015). Low quality of free coaching apps with respect to the American College of Sports Medicine Guidelines: A review of current mobile apps. *JMIR mHealth and uHealth*, 3(3), Article e77. https://doi.org/10.2196/mhealth.4669

Molyneaux, E., Trevillion, K., & Howard, L. M. (2015). Antidepressant treatment for postnatal depression. *JAMA*, 313(19), 1965–1966. https://doi.org/10.1001/jama.2015.2276

Moncada, L. V. V., & Mire, L. G. (2017). Preventing falls in older persons. *American Family Physician*, 96(4), 240–247. https://www.aafp.org/content/dam/brand/aafp/pubs/afp/issues/2017/0815/p240.pdf

Monroe Carell Jr. Children's Hospital. (n.d.). *Play nicely: The healthy discipline program*. https://www.childrenshospitalvanderbilt.org/information/play-nicely-healthy-discipline-program

Monteleone, P., Mascagni, G., Giannini, A., Genazzani, A. R., & Simoncini, T. (2018). Symptoms of menopause—Global prevalence, physiology and implications. *Nature Reviews Endocrinology*, 14(4), 199–215. https://doi.org/10.1038/nrendo.2017.180

Morin, C. M., Bootzin, R. R., Buysse, D. J., Edinger, J. D., Espie, C. A., & Lichstein, K. L. (2006). Psychological and behavioral treatment of insomnia: Update of the recent evidence (1998–2004). *Sleep*, 29(11), 1398–1414. https://doi.org/10.1093/sleep/29.11.1398

Morin, C. M., Drake, C. L., Harvey, A. G., Krystal, A. D., Manber, R., Riemann, D., & Spiegelhalder, K. (2015). Insomnia disorder. *Nature Reviews Disease Primers*, 1(1), Article 15026. https://doi.org/10.1038/nrdp.2015.26

Morin, C. M., & Espie, C. A. (2003). *Insomnia: A clinical guide to assessment and treatment*. Kluwer Academic/Plenum Publishers.

Morin, C. M., Jarrin, D. C., Ivers, H., Mérette, C., LeBlanc, M., & Savard, J. (2020). Incidence, persistence, and remission rates of insomnia over 5 years. *JAMA Network Open*, 3(11), Article e2018782. https://doi.org/10.1001/jamanetworkopen.2020.18782

Moseley, G. L. (2003). A pain neuromatrix approach to patients with chronic pain. *Manual Therapy*, 8(3), 130–140. https://doi.org/10.1016/s1356-689x(03)00051-1

Moye, J., Gurrera, R. J., Karel, M. J., Edelstein, B., & O'Connell, C. (2006). Empirical advances in the assessment of the capacity to consent to medical treatment: Clinical implications and research needs. *Clinical Psychology Review*, 26(8), 1054–1077. https://doi.org/10.1016/j.cpr.2005.04.013

Moye, J., Karel, M. J., Stamm, K. E., Qualls, S. H., Segal, D. L., Tazeau, Y. N., & DiGilio, D. A. (2019). Workforce analysis of psychological practice with older adults: Growing crisis requires urgent action. *Training and Education in Professional Psychology*, 13(1), 46–55. https://doi.org/10.1037/tep0000206

Moyer, V. A. (2013). Screening and behavioral counseling interventions in primary care to reduce alcohol misuse: U.S. Preventive Services Task Force recommendation statement. *Annals of Internal Medicine, 159*(3), 210–218. https://doi.org/10.7326/0003-4819-159-3-201308060-00652

Murphy, J. (2011). *Assertiveness: How to stand up for yourself and still win the respect of others.* CreateSpace Independent Publishing Platform.

Nasir, A., & Nasir, L. (2015). Counseling on early childhood concerns: Sleep issues, thumb-sucking, picky eating, school readiness, and oral health. *American Family Physician, 92*(4), 274–278. https://www.aafp.org/content/dam/brand/aafp/pubs/afp/issues/2015/0815/p274.pdf

Nasreddine, Z. S., Phillips, N. A., Bédirian, V., Charbonneau, S., Whitehead, V., Collin, I., Cummings, J. L., & Chertkow, H. (2005). The Montreal Cognitive Assessment, MoCA: A brief screening tool for mild cognitive impairment. *Journal of the American Geriatrics Society, 53*(4), 695–699. https://doi.org/10.1111/j.1532-5415.2005.53221.x

Nathan, D. M., Genuth, S., Lachin, J., Cleary, P., Crofford, O., Davis, M., Rand, L., Siebert, C., & the Diabetes Control and Complications Trial Research Group. (1993). The effect of intensive treatment of diabetes on the development and progression of long-term complications in insulin-dependent diabetes mellitus. *The New England Journal of Medicine, 329*(14), 977–986. https://doi.org/10.1056/NEJM199309303291401

National Assembly for Wales. (1999). *An introduction to clinical pathways.* Putting Clients First.

National Center for Health Statistics. (n.d.). *Percentage of regularly had feelings of worry, nervousness, or anxiety for adults aged 18 and over, United States, 2019, Jan–Jun—2022, Jan–Jun.* National Health Interview Survey. https://wwwn.cdc.gov/NHISDataQueryTool/SHS_adult/index.html

National Committee for Quality Assurance. (n.d.). *Distinction in behavioral health integration.* https://www.ncqa.org/programs/health-care-providers-practices/patient-centered-medical-home-pcmh/distinction-in-behavioral-health-integration/

National Committee for Quality Assurance. (2017). *NCQA PCMH recognition standards and guidelines, appendix 4, PCMH distinction in behavioral health integration.* https://www.chcanys.org/sites/default/files/2022-03/6.%20PCMH%20Recognition_Appendix%204_Distinction%20in%20Behavioral%20Health%20Integration%20Version%207.1.pdf

National Committee for Quality Assurance. (2019). *Latest evidence: Benefits of NCQA patient-centered medical home recognition.* https://www.ncqa.org/programs/health-care-providers-practices/patient-centered-medical-home-pcmh/benefits-support/pcmh-evidence/

National Committee for Quality Assurance & Janssen. (2019). *Population health management: Roadmap for integrated delivery networks.* https://www.ncqa.org/wp-content/uploads/2019/11/20191216_PHM_Roadmap.pdf

National Heart, Lung, and Blood Institute. (n.d.-a). *Calculate your body mass index.* National Institutes of Health. https://www.nhlbi.nih.gov/health/educational/lose_wt/BMI/bmicalc.htm

National Heart, Lung, and Blood Institute. (n.d.-b). *Health disparities and inequities.* National Institutes of Health. https://www.nhlbi.nih.gov/science/health-disparities-and-inequities

National Heart, Lung, and Blood Institute. (2020). *Asthma action plan.* https://www.nhlbi.nih.gov/resources/asthma-action-plan-2020

National Heart, Lung, and Blood Institute. (2021, December 29). *DASH eating plan.* National Institutes of Health. https://www.nhlbi.nih.gov/education/dash-eating-plan

National Institute for Children's Health Quality. (n.d.). *NICHQ Vanderbilt Assessment Scales.* NICHQ, American Academy of Pediatrics, McNeil. https://www.nichq.org/resource/nichq-vanderbilt-assessment-scales

National Institute for Health and Care Excellence. (n.d.). *Shared decision making.* https://www.nice.org.uk/about/what-we-do/our-programmes/nice-guidance/nice-guidelines/shared-decision-making

National Institute for Health and Care Excellence. (2011). *Generalised anxiety disorder and panic disorder (with or without agoraphobia) in adults: Management* (National Clinical Practice Guideline No. 113). https://www.nice.org.uk/guidance/cg113/chapter/guidance

National Institute for Health and Care Excellence. (2018). *Post-traumatic stress disorder* (National Clinical Practice Guideline No. NG116). https://www.nice.org.uk/guidance/ng116

National Institute for Health and Care Excellence. (2019). *Urinary incontinence and pelvic organ prolapse in women: Management* (National Practice Guideline No. 123). https://www.nice.org.uk/guidance/ng123

National Institute of Diabetes and Digestive and Kidney Diseases. (n.d.-a). *Body weight planner: Balancing your food and activity.* U.S. Department of Health and Human Services. https://www.niddk.nih.gov/bwp

National Institute of Diabetes and Digestive and Kidney Diseases. (n.d.-b). *Erectile dysfunction (ED).* https://www.niddk.nih.gov/health-information/urologic-diseases/erectile-dysfunction/all-content

National Institute of Mental Health. (2021a). *Ask Suicide-Screening Questions (ASQ) toolkit.* https://www.nimh.nih.gov/research/research-conducted-at-nimh/asq-toolkit-materials

National Institute of Mental Health. (2021b). *Attention-deficit/hyperactivity disorder in adults: What you need to know* (NIH Publication No. 21-MH-3572). National Institutes of Health. https://www.nimh.nih.gov/health/publications/adhd-what-you-need-to-know

National Institute on Aging. (n.d.). *Elder abuse.* National Institutes of Health. https://www.nia.nih.gov/health/topics/elder-abuse

National Institute on Alcohol Abuse and Alcoholism. (2007). *Helping patients who drink too much: A clinician's guide* (NIH Publication No. 07-3769). U.S. Department of Health and Human Services. https://pubs.niaaa.nih.gov/publications/clinicianGuide/guide/intro/data/resources/Clinicians%20Guide.pdf

National Institute on Alcohol Abuse and Alcoholism. (2015). *Alcohol use disorder: A comparison between* DSM-IV *and* DSM-5. National Institutes of Health. https://pubs.niaaa.nih.gov/publications/dsmfactsheet/dsmfact.pdf

National Institute on Alcohol Abuse and Alcoholism. (2022). *Rethinking drinking: Alcohol and your health.* https://www.niaaa.nih.gov/sites/default/files/publications/NIAAA_RethinkingDrinking.pdf

National Institute on Drug Abuse. (2011). *Screening for drug use in general medical settings: Quick reference guide.* https://nida.nih.gov/sites/default/files/pdf/screening_qr.pdf

National Institute on Drug Abuse. (2020). *Misuse of prescription drugs research report.* https://nida.nih.gov/download/37630/misuse-prescription-drugs-research-report.pdf

National Institutes of Health. (2007). *Expert panel report 3: Guidelines for the diagnosis and management of asthma 2007 (EPR-3).* https://www.nhlbi.nih.gov/health-pro/guidelines/current/asthma-guidelines

National Institutes of Health. (2012). *Asthma care quick reference: Diagnosing and managing asthma* (NIH Publication No. 12-5075). https://www.nhlbi.nih.gov/files/docs/guidelines/asthma_qrg.pdf

Neppl, T. K., Senia, J. M., & Donnellan, M. B. (2016). Effects of economic hardship: Testing the family stress model over time. *Journal of Family Psychology, 30*(1), 12–21. https://doi.org/10.1037/fam0000168

New Harbinger Publications. (2020). *The pain management workbook* [Cover copy]. https://www.newharbinger.com/9781684036462/the-pain-management-workbook/

Nguyen, T. P., Karney, B. R., & Bradbury, T. N. (2017). Childhood abuse and later marital outcomes: Do partner characteristics moderate the association? *Journal of Family Psychology, 31*(1), 82–92. https://doi.org/10.1037/fam0000208

Nicholas, M. K., McGuire, B. E., & Asghari, A. (2015). A 2-item short form of the Pain Self-Efficacy Questionnaire: Development and psychometric evaluation of PSEQ-2. *The Journal of Pain, 16*(2), 153–163. https://doi.org/10.1016/j.jpain.2014.11.002

Nicholas, R. A. (2016). *Bereavement, grief, and mourning* [Unpublished handout].

Nichter, B., Maguen, S., Monteith, L. L., Kachadourian, L., Norman, S. B., Hill, M. L., Herzog, S., & Pietrzak, R. H. (2021). Factors associated with multiple suicide attempts in a nationally representative study of U.S. military veterans. *Journal of Psychiatric Research, 140,* 295–300. https://doi.org/10.1016/j.jpsychires.2021.06.012

Nielsen, M., Gibson, A., Buelt, L., Grundy, P., & Grumbach, K. (2015). *The patient-centered medical home's impact on cost and quality: Annual review of the evidence, 2013–2014.* Primary Care Collaborative. https://www.pcpcc.org/resource/patient-centered-medical-homes-impact-cost-and-quality

Nieuwlaat, R., Wilczynski, N., Navarro, T., Hobson, N., Jeffery, R., Keepanasseril, A., Agoritsas, T., Mistry, N., Iorio, A., Jack, S., Sivaramalingam, B., Iserman, E., Mustafa, R. A., Jedraszewski, D., Cotoi, C., & Haynes, R. B. (2014, November 20). Interventions for enhancing medication adherence. *Cochrane Database of Systematic Reviews, 11,* Article CD000011. https://doi.org/10.1002/14651858.CD000011.pub4

Nigg, J. T. (2013). Attention-deficit/hyperactivity disorder and adverse health outcomes. *Clinical Psychology Review, 33*(2), 215–228. https://doi.org/10.1016/j.cpr.2012.11.005

Noffsinger, E. B. (1999). Will drop-in group medical appointments (DIGMAs) work in practice? *The Permanente Journal, 3*(3), 58–67. https://www.thepermanentejournal.org/doi/pdf/10.7812/TPP/99.952

Noffsinger, E. B. (2009). *Running group visits in your practice.* Springer. https://doi.org/10.1007/b106441

Noffsinger, E. B. (2013). *The ABCs of group visits: An implementation manual for your practice.* Springer. https://doi.org/10.1007/978-1-4614-3526-6

Noffsinger, E. B., & Scott, J. C. (2000a). Potential abuses of group visits. *The Permanente Journal, 4,* 87–98. https://www.thepermanentejournal.org/doi/pdf/10.7812/TPP/00.968

Noffsinger, E. B., & Scott, J. C. (2000b). Understanding today's group visit models. *The Permanente Journal, 4,* 99–112. https://www.thepermanentejournal.org/doi/pdf/10.7812/TPP/00.967

Norris, S. L., Zhang, X., Avenell, A., Gregg, E., Schmid, C. H., & Lau, J. (2005). Long-term non-pharmacological weight loss interventions for adults with prediabetes. *Cochrane Database of Systematic Reviews, 2,* Article CD005270. https://doi.org/10.1002/14651858.CD005270

North American Spine Society. (2020). *Evidence based clinical guidelines for multidisciplinary spine care: Diagnosis and treatment of low back pain.* https://www.spine.org/Portals/0/assets/downloads/ResearchClinicalCare/Guidelines/LowBackPain.pdf

Nouwen, A., Adriaanse, M. C., van Dam, K., Iversen, M. M., Viechtbauer, W., Peyrot, M., Caramlau, I., Kokoszka, A., Kanc, K., de Groot, M., Nefs, G., Pouwer, F., & the European Depression in Diabetes (EDID) Research Consortium. (2019). Longitudinal associations between depression and diabetes complications: A systematic review and meta-analysis. *Diabetic Medicine, 36*(12), 1562–1572. https://doi.org/10.1111/dme.14054

Noya, C. E., Chesla, C., Waters, C., & Alkon, A. (2019). Shared medical appointments: An innovative model to reduce health disparities among Latinxs with Type-2 diabetes. *Western Journal of Nursing Research, 42*(2), 117–124. https://doi.org/10.1177/0193945919845677

Nurmagambetov, T., Kuwahara, R., & Garbe, P. (2018). The economic burden of asthma in the United States, 2008–2013. *Annals of the American Thoracic Society, 15*(3), 348–356. https://doi.org/10.1513/AnnalsATS.201703-259OC

Nusbaum, M. R. H., & Hamilton, C. D. (2002). The proactive sexual health history. *American Family Physician, 66*(9), 1705–1712. https://www.aafp.org/content/dam/brand/aafp/pubs/afp/issues/2002/1101/p1705.pdf

Nyström, M. B., Neely, G., Hassmén, P., & Carlbring, P. (2015). Treating major depression with physical activity: A systematic overview with recommendations. *Cognitive Behaviour Therapy, 44*(4), 341–352. https://doi.org/10.1080/16506073.2015.1015440

O'Connor, E. A., Perdue, L. A., Senger, C. A., Rushkin, M., Patnode, C. D., Bean, S. I., & Jonas, D. E. (2018). *Screening and behavioral counseling interventions to reduce unhealthy alcohol use in adolescents and adults: An updated systematic review for the U.S. Preventive Services Task Force* (Synthesis No. 171, AHRQ Publication No. 18-05242-EF-1). Agency for Healthcare Research and Quality. https://www.ncbi.nlm.nih.gov/books/NBK534916/pdf/Bookshelf_NBK534916.pdf

O'Connor, E. A., Rossom, R. C., Henninger, M., Groom, H. C., Burda, B. U., Henderson, J. T., Bigler, K. D., & Whitlock, E. P. (2016). *Screening for depression in adults: An updated systematic evidence review for the U.S. Preventive Services Task Force* (Synthesis No. 128, AHRQ Publication No. 14-05208-EF-1). https://www.ncbi.nlm.nih.gov/books/n/es128/pdf/

O'Connor, E. A., Whitlock, E. P., Gaynes, B., & Beil, T. L. (2009). *Screening for depression in adults and older adults in primary care: An updated systematic review* (Evidence Synthesis No. 75, AHRQ Publication No. 10-05143-EF-1). Agency for Healthcare Research and Quality. https://www.ncbi.nlm.nih.gov/books/n/es75/pdf/

O'Conor, R., Muellers, K., Arvanitis, M., Vicencio, D. P., Wolf, M. S., Wisnivesky, J. P., & Federman, A. D. (2019). Effects of health literacy and cognitive abilities on COPD self-management behaviors: A prospective cohort study. *Respiratory Medicine, 160*, Article 105630. https://doi.org/10.1016/j.rmed.2019.02.006

O'Donnell, C. J., Schwartz Longacre, L., Cohen, B. E., Fayad, Z. A., Gillespie, C. F., Liberzon, I., Pathak, G. A., Polimanti, R., Risbrough, V., Ursano, R. J., Vander Heide, R. S., Yancy, C. W., Vaccarino, V., Sopko, G., & Stein, M. B. (2021). Posttraumatic stress disorder and cardiovascular disease: State of the science, knowledge gaps, and research opportunities. *JAMA Cardiology, 6*(10), 1207–1216. https://doi.org/10.1001/jamacardio.2021.2530

Ogbeide, S., Stermensky, G., & Rolin, S. (2016). Integrated primary care behavioral health for the rural older adult. *Practice Innovations, 1*(3), 145–153. https://doi.org/10.1037/pri0000022

Ogbeide, S. A., Young, A., Houston, B., & Knight, C. (2021). Treating post-traumatic stress disorder with a prolonged exposure protocol within primary care behavioral health: A case example. *Journal of Clinical Psychology in Medical Settings, 28*(3), 575–583. https://doi.org/10.1007/s10880-020-09747-z

Ogunmoroti, O., Osibogun, O., Spatz, E. S., Okunrintemi, V., Mathews, L., Ndumele, C. E., & Michos, E. D. (2022). A systematic review of the bidirectional relationship between depressive symptoms and cardiovascular health. *Preventive Medicine, 154*, Article 106891. https://doi.org/10.1016/j.ypmed.2021.106891

O'Hara, M. W., & McCabe, J. E. (2013). Postpartum depression: Current status and future directions. *Annual Review of Clinical Psychology, 9*(1), 379–407. https://doi.org/10.1146/annurev-clinpsy-050212-185612

Oja, P., Kelly, P., Murtagh, E. M., Murphy, M. H., Foster, C., & Titze, S. (2018). Effects of frequency, intensity, duration and volume of walking interventions on CVD risk factors: A systematic review and meta-regression analysis of randomised controlled trials among inactive healthy adults. *British Journal of Sports Medicine, 52*(12), 769–775. https://doi.org/10.1136/bjsports-2017-098558

Olariu, E., Forero, C. G., Castro-Rodriguez, J. I., Rodrigo-Calvo, M. T., Álvarez, P., Martín-López, L. M., Sánchez-Toto, A., Adroher, N. D., Blasco-Cubedo, M. J., Vilagut, G., Fullana, M. A., & Alonso, J. (2015). Detection of anxiety disorders in primary care: A meta-analysis of assisted and unassisted diagnoses. *Depression and Anxiety, 32*(7), 471–484. https://doi.org/10.1002/da.22360

Oliveira, C. B., Maher, C. G., Pinto, R. Z., Traeger, A. C., Lin, C. C., Chenot, J. F., van Tulder, M., & Koes, B. W. (2018). Clinical practice guidelines for the management of non-specific low back pain in primary care: An updated overview. *European Spine Journal, 27*(11), 2791–2803. https://doi.org/10.1007/s00586-018-5673-2

Oordt, M. S., Jobes, D. A., Fonseca, V. P., & Schmidt, S. M. (2009). Training mental health professionals to assess and manage suicidal behavior: Can provider confidence and practice behaviors be altered? *Suicide & Life-Threatening Behavior, 39*(1), 21–32. https://doi.org/10.1521/suli.2009.39.1.21

Oslin, D. W., Lynch, K. G., Maisto, S. A., Lantinga, L. J., McKay, J. R., Possemato, K., Ingram, E., & Wierzbicki, M. (2014). A randomized clinical trial of alcohol care management delivered in Department of Veterans Affairs primary care clinics versus specialty addiction treatment. *Journal of General Internal Medicine, 29,* 162–168. https://doi.org/10.1007/s11606-013-2625-8

Öst, L. G. (2014). The efficacy of Acceptance and Commitment Therapy: An updated systematic review and meta-analysis. *Behaviour Research and Therapy, 61,* 105–121. https://doi.org/10.1016/j.brat.2014.07.018

Osterberg, L., & Blaschke, T. (2005). Adherence to medication. *The New England Journal of Medicine, 353*(5), 487–497. https://doi.org/10.1056/NEJMra050100

Otto, M. W., Tolin, D. F., Nations, K. R., Utschig, A. C., Rothbaum, B. O., Hofmann, S. G., & Smits, J. A. (2012). Five sessions and counting: Considering ultra-brief treatment for panic disorder. *Depression and Anxiety, 29*(6), 465–470. https://doi.org/10.1002/da.21910

Owens, D. K., Davidson, K. W., Krist, A. H., Barry, M. J., Cabana, M., Caughey, A. B., Doubeni, C. A., Epling, J. W., Jr., Kubik, M., Landefeld, C. S., Mangione, C. M., Pbert, L., Silverstein, M., Simon, M. A., Tseng, C. W., Wong, J. B., & the U.S. Preventive Services Task Force. (2020). Screening for cognitive impairment in older adults: U.S. Preventive Services Task Force recommendation statement. *JAMA, 323*(8), 757–763. https://doi.org/10.1001/jama.2020.0435

Ozer, S., Young, J., Champ, C., & Burke, M. (2016). A systematic review of the diagnostic test accuracy of brief cognitive tests to detect amnestic mild cognitive impairment. *International Journal of Geriatric Psychiatry, 31*(11), 1139–1150. https://doi.org/10.1002/gps.4444

Pagoto, S., Schneider, K., Jojic, M., DeBiasse, M., & Mann, D. (2013). Evidence-based strategies in weight-loss mobile apps. *American Journal of Preventive Medicine, 45*(5), 576–582. https://doi.org/10.1016/j.amepre.2013.04.025

Pangarkar, S. S., Kang, D. G., Sandbrink, F., Bevevino, A., Tillisch, K., Konitzer, L., & Sall, J. (2019). VA/DoD clinical practice guideline: Diagnosis and treatment of low back pain. *Journal of General Internal Medicine, 34*(11), 2620–2629. https://doi.org/10.1007/s11606-019-05086-4

Park, S. H., & Han, K. S. (2017). Blood pressure response to meditation and yoga: A systematic review and meta-analysis. *Journal of Alternative and Complementary Medicine, 23*(9), 685–695. https://doi.org/10.1089/acm.2016.0234

Parkerson, G. R., Jr., Broadhead, W. E., & Tse, C. K. (1990). The Duke Health Profile. A 17-item measure of health and dysfunction. *Medical Care, 28*(11), 1056–1072. https://doi.org/10.1097/00005650-199011000-00007

Parkhurst, J. T., Ballard, R. R., Lavigne, J. V., Von Mach, T., Romba, C., Perez-Reisler, M., & Walkup, J. T. (2022). Extending collaborative care to independent primary care practices; A Chronic Care Model. *Clinical Practice in Pediatric Psychology, 10*(1), 32–43. https://doi.org/10.1037/cpp0000383

Patel, M. R., Piette, J. D., Resnicow, K., Kowalski-Dobson, T., & Heisler, M. (2016). Social determinants of health, cost-related nonadherence, and cost-reducing behaviors among adults with diabetes: Findings from the National Health Interview Survey. *Medical Care, 54*(8), 796–803. https://doi.org/10.1097/MLR.0000000000000565

Pateraki, E., & Morris, P. G. (2018). Effectiveness of cognitive behavioural therapy in reducing anxiety in adults and children with asthma: A systematic review. *The Journal of Asthma, 55*(5), 532–554. https://doi.org/10.1080/02770903.2017.1350967

Patnode, C. D., Henderson, J. T., Coppola, E. L., Melnikow, J., Durbin, S., & Thomas, R. G. (2021). Interventions for tobacco cessation in adults, including pregnant persons: Updated evidence report and systematic review for the U.S. Preventive Services Task Force. *JAMA, 325*(3), 280–298. https://doi.org/10.1001/jama.2020.23541

Patnode, C. D., Perdue, L. A., Rushkin, M., Dana, T., Blazina, I., Bougatsos, C., Grusing, S., O'Connor, E. A., Fu, R., & Chou, R. (2020). Screening for unhealthy drug use: Updated evidence report and systematic review for the U.S. Preventive Services Task Force. *JAMA, 323*(22), 2310–2338. https://doi.org/10.1001/jama.2019.21381

Patnode, C. D., Perdue, L. A., Rushkin, M., & O'Connor, E. A. (2020) *Screening for unhealthy drug use in primary care in adolescents and adults, including pregnant persons: Updated systematic review for the U.S. Preventive Services Task Force* (Evidence Synthesis No. 186). Agency for Healthcare Research and Quality. https://www.ncbi.nlm.nih.gov/books/NBK558174/pdf/Bookshelf_NBK558174.pdf

Patnode, C. D., Webber, E. M., Thomas, R. G., Guirguis-Blake, J., Chou, R., & Lin, J. S. (2021). *Primary care-relevant interventions to prevent opioid use disorder: Current research and evidence gaps* (AHRQ No. 21-05280-EF-1). Agency for Healthcare Research and Quality. https://www.uspreventiveservicestaskforce.org/uspstf/sites/default/files/inline-files/prevention-of-opioid-user-disorder-ehc-tech-brief.pdf

Paused for Thought. (n.d.). *Balance: The menopause support app.* https://www.pausedforthought.co.uk/

Pedersen, S. S., Nielsen, J. C., Wehberg, S., Jørgensen, O. D., Riahi, S., Haarbo, J., Philbert, B. T., Larsen, M. L., Johansen, J. B., & the DEFIB-WOMEN Investigators. (2021). New onset anxiety and depression in patients with an implantable cardioverter defibrillator during 24 months of follow-up (data from the national DEFIB-WOMEN study). *General Hospital Psychiatry, 72,* 59–65. https://doi.org/10.1016/j.genhosppsych.021.07.003

Peek, C. J. (2008). Planning care in the clinical, operational, and financial worlds. In R. Keesler & D. Stafford (Eds.), *Collaborative medicine case studies: Evidence in practice* (pp. 25–38). Springer. https://doi.org/10.1007/978-0-387-76894-6_3

Peek, C. J., & the National Integration Academy Council. (2013). *Lexicon for behavioral health and primary care integration: Concepts and definitions developed by expert consensus.* https://integrationacademy.ahrq.gov/sites/default/files/2020-06/Lexicon.pdf

Pennachio, D. L. (2003). Should you offer group visit? *Medical Economics, 80*(15), 70–74.

Pentel, K. Z., & Baucom, D. H. (2022). A clinical framework for sexual minority couple therapy. *Couple & Family Psychology, 11*(2), 177–191. https://doi.org/10.1037/cfp0000187

Perciavalle, V., Blandini, M., Fecarotta, P., Buscemi, A., Di Corrado, D., Bertolo, L., Fichera, F., & Coco, M. (2017). The role of deep breathing on stress. *Neurological Sciences, 38*(3), 451–458. https://doi.org/10.1007/s10072-016-2790-8

Perrin, N. E., Davies, M. J., Robertson, N., Snoek, F. J., & Khunti, K. (2017). The prevalence of diabetes-specific emotional distress in people with Type 2 diabetes: A systematic review and meta-analysis. *Diabetic Medicine, 34*(11), 1508–1520. https://doi.org/10.1111/dme.13448

Peterson, A. L., Brundige, A. R., & Houghton, D. (2015). Tobacco use. In F. Andrasik, J. L. Goodie, & A. L. Peterson (Eds.), *Biopsychosocial assessment in clinical health psychology* (pp. 61–86). Guilford Press.

Peterson, A. L., Raj, J., & Lancaster, C. L. (2014). Psychology and population health management. In C. M. Hunter, C. L. Hunter, & R. Kessler (Eds.), *Handbook of clinical psychology in medical settings: Evidence-based assessment and intervention* (pp. 3–18). Springer. https://doi.org/10.1007/978-0-387-09817-3_1

Peterson, A. L., Vander Weg, M. W., & Jaén, C. R. (2011). *Nicotine and tobacco dependence.* Hogrefe Publishing.

Petterson, S. M., Phillips, R. L., Jr., Bazemore, A. W., Dodoo, M. S., Zhang, X., & Green, L. A. (2008). Why there must be room for mental health in the medical home. *American Family Physician, 77*(6), 757. https://www.aafp.org/pubs/afp/issues/2008/0315/p757.html

Pfeiffer, E. (n.d.). *The Short Portable Mental Status Questionnaire (SPMSQ).* Stanford Medicine. https://geriatrics.stanford.edu/culturemed/overview/assessment/assessment_toolkit/spmsq.html

Pfeiffer, E. (1975). A short portable mental status questionnaire for the assessment of organic brain deficit in elderly patients. *Journal of the American Geriatrics Society, 23*(10), 433–441. https://doi.org/10.1111/j.1532-5415.1975.tb00927.x

Pfiffner, L. J., & Haack, L. M. (2015). Nonpharmacologic treatments for childhood attention-deficit/hyperactivity disorder and their combination with medications. In P. E. Nathan & J. M. Gorman (Eds.), *A guide to treatments that work* (4th ed., pp. 55–84). Oxford University Press.

Philip, S., Govier, D., & Pantely, S. (2019). *Patient-centered medical home: Developing the business case from a practice perspective.* Milliman. https://www.ncqa.org/wp-content/uploads/2019/06/06142019_WhitePaper_Milliman_BusinessCasePCMH.pdf

Physical Activity Guidelines Advisory Committee. (2018). *2018 Physical Activity Guidelines Advisory Committee scientific report.* https://health.gov/sites/default/files/2019-09/PAG_Advisory_Committee_Report.pdf

Piasecki, T. M. (2006). Relapse to smoking. *Clinical Psychology Review, 26*(2), 196–215. https://doi.org/10.1016/j.cpr.2005.11.007

Piercy, K. L., Troiano, R. P., Ballard, R. M., Carlson, S. A., Fulton, J. E., Galuska, D. A., George, S. M., & Olson, R. D. (2018). The physical activity guidelines for Americans. *JAMA, 320*(19), 2020–2028. https://doi.org/10.1001/jama.2018.14854

Pimenta, F., Leal, I., Maroco, J., & Ramos, C. (2011). Perceived control, lifestyle, health, socio-demographic factors and menopause: Impact on hot flashes and night sweats. *Maturitas, 69*(4), 338–342. https://doi.org/10.1016/j.maturitas.2011.05.005

Plummer, F., Manea, L., Trepel, D., & McMillan, D. (2016). Screening for anxiety disorders with the GAD-7 and GAD-2: A systematic review and diagnostic metaanalysis. *General Hospital Psychiatry, 39*, 24–31. https://doi.org/10.1016/j.genhosppsych.2015.11.005

Polanczyk, G. V., Salum, G. A., Sugaya, L. S., Caye, A., & Rohde, L. A. (2015). Annual research review: A meta-analysis of the worldwide prevalence of mental disorders in children and adolescents. *Journal of Child Psychology and Psychiatry, 56*(3), 345–365. https://doi.org/10.1111/jcpp.12381

Poleshuck, E. L., Gamble, S. A., Bellenger, K., Lu, N., Tu, X., Sörensen, S., Giles, D. E., & Talbot, N. L. (2014). Randomized controlled trial of interpersonal psychotherapy versus enhanced treatment as usual for women with co-occurring depression and pelvic pain. *Journal of Psychosomatic Research, 77*(4), 264–272. https://doi.org/10.1016/j.jpsychores.2014.07.016

Polomano, R. C., Galloway, K. T., Kent, M. L., Brandon-Edwards, H., Kwon, K. N., Morales, C., & Buckenmaier, C. T., III. (2016). Psychometric testing of the Defense and Veterans Pain Rating Scale (DVPRS): A new pain scale for military population. *Pain Medicine, 17*(8), 1505–1519. https://doi.org/10.1093/pm/pnw105

Polonsky, D. C. (2000). Premature ejaculation. In S. R. Leiblum & R. C. Rosen (Eds.), *Principles and practice of sex therapy* (3rd ed., pp. 305–332). Guilford Press.

Polonsky, W. H., Anderson, B. J., Lohrer, P. A., Welch, G., Jacobson, A. M., Aponte, J. E., & Schwartz, C. E. (1995). Assessment of diabetes-related distress. *Diabetes Care, 18*(6), 754–760. https://doi.org/10.2337/diacare.18.6.754

Polonsky, W. H., Fisher, L., Earles, J., Dudl, R. J., Lees, J., Mullan, J., & Jackson, R. A. (2005). Assessing psychosocial distress in diabetes: Development of the diabetes distress scale. *Diabetes Care, 28*(3), 626–631. https://doi.org/10.2337/diacare.28.3.626

Pool, A. C., Kraschnewski, J. L., Cover, L. A., Lehman, E. B., Stuckey, H. L., Hwang, K. O., Pollak, K. I., & Sciamanna, C. N. (2014). The impact of physician weight discussion on weight loss in U.S. adults. *Obesity Research & Clinical Practice, 8*(2), e131–e139. https://doi.org/10.1016/j.orcp.2013.03.003

Posadzki, P., & Ernst, E. (2011). Guided imagery for musculoskeletal pain: A systematic review. *The Clinical Journal of Pain, 27*(7), 648–653. https://doi.org/10.1097/AJP.0b013e31821124a5

Posner, K., Brown, G. K., Stanley, B., Brent, D. A., Yershova, K. V., Oquendo, M. A., Currier, G. W., Melvin, G. A., Greenhill, L., Shen, S., & Mann, J. J. (2011). The

Columbia–Suicide Severity Rating Scale: Initial validity and internal consistency findings from three multisite studies with adolescents and adults. *The American Journal of Psychiatry, 168*(12), 1266–1277. https://doi.org/10.1176/appi.ajp.2011.10111704

Possemato, K. (2011). The current state of intervention research for posttraumatic stress disorder within the primary care setting. *Journal of Clinical Psychology in Medical Settings, 18*(3), 268–280. https://doi.org/10.1007/s10880-011-9237-4

Pourdowlat, G., Hejrati, R., & Lookzadeh, S. (2019). The effectiveness of relaxation training in the quality of life and anxiety of patients with asthma. *Advances in Respiratory Medicine, 87*(3), 146–151. https://doi.org/10.5603/ARM.2019.0024

Poureslami, I., Nimmon, L., Doyle-Waters, M., Rootman, I., Schulzer, M., Kuramoto, L., & FitzGerald, J. M. (2012). Effectiveness of educational interventions on asthma self-management in Punjabi and Chinese asthma patients: A randomized controlled trial. *The Journal of Asthma, 49*(5), 542–551. https://doi.org/10.3109/02770903.2012.682125

Powers, M. A., Bardsley, J. K., Cypress, M., Funnell, M. M., Harms, D., Hess-Fischl, A., Hooks, B., Isaacs, D., Mandel, E. D., Maryniuk, M. D., Norton, A., Rinker, J., Siminerio, L. M., & Uelmen, S. (2020). Diabetes self-management education and support in adults with Type 2 diabetes: A consensus report of the American Diabetes Association, the Association of Diabetes Care & Education Specialists, the Academy of Nutrition and Dietetics, the American Academy of Family Physicians, the American Academy of PAs, the American Association of Nurse Practitioners, and the American Pharmacists Association. *Diabetes Care, 43*(7), 1636–1649. https://doi.org/10.2337/dci20-0023

Preston, R. (2022). Quality of life among LGBTQ older adults in the United States: A systematic review. *Journal of the American Psychiatric Nurses Association.* Advance online publication. https://doi.org/10.1177/10783903221127697

Prins, A., Bovin, M. J., Kimerling, R., Kaloupek, D. G., Marx, B. P., Pless Kaiser, A., & Schnurr, P. P. (2015). *The primary care PTSD screen for* DSM-5 *(PC-PTSD)*. U.S. Department of Veterans Affairs. https://www.ptsd.va.gov/professional/assessment/screens/pc-ptsd.asp

Prins, A., Bovin, M. J., Smolenski, D. J., Marx, B. P., Kimerling, R., Jenkins-Guarnieri, M. A., Kaloupek, D. G., Schnurr, P. P., Kaiser, A. P., Leyva, Y. E., & Tiet, Q. Q. (2016). The primary care PTSD screen for *DSM-5* (PC-PTSD-5): Development and evaluation within a veteran primary care sample. *Journal of General Internal Medicine, 31*(10), 1206–1211. https://doi.org/10.1007/s11606-016-3703-5

Prins, A., Ouimette, P., Kimerling, R., Cameron, R. P., Hugelshofer, D. S., Shaw-Hegwer, J., Thrailkill, A., Gusman, F. D., & Sheikh, J. I. (2003). The primary care PTSD screen (PC-PTSD): Development and operating characteristics. *Primary Care Psychiatry, 9*(1), 9–14.

Prochaska, J. O., & DiClemente, C. C. (1983). Stages and processes of self-change of smoking: Toward an integrative model of change. *Journal of Consulting and Clinical Psychology, 51*(3), 390–395. https://doi.org/10.1037/0022-006X.51.3.390

Prochaska, J. O., & Velicer, W. F. (1997). The transtheoretical model of health behavior change. *American Journal of Health Promotion, 12*(1), 38–48. https://doi.org/10.4278/0890-1171-12.1.38

Public Health Service. (2008). *Helping smokers quit: A guide for clinicians.* U.S. Department of Health and Human Services. https://www.ahrq.gov/sites/default/files/wysiwyg/professionals/clinicians-providers/guidelines-recommendations/tobacco/clinicians/references/clinhlpsmkqt/clinhlpsmksqt.pdf

Puente-Maestu, L., Calle, M., Rodríguez-Hermosa, J. L., Campuzano, A., de Miguel Díez, J., Álvarez-Sala, J. L., Puente-Andues, L., Pérez-Gutiérrez, M. J., & Lee, S. Y. (2016). Health literacy and health outcomes in chronic obstructive pulmonary disease. *Respiratory Medicine, 115*, 78–82. https://doi.org/10.1016/j.rmed.2016.04.016

Qaseem, A., Vijan, S., Snow, V., Cross, J. T., Weiss, K. B., Owens, D. K., & the Clinical Efficacy Assessment Subcommittee of the American College of Physicians. (2007). Glycemic control and Type 2 diabetes mellitus: The optimal hemoglobin A1c targets. A guidance statement from the American College of Physicians. *Annals of Internal Medicine, 147*(6), 417–422. https://doi.org/10.7326/0003-4819-147-6-200709180-00012

Qaseem, A., Wilt, T. J., McLean, R. M., Forciea, M. A., & Clinical Guidelines Committee of the American College of Physicians. (2017). Noninvasive treatments for acute, subacute, and chronic low back pain: A clinical practice guideline from the American College of Physicians. *Annals of Internal Medicine, 166*(7), 514–530. https://doi.org/10.7326/M16-2367

Quartana, P. J., Campbell, C. M., & Edwards, R. R. (2009). Pain catastrophizing: A critical review. *Expert Review of Neurotherapeutics, 9*(5), 745–758. https://doi.org/10.1586/ern.09.34

Rabasco, A., McKay, D., Smits, J. A., Powers, M. B., Meuret, A. E., & McGrath, P. B. (2022). Psychosocial treatment for panic disorder: An umbrella review of systematic reviews and meta-analyses. *Journal of Anxiety Disorders, 86*, Article 102528. https://doi.org/10.1016/j.janxdis.2022.102528

Racine, M. (2018). Chronic pain and suicide risk: A comprehensive review. *Progress in Neuro-Psychopharmacology & Biological Psychiatry, 87*(Pt. B), 269–280. https://doi.org/10.1016/j.pnpbp.2017.08.020

Raja, S. (2012). *Overcoming trauma and PTSD: A workbook integrating skills from ACT, DBT, and CBT.* New Harbinger Publications.

Ram, S., Seirawan, H., Kumar, S. K. S., & Clark, G. T. (2010). Prevalence and impact of sleep disorders and sleep habits in the United States. *Sleep and Breathing, 14*(1), 63–70. https://doi.org/10.1007/s11325-009-0281-3

Ratzan, S. C., & Parker, R. M. (2000). Introduction. In C. R. Selden, M. Zorn, S. C. Ratzan, & R. M. Parker (Eds.), *National Library of Medicine current bibliographies in medicine: Health literacy* (NLM Pub. No. CBM 2000-1, pp. v–vii). National Institutes of Health. https://www.nlm.nih.gov/archive/20061214/pubs/cbm/hliteracy.html#15

Ratzliff, A., Phillips, K. E., Sugarman, J. R., Unützer, J., & Wagner, E. H. (2017). Practical approaches for achieving integrated behavioral health care in primary care settings. *American Journal of Medical Quality, 32*(2), 117–121. https://doi.org/10.1177/1062860615618783

Raue, P. J., Ghesquiere, A. R., & Bruce, M. L. (2014). Suicide risk in primary care: Identification and management in older adults. *Current Psychiatry Reports, 16*(9), 466. https://doi.org/10.1007/s11920-014-0466-8

Reavell, J., Hopkinson, M., Clarkesmith, D., & Lane, D. A. (2018). Effectiveness of cognitive behavioral therapy for depression and anxiety in patients with cardiovascular disease: A systematic review and meta-analysis. *Psychosomatic Medicine, 80*(8), 742–753. https://doi.org/10.1097/PSY.0000000000000626

Rehm, J., Anderson, P., Manthey, J., Shield, K. D., Struzzo, P., Wojnar, M., & Gual, A. (2016). Alcohol use disorders in primary health care: What do we know and where do we go? *Alcohol and Alcoholism, 51*(4), 422–427. https://doi.org/10.1093/alcalc/agv127

Rehm, J., Mathers, C., Popova, S., Thavorncharoensap, M., Teerawattananon, Y., & Patra, J. (2009). Global burden of disease and injury and economic cost attributable to alcohol use and alcohol-use disorders. *The Lancet, 373*(9682), 2223–2233. https://doi.org/10.1016/S0140-6736(09)60746-7

Reijnders, J., van Heugten, C., & van Boxtel, M. (2013). Cognitive interventions in healthy older adults and people with mild cognitive impairment: A systematic review. *Ageing Research Reviews, 12*(1), 263–275. https://doi.org/10.1016/j.arr.2012.07.003

Reiter, J. T., Dobmeyer, A. C., & Hunter, C. L. (2018). The primary care behavioral health (PCBH) model: An overview and operational definition. *Journal of Clinical Psychology in Medical Settings, 25*(2), 109–126. https://doi.org/10.1007/s10880-017-9531-x

Ribisl, K. M., D'Angelo, H., Feld, A. L., Schleicher, N. C., Golden, S. D., Luke, D. A., & Henriksen, L. (2017). Disparities in tobacco marketing and product availability at the point of sale: Results of a national study. *Preventive Medicine, 105,* 381–388. https://doi.org/10.1016/j.ypmed.2017.04.010

Riblet, N. B. V., Shiner, B., Young-Xu, Y., & Watts, B. V. (2017). Strategies to prevent death by suicide: Meta-analysis of randomised controlled trials. *The British Journal of Psychiatry, 210*(6), 396–402. https://doi.org/10.1192/bjp.bp.116.187799

Richard, D. C. S., & Lauterbach, D. (2007). *Handbook of exposure therapies.* Academic Press.

Richardson, H. L., & Damashek, A. (2022). Examining the use of a brief online intervention in primary care for changing low-income caregivers' attitudes toward spanking. *Journal of Interpersonal Violence, 37*(21–22), NP20409–NP20427. https://doi.org/10.1177/08862605211054101

Rikard, S. M., Strahan, A. E., Schmit, K. M., & Guy, G. P., Jr (2023). Chronic pain among adults—United States, 2019–2021. *Morbidity and Mortality Weekly Report, 72*(15), 379–385. https://doi.org/10.15585/mmwr.mm7215a1

Rittenhouse, D. R., & Shortell, S. M. (2009). The patient-centered medical home: Will it stand the test of health reform? *JAMA, 301*(19), 2038–2040. https://doi.org/10.1001/jama.2009.691

Ritz, T., Meuret, A. E., Trueba, A. F., Fritzsche, A., & von Leupoldt, A. (2013). Psychosocial factors and behavioral medicine interventions in asthma. *Journal of Consulting and Clinical Psychology, 81*(2), 231–250. https://doi.org/10.1037/a0030187

Robinson, P. J. (2019). *Basics of behavior change in primary care.* Springer. https://doi.org/10.1007/978-3-030-32050-8

Robinson, P. J., Gould, D. A., & Strosahl, K. D. (2011). *Real behavior change in primary care: Improving patient outcomes and increasing job satisfaction.* New Harbinger Publications.

Robinson, P. J., & Reiter, J. (2016). *Behavioral consultation and primary care: A guide to integrating services* (2nd ed.). Springer International Publishing. https://doi.org/10.1007/978-3-319-13954-8

Robinson, P. J., Von Korff, M., Bush, T., Lin, E. H. B., & Ludman, E. J. (2020). The impact of primary care behavioral health services on patient behaviors: A randomized controlled trial. *Families, Systems, & Health, 38*(1), 6–15. https://doi.org/10.1037/fsh0000474

Robles, T. F. (2014). Marital quality and health: Implications for marriage in the 21st century. *Current Directions in Psychological Science, 23*(6), 427–432. https://doi.org/10.1177/0963721414549043

Robles, T. F., Slatcher, R. B., Trombello, J. M., & McGinn, M. M. (2014). Marital quality and health: A meta-analytic review. *Psychological Bulletin, 140*(1), 140–187. https://doi.org/10.1037/a0031859

Roddy, M. K., Walsh, L. M., Rothman, K., Hatch, S. G., & Doss, B. D. (2020). Meta-analysis of couple therapy: Effects across outcomes, designs, timeframes, and other moderators. *Journal of Consulting and Clinical Psychology, 88*(7), 583–596. https://doi.org/10.1037/ccp0000514

Rodriguez, L. M., Neighbors, C., & Knee, C. R. (2014). Problematic alcohol use and marital distress: An interdependence theory perspective. *Addiction Research and Theory, 22*(4), 294–312. https://doi.org/10.3109/16066359.2013.841890

Rojewski, A. M., Bailey, S. R., Bernstein, S. L., Cooperman, N. A., Gritz, E. R., Karam-Hage, M. A., Piper, M. E., Rigotti, N. A., & Warren, G. W. (2019). Considering systemic barriers to treating tobacco use in clinical settings in the United States. *Nicotine & Tobacco Research, 21*(11), 1453–1461. https://doi.org/10.1093/ntr/nty123

Rollnick, S., Miller, W. R., & Bulter, C. C. (2022). *Motivational interviewing in healthcare: Helping patients change behavior* (2nd ed.). Guilford Press.

Romeo, A., Edney, S., Plotnikoff, R., Curtis, R., Ryan, J., Sanders, I., Crozier, A., & Maher, C. (2019). Can smartphone apps increase physical activity? Systematic review and meta-analysis. *Journal of Medical Internet Research, 21*(3), Article e12053. https://doi.org/10.2196/12053

Ronksley, P. E., Brien, S. E., Turner, B. J., Mukamal, K. J., & Ghali, W. A. (2011). Association of alcohol consumption with selected cardiovascular disease outcomes: A systematic review and meta-analysis. *BMJ, 342*, Article d671. https://doi.org/10.1136/bmj.d671

Rosas-Salazar, C., Apter, A. J., Canino, G., & Celedón, J. C. (2012). Health literacy and asthma. *The Journal of Allergy and Clinical Immunology, 129*(4), 935–942. https://doi.org/10.1016/j.jaci.2012.01.040

Rosqvist, J. (2005). *Exposure treatments for anxiety disorders: A practitioner's guide to concepts, methods, and evidence-based practice.* Routledge.

Ross, L. E., Grigoriadis, S., Mamisashvili, L., Vonderporten, E. H., Roerecke, M., Rehm, J., Dennis, C.-L., Koren, G., Steiner, M., Mousmanis, P., & Cheung, A. (2013). Selected pregnancy and delivery outcomes after exposure to antidepressant medication: A systematic review and meta-analysis. *JAMA Psychiatry, 70*(4), 436–443. https://doi.org/10.1001/jamapsychiatry.2013.684

Rowland, D. L., & Kolba, T. N. (2018). The burden of sexual problems: Perceived effects on men's and women's sexual partners. *Journal of Sex Research, 55*(2), 226–235. https://doi.org/10.1080/00224499.2017.1332153

Roy-Byrne, P. P., Craske, M. G., Sullivan, G., Rose, R. D., Edlund, M. J., Lang, A. J., Bystritsky, A., Welch, S. S., Chavira, D. A., Golinelli, D., Campbell-Sills, L., Sherbourne, C. D., & Stein, M. B. (2010). Delivery of evidence-based treatment for multiple anxiety disorders in primary care: A randomized controlled trial. *JAMA, 303*(19), 1921–1928. https://doi.org/10.1001/jama.2010.608

Roy-Byrne, P. P., Davidson, K. W., Kessler, R. C., Asmundson, G. J. G., Goodwin, R. D., Kubzansky, L., Lydiard, R. B., Massie, M. J., Katon, W., Laden, S. K., & Stein, M. B. (2008). Anxiety disorders and comorbid medical illness. *General Hospital Psychiatry, 30*(3), 208–225. https://doi.org/10.1016/j.genhosppsych.2007.12.006

Roy-Byrne, P. P., Veitengruber, J. P., Bystritsky, A., Edlund, M. J., Sullivan, G., Craske, M. G., Welch, S. S., Rose, R., & Stein, M. B. (2009). Brief intervention for anxiety in primary care patients. *Journal of the American Board of Family Medicine, 22*(2), 175–186. https://doi.org/10.3122/jabfm.2009.02.080078

Rudd, M. D., Joiner, T., & Rajab, M. H. (1996). Relationships among suicide ideators, attempters, and multiple attempters in a young-adult sample. *Journal of Abnormal Psychology, 105*(4), 541–550. https://doi.org/10.1037/0021-843X.105.4.541

Runyan, C. N., Carter-Henry, S., & Ogbeide, S. (2018). Ethical challenges unique to the primary care behavioral health (PCBH) model. *Journal of Clinical Psychology in Medical Settings, 25*(2), 224–236. https://doi.org/10.1007/s10880-017-9502-2

Runyan, C. N., Robinson, P., & Gould, D. A. (2013). Ethical issues facing providers in collaborative primary care settings: Do current guidelines suffice to guide the future of team based primary care? *Families, Systems, & Health, 31*(1), 1–8. https://doi.org/10.1037/a0031895

Rushforth, B., McCrorie, C., Glidewell, L., Midgley, E., & Foy, R. (2016). Barriers to effective management of Type 2 diabetes in primary care: Qualitative systematic review. *British Journal of General Practice, 66*(643), e114–e127. https://doi.org/10.3399/bjgp16X683509

Saitz, R. (2005). Clinical practice: Unhealthy alcohol use. *The New England Journal of Medicine, 352*(6), 596–607. https://doi.org/10.1056/NEJMcp042262

Salinas, G. D., Glauser, T. A., Williamson, J. C., Rao, G., & Abdolrasulnia, M. (2011). Primary care physician attitudes and practice patterns in the management of obese adults: Results from a national survey. *Postgraduate Medicine, 123*(5), 214–219. https://doi.org/10.3810/pgm.2011.09.2477

Salthouse, T. A. (2019). Trajectories of normal cognitive aging. *Psychology and Aging*, *34*(1), 17–24. https://doi.org/10.1037/pag0000288

Samdal, G. B., Eide, G. E., Barth, T., Williams, G., & Meland, E. (2017). Effective behaviour change techniques for physical activity and healthy eating in overweight and obese adults; systematic review and meta-regression analyses. *The International Journal of Behavioral Nutrition and Physical Activity*, *14*(1), Article 42. https://doi.org/10.1186/s12966-017-0494-y

Sanders, M. R. (2012). Development, evaluation, and multinational dissemination of the Triple P-Positive Parenting Program. *Annual Review of Clinical Psychology*, *8*(1), 345–379. https://doi.org/10.1146/annurev-clinpsy-032511-143104

Sanders, M. R., Kirby, J. N., Tellegen, C. L., & Day, J. J. (2014). The Triple P-Positive Parenting Program: A systematic review and meta-analysis of a multi-level system of parenting support. *Clinical Psychology Review*, *34*(4), 337–357. https://doi.org/10.1016/j.cpr.2014.04.003

Sanders, M. R., & Murphey-Brennan, M. (2010). The international dissemination of the Triple P-Positive Parenting Program. In J. R. Weisz & A. E. Kazdin (Eds.), *Evidence-based psychotherapies for children and adolescents* (2nd ed., pp. 519–537). Guilford Press.

Santo, L., & Okeyode, T. (2018). *National ambulatory medical care survey: 2018 national summary tables*. U.S. Department of Health and Human Services, Centers for Disease Control and Prevention, National Center for Health Statistics. https://www.cdc.gov/nchs/data/ahcd/namcs_summary/2018-namcs-web-tables-508.pdf

Santoro, N., Roeca, C., Peters, B. A., & Neal-Perry, G. (2021). The menopause transition: Signs, symptoms, and management options. *The Journal of Clinical Endocrinology and Metabolism*, *106*(1), 1–15. https://doi.org/10.1210/clinem/dgaa764

Sara, J. D. S., Toya, T., Ahmad, A., Clark, M. M., Gilliam, W. P., Lerman, L. O., & Lerman, A. (2022). Mental stress and its effects on vascular health. *Mayo Clinic Proceedings*, *97*(5), 951–990. https://doi.org/10.1016/j.mayocp.2022.02.004

Sathianathen, N. J., Hwang, E. C., Mian, R., Bodie, J. A., Soubra, A., Lyon, J. A., Sultan, S., & Dahm, P. (2021). Selective serotonin re-uptake inhibitors for premature ejaculation in adult men: A Cochrane systematic review. *The World Journal of Men's Health*, *40*(2), 257–263. https://doi.org/10.5534/wjmh.210155

Saunders, J. B., Aasland, O. G., Babor, T. F., de la Fuente, J. R., & Grant, M. (1993). Development of the Alcohol Use Disorders Identification Test (AUDIT): WHO collaborative project on early detection of persons with harmful alcohol consumption-II. *Addiction*, *88*(6), 791–804. https://doi.org/10.1111/j.1360-0443.1993.tb02093.x

Sayed, S., Iacoviello, B. M., & Charney, D. S. (2015). Risk factors for the development of psychopathology following trauma. *Current Psychiatry Reports*, *17*(8), Article 70. https://doi.org/10.1007/s11920-015-0612-y

Saynisch, P. A., David, G., Ukert, B., Agiro, A., Scholle, S. H., & Oberlander, T. (2021). Model homes: Evaluating approaches to patient-centered medical home implementation. *Medical Care*, *59*(3), 206–212. https://doi.org/10.1097/MLR.0000000000001497

Schein, J., Houle, C., Urganus, A., Cloutier, M., Patterson-Lomba, O., Wang, Y., King, S., Levinson, W., Guérin, A., Lefebvre, P., & Davis, L. L. (2021). Prevalence of post-traumatic stress disorder in the United States: A systematic literature review. *Current Medical Research and Opinion*, *37*(12), 2151–2161. https://doi.org/10.1080/03007995.2021.1978417

Schmidt, H. M., Munder, T., Gerger, H., Frühauf, S., & Barth, J. (2014). Combination of psychological intervention and phosphodiesterase-5 inhibitors for erectile dysfunction: A narrative review and meta-analysis. *Journal of Sexual Medicine*, *11*(6), 1376–1391. https://doi.org/10.1111/jsm.12520

Schmidt, S., Andersen Nexø, M., Norgaard, O., Willaing, I., Pedersen-Bjergaard, U., Skinner, T. C., & Nørgaard, K. (2020). Psychosocial factors associated with HbA1c in adults with insulin pump-treated Type 1 diabetes: A systematic review. *Diabetic Medicine*, *37*(9), 1454–1462. https://doi.org/10.1111/dme.14347

Schmidt, S., Madsen, K. P., Pedersen-Bjergaard, U., Rytter, K., Hommel, E., Cleal, B., Willaing, I., Andersen, H. U., & Nørgaard, K. (2023). Associations between clinical and psychosocial factors and HbA1c in adult insulin pump users with Type 1 diabetes. *Acta Diabetologica, 60*(8), 1089–1097. https://doi.org/10.1007/s00592-023-02081-4

Schmitt, A., Gahr, A., Hermanns, N., Kulzer, B., Huber, J., & Haak, T. (2013). The Diabetes Self-Management Questionnaire (DSMQ): Development and evaluation of an instrument to assess diabetes self-care activities associated with glycaemic control. *Health and Quality of Life Outcomes, 11*(1), Article 138. https://doi.org/10.1186/1477-7525-11-138

Schmitt, A., Kulzer, B., Ehrmann, D., Haak, T., & Hermanns, N. (2022). A self-report measure of diabetes self-management for Type 1 and Type 2 diabetes: The Diabetes Self-Management Questionnaire-Revised (DSMQ-R)—Clinimetric evidence from five studies. *Frontiers in Clinical Diabetes and Healthcare, 2*, Article 30. https://doi.org/10.3389/fcdhc.2021.823046

Schmitt, A., Reimer, A., Hermanns, N., Huber, J., Ehrmann, D., Schall, S., & Kulzer, B. (2016). Assessing diabetes self-management with the Diabetes Self-Management Questionnaire (DSMQ) can help analyse behavioural problems related to reduced glycaemic control. *PLOS ONE, 11*(3), Article e0150774. https://doi.org/10.1371/journal.pone.0150774

Schneider, E. C., Shah, A., Doty, M. M., Tikkanen, R., Fields, K., & Williams, R. D., II. (2021). *Mirror, mirror 2021 reflecting poorly: Health care in the U.S. compared to other high-income countries.* https://www.commonwealthfund.org/publications/fund-reports/2021/aug/mirror-mirror-2021-reflecting-poorly

Seelert, K. R., Hill, R. D., Rigdon, M. A., & Schwenzfeier, E. (1999). Measuring patient distress in primary care. *Family Medicine, 31*(7), 483–487.

Seesing, F. M., Drost, G., Groenewoud, J., van der Wilt, G. J., & van Engelen, B. G. M. (2014). Shared medical appointments improve QOL in neuromuscular patients: A randomized controlled trial. *Neurology, 83*(3), 240–246. https://doi.org/10.1212/WNL.0000000000000588

Seitz, D. P. (2005). Screening mnemonic for generalized anxiety disorder. *Canadian Family Physician, 51*(10), 1340–1342. https://www.ncbi.nlm.nih.gov/pmc/articles/PMC1479789/

Selph, S. S., & McDonagh, M. S. (2019). Depression in children and adolescents: Evaluation and treatment. *American Family Physician, 100*(10), 609–617. https://pubmed.ncbi.nlm.nih.gov/31730312/

Semans, J. H. (1956). Premature ejaculation: A new approach. *Southern Medical Journal, 49*(4), 353–358. https://pubmed.ncbi.nlm.nih.gov/13311629/

Semper, H. M., Povey, R., & Clark-Carter, D. (2016). A systematic review of the effectiveness of smartphone applications that encourage dietary self-regulatory strategies for weight loss in overweight and obese adults. *Obesity Reviews, 17*(9), 895–906. https://doi.org/10.1111/obr.12428

Serrano, N., Cordes, C., Cubic, B., & Daub, S. (2018). The state and future of the primary care behavioral health model of service delivery workforce. *Journal of Clinical Psychology in Medical Settings, 25*(2), 157–168. https://doi.org/10.1007/s10880-017-9491-1

Seshadri, A., Orth, S. S., Adaji, A., Singh, B., Clark, M. M., Frye, M. A., McGillivray, J., & Fuller-Tyszkiewicz, M. (2021). Mindfulness-based cognitive therapy, acceptance and commitment therapy, and positive psychotherapy for major depression. *American Journal of Psychotherapy, 74*(1), 4–12. https://doi.org/10.1176/appi.psychotherapy.20200006

Shadish, W. R., & Baldwin, S. A. (2005). Effects of behavioral marital therapy: A meta-analysis of randomized controlled trials. *Journal of Consulting and Clinical Psychology, 73*(1), 6–14. https://doi.org/10.1037/0022-006X.73.1.6

Shaeer, O., & Shaeer, K. (2012). The Global Online Sexuality Survey (GOSS): The United States of America in 2011. Chapter I: Erectile dysfunction among English-speakers. *Journal of Sexual Medicine, 9*(12), 3018–3027. https://doi.org/10.1111/j.1743-6109.2012.02976.x

Shapiro, L. E. (2022). *Generalized anxiety disorder workbook: CBT activities to manage anxiety, cope with uncertainty, and overcome stress.* PESI Publishing.

Sharpe, L., Dudeney, J., Williams, A. C. C., Nicholas, M., McPhee, I., Baillie, A., Welgampola, M., & McGuire, B. (2019). Psychological therapies for the prevention of migraine in adults. *Cochrane Database of Systematic Reviews, 7,* Article CD012295. https://doi.org/10.1002/14651858.CD012295.pub2

Shaw, E., Levitt, C., Wong, S., Kaczorowski, J., & the McMaster University Postpartum Research Group. (2006). Systematic review of the literature on postpartum care: Effectiveness of postpartum support to improve maternal parenting, mental health, quality of life, and physical health. *Birth, 33*(3), 210–220. https://doi.org/10.1111/j.1523-536X.2006.00106.x

Shear, M. K. (2015). Clinical practice: Complicated grief. *The New England Journal of Medicine, 372*(2), 153–160. https://doi.org/10.1056/NEJMcp1315618

Shear, M. K., Simon, N., Wall, M., Zisook, S., Neimeyer, R., Duan, N., Reynolds, C., Lebowitz, B., Sung, S., Ghesquiere, A., Gorscak, B., Clayton, P., Ito, M., Nakajima, S., Konishi, T., Melhem, N., Meert, K., Schiff, M., O'Connor, M. F., . . . Keshaviah, A. (2011). Complicated grief and related bereavement issues for *DSM-5. Depression and Anxiety, 28*(2), 103–117. https://doi.org/10.1002/da.20780

Shepardson, R. L., Buchholz, L. J., Weisberg, R. B., & Funderburk, J. S. (2018). Psychological interventions for anxiety in adult primary care patients: A review and recommendations for future research. *Journal of Anxiety Disorders, 54,* 71–86. https://doi.org/10.1016/j.janxdis.2017.12.004

Sherin, K. M. (n.d.). *Hurt, Insult, Threaten, Scream (HITS) score.* MDCalc. https://www.mdcalc.com/calc/10417/hurt-insult-threaten-scream-hits-score

Sherin, K. M., Sinacore, J. M., Li, X. Q., Zitter, R. E., & Shakil, A. (1998). HITS: A short domestic violence screening tool for use in a family practice setting. *Family Medicine, 30*(7), 508–512. https://www.researchgate.net/publication/13616105

Shield, K. D., Parry, C., & Rehm, J. (2014). Chronic diseases and conditions related to alcohol use. *Alcohol Research: Current Reviews, 35*(2), 155–173. https://www.ncbi.nlm.nih.gov/pmc/articles/PMC3908707/pdf/arcr-35-2-155.pdf

Shiina, A., Nakazato, M., Mitsumori, M., Koizumi, H., Shimizu, E., Fujisaki, M., & Iyo, M. (2005). An open trial of outpatient group therapy for bulimic disorders: Combination program of cognitive behavioral therapy with assertive training and self-esteem enhancement. *Psychiatry and Clinical Neurosciences, 59*(6), 690–696. https://doi.org/10.1111/j.1440-1819.2005.01438.x

Shulman, K. I. (2000). Clock-drawing: Is it the ideal cognitive screening test? *International Journal of Geriatric Psychiatry, 15*(6), 548–561. https://doi.org/10.1002/1099-1166(200006)15:6<548::aid-gps242>3.0.co;2-u

Sibley, M. H., Kuriyan, A. B., Evans, S. W., Waxmonsky, J. G., & Smith, B. H. (2014). Pharmacological and psychosocial treatments for adolescents with ADHD: An updated systematic review of the literature. *Clinical Psychology Review, 34*(3), 218–232. https://doi.org/10.1016/j.cpr.2014.02.001

Silberman, S. A. (2008). *The insomnia workbook: A comprehensive guide to getting the sleep you need.* New Harbinger Publications.

Silverstein, M., Hironaka, L. K., Walter, H. J., Feinberg, E., Sandler, J., Pellicer, M., Chen, N., & Cabral, H. (2015). Collaborative care for children with ADHD symptoms: A randomized comparative effectiveness trial. *Pediatrics, 135*(4), e858–e867. https://doi.org/10.1542/peds.2014-3221

Simon, G. E., Katon, W. J., Lin, E. H., Rutter, C., Manning, W. G., Von Korff, M., Ciechanowski, P., Ludman, E. J., & Young, B. A. (2007). Cost-effectiveness of systematic depression treatment among people with diabetes mellitus. *Archives of General Psychiatry, 64*(1), 65–72. https://doi.org/10.1001/archpsyc.64.1.65

Simon & Schuster. (2020). *The postpartum depression workbook* [Cover copy]. https://www.simonandschuster.com/books/The-Postpartum-Depression-Workbook/Abigail-Burd/9781647398378

Siqueira, G. S. A., Hagemann, P. M. S., Coelho, D. S., Santos, F. H. D., & Bertolucci, P. H. F. (2019). Can MoCA and MMSE be interchangeable cognitive screening tools? A systematic review. *The Gerontologist, 59*(6), e743–e763. https://doi.org/10.1093/geront/gny126

Siu, A. L., Bibbins-Domingo, K., Grossman, D. C., Baumann, L. C., Davidson, K. W., Ebell, M., García, F. A., Gillman, M., Herzstein, J., Kemper, A. R., Krist, A. H., Kurth, A. E., Owens, D. K., Phillips, W. R., Phipps, M. G., & Pignone, M. P. (2016). Screening for depression in adults: U.S. Preventive Services Task Force recommendation statement. *JAMA, 315*(4), 380–387. https://doi.org/10.1001/jama.2015.18392

Skinner, T. C., Joensen, L., & Parkin, T. (2020). Twenty-five years of diabetes distress research. *Diabetic Medicine, 37*(3), 393–400. https://doi.org/10.1111/dme.14157

Slee, A., Nazareth, I., Bondaronek, P., Liu, Y., Cheng, Z., & Freemantle, N. (2019). Pharmacological treatments for generalised anxiety disorder: A systematic review and network meta-analysis. *The Lancet, 393*(10173), 768–777. https://doi.org/10.1016/S0140-6736(18)31793-8

Slobodin, O., & Masalha, R. (2020). Challenges in ADHD care for ethnic minority children: A review of the current literature. *Transcultural Psychiatry, 57*(3), 468–483. https://doi.org/10.1177/1363461520902885

Smit, E. S., Hoving, C., Schelleman-Offermans, K., West, R., & de Vries, H. (2014). Predictors of successful and unsuccessful quit attempts among smokers motivated to quit. *Addictive Behaviors, 39*(9), 1318–1324. https://doi.org/10.1016/j.addbeh.2014.04.017

Smith, J. D., Cruden, G. H., Rojas, L. M., Van Ryzin, M., Fu, E., Davis, M. M., Landsverk, J., & Brown, C. H. (2020). Parenting interventions in pediatric primary care: A systematic review. *Pediatrics, 146*(1), Article e20193548. https://doi.org/10.1542/peds.2019-3548

Smith, K. J., Deschênes, S. S., & Schmitz, N. (2018). Investigating the longitudinal association between diabetes and anxiety: A systematic review and meta-analysis. *Diabetic Medicine, 35*(6), 677–693. https://doi.org/10.1111/dme.13606

Smith, L., Shin, J. I., Carmichael, C., Oh, H., Jacob, L., López Sánchez, G. F., Tully, M. A., Barnett, Y., Butler, L., McDermott, D. T., & Koyanagi, A. (2021). Prevalence and correlates of multiple suicide attempts among adolescents aged 12–15 years from 61 countries in Africa, Asia, and the Americas. *Journal of Psychiatric Research, 144*, 45–53. https://doi.org/10.1016/j.jpsychires.2021.09.047

Smith, P. C., Schmidt, S. M., Allensworth-Davies, D., & Saitz, R. (2009). Primary care validation of a single-question alcohol screening test. *Journal of General Internal Medicine, 24*(7), 783–788. https://doi.org/10.1007/s11606-009-0928-6

Smith, P. C., Schmidt, S. M., Allensworth-Davies, D., & Saitz, R. (2010). A single-question screening test for drug use in primary care. *Archives of Internal Medicine, 170*(13), 1155–1160. https://doi.org/10.1001/archinternmed.2010.140

Smith, T. B., & Trimble, J. E. (2016). *Foundations of multicultural psychology: Research to inform effective practice.* American Psychological Association. https://doi.org/10.1037/14733-000

Sockol, L. E., Epperson, C. N., & Barber, J. P. (2011). A meta-analysis of treatments for perinatal depression. *Clinical Psychology Review, 31*(5), 839–849. https://doi.org/10.1016/j.cpr.2011.03.009

Sofianou, A., Martynenko, M., Wolf, M. S., Wisnivesky, J. P., Krauskopf, K., Wilson, E. A., Goel, M. S., Leventhal, H., Halm, E. A., & Federman, A. D. (2013). Asthma beliefs are associated with medication adherence in older asthmatics. *Journal of General Internal Medicine, 28*(1), 67–73. https://doi.org/10.1007/s11606-012-2160-z

Sohal, H. (n.d.). *Humiliation, afraid, rape, kick (HARK).* MDCalc. https://www.mdcalc.com/calc/10420/humiliation-afraid-rape-kick-hark

Sohal, H., Eldridge, S., & Feder, G. (2007). The sensitivity and specificity of four questions (HARK) to identify intimate partner violence: A diagnostic accuracy study in general practice. *BMC Family Practice, 8*(1), Article 49. https://doi.org/10.1186/1471-2296-8-49

Soones, T. N., Lin, J. L., Wolf, M. S., O'Conor, R., Martynenko, M., Wisnivesky, J. P., & Federman, A. D. (2017). Pathways linking health literacy, health beliefs, and cognition to medication adherence in older adults with asthma. *The Journal of Allergy and Clinical Immunology, 139*(3), 804–809. https://doi.org/10.1016/j.jaci.2016.05.043

Spanier, G. B. (1976). Measuring dyadic adjustment: New scales for assessing the quality of marriage and similar dyads. *Journal of Marriage and Family, 38*(1), 15–28. https://doi.org/10.2307/350547

Spann, S. J., Nutting, P. A., Galliher, J. M., Peterson, K. A., Pavlik, V. N., Dickinson, L. M., & Volk, R. J. (2006). Management of Type 2 diabetes in the primary care setting: A practice-based research network study. *Annals of Family Medicine, 4*(1), 23–31. https://doi.org/10.1370/afm.420

Spithoff, S., & Kahan, M. (2015). Primary care management of alcohol use disorder and at-risk drinking: Part 2: Counsel, prescribe, connect. *Canadian Family Physician, 61*(6), 515–521. https://www.ncbi.nlm.nih.gov/pmc/articles/PMC4463892/

Spitzer, R. L., Kroenke, K., & Williams, J. B. (1999). Validation and utility of a self-report version of PRIME-MD: The PHQ primary care study. *JAMA, 282*(18), 1737–1744. https://doi.org/10.1001/jama.282.18.1737

Spitzer, R. L., Kroenke, K., Williams, J. B. W., & Löwe, B. (2006). A brief measure for assessing generalized anxiety disorder: The GAD-7. *Archives of Internal Medicine, 166*(10), 1092–1097. https://doi.org/10.1001/archinte.166.10.1092

Spitzer, R. L., Williams, J. B. W., & Kroenke, K. (2016). *Patient Health Questionnaire (PHQ)*. https://www.phqscreeners.com/images/sites/g/files/g10060481/f/201412/English_0.pdf

Stanley, M. A., Hopko, D. R., Diefenbach, G. J., Bourland, S. L., Rodriguez, H., & Wagener, P. (2003). Cognitive-behavior therapy for late-life generalized anxiety disorder in primary care: Preliminary findings. *The American Journal of Geriatric Psychiatry, 11*(1), 92–96.

Stead, L. F., Perera, R., Bullen, C., Mant, D., Hartmann-Boyce, J., Cahill, K., & Lancaster, T. (2012). Nicotine replacement therapy for smoking cessation. *Cochrane Database of Systematic Reviews, 11*, Article CD000146. https://doi.org/10.1002/14651858.CD000146.pub4

Stein, A. T., Carl, E., Cuijpers, P., Karyotaki, E., & Smits, J. A. J. (2021). Looking beyond depression: A meta-analysis of the effect of behavioral activation on depression, anxiety, and activation. *Psychological Medicine, 51*(9), 1491–1504. https://doi.org/10.1017/S0033291720000239

Steinman, L. E., Frederick, J. T., Prohaska, T., Satariano, W. A., Dornberg-Lee, S., Fisher, R., Graub, P. B., Leith, K., Presby, K., Sharkey, J., Snyder, S., Turner, D., Wilson, N., Yagoda, L., Unutzer, J., Snowden, M., & the Late Life Depression Special Interest Project (SIP) Panelists. (2007). Recommendations for treating depression in community-based older adults. *American Journal of Preventive Medicine, 33*(3), 175–181. https://doi.org/10.1016/j.amepre.2007.04.034

Stephenson, K. R., Truong, L., & Shimazu, L. (2018). Why is impaired sexual function distressing to men? Consequences of impaired male sexual function and their associations with sexual well-being. *Journal of Sexual Medicine, 15*(9), 1336–1349. https://doi.org/10.1016/j.jsxm.2018.07.014

Stewart, J. C., Perkins, A. J., & Callahan, C. M. (2014). Effect of collaborative care for depression on risk of cardiovascular events: Data from the IMPACT randomized controlled trial. *Psychosomatic Medicine, 76*(1), 29–37. https://doi.org/10.1097/PSY.0000000000000022

Stierman, B., Afful, J., Carroll, M. D., Chen, T.-C., Davy, O., Fink, S., Fryar, C. D., Gu, Q., Hales, C. M., Hughes, J. P., Ostchega, Y., Storandt, R. J., & Akinbami, L. J. (2021). National health and nutrition examination survey 2017–March 2020 prepandemic data files—Development of files and prevalence estimates for selected health outcomes. *National Health Statistics Reports, 158*.

Strosahl, K. D., & Robinson, P. J. (2008). The primary care behavioral health model: Applications to prevention, acute care and chronic condition management. In R. Keesler & D. Stafford (Eds.), *Collaborative medicine case studies: Evidence in practice* (pp. 85–95). Springer. https://doi.org/10.1007/978-0-387-76894-6_8

Strosahl, K. D., & Robinson, P. J. (2017). *The mindfulness and acceptance workbook for depression: Using acceptance and commitment therapy to move through depression and create a life worth living* (2nd ed.). New Harbinger Publications.

Strosahl, K. D., Robinson, P. J., & Gustavsson, T. (2012). *Brief interventions for radical change: Principles and practice of focused acceptance and commitment therapy.* New Harbinger Publications.

Stubbs, B., & Rosenbaum, S. (2018). *Exercise-based interventions for mental illness: Physical activity as part of clinical treatment.* Academic Press.

Styne, D. M., Arslanian, S. A., Connor, E. L., Farooqi, I. S., Murad, M. H., Silverstein, J. H., & Yanovski, J. A. (2017). Pediatric obesity—Assessment, treatment, and prevention: An Endocrine Society clinical practice guideline. *The Journal of Clinical Endocrinology and Metabolism, 102*(3), 709–757. https://doi.org/10.1210/jc.2016-2573

Substance Abuse and Mental Health Services Administration. (2014). *Advancing behavioral health integration within NCQA recognized patient-centered medical homes.* SAMHSA-HRSA Center for Integrated Health Solutions. https://brsstacs.center4si.com/Behavioral_Health_Integration.pdf

Substance Abuse and Mental Health Services Administration. (2016). *Preventing prescription drug misuse: Understanding who is at risk.* https://www.michigan.gov/documents/mdhhs/UnderstandingWhoIsAtRisk_547024_7.pdf

Substance Abuse and Mental Health Services Administration. (2018a). *Key substance use and mental health indicators in the United States: Results from the 2017 National Survey on Drug Use and Health* (HHS Publication No. SMA 18-5068, NSDUH Series H-53). https://www.samhsa.gov/data/sites/default/files/cbhsq-reports/NSDUHFFR2017/NSDUHFFR2017.pdf

Substance Abuse and Mental Health Services Administration. (2018b). *National survey on drug use and health: Detailed tables. Table 2.51B—Alcohol use in lifetime, past year, and past month and binge and heavy alcohol use in past month among persons aged 21 or older, by demographic characteristics: Percentages, 2016 and 2017.* https://www.samhsa.gov/data/sites/default/files/cbhsq-reports/NSDUHDetailedTabs2017/NSDUHDetailedTabs2017.htm#tab2-51B

Substance Abuse and Mental Health Services Administration. (2021a). *Key substance use and mental health indicators in the United States: Results from the 2020 National Survey on Drug Use and Health* (HHS Publication No. PEP21-07-01-003, NSDUH Series H-56). Center for Behavioral Health Statistics and Quality, Substance Abuse and Mental Health Services Administration. https://www.samhsa.gov/data/report/2020-nsduh-annual-national-report

Substance Abuse and Mental Health Services Administration. (2021b). *Medications for opioid use disorder: For healthcare and addiction professionals, policymakers, patients, and families* (TIP 63, Publication No. PEP21-02-01-002). https://store.samhsa.gov/sites/default/files/pep21-02-01-002.pdf

Substance Abuse and Mental Health Services Administration. (2022, August 12). *Screening, brief intervention, and referral to treatment (SBIRT).* https://www.samhsa.gov/sbirt

Sundquist, J., Lilja, Å., Palmér, K., Memon, A. A., Wang, X., Johansson, L. M., & Sundquist, K. (2015). Mindfulness group therapy in primary care patients with depression, anxiety and stress and adjustment disorders: Randomised controlled trial. *The British Journal of Psychiatry, 206*(2), 128–135. https://doi.org/10.1192/bjp.bp.114.150243

Sveinsdottir, V., Eriksen, H. R., & Reme, S. E. (2012). Assessing the role of cognitive behavioral therapy in the management of chronic nonspecific back pain. *Journal of Pain Research, 5,* 371–380. https://doi.org/10.2147/JPR.S25330

Swanson, S. A., Eyllon, M., Sheu, Y. H., & Miller, M. (2021). Firearm access and adolescent suicide risk: Toward a clearer understanding of effect size. *Injury Prevention*, 27(3), 264–270. https://doi.org/10.1136/injuryprev-2019-043605

Swartz, K., & Collins, L. G. (2019). Caregiver care. *American Family Physician*, 99(11), 699–706. https://www.aafp.org/dam/brand/aafp/pubs/afp/issues/2019/0601/p699.pdf

Swift, D. L., Johannsen, N. M., Lavie, C. J., Earnest, C. P., & Church, T. S. (2014). The role of exercise and physical activity in weight loss and maintenance. *Progress in Cardiovascular Diseases*, 56(4), 441–447. https://doi.org/10.1016/j.pcad.2013.09.012

Symonds, T., Perelman, M. A., Althof, S., Giuliano, F., Martin, M., May, K., Abraham, L., Crossland, A., & Morris, M. (2007). Development and validation of a premature ejaculation diagnostic tool. *European Urology*, 52(2), 565–573. https://doi.org/10.1016/j.eururo.2007.01.028

Tariq, S. H., Tumosa, N., Chibnall, J. T., Perry, H. M., III, & Morley, J. E. (2006). *The Saint Louis University (SLU) Mental Status Exam*. Saint Louis University School of Medicine. https://www.slu.edu/medicine/internal-medicine/geriatric-medicine/aging-successfully/assessment-tools/mental-status-exam.php

Tavares, I. M., Laan, E. T. M., & Nobre, P. J. (2018). Sexual inhibition is a vulnerability factor for orgasm problems in women. *Journal of Sexual Medicine*, 15(3), 361–372. https://doi.org/10.1016/j.jsxm.2017.12.015

Taylor, S. J. C., Pinnock, H., Epiphaniou, E., Pearce, G., Parke, H. L., Schwappach, A., Purushotham, N., Jacob, S., Griffiths, C. J., Greenhalgh, T., & Sheikh, A. (2014). A rapid synthesis of the evidence on interventions supporting self-management for long-term conditions: PRISMS—Practical systematic review of self-management support for long-term conditions. *Health Services and Delivery Research*, 2(53), 1–580. https://doi.org/10.3310/hsdr02530

Taylor & Francis Group. (2020). *Managing hot flushes and night sweats* [Cover copy]. https://www.taylorfrancis.com/books/mono/10.4324/9781003000761/managing-hot-flushes-night-sweats-myra-hunter-melanie-smith

Tchero, H., Kangambega, P., Briatte, C., Brunet-Houdard, S., Retali, G. R., & Rusch, E. (2019). Clinical effectiveness of telemedicine in diabetes mellitus: A meta-analysis of 42 randomized controlled trials. *Telemedicine Journal and e-Health*, 25(7), 569–583. https://doi.org/10.1089/tmj.2018.0128

Telch, M. J., & Pujols, Y. (2013). The Erectile Performance Anxiety Index: Scale development and psychometric properties. *Journal of Sexual Medicine*, 10(12), 3019–3028. https://doi.org/10.1111/jsm.12305

Thomas, R., Abell, B., Webb, H. J., Avdagic, E., & Zimmer-Gembeck, M. J. (2017). Parent–child interaction therapy: A meta-analysis. *Pediatrics*, 140(3), Article e20170352. https://doi.org/10.1542/peds.2017-0352

Thomas, R., & Zimmer-Gembeck, M. J. (2007). Behavioral outcomes of parent–child interaction therapy and Triple P—Positive Parenting Program: A review and meta-analysis. *Journal of Abnormal Child Psychology*, 35, 475–495. https://doi.org/10.1007/s10802-007-9104-9

Thompson, E. M., Destree, L., Albertella, L., & Fontenelle, L. F. (2021). Internet-based acceptance and commitment therapy: A transdiagnostic systematic review and meta-analysis for mental health outcomes. *Behavior Therapy*, 52(2), 492–507. https://doi.org/10.1016/j.beth.2020.07.002

Tolin, D. (2012). *Face your fears: A proven plan to beat anxiety, panic, phobias, and obsessions*. Turner Publishing Company.

Tomaszewski, M., White, C., Patel, P., Masca, N., Damani, R., Hepworth, J., Samani, N. J., Gupta, P., Madira, W., Stanley, A., & Williams, B. (2014). High rates of non-adherence to antihypertensive treatment revealed by high-performance liquid chromatography-tandem mass spectrometry (HP LC-MS/MS) urine analysis. *Heart*, 100(11), 855–861. https://doi.org/10.1136/heartjnl-2013-305063

Topolski, T. D., LoGerfo, J., Patrick, D. L., Williams, B., Walwick, J., & Patrick, M. B. (2006). The Rapid Assessment of Physical Activity (RAPA) among older adults. *Pre-*

venting Chronic Disease, *3*(4), Article A118. https://www.ncbi.nlm.nih.gov/pubmed/16978493

Townend, J., Minelli, C., Mortimer, K., Obaseki, D. O., Al Ghobain, M., Cherkaski, H., Denguezli, M., Gunesekera, K., Hafizi, H., Koul, P. A., Loh, L. C., Nejjari, C., Patel, J., Sooronbayev, T., Buist, S. A., & Burney, P. G. J. (2017). The association between chronic airflow obstruction and poverty in 12 sites of the multinational BOLD study. *The European Respiratory Journal*, *49*(6), Article 1601880. https://doi.org/10.1183/13993003.01880-2016

Trauer, J. M., Qian, M. Y., Doyle, J. S., Rajaratnam, S. M., & Cunnington, D. (2015). Cognitive behavioral therapy for chronic insomnia: A systematic review and meta-analysis. *Annals of Internal Medicine*, *163*(3), 191–204. https://doi.org/10.7326/M14-2841

Trevor Project. (2022). *2022 national survey on LGBTQ youth mental health*. https://www.thetrevorproject.org/survey-2022/

Troxel, W. M., Germain, A., & Buysse, D. J. (2012). Clinical management of insomnia with brief behavioral treatment (BBTI). *Behavioral Sleep Medicine*, *10*(4), 266–279. https://doi.org/10.1080/15402002.2011.607200

Tsao, C. W., Aday, A. W., Almarzooq, Z. I., Alonso, A., Beaton, A. Z., Bittencourt, M. S., Boehme, A. K., Buxton, A. E., Carson, A. P., Commodore-Mensah, Y., Elkind, M. S. V., Evenson, K. R., Eze-Nliam, C., Ferguson, J. F., Generoso, G., Ho, J. E., Kalani, R., Khan, S. S., Kissela, B. R., . . . Martin, S. S. (2022). Heart disease and stroke statistics—2022 update: A report from the American Heart Association. *Circulation*, *145*(8), e153–e639. https://doi.org/10.1161/CIR.0000000000001052

Tully, P. J., Harrison, N. J., Cheung, P., & Cosh, S. (2016). Anxiety and cardiovascular disease risk: A review. *Current Cardiology Reports*, *18*(12), Article 120. https://doi.org/10.1007/s11886-016-0800-3

Turk, D. C., Fillingim, R. B., Ohrbach, R., & Patel, K. V. (2016). Assessment of psychosocial and functional impact of chronic pain. *The Journal of Pain*, *17*(9, Suppl.), T21–T49. https://doi.org/10.1016/j.jpain.2016.02.006

Twiddy, H., Lane, N., Chawla, R., Johnson, S., Bradshaw, A., Aleem, S., & Mawdsley, L. (2015). The development and delivery of a female chronic pelvic pain management programme: A specialised interdisciplinary approach. *British Journal of Pain*, *9*(4), 233–240. https://doi.org/10.1177/2049463715584408

Uchendu, C., & Blake, H. (2017). Effectiveness of cognitive-behavioural therapy on glycaemic control and psychological outcomes in adults with diabetes mellitus: A systematic review and meta-analysis of randomized controlled trials. *Diabetic Medicine*, *34*(3), 328–339. https://doi.org/10.1111/dme.13195

Ulmer, C. S., Bosworth, H. B., Beckham, J. C., Germain, A., Jeffreys, A. S., Edelman, D., Macy, S., Kirby, A., & Voils, C. I. (2017). Veterans Affairs primary care provider perceptions of insomnia treatment. *Journal of Clinical Sleep Medicine*, *13*(8), 991–999. https://doi.org/10.5664/jcsm.6702

University of Wisconsin Population Health Institute. (2014). *County health rankings model*. County Health Rankings & Roadmaps. https://www.countyhealthrankings.org/explore-health-rankings/measures-data-sources/county-health-rankings-model

Uphoff, E., Ekers, D., Robertson, L., Dawson, S., Sanger, E., South, E., Samaan, Z., Richards, D., Meader, N., & Churchill, R. (2020). Behavioural activation therapy for depression in adults. *Cochrane Database of Systematic Reviews*, *7*, Article CD013305. https://doi.org/10.1002/14651858.CD013305.pub2

Upside Health. (n.d.). *Get the branch health app*. https://upside.health/patients/

Urology Care Foundation. (2014). *Diagnosing erectile dysfunction: What you should know*.

U.S. Department of Agriculture & U.S. Department of Health and Human Services. (2020). *Dietary guidelines for Americans, 2020–2025* (9th ed.). https://www.dietaryguidelines.gov/sites/default/files/2021-03/Dietary_Guidelines_for_Americans-2020-2025.pdf

U.S. Department of Health and Human Services. (2000). *The practical guide: Identification, evaluation, and treatment of overweight and obesity in adults* (NIH Publication No. 00-

4084). National Institutes of Health. https://www.nhlbi.nih.gov/guidelines/obesity/prctgd_c.pdf

U.S. Department of Health and Human Services. (2003). *Your guide to lowering blood pressure* (NIH Publication No. 03-5232). National Institutes of Health. https://www.nhlbi.nih.gov/files/docs/public/heart/hbp_low.pdf

U.S. Department of Health and Human Services. (2006). *Your guide to lowering your blood pressure with DASH* (NIH Publication No. 06-4082). National Institutes of Health. https://www.nhlbi.nih.gov/files/docs/public/heart/new_dash.pdf

U.S. Department of Health and Human Services. (2013). *Managing overweight and obesity in adults: Systematic evidence review from the obesity expert panel, 2013*. https://www.nhlbi.nih.gov/sites/default/files/media/docs/obesity-evidence-review.pdf

U.S. Department of Health and Human Services. (2016). *Facing addiction in America: The Surgeon General's report on alcohol, drugs, and health*. https://addiction.surgeongeneral.gov/sites/default/files/surgeon-generals-report.pdf

U.S. Department of Health and Human Services. (2020). *Smoking cessation: A report of the Surgeon General*. Office on Smoking and Health, National Center for Chronic Disease Prevention and Health Promotion. https://www.cdc.gov/tobacco/sgr/2020-smoking-cessation/index.html#full-report

U.S. Department of Veterans Affairs and Department of Defense. (2017). *VA/DoD clinical practice guideline for the management of posttraumatic stress disorder and acute stress disorder*. https://www.healthquality.va.gov/guidelines/MH/ptsd/VADoDPTSDCPGFinal012418.pdf

U.S. Department of Veterans Affairs and Department of Defense. (2019a). *VA/DoD clinical practice guideline for the assessment and management of patients at risk for suicide*. https://www.healthquality.va.gov/guidelines/MH/srb/VADoDSuicideRiskFullCPGFinal5088212019.pdf

U.S. Department of Veterans Affairs and Department of Defense. (2019b). *VA/DoD clinical practice guideline for the primary care management of asthma*. https://www.healthquality.va.gov/guidelines/CD/asthma/VADoDAsthmaCPGFinal121019.pdf

U.S. Department of Veterans Affairs and Department of Defense. (2021). *VA/DoD clinical practice guideline for the management of chronic obstructive pulmonary disease*. https://www.healthquality.va.gov/guidelines/CD/copd/VADoDCOPDCPG.pdf

U.S. Department of Veterans Affairs and Department of Defense. (2022). *VA/DoD clinical practice guideline for the management of major depressive disorder*. https://www.healthquality.va.gov/guidelines/MH/mdd/VADoDMDDCPGFinal508.pdf

U.S. Food and Drug Administration. (2022). *Sodium in your diet: Use the nutrition facts label and reduce your intake*. https://www.fda.gov/food/nutrition-education-resources-materials/sodium-your-diet

Valero-Aguayo, L., Rodríguez-Bocanegra, M., Ferro-García, R., & Ascanio-Velasco, L. (2021). Meta-analysis of the efficacy and effectiveness of parent child interaction therapy (PCIT) for child behaviour problems. *Psicothema, 33*(4), 544–555. https://doi.org/10.7334/psicothema2021.70

van Boeijen, C. A., van Oppen, P., van Balkom, A. J. L. M., Visser, S., Kempe, P. T., Blankenstein, N., & van Dyck, R. (2005). Treatment of anxiety disorders in primary care practice: A randomised controlled trial. *The British Journal of General Practice, 55*(519), 763–769. https://www.ncbi.nlm.nih.gov/pmc/articles/PMC1562341/

Vancampfort, D., Rosenbaum, S., Ward, P. B., Steel, Z., Lederman, O., Lamwaka, A. V., Richards, J. W., & Stubbs, B. (2016). Type 2 diabetes among people with posttraumatic stress disorder: Systematic review and meta-analysis. *Psychosomatic Medicine, 78*(4), 465–473. https://doi.org/10.1097/PSY.0000000000000297

van der Zweerde, T., Bisdounis, L., Kyle, S. D., Lancee, J., & van Straten, A. (2019). Cognitive behavioral therapy for insomnia: A meta-analysis of long-term effects in controlled studies. *Sleep Medicine Reviews, 48*, Article 101208. https://doi.org/10.1016/j.smrv.2019.08.002

Vande Walle, J., Rittig, S., Bauer, S., Eggert, P., Marschall-Kehrel, D., & Tekgul, S. (2012). Practical consensus guidelines for the management of enuresis. *European Journal of Pediatrics, 171*(6), 971–983. https://doi.org/10.1007/s00431-012-1687-7

Van Durme, T., Macq, J., Jeanmart, C., & Gobert, M. (2012). Tools for measuring the impact of informal caregiving of the elderly: A literature review. *International Journal of Nursing Studies, 49*(4), 490–504. https://doi.org/10.1016/j.ijnurstu.2011.10.011

Vangeli, E., Stapleton, J., Smit, E. S., Borland, R., & West, R. (2011). Predictors of attempts to stop smoking and their success in adult general population samples: A systematic review. *Addiction, 106*(12), 2110–2121. https://doi.org/10.1111/j.1360-0443.2011.03565.x

Van Herzeele, C., De Bruyne, P., De Bruyne, E., & Walle, J. V. (2015). Challenging factors for enuresis treatment: Psychological problems and non-adherence. *Journal of Pediatric Urology, 11*(6), 308–313. https://doi.org/10.1016/j.jpurol.2015.04.035

Van Hoecke, E., Baeyens, D., Vanden Bossche, H., Hoebeke, P., & Vande Walle, J. (2007). Early detection of psychological problems in a population of children with enuresis: Construction and validation of the Short Screening Instrument for Psychological Problems in Enuresis. *The Journal of Urology, 178*(6), 2611–2615. https://doi.org/10.1016/j.juro.2007.08.025

van Hooff, M. L., Ter Avest, W., Horsting, P. P., O'Dowd, J., de Kleuver, M., van Lankveld, W., & van Limbeek, J. (2012). A short, intensive cognitive behavioral pain management program reduces health-care use in patients with chronic low back pain: Two-year follow-up results of a prospective cohort. *European Spine Journal, 21*(7), 1257–1264. https://doi.org/10.1007/s00586-011-2091-0

van Schaik, D. J. F., Klijn, A. F., van Hout, H. P. J., van Marwijk, H. W. J., Beekman, A. T. F., de Haan, M., & van Dyck, R. (2004). Patients' preferences in the treatment of depressive disorder in primary care. *General Hospital Psychiatry, 26*(3), 184–189. https://doi.org/10.1016/j.genhosppsych.2003.12.001

Vasiliou, V. S., Karademas, E. C., Christou, Y., Papacostas, S., & Karekla, M. (2021). Acceptance and commitment therapy for primary headache sufferers: A randomized controlled trial of efficacy. *The Journal of Pain, 22*(2), 143–160. https://doi.org/10.1016/j.jpain.2020.06.006

Vicard-Olagne, M., Pereira, B., Rougé, L., Cabaillot, A., Vorilhon, P., Lazimi, G., & Laporte, C. (2022). Signs and symptoms of intimate partner violence in women attending primary care in Europe, North America and Australia: A systematic review and meta-analysis. *Family Practice, 39*(1), 190–199. https://doi.org/10.1093/fampra/cmab097

Vilchinsky, N., Ginzburg, K., Fait, K., & Foa, E. B. (2017). Cardiac-disease-induced PTSD (CDI-PTSD): A systematic review. *Clinical Psychology Review, 55*, 92–106. https://doi.org/10.1016/j.cpr.2017.04.009

Vincent, K., & Moore, J. (2010). Pelvic pain in females. In S. Fishman, J. Ballantyne, & J. Rathmell (Eds.), *Bonica's management of pain* (4th ed., pp. 925–941). Lippincott Williams & Wilkins.

Vinson, D. C., Manning, B. K., Galliher, J. M., Dickinson, L. M., Pace, W. D., & Turner, B. J. (2010). Alcohol and sleep problems in primary care patients: A report from the AAFP National Research Network. *Annals of Family Medicine, 8*(6), 484–492. https://doi.org/10.1370/afm.1175

Visser, S. N., Danielson, M. L., Bitsko, R. H., Holbrook, J. R., Kogan, M. D., Ghandour, R. M., Perou, R., & Blumberg, S. J. (2014). Trends in the parent-report of health care provider-diagnosed and medicated attention-deficit/hyperactivity disorder: United States, 2003–2011. *Journal of the American Academy of Child & Adolescent Psychiatry, 53*(1), 34–46.e2. https://doi.org/10.1016/j.jaac.2013.09.001

Vitiello, M. V., McCurry, S. M., Shortreed, S. M., Balderson, B. H., Baker, L. D., Keefe, F. J., Rybarczyk, B. D., & Von Korff, M. (2013). Cognitive-behavioral treatment for comorbid insomnia and osteoarthritis pain in primary care: The lifestyles randomized controlled trial. *Journal of the American Geriatrics Society, 61*(6), 947–956. https://doi.org/10.1111/jgs.12275

Volkow, N. D., & McLellan, A. T. (2016). Opioid abuse in chronic pain—Misconceptions and mitigation strategies. *The New England Journal of Medicine, 374*(13), 1253–1263. https://doi.org/10.1056/NEJMra1507771

Vollebregt, M. A., van Dongen-Boomsma, M., Buitelaar, J. K., & Slaats-Willemse, D. (2014). Does EEG-neurofeedback improve neurocognitive functioning in children with attention-deficit/hyperactivity disorder? A systematic review and a double-blind placebo-controlled study. *Journal of Child Psychology and Psychiatry, 55*(5), 460–472. https://doi.org/10.1111/jcpp.12143

Vosoughi, K., Salman Roghani, R., & Camilleri, M. (2022). Effects of GLP-1 agonists on proportion of weight loss in obesity with or without diabetes: Systematic review and meta-analysis. *Obesity Medicine, 35*, Article 100456. https://doi.org/10.1016/j.obmed.2022.100456

Vowles, K. E., McEntee, M. L., Julnes, P. S., Frohe, T., Ney, J. P., & Van Der Goes, D. N. (2015). Rates of opioid misuse, abuse, and addiction in chronic pain: A systematic review and data synthesis. *Pain, 156*(4), 569–576. https://doi.org/10.1097/01.j.pain.0000460357.01998.f1

Wadden, T. A., Butryn, M. L., Hong, P. S., & Tsai, A. G. (2014). Behavioral treatment of obesity in patients encountered in primary care settings: A systematic review. *JAMA, 312*(17), 1779–1791. https://doi.org/10.1001/jama.2014.14173

Wadsworth, K. H., Archibald, T. G., Payne, A. E., Cleary, A. K., Haney, B. L., & Hoverman, A. S. (2019). Shared medical appointments and patient-centered experience: A mixed-methods systematic review. *BMC Family Practice, 20*(1), Article 97. https://doi.org/10.1186/s12875-019-0972-1

Wallace, E., Salisbury, C., Guthrie, B., Lewis, C., Fahey, T., & Smith, S. M. (2015). Managing patients with multimorbidity in primary care. *BMJ, 350*, Article h176. https://doi.org/10.1136/bmj.h176

Walser, R. D., & Westrup, D. (2007). *Acceptance and commitment therapy for the treatment of post-traumatic stress disorder and trauma-related problems: A practitioner's guide to using mindfulness and acceptance strategies.* New Harbinger Publications.

Wang, X., Yang, X., Cai, Y., Wang, S., & Weng, W. (2018). High prevalence of erectile dysfunction in diabetic men with depressive symptoms: A meta-analysis. *Journal of Sexual Medicine, 15*(7), 935–941. https://doi.org/10.1016/j.jsxm.2018.05.007

Watson, S. M. R., Richels, C., Michalek, A. P., & Raymer, A. (2015). Psychosocial treatments for ADHD: A systematic appraisal of the evidence. *Journal of Attention Disorders, 19*(1), 3–10. https://doi.org/10.1177/1087054712447857

Webb, R. T., Kontopantelis, E., Doran, T., Qin, P., Creed, F., & Kapur, N. (2012). Suicide risk in primary care patients with major physical diseases: A case-control study. *Archives of General Psychiatry, 69*(3), 256–264. https://doi.org/10.1001/archgenpsychiatry.2011.1561

Wehry, A. M., Beesdo-Baum, K., Hennelly, M. M., Connolly, S. D., & Strawn, J. R. (2015). Assessment and treatment of anxiety disorders in children and adolescents. *Current Psychiatry Reports, 17*(7), Article 52. https://doi.org/10.1007/s11920-015-0591-z

Weiner, L., & Avery-Clark, C. (2017). *Sensate focus in sex therapy: The illustrated manual.* Routledge. https://doi.org/10.4324/9781315630038

Weiss, J. M. (2019). *Breaking through chronic pelvic pain: A holistic approach for relief.* Jerome M. Weiss.

Weitzman, C., Wegner, L., Blum, N. J., Macias, M. M., Bauer, N. S., Bridgemohan, C., Goldson, E., McGuinn, L. J., Weitzman, C., Siegel, B. S., Yogman, M. W., Gambon, T. B., Lavin, A., Lemmon, K. M., Mattson, G., McGuinn, L. J., Rafferty, J. R., Wissow, L. S., Donoghue, E., . . . Wildman, B. (2015). Promoting optimal development: Screening for behavioral and emotional problems. *Pediatrics, 135*(2), 384–395. https://doi.org/10.1542/peds.2014-3716

Welton, S., Minty, R., O'Driscoll, T., Willms, H., Poirier, D., Madden, S., & Kelly, L. (2020). Intermittent fasting and weight loss: Systematic review. *Canadian Family Physician, 66*(2), 117–125. https://pubmed.ncbi.nlm.nih.gov/32060194/

Wetherell, J. L., Sorrell, J. T., Thorp, S. R., & Patterson, T. L. (2005). Psychological interventions for late-life anxiety: A review and early lessons from the CALM study. *Journal of Geriatric Psychiatry and Neurology, 18*(2), 72–82. https://doi.org/10.1177/0891988705276058

Whalley, B., Thompson, D. R., & Taylor, R. S. (2014). Psychological interventions for coronary heart disease: Cochrane systematic review and meta-analysis. *International Journal of Behavioral Medicine, 21,* 109–121. https://doi.org/10.1007/s12529-012-9282-x

Wheeler, L. J., & Guntupalli, S. R. (2020). Female sexual dysfunction: Pharmacologic and therapeutic interventions. *Obstetrics and Gynecology, 136*(1), 174–186. https://doi.org/10.1097/AOG.0000000000003941

Whelton, P. K., Carey, R. M., Aronow, W. S., Casey, D. E., Jr., Collins, K. J., Dennison Himmelfarb, C., DePalma, S. M., Gidding, S., Jamerson, K. A., Jones, D. W., MacLaughlin, E. J., Muntner, P., Ovbiagele, B., Smith, S. C., Jr., Spencer, C. C., Stafford, R. S., Taler, S. J., Thomas, R. J., Williams, K. A., Sr., . . . Wright, J. T., Jr. (2018). 2017 ACC/AHA/AAPA/ABC/ACPM/AGS/APhA/ASH/ASPC/NMA/PCNA guideline for the prevention, detection, evaluation, and management of high blood pressure in adults: A report of the American College of Cardiology/American Heart Association Task Force on Clinical Practice Guidelines. *Hypertension, 71*(6), e13–e115. https://doi.org/10.1161/HYP.0000000000000066

Whelton, P. K., He, J., Appel, L. J., Cutler, J. A., Havas, S., Kotchen, T. A., Roccella, E. J., Stout, R., Vallbona, C., Winston, M. C., Karimbakas, J., & the National High Blood Pressure Education Program Coordinating Committee. (2002). Primary prevention of hypertension: Clinical and public health advisory from The National High Blood Pressure Education Program. *JAMA, 288*(15), 1882–1888. https://doi.org/10.1001/jama.288.15.1882

White, A. R., Rampes, H., Liu, J. P., Stead, L. F., & Campbell, J. (2014). Acupuncture and related interventions for smoking cessation. *Cochrane Database of Systematic Reviews, 1,* Article CD000009. https://doi.org/10.1002/14651858.CD000009.pub4

Whitlock, E. P., Orleans, C. T., Pender, N., & Allan, J. (2002). Evaluating primary care behavioral counseling interventions: An evidence-based approach. *American Journal of Preventive Medicine, 22*(4), 267–284. https://doi.org/10.1016/S0749-3797(02)00415-4

Wilde, B. E., Sidman, C. L., & Corbin, C. B. (2001). A 10,000-step count as a physical activity target for sedentary women. *Research Quarterly for Exercise and Sport, 72*(4), 411–414. https://doi.org/10.1080/02701367.2001.10608977

Wilfley, D. E., Kolko, R. P., & Kass, A. E. (2011). Cognitive-behavioral therapy for weight management and eating disorders in children and adolescents. *Child and Adolescent Psychiatric Clinics of North America, 20*(2), 271–285. https://doi.org/10.1016/j.chc.2011.01.002

Wilfong, K. (2021). *The impact of cardiovascular disease and intervention through modifiable risk factors in the primary care behavioral health (PCBH) model* [Doctoral dissertation, Uniformed Services University of the Health Sciences]. Defense Technical Information Center. https://apps.dtic.mil/sti/citations/trecms/AD1186137

Wilfong, K. M., Goodie, J. L., Curry, J. C., Hunter, C. L., & Kroke, P. C. (2022). The impact of brief interventions on functioning among those demonstrating anxiety, depressive, and adjustment disorder symptoms in primary care: The effectiveness of the primary care behavioral health (PCBH) model. *Journal of Clinical Psychology in Medical Settings, 29*(2), 318–331. https://doi.org/10.1007/s10880-021-09826-9

Willgoss, T. G., & Yohannes, A. M. (2013). Anxiety disorders in patients with COPD: A systematic review. *Respiratory Care, 58*(5), 858–866. https://doi.org/10.4187/respcare.01862

Williams, C. (2017). *Overcoming depression and low mood: A five areas approach* (4th ed.). CRC Press.

Williams, M. B., & Poijula, S. (2016). *The PTSD workbook: Simple, effective techniques for overcoming traumatic stress symptoms.* New Harbinger Publications.

Williamson, M. L. C., Stickley, M. M., Armstrong, T. W., Jackson, K., & Console, K. (2022). Diagnostic accuracy of the Primary Care PTSD Screen for *DSM-5* (PC-PTSD-5) within a civilian primary care sample. *Journal of Clinical Psychology, 78*(11), 2299–2308. https://doi.org/10.1002/jclp.23405

Wilson, J. F. (2007). Posttraumatic stress disorder needs to be recognized in primary care. *Annals of Internal Medicine, 146*(8), 617–620. https://doi.org/10.7326/0003-4819-146-8-200704170-00025

Wing, R. R., Bolin, P., Brancati, F. L., Bray, G. A., Clark, J. M., Coday, M., Crow, R. S., Curtis, J. M., Egan, C. M., Espeland, M. A., Evans, M., Foreyt, J. P., Ghazarian, S., Gregg, E. W., Harrison, B., Hazuda, H. P., Hill, J. O., Horton, E. S., Hubbard, V. S., . . . Yanovski, S. Z. (2013). Cardiovascular effects of intensive lifestyle intervention in Type 2 diabetes. *The New England Journal of Medicine, 369*(2), 145–154. https://doi.org/10.1056/NEJMoa1212914

Winston, S. (2010). *Women's anatomy of arousal: Secret maps to buried pleasure.* Mango Garden Press.

Witkiewitz, K., Litten, R. Z., & Leggio, L. (2019). Advances in the science and treatment of alcohol use disorder. *Science Advances, 5*(9), Article eaax4043. https://doi.org/10.1126/sciadv.aax4043

Wolff, L. S., Flynn, A., Xuan, Z., Errichetti, K. S., Tapia Walker, S., & Brodesky, M. K. (2021). The effect of integrating primary care and mental health services on diabetes and depression: A multi-site impact evaluation on the U.S.–Mexico border. *Medical Care, 59*(1), 67–76. https://doi.org/10.1097/MLR.0000000000001429

Wolitzky-Taylor, K. B., Castriotta, N., Lenze, E. J., Stanley, M. A., & Craske, M. G. (2010). Anxiety disorders in older adults: A comprehensive review. *Depression and Anxiety, 27*(2), 190–211. https://doi.org/10.1002/da.20653

Wolraich, M. L., Hagan, J. F., Allan, C., Chan, E., Davison, D., Earls, M., Evans, S. W., Flinn, S. K., Froehlich, T., Frost, J., Holbrook, J. R., Lehmann, C. U., Lessin, H. R., Okechukwu, K., Pierce, K. L., Winner, J. D., Zurhellen, W., & Subcommittee on Children and Adolescents with Attention-Deficit/Hyperactivity Disorder. (2019). Clinical practice guideline for the diagnosis, evaluation, and treatment of attention-deficit/hyperactivity disorder in children and adolescents. *Pediatrics, 144,* Article e20192528. https://doi.org/10.1542/peds.2019-2528

Workman. (2018). *The menopause book* [Cover copy]. https://www.workman.com/products/the-menopause-book/paperback

World Health Organization. (n.d.). *Primary care.* https://www.who.int/teams/integrated-health-services/clinical-services-and-systems/primary-care

World Health Organization. (2010). *The Alcohol, Smoking and Substance Involvement Screening Test (ASSIST) manual for use in primary care.* https://www.who.int/publications/i/item/978924159938-2

World Health Organization. (2016). Mental and behavioral disorders due to use of alcohol: Harmful use. In *International statistical classification of diseases and related health problems* (10th ed.). https://icd.who.int/browse10/2010/en#/F10.1

Wu, F. L., Lin, C. H., Lin, C. L., & Juang, J. H. (2021). Effectiveness of a problem-solving program in improving problem-solving ability and glycemic control for diabetics with hypoglycemia. *International Journal of Environmental Research and Public Health, 18*(18), Article 9559. https://doi.org/10.3390/ijerph18189559

Wu, L. T., McNeely, J., Subramaniam, G. A., Brady, K. T., Sharma, G., VanVeldhuisen, P., Zhu, H., & Schwartz, R. P. (2017). *DSM-5* substance use disorders among adult primary care patients: Results from a multisite study. *Drug and Alcohol Dependence, 179,* 42–46. https://doi.org/10.1016/j.drugalcdep.2017.05.048

Wynne, B., McHugh, L., Gao, W., Keegan, D., Byrne, K., Rowan, C., Hartery, K., Kirschbaum, C., Doherty, G., Cullen, G., Dooley, B., & Mulcahy, H. E. (2019). Acceptance and commitment therapy reduces psychological stress in patients with inflammatory bowel diseases. *Gastroenterology, 156*(4), 935–945.e1. https://doi.org/10.1053/j.gastro.2018.11.030

Xi, B., Veeranki, S. P., Zhao, M., Ma, C., Yan, Y., & Mi, J. (2017). Relationship of alcohol consumption to all-cause, cardiovascular, and cancer-related mortality in U.S. adults.

Journal of the American College of Cardiology, 70(8), 913–922. https://doi.org/10.1016/j.jacc.2017.06.054

Xu, J. Q., Murphy, S. L., Kochanek, K. D., & Arias, E. (2020). *Mortality in the United States, 2018* (NCHS Data Brief No. 335). National Center for Health Statistics. https://www.cdc.gov/nchs/data/databriefs/db355-h.pdf

Yamamoto, S., Mogi, N., Umegaki, H., Suzuki, Y., Ando, F., Shimokata, H., & Iguchi, A. (2004). The clock drawing test as a valid screening method for mild cognitive impairment. *Dementia and Geriatric Cognitive Disorders, 18*(2), 172–179. https://doi.org/10.1159/000079198

Yesavage, J. A., Brink, T. L., Rose, T. L., Lum, O., Huang, V., Adey, M., & Leirer, V. O. (1982–1983). Development and validation of a geriatric depression screening scale: A preliminary report. *Journal of Psychiatric Research, 17*(1), 37–49. https://doi.org/10.1016/0022-3956(82)90033-4

Yohannes, A. M., Kaplan, A., & Hanania, N. A. (2018). Anxiety and depression in chronic obstructive pulmonary disease: Recognition and management. *The Journal of Family Practice, 67*(2 Suppl. 1), S11–S18. https://doi.org/10.3949/ccjm.85.s1.03

Young, H. M., & Nesbitt, T. S. (2017). Increasing the capacity of primary care through enabling technology. *Journal of General Internal Medicine, 32*(4), 398–403. https://doi.org/10.1007/s11606-016-3952-3

Young, J., Angevaren, M., Rusted, J., & Tabet, N. (2015). Aerobic exercise to improve cognitive function in older people without known cognitive impairment. *Cochrane Database of Systematic Reviews, 4*, Article CD005381. https://doi.org/10.1002/14651858.CD005381.pub4

Zamboni, L., Centoni, F., Fusina, F., Mantovani, E., Rubino, F., Lugoboni, F., & Federico, A. (2021). The effectiveness of cognitive behavioral therapy techniques for the treatment of substance use disorders: A narrative review of evidence. *Journal of Nervous and Mental Disease, 209*(11), 835–845. https://doi.org/10.1097/NMD.0000000000001381

Zarit, S. H., Orr, N. K., & Zarit, J. M. (1985). *The hidden victims of Alzheimer's disease: Families under stress.* University Press.

Zech, N., Hansen, E., Bernardy, K., & Häuser, W. (2017). Efficacy, acceptability and safety of guided imagery/hypnosis in fibromyalgia—A systematic review and meta-analysis of randomized controlled trials. *European Journal of Pain, 21*(2), 217–227. https://doi.org/10.1002/ejp.933

Zhang, F., Zhang, Y., Jiang, N., Zhai, Q., Hu, J., & Feng, J. (2021). Influence of mindfulness and relaxation on treatment of essential hypertension: Meta-analysis. *Journal of Healthcare Engineering, 2021*, Article 2272469. https://doi.org/10.1155/2021/2272469

Zhang, M. W., Ho, R. C., Cheung, M. W., Fu, E., & Mak, A. (2011). Prevalence of depressive symptoms in patients with chronic obstructive pulmonary disease: A systematic review, meta-analysis and meta-regression. *General Hospital Psychiatry, 33*(3), 217–223. https://doi.org/10.1016/j.genhosppsych.2011.03.009

Zhang, Y., Ren, R., Yang, L., Zhang, H., Shi, Y., Shi, J., Sanford, L. D., Lu, L., Vitiello, M. V., & Tang, X. (2022). Comparative efficacy and acceptability of psychotherapies, pharmacotherapies, and their combination for the treatment of adult insomnia: A systematic review and network meta-analysis. *Sleep Medicine Reviews, 65*, Article 101687. https://doi.org/10.1016/j.smrv.2022.101687

Zilbergeld, B., & Zilbergeld, G. (2010). *Sex and love at midlife: It's better than ever.* Crown House Publishing.

Zisser, A., & Eyberg, S. M. (2010). Parent–child interaction therapy and treatment of disruptive behavior disorders. In J. R. Weisz & A. E. Kazdin (Eds.), *Evidence-based psychotherapies for children and adolescents* (2nd ed., pp. 179–193). Guilford Press.

Zoffness, R. (2020). *The pain management workbook: Powerful CBT and mindfulness skills to take control of pain and reclaim your life.* New Harbinger Publications.

INDEX

A

AAFP. *See* American Academy of Family Physicians (AAFP)
ABA (American Bar Association), 333
ABC model, 93–94
Abilify, 390
ACC/AHA (American College of Cardiology/ American Heart Association), 228
Acceptance and Avoidance Questionnaire, Version 2, 84
Acceptance and commitment therapy (ACT), 84–85
    advise phase, 84–85
    agree phase, 85
    arrange phase, 85
    assess phase, 84
    assist phase, 85
    techniques, 65
Acceptance-based interventions, 84
Accountable Health Communities Health-Related Social Needs Screening Tool, 251
Acetaminophen, 287
ACT. *See* Acceptance and commitment therapy (ACT)
Activities of daily living (ADLs), 332
Acute bronchitis, 199
Acute grief, 345
Acute myocardial infarctions, 227
Acute pain, 251. *See also* Chronic pain; Pain; Pain disorders
ADAPPC (American Diabetes Association Professional Practice Committee), 177

Adaptation, 8–9
Adderall XR, 390
Addressing Alcohol Use Practice Manual: An Alcohol Screening and Brief Intervention Program, 274
ADHD. *See* Attention-deficit/hyperactivity disorder (ADHD)
ADLs (activities of daily living), 332
Adult-onset diabetes. *See* Type 2 diabetes
Advise phase, 10
    acceptance and commitment therapy (ACT), 84–85
    assertive communication, 98
    asthma, 218–219
    attention-deficit/hyperactivity disorder (ADHD), 392
    bed-wetting, 385–386
    behavior management of children and adolescents, 378
    cardiovascular disease (CVD), 240
    chronic obstructive pulmonary disease (COPD), 205–207
    chronic pain, 255–257
    chronic pelvic pain (CPP), 360–361
    cognitive disputation, 80
    cognitive impairment, 334
    couple distress, 402–403
    depression, 109–110
    diabetes, 188–189
    enhancing motivation to change and adhere to treatment regimens, 88–89
    erectile disorder (ED), 306
    5As model, 10

Advise phase (*continued*)
  generalized anxiety disorder (GAD),
    117–118
  goal setting, 77–78
  incontinence, 339
  insomnia, 139–140
  menopause, 367–368
  mindfulness exercises, 75
  orgasmic disorder (OD), 323
  overweight and obesity, 160–161
  pain disorders, 255–257
  panic disorder, 123–124
  peripartum depression, 353–354
  physical inactivity, 172–173
  posttraumatic stress disorder (PTSD), 131
  premature ejaculation (PE), 316, 316–317
  relaxation training, 67–68
  stimulus control, 95
  suicide, 430
  tobacco use, 150
  unhealthy alcohol use, 278, 279–281
Age
  chronic obstructive pulmonary disease
    (COPD) and, 203
  degeneration and, 228
  erectile disorder (ED) and, 303
  suicide and, 423
Agency for Healthcare Research and Quality,
    25, 444
Agree phase, 10–11
  acceptance and commitment therapy
    (ACT), 85
  assertive communication, 98
  asthma, 219–220
  attention-deficit/hyperactivity disorder
    (ADHD), 393
  bed-wetting, 387
  behavior management of children and
    adolescents, 378–379
  cardiovascular disease (CVD), 240–243
  chronic obstructive pulmonary disease
    (COPD), 207
  chronic pain, 257–258
  chronic pelvic pain (CPP), 361
  cognitive disputation, 80
  cognitive impairment, 334–335
  couple distress, 403–404
  depression, 112
  diabetes, 189–190
  enhancing motivation to change and
    adhere to treatment regimens, 89
  erectile disorder (ED), 306
  5As model, 10–11
  generalized anxiety disorder (GAD), 119
  goal setting, 78
  incontinence, 339
  insomnia, 140
  menopause, 369
  mindfulness exercises, 76

  orgasmic disorder (OD), 323–324
  overweight and obesity, 161
  pain disorders, 257–258
  panic disorder, 124
  peripartum depression, 354
  physical inactivity, 173
  posttraumatic stress disorder (PTSD),
    133–135
  premature ejaculation (PE), 317
  relaxation training, 68, 119
  shared decision making and, 11
  stimulus control, 95
  suicide, 430
  tobacco use, 150–151
  unhealthy alcohol use, 278–279
AHA diet, 229
Aid to Capacity Evaluation, 333
Alcohol. *See* Unhealthy alcohol use
Alcohol misuse. *See* Unhealthy alcohol use
Alcohol, Smoking and Substance
    Involvement Screening Test, 289
Alcohol use disorder (AUD), 271–285. *See
    also* Unhealthy alcohol use
  assessment, 276–277
  couple distress and, 396
  diagnosis, 275–277
Alcohol Use Disorders Identification Test, 41
Alcohol Use Disorders Identification
    Test-Consumption (AUDIT-C), 274
ALDEA (Latinxs con Diabetes en Acción),
    453
Aldosterone, 233
Alpha-1 antitrypsin, 201
Alpha-2 receptor agonists, 390
Alprazolam, 118, 287
Alzheimer's Association, 334
Alzheimer's disease, 329
Ambien, 287
American Academy of Family Physicians
    (AAFP), 258, 273, 373
  primary care, definition of, 4
American Academy of Pediatrics, 158, 373
  clinical practice guidelines for
    attention-deficit/hyperactivity disorder
    (ADHD), 391
American Association of Suicidology, 423
American Bar Association (ABA), 333
American College of Cardiology/American
    Heart Association (ACC/AHA), 228
American College of Physicians Foundation,
    334
American College of Sports Medicine, 170
American Diabetes Association Professional
    Practice Committee (ADAPPC), 177
American Lung Association, 147
American Psychological Association (APA),
    25, 333
  capacity evaluations and, 333
Amphetamines, 390

Amylin mimetic, 180
AND I C REST mnemonic device, 117, 118
Aneurism, 227
Angina pectoris, 227
Anhedonia, 201
Antidepressants, 109
Anxiety, 105, 232
    asthma and, 213
    Beck Index, 342
    cardiovascular disease (CVD) and, 232,
        247
    chronic obstructive pulmonary disease
        (COPD) and, 201
    Crohn's disease and, 269
    diabetes and, 180, 196
    erectile disorder (ED) and, 303, 312
    irritable bowel syndrome (IBS) and, 269
    menopause and, 364
    older adults and, 327, 342–343
    orgasmic disorder (OD) and, 325
    premature ejaculation (PE) and, 314
    questions, 123
    resources for, 129
    suicide and, 421
Anxiety disorders, 114–116. *See also* Anxiety;
    Generalized anxiety disorder (GAD)
    prevalence of, 114–115
Anxiety–dyspnea cycle, 201, 208–209
Anxious worry handout, 120
APA. *See* American Psychological Association
    (APA)
Appointments. *See* Consultations
Appointment template form, 39
Area Agency on Aging, 334
Aripiprazole, 390
Arrange phase, 11
    acceptance and commitment therapy
        (ACT), 85
    assertive communication, 100
    asthma, 223–225
    attention-deficit/hyperactivity disorder
        (ADHD), 393
    bed-wetting, 388
    behavior management of children and
        adolescents, 382
    cardiovascular disease (CVD), 248
    chronic obstructive pulmonary disease
        (COPD), 209, 209–210
    chronic pain, 264–266
    chronic pelvic pain (CPP), 361
    cognitive disputation, 82
    cognitive impairment, 337
    couple distress, 413–414
    depression, 114
    diabetes, 197
    enhancing motivation to change and
        adhere to treatment regimens, 94
    erectile disorder (ED), 313
    5As model, 11

generalized anxiety disorder (GAD), 121
goal setting, 78
incontinence, 340
insomnia, 143–144
menopause, 370
mindfulness exercises, 76
orgasmic disorder (OD), 325
overweight and obesity, 166–167
pain disorders, 264–266
panic disorder, 128–129
peripartum depression, 355
physical activity, 176
posttraumatic stress disorder (PTSD), 134
premature ejaculation (PE), 319
relaxation training, 74
stimulus control, 95
suicide, 437–439
tobacco use, 155–156
unhealthy alcohol use, 283
unhealthy drug use, 296–298
Arteriosclerosis, 227
Ask Suicide Screening Questions (ASQ), 427
ASQ Suicide Risk Screening Tool, 428
Assertive communication, 65, 95–100, 404
    advise phase, 98
    agree phase, 98
    arrange phase, 100
    assess phase, 98
    assist phase, 98–100
    handout, 99
    HARD acronym (honest, appropriate,
        respectful, direct) and, 98–99
    irritable bowel syndrome (IBS) and, 269
    orgasmic disorder (OD) and, 325
    XYZ* formula and, 99, 100
Assessments, 46–47, 63
    areas for, 56
    asthma, 212
    bed-wetting, 384
    Behavioral Health Measure-20, 41
    cardiovascular disease (CVD), 236–240
    chronic pain, 249–250
    COPD Assessment Test, 205
    couple distress, 401–402
    for diabetes, 184
    Duke Health Profile, 41
    erectile disorder (ED), 304
    evaluations, 80
    expectations, 80
    5As model and, 9–11
    follow-up appointments and, 63
    functional, 55–60
    global assessment measures, 41
    Hopkins Competency Assessment Test,
        333
    incontinence, 338
    menopause, 365–366
    Montreal Cognitive Assessment, 205
    orgasmic disorder (OD), 322

Assessments (*continued*)
  Outcome Questionnaire Short Form, 41
  Pikes Peak Geropsychology Knowledge
    and Skill Assessment Tool, 328
  predictions, 80
  premature ejaculation (PE), 315–316
  primary care and, 52
  Primary Care Behavioral Health Provider
    Adherence Questionnaire (PPAQ-2),
    46
  sleep, 136–138
  structure for in primary care, 79–80
  suicide, 425–429
  unhealthy alcohol use, 277
Assess phase, 10, 63
  acceptance and commitment therapy
    (ACT), 84
  assertive communication, 98
  asthma, 216–218
  attention-deficit/hyperactivity disorder
    (ADHD), 391–392
  bed-wetting, 384–385
  behavior management of children and
    adolescents, 377–378
  cardiovascular disease (CVD), 235–239
  chronic obstructive pulmonary disease
    (COPD), 204–205
  chronic pain, 254–255
  chronic pelvic pain (CPP), 358–360
  cognitive disputation, 79–83
  cognitive impairment, 329–333
  couple distress, 400–402
  depression, 107–109
  diabetes, 184–187
  enhancing motivation to change and
    adhere to treatment regimens, 86–88
  erectile disorder (ED), 304–305
  5As model, 10
  generalized anxiety disorder (GAD), 117
  goal setting, 77
  incontinence, 338
  insomnia, 136–139
  menopause, 365–366
  mindfulness exercises, 75
  orgasmic disorder (OD), 322–323
  overweight and obesity, 158–160
  pain disorders, 254–255
  panic disorder, 122–123
  peripartum depression, 351–352
  physical inactivity, 170–172
  posttraumatic stress disorder (PTSD), 131
  premature ejaculation (PE), 315–316
  relaxation training, 67
  stimulus control, 94–95
  suicide, 424–429
  tobacco use, 148–150
  unhealthy alcohol use, 274–277
  unhealthy drug use, 289–296

Assist phase, 11
  acceptance and commitment therapy
    (ACT), 85
  assertive communication, 98–100
  asthma, 220–223
  attention-deficit/hyperactivity disorder
    (ADHD), 393–394
  bed-wetting, 387–388
  behavior management of children and
    adolescents, 379–382
  cardiovascular disease (CVD), 243–248
  chronic obstructive pulmonary disease
    (COPD), 207–209
  chronic pain, 258–264
  chronic pelvic pain (CPP), 361
  cognitive disputation, 80–82
  cognitive impairment, 335–337
  couple distress, 404–413
  depression, 112–114
  diabetes, 189–196
  enhancing motivation to change and
    adhere to treatment regimens, 89–94
  erectile disorder (ED), 306–312
  5As model, 11
  generalized anxiety disorder (GAD),
    119–121
  goal setting, 78
  incontinence, 339–340
  insomnia, 140–143
  menopause, 370–372
  mindfulness exercises, 76
  orgasmic disorder (OD), 324–325
  overweight and obesity, 162–166
  pain disorders, 258–264
  panic disorder, 124–128
  peripartum depression, 354–355
  physical inactivity, 173–175
  posttraumatic stress disorder (PTSD), 133
  premature ejaculation (PE), 317
  relaxation training, 68–74
  stimulus control, 95
  suicide, 430–437
  tobacco use, 151–155
  unhealthy alcohol use, 281–286
  unhealthy drug use, 298–299
Asthma, 199, 210–225
  action plan, 221
  acute exacerbations management,
    220–221
  advise phase, 218–219
  agree phase, 219–220
  anxiety and, 213
  arrange phase, 223–225
  assessments, 212
  assess phase, 216–218
  assist phase, 220–223
  behavioral factors, 214
  behavioral health consultants (BHCs)
    and, 215–216

behavioral health in primary care, 215–216
cognitive behavioral interventions for
anxiety from, 200
controller medication, 213, 222
cultural and diversity considerations,
214–215
definition of, 210
depression and, 213
education, 215
emotional and cognitive factors, 213–214
environmental factors, 214
exercise induced, 213, 214, 223
Factors That May Worsen Asthma
handout, 223
family and management of, 220
gender and, 210
healthcare burden of, 210
health literacy and, 213
inhalers and, 213, 221
management of, 200
medication adherence and, 214, 216,
221–222
medications and, 212–213, 222
peak flow and, 212, 216, 220
physical activity and, 223
physical factors, 212–213
prevalence of, 210
primary care adaptation, 216–225
race and, 210, 214
reliever medication, 213
resources for, 225
risk factors for, 218
Shortness of Breath Cycle for COPD and
Asthma handout, 202
side effects of medications for, 213
smoking and, 214
specialty behavioral medicine treatment,
215
symptoms of, 210
tobacco cessation and, 222
treatment of, 213, 215
triggering factors, 210, 222
Asthma allergen and exposure checklist
patient handout, 223
Asthma assessment questions handout, 217
Asthma Monitoring Form handout, 221
Atherosclerosis, 227, 229
Atomoxetine, 390
Attention-deficit/hyperactivity disorder
(ADHD), 373, 389–394
Academy of Pediatrics clinical practice
guidelines for, 391
advise phase, 392
agree phase, 393
arrange phase, 393
assess phase, 391–392
assist phase, 393–394
behavioral health in primary care, 391
behavioral treatments for, 390, 391
controlled playdates and, 393
criteria for, 389
cultural and diversity considerations, 389
*Diagnostic and Statistical Manual of Mental
Disorders, Text Revision (DSM-5-TR)*, 389
electroencephalogram (EEG)
neurofeedback and, 390
interventions for, 390
medications for, 390
motivational interviewing and, 393
presentations of, 389
prevalence of, 389
primary care adaptation, 391–394
resources for, 392
screening for, 392
Section 504 of the Rehabilitation Act and,
393
specialty mental health, 390
stimulant medication for, 389
AUD. *See* Alcohol use disorder (AUD)
AUDIT-C (Alcohol Use Disorders
Identification Test-Consumption), 274
Avanafil, 302
Aversive smoking, 153–154
Avoidance, 126

B

B12 deficiency, 180
Baby stroller walking group, 354
BCBT-CP. *See* Brief cognitive behavioral
therapy for chronic pain (BCBT-CP)
Beck Anxiety Index, 342
Beck Depression Inventory-II, 342
Bed-wetting, 373, 382–388
advise phase, 385–386
agree phase, 387
alarm for, 383, 387
arrange phase, 388
assessments, 384
assess phase, 384–385
assist phase, 387–388
behavioral health in primary care, 383
cultural and diversity considerations, 383
desmopressin (DDAVP) for, 383
*Diagnostic and Statistical Manual of Mental
Disorders, Text Revision (DSM-5-TR)* and,
382
interventions for, 383, 387
monitoring chart for, 386
prevalence of, 382–383
primary care adaptation, 383–388
resources for, 388
specialty mental health, 383
Behavioral activation, 113, 354
depression and, 113
suicide and, 436
Behavioral classroom management/
interventions, 390

Behavioral counseling interventions and
    cardiovascular disease (CVD), 235
Behavioral health
  assessment and intervention, 7
  definition of, 12
Behavioral health consultants (BHCs), 3,
    5–6, 7, 51, 65
  activities of daily living (ADLs) and, 332
  additional training for, 47–49
  assessment against core competencies,
    46–47
  assessment/intervention feedback for
    primary care providers (PCPs) and, 34,
    236
  asthma and, 215–216
  availability and responsiveness, 7, 38
  availability of, 38
  being part of the clinic team, 36
  best practices, 38–40
  building key relationships, 36–37
  cardiovascular disease (CVD) and,
    235–248
  as caregiver of the staff, 40
  chronic pain and, 252–253
  clinical pathways and, 20
  clinical practice management skills and,
    25–30
  clinic priorities identification and, 41
  collaboration and, 32
  as consultants to primary care providers
    (PCPs), 33–34
  consultation skills and, 30–40
  core competencies and, 25–30
  daily check-ins and, 37
  depression and, 106
  diabetes and, 184
  documentation and, 42
  drop-in group medical appointment
    (DIGMA) and, 445
  electronic health record (EHR) and, 52
  ethical considerations in primary care
    settings for, 8
  feedback and, 34
  flexibility and, 31
  funding and, 30
  GATHER and, 6
  informal leaders and, 36
  instrumental activities of daily living
    (IADLs) and, 332
  integrating into primary care, 29
  interventions, 38
  introducing the service to patients, 53
  learning the primary care culture, 38–40
  marketing of, 31, 36–37
  marketing survey, 33
  note example, 44–45
  number of appointments with, 6
  older adults and, 329
  onboarding activities and, 31

  pain assessment and treatment by, 250
  patient progress and, 6
  population health approach to primary
    care and, 20
  primary care environment and, 7–8
  primary care provider (PCP) and, 33–34
  primary care providers (PCPs) and, 5
  primary care settings adaptations, 7–8
  primary care team as the internal
    customer, 31
  schedule template, 39
  scope and competency and, 32
  shared decision making and, 11, 40
  specialty referrals and, 40
  team-based primary care and, 21
  as a team member, 32–34
  team performance and, 30–40
  Type 2 diabetes awareness and, 179
  unhealthy alcohol use and, 274
  unhealthy drug use and, 297–299
  warm handoffs and, 37
  women's health clinics and, 349
Behavioral health consultation service
    handout, 54
Behavioral Health Measure-20, 41
Behavioral health professionals. *See*
    Behavioral health consultants (BHCs)
Behavioral health provider. *See* Behavioral
    health consultants (BHCs)
Behavioral interventions, 65. *See also*
    Interventions
  acceptance and commitment techniques,
    65
  asthma, 216–225
  chronic obstructive pulmonary disease
    (COPD) and, 203
  cognitive disputation, 65
  desired behavior and, 410–411
  goal setting, 65
  insomnia and, 140
  mindfulness exercises, 65
  relaxation training, 65
Behavioral marital therapy (BMT), 398
Behavioral pain management, 258
Behavioral parent training, 390
Behavioral self-analysis, 92–94
  ABC model and, 93–94
Behavior change interventions, 410–411
Behavior exchange, 411–412
  handout, 412
Behavior management of children and
    adolescents, 373, 374–382
  advise phase, 378
  agree phase, 378–379
  arrange phase, 382
  assess phase, 377–378
  assist phase, 379–382
  aversive consequences and, 381–382

behavioral health in primary care, 376–377
caregivers and, 379
consequences timing, 379
consistency between parents and caregivers, 379
cultural and diversity considerations, 375
cultural norms and, 375
discipline, age-appropriate techniques for, 379
high-risk situations for unwanted behaviors plan for, 380
interventions and, 376, 378
labeled praise and, 380
monitor progress, 381
parent–child interaction therapy (PCIT) and, 375
parent emotions and, 381
positive attention and, 380
primary care adaptation, 377–382
resources for, 374
shape and practice desired behavior, 380
spanking and, 381
specialty mental health, 375–376
threats and, 381
time-outs and, 380–381
Triple P (Positive Parenting Program) and, 375–376
Behavior prescription pad, 62
Behavior prescription pad form, 62
Behavior therapy for attention-deficit/hyperactivity disorder (ADHD), 391
Benzodiazepines, 123
Bereavement, Grief, and Mourning handout, 347
BHC. *See* Behavioral health consultants (BHCs)
Biguanides, 180
Bile acid sequestrants, 180
Binge-eating disorder, 159
Bingeing, 160
Biofeedback
for chronic pain, 258
for migraines, 267
Biopsychosocial formulation, 64
Bipolar disorder and depression, 106
Bladder training, 340
Bladder wall injection, 340
Blood pressure
cardiovascular disease (CVD) mortality and, 235
categories of, 228
classifications of in adults, 228
diastolic and heart disease, 228
relaxation techniques and, 246
systolic and heart disease, 228
BMI (body mass index), 158
BMT (behavioral marital therapy), 398
Body mass index (BMI), 158

Body Weight Planner, 163
Brand switching, 153, 154
Breathing retraining, 126
Brief cognitive behavioral therapy (BCBT) for chronic obstructive pulmonary disease (COPD), 204
Brief cognitive behavioral therapy for chronic pain (BCBT-CP), 252
efficacy of, 253
Brief contact interventions for suicide, 435–436
Brief intervention, 273
Brief Interventions for Radical Change, 84
Bronchiectasis, 199
Bronchiolitis, 200
Bronchitis, 200
acute, 199
Bruxism, 139
Bulimia nervosa, 159
Buprenorphine, 266, 295
Bupropion, 320, 390
Bupropion SR, 147
Burdensomeness, 422

C

Calorie education, 163
C.A.M.E.S. (CUT—ADD—MOVE—ELIMINATE—SUBSTITUTE)
approach, 164
principle for improvement handout, 165
Capacity evaluations, 333
clinical judgment and, 333
older adults and, 333
tests for, 333
Carbamazepine, 390
Carbohydrates, 181
diabetes and, 181, 196
Cardiac rehabilitation programs, 234
Cardiomyopathy, 227, 228
Cardiovascular disease (CVD), 168
acute stressors and, 232
advise phase, 240
agree phase, 240–243
AHA diet and, 229
alcohol and, 230–231, 246
anxiety and, 232, 247
arrange phase, 248
assessments and, 236–240
assess phase, 235–239
assist phase, 243–248
behavioral counseling interventions and, 235
behavioral factors, 229–231, 237–238, 244–246
behavioral health consultants (BHCs) and, 235–248

Cardiovascular disease (CVD) (*continued*)
  behavioral health in primary care,
    234–235
  blood pressure and, 235
  cardiac rehabilitation programs and, 234
  cholesterol and, 228
  chronic stressors and, 232
  cognitive factors, 231–233
  cost of, 227
  cultural and diversity considerations,
    233–234
  deaths from, 227
  depression and, 232, 247
  description of, 227
  diabetes and, 228
  diet and, 238, 244
  Dietary Approaches to Stop Hypertension
    (DASH) eating plan for, 229
  dietary nutrients and, 229
  emotional factors, 231–233, 239, 246–247
  emotional reactivity and, 246
  environmental factors, 233, 247–248
  excess weight and, 244
  health behaviors and, 237–238
  high blood pressure and, 228
  high cholesterol and, 228
  interventions for, 234
  medication adherence and, 231, 238, 246
  medications and, 235
  Mediterranean diet for, 229
  negative mood assessment and, 239
  physical activity and, 234, 244–246, 248
  physical factors, 228–229, 237
  physical inactivity and, 169
  posttraumatic stress disorder (PTSD) and,
    231, 232–233, 247
  prevalence of, 233
  primary care adaptation, 235–248
  relaxation techniques, 246
  resources for, 230
  risk reductions and, 234
  social isolation and, 233
  social support and, 247–248
  specialty mental health, 234
  stress and, 246
  stressors and, 232
  tobacco use and, 244
  treatments and emotional distress, 232
  weight and, 244
Care facilitation model. *See* Collaborative
    care
Caregiver burden, 340–342
  assessment, 340–341
  psychoeducational interventions for, 341
  therapies for, 341
Care management model. *See* Collaborative
    care
Care map. *See* Clinical pathways
Care pathway. *See* Clinical pathways

Catapres, 390
CBCL (Child Behavior Checklist), 392
CBCT (cognitive behavioral couple therapy),
    398
CBT. *See* Cognitive behavioral therapy (CBT)
CCM. *See* Collaborative care management
    (CCM)
CDC. *See* Centers for Disease Control and
    Prevention (CDC)
Center for Epidemiologic Studies Depression
    Scale-Revised, 107
Centers for Disease Control and Prevention
    (CDC), 169, 177, 251, 273
  suicide rates, 420
Centers for Medicare and Medicaid
    Innovation, 251
Cerebrovascular diseases, 329
Change
  confidence and, 90
  difficulty of, 89
  importance of, 90
  pros and cons of, 90–91
  readiness for, 90
  readiness-to-change ruler, 90
Change plan, 51
  creation of, 62–63
  options, 61
Changing thinking and depression, 113–114
CHCC. *See* Cooperative health care clinic
    (CHCC)
Cherokee Health System, 6, 30
Chest discomfort, 227
Child Behavior Checklist (CBCL), 392
Childhood discipline, age-appropriate
    techniques for, 379
Child maltreatment, 377
Child sexual abuse and premature
    ejaculation (PE), 314
Child skills training, 390
Chinese finger trap, 126
Cholesterol
  cardiovascular disease (CVD) and, 228
  forms of, 229
  lowering, 229
  race and, 233
  statin therapy and, 229
Chronic obstructive pulmonary disease
    (COPD), 199, 200–210
  advise phase, 205–207
  age and, 203
  agree phase, 207
  anxiety and, 201
  anxiety–dyspnea cycle and, 201, 208–209
  arrange phase, 209–210
  assessment questions, 206
  assess phase, 204–205
  assist phase, 207–209
  behavioral factors, 202
  behavioral health interventions for, 203

clinical practice guideline (CPG)
recommendations for, 199
COPD Assessment Test, 205
coronavirus disease-2019 (COVID-19)
and, 200
definition of, 200
depression and, 201
diaphragmatic breathing and, 208
emotional and cognitive factors, 201–202
environmental factors, 202–203
exercise training and, 207–208
fatigue and, 200
functional impact of, 200
gender and, 203
genetics and, 201
health literacy and, 203
management of, 199
medical treatment of, 201
morbidity from, 200
nicotine use and, 202
oxygen therapy and, 201
physical factors, 201
physical inactivity and, 202
prevalence of, 200
primary care adaptations, 204–209
pursed-lip breathing and, 208
relaxation training for, 208
resources for, 211
self-management interventions for,
203–204
Shortness of Breath Cycle for COPD and
Asthma handout, 202
smoking and, 201
socioeconomic status and, 203
specialty behavioral medicine treatment,
203–204
surgical treatments for, 201
symptoms of, 200
tobacco cessation and, 199, 202, 204, 208
vaccines recommended for patients with,
201
weight loss and, 200
Chronic pain. *See also* Acute pain; Chronic
pelvic pain (CPP); Pain; Pain disorders
advise phase, 255–257
agree phase, 257–258
arrange phase, 264–266
assessments, 249–250
assess phase, 254–255
assist phase, 258–264
behavioral health consultants (BHCs)
and, 252–253
biofeedback for, 258
cognitive behavioral interventions for,
251–252
coping with intense episodes, 262
Crohn's disease and, 268
deep breathing and, 263

Defense and Veterans Pain Rating Scale
and, 253
definition of, 251
distraction and, 263
high-impact, 249
imagery and, 263
irritable bowel syndrome (IBS) and,
268–269
managing your thinking about, 263
medications for, 250, 263
mindfulness-based stress reduction for,
258
muscle tension and, 260, 262
nonpharmacological approaches to
treating, 258
opioids and, 250, 258
overactivity and underactivity cycle, 259
pacing activities and, 259–261
prevalence of, 249
primary care adaptation, 253–266
psychogenic pain vs., 249–250
psychological components of, 255–256
relaxation training for, 258, 262, 263
resources for, 265
stepped care models for, 264
suicide and, 421
support networks and, 264
time-based pacing for, 260
treatment guidelines for, 252
treatment of, 249–250
Chronic pelvic pain (CPP), 349, 355–361. *See
also* Chronic pain; Pain; Pain disorder
advise phase, 360–361
agree phase, 361
arrange phase, 361
assessment areas, 358
assess phase, 358–360
assist phase, 361
causes of, 357
conditions relating to, 357
cultural and diversity considerations, 358
definition of, 355
interventions for, 360–361
pain management and, 361
prevalence of, 357
primary care adaptation, 358–361
resources for, 362–363
sexual and physical abuse and, 359
sexual dysfunction and, 359–361
specialty mental health, 358
Chronic prostatitis and premature
ejaculation (PE), 313
Chronic renal insufficiency and premature
ejaculation (PE), 313
Chronic stressors, 232
Cialis, 302
Circumstances That Protect Against Suicide
Risk handout, 425–426
Citalopram, 122

Clinic team, being part of, 36
Clinical pathways, 20, 442–443
  behavioral health consultants (BHCs)
    and, 20
  clinical practice guidelines vs., 442
  operational definition of, 442
  use of, 442
  using behavioral health consultants
    (BHCs), 441
*Clinical Practice Guideline for the Management of
  Major Depressive Disorder*, 353
Clinical practice guidelines (CPGs)
  chronic obstructive pulmonary disease
    (COPD) recommendations, 199
  clinical pathways vs., 442
  definition of, 442
Clock Drawing Test, 330
  measures of, 330–331
Clomipramine, 123
Cocaine, 287
Cochrane systematic reviews of tobacco use,
    147
Cognition monitoring form, 82
Cognitive behavioral couple therapy
    (CBCT), 398
Cognitive behavioral interventions
  for anxiety from asthma, 200
  for chronic pain, 251–252
  mobile apps to support, 101
Cognitive behavioral therapy (CBT)
  for Crohn's disease, 269
  generalized anxiety disorder (GAD) and,
    116
  for insomnia, 135, 136
  for irritable bowel syndrome (IBS), 269
  for menopause, 365
  for migraines, 267
  pain catastrophizing and, 268
  for peripartum depression, 351
  for suicide, 435
Cognitive disputation, 65, 79–83, 354
  advise phase, 80
  agree phase, 80
  arrange phase, 82
  assess phase, 79–80
  assist phase, 80–82
  behavioral interventions for, 65
  common patterns of unhealthy thinking
    and, 82
  diabetes and, 196
  scripts for, 81
Cognitive disputation patient education
    handout, 79
Cognitive exercises, 336
Cognitive functioning
  cardiorespiratory fitness and, 336
  depression and, 332–333
  depression vs. dementia, 332
  leisure cognitive activity and, 336

medical problems and, 333
  physical activity and, 336
  relaxation techniques and, 336
Cognitive impairment
  advise phase, 334
  agree phase, 334–335
  arrange phase, 337
  assess phase, 329–333
  assist phase, 335–337
  older adults and, 329–337
Collaboration, 32
Collaborative care, 5, 7
  colocated care and, 5
  coordinated care and, 5
  definition of, 5
  depression and, 5, 107
  ethics in, 8
  integrated care vs., 4–5
  models of, 5
Collaborative care management (CCM), 46
  domains, 46–47
Colocated care, 5, 7
Columbia Lighthouse Project, 427
Columbia-Suicide Severity Rating Scale, 427
Common Mistakes and Assumptions About
    Alcohol handout, 279–280
Common pain beliefs handout, 259
Communication
  assertive, 404
  effective, 405
Communication training, 404–406
  couple distress and, 404
  for erectile disorder (ED), 311–312
  for peripartum depression, 354
Community Preventive Services Task Force,
    169
Complicated grief, 345
Conceptual statements, 56, 60
Concerta, 390
Congenital abnormalities, 228
Consequences, 379
Consultations. *See also* Follow-up
    appointments; Initial consultations
  Consultation Request form, 35
  empathic or reflective statements and
    restatement, 56
  focused vs. open-ended questions and,
    55–56
  information gathering and, 55
  interventions and, 63
  note example, 44–45
  primary care screening or assessment
    measures and, 52
  reason for, 55
  steps to follow, 51
  summary statements after, 56
Consultative model, 420
Contextual interview, 60
Continuity consultations, 39

Cooperative health care clinic (CHCC), 451–452. *See also* Shared Medical Appointments (SMAs)
  components of, 452
  duration of, 451
  group size, 451
  stages of, 452
Coordinated care, 5
COPD. *See* Chronic obstructive pulmonary disease (COPD)
COPD Assessment Test, 205
Coping cards, 436
Core competencies, 46–47
Coronary heart disease, 227
Coronavirus disease-2019 (COVID-19) and chronic obstructive pulmonary disease (COPD), 200
Corticosteroids, 213
Cough, 200
County health rankings model, 18
Couple distress
  advise phase, 402–403
  agree phase, 403–404
  alcohol use disorder (AUD) and, 396
  arrange phase, 413–414
  assessment at BHC appointments, 401
  assess phase, 400–402
  assist phase, 404–413
  behavioral factors, 396–397
  behavioral health in primary care, 399
  behavioral interventions for increasing desired behavior, 410–411
  behavioral marital therapy (BMT) and, 398
  behavior exchange and, 411–412
  communication training and, 404
  couples interventions and, 399
  couple therapy and, 398
  cultural and diversity considerations, 397
  emotional and cognitive factors, 396
  environmental factors, 397
  interventions for, 398–399
  motivational enhancement strategies and, 408–410
  motivational interviewing and, 403
  physical factors, 396
  primary care adaptation, 400–414
  problem-solving training and, 407–408
  resources for, 415–416
  safety and, 412–413
  screenings, 400
  sexual and gender minority populations and, 399
  Socratic questioning and, 403
  specialty mental health intervention, 398–399
  violence and, 396
Couple therapy
  for couple distress, 398
  emotionally focused, 398
  for sexual and gender minority populations, 398–399
Couples Guidelines for Problem Solving handout, 409
Couples interventions, 399
CPGs. *See* Clinical practice guidelines (CPGs)
CPP. *See* Chronic pelvic pain (CPP)
Crisis Response Plan handout, 434
Crisis response planning worksheet, 434
Critical pathway. *See* Clinical pathways
Crohn's disease, 268
  anxiety and, 269
  chronic pain and, 268
  cognitive behavioral therapy and, 269
  depression and, 269
  symptoms of, 269
Cryoablation, 314
Cue-controlled relaxation, 65, 70–71
  deep breathing handout, 70
  examples of cues, 70
  external and internal cues, 71
Cultural adaptation/tailoring, 8–9
Cultural and diversity considerations
  chronic pelvic pain (CPP), 358
  insomnia, 135
  menopause, 364–365
  older adults, 328
  orgasmic disorder (OD), 321
  overweight and obesity, 157
  pain disorders, 251
  peripartum depression, 350–351
  physical inactivity, 168–169
  posttraumatic stress disorder (PTSD), 130
  premature ejaculation (PE), 314
  shared medical appointments (SMAs), 453
  suicide, 423–424
  tobacco use, 146
  treatment regimes, 87–88
  unhealthy alcohol use, 272
  unhealthy drug use, 288
Cultural sensitivity, 8–9
CVD. *See* Cardiovascular disease (CVD)
Cystic fibrosis, 199

D

Daily check-ins, 37
DASH (Dietary Approaches to Stop Hypertension), 229
DDAVP (desmopressin), 383
Deep breathing, 65, 69–71, 246, 263
  chronic obstructive pulmonary disease (COPD) and, 208
  handout, 70
Defense and Veterans Pain Rating Scale, 253
Dementia, 329, 332
  discussing a diagnosis of, 334

Department of Defense Medical Health
    System, 6
Depression, 5, 105–114, 232. *See also*
    Peripartum depression
    advise phase, 109–110
    agree phase, 112
    antidepressants and, 109
    arrange phase, 114
    assess phase, 107–109
    assist phase, 112–114
    asthma and, 213
    Beck Depression Inventory-II, 342
    behavioral activation and, 113
    behavioral health consultants (BHCs)
        and, 106
    behavioral health in primary care, 107
    bipolar disorder and, 106
    cardiovascular disease (CVD) and, 232,
        247
    care managers, 183
    Center for Epidemiologic Studies
        Depression Scale-Revised and, 107
    changing thinking and, 113–114
    chronic obstructive pulmonary disease
        (COPD) and, 201
    cognitive functioning and, 332–333
    collaborative care models and, 5, 107
    Crohn's disease and, 269
    cultural and diversity considerations, 106
    definition of, 106
    Depression Spiral handout, 110–112
    diabetes and, 180, 183, 196
    economic burden of, 105
    erectile disorder (ED) and, 303
    5As model of, 107–114
    functional assessment and, 108–109
    irritable bowel syndrome (IBS) and, 269
    medications and, 109
    menopause and, 364
    older adults and, 327, 342–343
    orgasmic disorder (OD) and, 323
    Patient Health Questionnaire-2 (PHQ-2)
        and, 108
    physical activity or exercise and, 113
    prevalence of, 105–106
    primary care adaptation, 107–114
    primary care behavioral health (PCBH)
        model and, 107
    primary care provider (PCP) and, 107
    problem solving and, 114
    resources for, 115
    screening for, 107–109
    screening for in older adults, 342
    specialty mental health, 106–107
    stepped-care approach to, 109
    therapies for treatment of, 106–107
Depression Spiral handout, 110–112
Desipramine, 313
Desmopressin (DDAVP), 383

Detrol, 340
Developing Helpful Beliefs for Enhancing
    Arousal and Orgasm handout, 324
Dexedrine, 287
Dextroamphetamine, 287
Diabetes, 177–198
    advise phase, 188–189
    agree phase, 189–190
    anxiety and, 180, 196
    arrange phase, 197
    assessment of, 184
    assess phase, 184–187
    assist phase, 189–196
    associated problems, 180
    behavioral factors, 181, 186–187
    behavioral health consultants (BHCs)
        and, 184
    behavioral health in primary care, 183
    behavior changes and, 188
    biopsychosocial factors, 179–183
    blindness and, 181
    blood glucose monitoring and, 181
    carbohydrates and, 181, 196
    cardiovascular disease (CVD) and, 228
    classifications of, 178
    cognitive disputation and, 196
    complications from, 177, 179
    cultural and diversity considerations, 182
    depression and, 180, 183, 196
    depression care managers and, 183
    Diabetes Goals handout, 191
    diagnosis of, 178
    distress, 180–181
    eating habits and, 195–196
    emotional and cognitive factors, 180–181,
        185–186
    environmental factors, 181–182, 187
    erectile disorder (ED) and, 303, 312
    family and, 187, 196
    Fasting Plasma Glucose Test for, 178
    foot care and, 181
    gestational, 178
    glycemic response and, 181
    goal setting and, 189
    hemoglobin A1C test (HbA1C) for
        detecting, 178
    hypoglycemia and, 179
    individualized eating plans and, 195
    insulin and, 180
    insulin resistance and, 178
    interventions for, 182–183, 183, 189
    kidney disease and, 181
    macrovascular and microvascular diseases
        and, 179
    management goals, 187
    medications for, 180
    metformin for, 180
    modifiable biopsychosocial factors,
        184–187

nutritional intake and, 181
Oral Glucose Tolerance Test for, 178
physical activity and, 195–196
physical factors, 179–180, 184
posttraumatic stress disorder (PTSD) and, 180
prediabetes, 177
prevalence of, 177
primary care adaptation, 184–197
primary care settings and, 183
random blood glucose test for, 178
relaxation training and, 196
resources for, 193–194
screening for, 185
social support and, 181–182, 196
specialty behavioral medicine treatment, 182–183
stress and, 196
telemedicine and, 183
Type 1, 178
Type 2, 178
weight loss and, 179
Diabetes Distress Scale 2, 185
Diabetes Distress Scale 17, 185
Diabetes Goals handout, 191
Diabetes self-management education and support (DSMES), 182–183
Diabetes Self-Management Questionnaire (DSMQ), 186
Diabetes Self-Management Questionnaire, Revised (DSMQ-R), 186
Diabetes Self-Monitoring handout, 192
Diabetic retinopathy, 181
Diagnostic and Statistical Manual of Mental Disorders, Text Revision (DSM-5-TR), 250
    attention-deficit/hyperactivity disorder (ADHD), 389
    bed-wetting, 382
    erectile disorder (ED), 302
    generalized anxiety disorder (GAD), 116
    grief disorder, 345
    insomnia, 135
    major depressive episode, 106
    panic disorder, 122
    posttraumatic stress disorder (PTSD), 129–130
Dialectical behavior therapy, 435
Diaphragmatic breathing. *See* Deep breathing
Diastolic blood pressure, 228
Diazepam, 287
Dietary Approaches to Stop Hypertension (DASH), 229
Dietary nutrients, 229
Diet Change handout, 245
Diets, 160
    cardiovascular disease (CVD) and, 238, 244
DIGMA. *See* Drop-in group medical appointment (DIGMA)

Disease management, 65
Distraction and chronic pain, 263
Ditropan, 340
Documentation, 42
DoD. *See* U.S. Department of Defense (DoD)
Dopamine-2 agonists, 180
DPP-4 inhibitors, 180
Drinking goals, 281. *See also* Unhealthy alcohol use
Drop-in group medical appointment (DIGMA), 444–449. *See also* Shared medical appointments (SMAs)
    appointment introduction, 447
    behavioral health consultants (BHCs) roles in, 445
    goals of, 444
    session profile, 446–448
    size of, 444
    skills behavioral health consultants (BHCs) need to develop for, 448–449
    subtypes, 444
    success factors, 445–446
    timing of, 444
DSMES (Diabetes self-management education and support), 182–183
DSMQ (Diabetes Self-Management Questionnaire), 186
DSMQ-R (Diabetes Self-Management Questionnaire, Revised), 186
Dual relationships, 40
Duke Health Profile Assessment, 41
Dulaglutide, 161
Duloxetine, 118
Dyadic Adjustment Scale, 400, 401
Dysphonia, 213
Dyspnea, 200–202

E

Eating disorders, 159
EBT (evidence-based treatment), 8–9
ED. *See* Erectile disorder (ED)
Edinburgh Postnatal Depression Scale (EPDS), 352
EEG (electroencephalogram) neurofeedback, 390
Effective communication, 405
    listening and, 405
EHR. *See* Electronic health record (EHR)
Ejaculation, 317
    stages of, 317
Elder abuse, 329
Electroencephalogram (EEG) neurofeedback, 390
Electronic health record (EHR), 41, 51, 304
    behavioral health consultants (BHCs) and, 52
    review of, 52
Emission, 317

Emotional distress
  cardiovascular disease (CVD) and, 232
  suicide and, 421
Empathic statements, 56
Emphysema, 200
Enhancing motivation to change and adhere
    to treatment regimens. *See* Treatment
    regimens, enhancing motivation to
    change and adhere to
EPDS (Edinburgh Postnatal Depression
    Scale), 352
Ephedrine, 313
Epilepsy and premature ejaculation (PE),
    313
Erectile disorder (ED), 301–313
  advise phase, 306
  age and, 303
  agree phase, 306
  anxiety and, 303, 312
  arrange phase, 313
  assessment questions for, 304
  assess phase, 304–305
  assist phase, 306–312
  behavioral factors, 303
  behavioral health in primary care, 304
  behavioral interventions for, 303
  cognitive restructuring and, 312
  communication training for, 311–312
  cultural and diversity considerations, 303
  depression and, 303
  description of, 301–302
  diabetes and, 303, 312
  *Diagnostic and Statistical Manual of Mental
    Disorders, Text Revision* (*DSM-5-TR*) and,
    302
  education and, 306
  emotional and cognitive factors, 302–303
  environmental factors, 303
  hypertension and, 303, 312
  interventions for, 306
  lifestyle habits and, 312
  medical intervention for, 306–309
  medications contributing to, 302
  mental health interventions for, 304
  older adults and, 344
  performance anxiety and, 312
  physical factors, 302
  prevalence of, 302
  primary care adaptation, 304–313
  relaxation training and, 312
  resources for, 308–309
  sensate focus and, 309–311
  specialty mental health, 303–304
  testosterone and, 302
  treatment of, 302
  weight and, 312
Erectile Dysfunction handout, 307
Erectile Performance Anxiety Index, 305
Escape plans, 412

Escitalopram, 117, 118, 122
"Ethical Challenges Unique to the Primary
    Care Behavioral Health (PCBH)
    Model", 8
European Society of Sexual Medicine, 303
Evaluations, 80
The Everyday Parenting Toolkit, 382
Evidence-based treatment (EBT), 8–9
Exacerbations, 200
Exercise. *See* Physical activity
*Exercise-Based Interventions for Mental Illness:
    Physical Activity as Part of Clinical
    Treatment*, 169
Expectations, 80
Expulsion, 317

F

Fading, 153
Fagerstrom Test for Nicotine Dependence,
    148
Fall risk and older adults, 344
Families, Systems, & Health, 8
Fasting Plasma Glucose Test, 178
Fatigue and chronic obstructive pulmonary
    disease (COPD), 200
Feedback, 34, 40
Fibromyalgia, 267–268
  guided imagery and, 268
  hypnosis and, 268
  progressive muscle relaxation training
    and, 268
*Financing the Primary Care Behavioral Health
    model*, 30
Firearms and suicide, 423
5As model, 9–11
  advise phase, 10
  agree phase, 10–11
  arrange phase, 11
  assessments, 9–11
  assess phase, 10
  assist phase, 11
  depression and, 107–114
  generalized anxiety disorder (GAD) and,
    117–121
  insomnia and, 136–143
  interventions and, 9–11
  obesity, 157
  obesity and, 158–168
  panic disorder and, 122–129
  physical inactivity and, 170–176
  posttraumatic stress disorder (PTSD) and,
    131–134
  primary care and, 10
  30-minute time frame and, 51
  tobacco use and, 148–156
Five Facet Mindfulness Scale-Short Form,
    75

Five Steps for Managing Intense Pain Episodes handout, 262
Fluoxetine, 130
Flushes, 363
Focused ACT, 84
Follow-up appointments. *See also* Consultations
  assessment and, 63
  global or problem-specific measures and, 52
  interventions and, 63
  multiple problems and, 55
  shared decision making and, 63
  structure of, 63–64
Formoterol, 213
Forms. *See also* Handouts; Questionnaires; Surveys; Worksheets
  appointment template, 39
  Asthma Monitoring, 221
  bed-wetting monitoring chart, 386
  behavior prescription pad, 62
  cognition monitoring, 82
  consultation note example, 44–45
  Consultation Request, 35
  disputing/challenging thoughts and beliefs, 83
  functional assessment of the problem, 57–59
  Geriatric Depression Scale 5/15, 343
  headache monitoring, 268
  hot flash symptom diary, 368
  managing menopausal hot flashes with reassuring thinking, 368, 369
  Monitoring Pain, 266
  primary care PTSD-5 screen, 132–133
  Short Screening Instrument for Psychological Problems in Enuresis (SSIPPE), 385
  strategies to improve motivation to change, 91
Four As for Managing Alcohol Consumption handout, 284
Four As guide for tobacco use, 154
Freedom From Smoking, 147
Functional assessment, 55
  conceptualization statements after, 56
  conducting, 55–60
  contextual interview strategy for, 60
  depression and, 108–109
  example questions for, 57–59
  generalized anxiety disorder (GAD) and, 117
  panic disorder and, 123
  problem conceptualization and, 60–61
  summarization and, 60–61

G

GAD. *See* Generalized anxiety disorder (GAD)
GAD-7. *See* Generalized Anxiety Disorder-7 (GAD-7)
Gastrointestinal disorders, 268–269
Gate control theory of pain, 250
GATHER acronym, 5
  behavioral health consultants (BHCs) and, 6
GDS (Geriatric Depression Scale), 342
Gender
  asthma and, 210
  chronic obstructive pulmonary disease (COPD) and, 203
  hypertension and, 233
  suicide and, 423
Generalized Anxiety Disorder-7 (GAD-7), 41, 117, 342
Generalized anxiety disorder (GAD), 115, 116–121
  advise phase, 117–118
  agree phase, 119
  arrange phase, 121
  assess phase, 117
  assist phase, 119–121
  behavioral health in primary care, 116–117
  cognitive behavioral therapy (CBT) and, 116
  Diagnostic and Statistical Manual of Mental Disorders, Text Revision (DSM-5-TR) and, 116
  5As model and, 117–121
  functional assessment of, 117
  medications for, 117–118
  prevalence of, 116
  primary care adaptation, 117–121
  relaxation exercises for, 119
  selective serotonin reuptake inhibitors (SSRIs) and, 117
  serotonin and norepinephrine reuptake inhibitors (SNRIs) and, 117
  specialty mental health, 116
Geriatric Anxiety Inventory, 342
Geriatric Anxiety Inventory-Short Form, 342
Geriatric Anxiety Scale, 342
Geriatric Anxiety Scale-10, 342
Geriatric Depression Scale 5/15 form, 343
Geriatric Depression Scale (GDS), 342
Geropsychology, 328
Gestational diabetes, 178. *See also* Diabetes
Global assessment measures, 41
Global Initiative for Chronic Obstructive Lung Disease (GOLD), 199
Glucagon-like peptide-1 (GLP-1), 161
  receptor agonists, 180

Glycemic response, 181
Goals
    drop-in group medical appointment
        (DIGMA) and, 444
    patient's realm of control or influence
        and, 78
    personally important, 78
    prioritization of, 78
    realistic and achievable, 77–78
    subgoals, 78
    well-defined, 77
Goal setting, 65, 76–78
    advise phase, 77–78
    agree, assist, and arrange phases, 78
    assess phase, 77
    behavioral interventions for, 65
    SMART acronym (specific, measurable,
        achievable, relevant, and time-bound)
        and, 77–78
GOLD (Global Initiative for Chronic
    Obstructive Lung Disease), 199
Grief
    acute, 345
    complicated, 345
    older adults and, 345
Grief disorder, 345
Guided imagery, 73–74, 246
    for fibromyalgia, 268

H

Hallucinogens, 287
Handouts, 70. *See also* Forms;
        Questionnaires; Surveys; Worksheets
    anxiety questions, 123
    anxious worry, 120
    assertive communication, 99
    Assertiveness Is Simple but HARD, 99
    asthma allergen and exposure checklist,
        223
    asthma assessment questions, 217
    Asthma Monitoring Form, 221
    behavioral health consultation service, 54
    behavior exchange, 412
    Bereavement, Grief, and Mourning, 347
    C.A.M.E.S. principle for improvement,
        165
    Circumstances That Protect Against
        Suicide Risk, 425–426
    cognitive disputation patient education,
        79
    Common Mistakes and Assumptions
        About Alcohol Patient, 279–280
    common pain beliefs, 259
    Common Symptoms of Anxious Worry,
        120
    Couples Guidelines for Problem Solving,
        409
    Crisis Response Plan, 434

cue-controlled relaxation, 70
deep breathing, 70
Depression Spiral, 110–112
Developing Helpful Beliefs for Enhancing
    Arousal and Orgasm, 324
Diabetes Goals, 191
Diabetes Self-Monitoring, 192
Diet Change, 245
Erectile Dysfunction, 307
Factors That May Worsen Asthma, 223
Five Steps for Managing Intense Pain
    Episodes, 262
Four As for Managing Alcohol
    Consumption, 284
High Blood Pressure, 241–243
Home Practice Plan for Improving
    Communication, 406
Improving Communication Through
    Effective Listening, 405
Improving Premature Ejaculation, 318
Improving Sleep Through Behavior
    Change, 141
increasing physical activity, 174
modifying eating habits, 165
Monitoring Pain, 266
Pacing Activities, 261
Panic Disorder, 125–126
problem of the week, 37
protective and risk factors for suicide,
    425–426
Pursed-Lip Breathing for Asthma and
    COPD, 209
Sample Assessment Questions for
    Asthma, 217
Sample Assessment Questions for Female
    Orgasmic Disorder, 322
Sexual Problems and Self-Management
    Interventions, 310–311
Shortness of Breath Cycle for COPD and
    Asthma, 202
Situational Exposure Hierarchy, 127–128
Sleep Restriction, 143
Taking Action to Show Your Partner You
    Care, 412
tobacco cessation, 151–152
understanding chronic pain, 257
weight maintenance, 168
what is a standard drink, 282
Worry Management, 121
HARD acronym (honest, appropriate,
    respectful, direct), 98–99
Hardening of the arteries. *See* Atherosclerosis
Harmful alcohol consumption, 272. *See also*
        Unhealthy alcohol use
HbA1C (hemoglobin A1C test), 178
Headache Monitoring form, 268
Headaches, 267. *See also* Migraines
    tension-type, 267
    triggers for, 267

Health care team well-being, 21
Health Insurance Portability and
    Accountability Act, 452
Health literacy, 203
    asthma and, 213
Health outcomes factors, 18–19
Health-related behavior, 89–90
Heart attacks, 227
Heart failure, 228
Heavy Smoking Index, 148
Helping Patients Who Drink Too Much: A
    Clinician's Guide, 274
Hemoglobin A1C test (HbA1C), 178
Heroin, 287
High blood pressure, 227, 228
    cardiovascular disease (CVD) and, 228
High Blood Pressure handout, 241–243
Holistic interventions. *See also* Behavioral
    interventions; Interventions
    assertive communication and, 66
    stimulus control and, 66
Home Practice Plan for Improving
    Communication handout, 406
Homework, Organization, and Planning
    Skills program, 390
Hopkins Competency Assessment Test, 333
Hormone replacement therapy (HRT), 364
Hot flashes, 363
    reassuring thinking for managing
        menopausal, 369
    symptom diary, 368
HRT (hormone replacement therapy), 364
Humiliation, Afraid, Rape, Kick measure,
    401
Hurt, Insult, Threaten, Scream measure, 400
Hydrocodone, 287
Hyperarousability, 313
Hypercholesterolemia, 229
Hyperglycemia, 179
    complications from, 179
    responses to, 194
Hypertension, 229, 235
    erectile disorder (ED) and, 303, 312
    gender and, 233
    prevalence of, 233
    race and, 233
    stressors and, 232
Hyperthyroidism and premature ejaculation
    (PE), 313
Hyperventilation, 126, 213
Hypnosis, 74
    for fibromyalgia, 268
Hypoglycemia, 179
    responses to, 194
    symptoms of, 195

I

IADLs. *See* instrumental activities of daily
    living (IADLs)
IBCT (integrative behavioral couple
    therapy), 398
IBS. *See* Irritable bowel syndrome (IBS)
ICD-10 (International Statistical Classification of
    Diseases and Related Health Problems),
    272
ICD (implantable cardioverter defibrillator),
    232
Imagery and chronic pain, 263
Imipramine, 123
Implantable cardioverter defibrillator (ICD),
    232
Improving Communication Through
    Effective Listening handout, 405
Improving Premature Ejaculation handout,
    318
Improving Sleep Through Behavior Change
    handout, 141
In-bed behaviors, 138
Incontinence, 337–340
    advise phase, 339
    agree phase, 339
    arrange phase, 340
    assess phase, 338
    assist phase, 339–340
    behavioral interventions for, 338
    bladder training for, 340
    bladder wall injection for, 340
    functional, 338
    interventions for, 338
    Kegel exercises for, 338
    mixed, 338
    overflow, 338
    pelvic floor muscle training (PFMT) for,
        338
    percutaneous sacral nerve stimulation for,
        340
    pharmacological interventions for, 339
    from physical exertion, 338
    prevalence of, 337
    stress, 338
    urge, 338
Increasing physical activity handout, 174
Influenza, 199
Informal leaders, 36
Informant Questionnaire on Cognitive
    Decline in the Elderly, 331
Information gathering, 55
Inhalants, 287
Inhalers, 214, 221
    budesonide, 222
    training in correct use of, 215
Initial consultation, 52. *See also*
    Consultations

Insomnia, 105
    advise phase, 139–140
    agree phase, 140
    arrange phase, 143–144
    assess phase, 136–139
    assist phase, 140–143
    behavioral health in primary care, 136
    behavioral interventions for, 140
    cognitive behavioral therapy (CBT) for,
        135–136
    consequences of, 138
    cultural and diversity considerations, 135
    *Diagnostic and Statistical Manual of Mental
        Disorders, Text Revision (DSM-5-TR)*
        definition of, 135
    exclusions, 139
    5As model and, 136–143
    in-bed behaviors and, 138
    interventions for, 135, 136, 140
    medication for, 139
    presleep behaviors and, 138
    prevalence of, 135–136
    primary care adaptation, 136–143
    relaxation and, 142
    resources for, 144
    sleep diaries and, 136
    sleep environment and, 138
    sleep hygiene and, 135, 141, 142
    sleep restriction and, 142
    specialty mental health, 135–136
    stimulus control and, 135, 142
    therapies for, 135–136
Insomnia Severity Index, 136, 137
Institute of Medicine Committee on
        Standards for Developing Trustworthy
        Clinical Practice Guideline, 442
Instrumental activities of daily living
        (IADLs), 329
    behavioral health consultants (BHCs)
        and, 332
Insulin, 180
    resistance, 178
Insulin-dependent diabetes mellitus. *See*
        Type 1 diabetes
Integrated behavioral health care, 7
    benefits of, 30
    creation of, 7–8
    patient-centered medical home (PCMH)
        and, 17
    population health and, 17
Integrated behavioral health services
    competency domains of, 25–27
    funding for, 30
    patient-centered medical home (PCMH)
        and, 3
Integrated care, 4–6
    collaborative care vs., 4–5
    models, 5, 6–7
    patient-centered care and, 5

*Integrated Care Pathways: A Guide to Good
    Practice*, 443
Integrated care providers. *See* Integrated
    behavioral health care
Integrated clinical pathway. *See* Clinical
    pathways
*Integrating Behavioral Health into the Medical
    Home: A Rapid Implementation Guide*, 30
Integrative behavioral couple therapy
    (IBCT), 398
Intermittent fasting, 160
International Society for Sexual Medicine,
    315, 317
*International Statistical Classification of Diseases
    and Related Health Problems (ICD-10)*,
    272
Interoceptive exposure, 127
Interventions, 38, 65, 399. *See also*
        Behavioral interventions; Holistic
        interventions; Motivational
        interventions; Relaxation training
    acceptance-based, 84
    adaptation for primary care, 66
    attention-deficit/hyperactivity disorder
        (ADHD), 390
    bed-wetting, 383, 387
    behavior change, 410–411
    behavior management of children and
        adolescents, 376, 378
    biopsychosocial formulation and, 64
    brief, 273
    brief contact for suicide, 435–436
    cardiovascular disease (CVD), 234
    caregiver burden, 341
    cognitive behavior, mobile apps to
        support, 101
    cognitive functioning, 335–336
    communication training, 404–406
    consultations and, 63
    couple distress, 398–399
    couples, 399
    diabetes, 182–183, 189
    e-cigarette cessation, 148
    enhancing motivation to change and
        adhere to treatment regimens, 86
    erectile disorder (ED), 306
    evidence-based, 19
    5As model and, 9–11
    follow-up appointments and, 63
    incontinence, 338
    insomnia, 135, 136, 140
    intimate partner violence (IPV), 399,
        412–413
    irritable bowel syndrome (IBS), 269
    medication adherence and, 231
    menopause, 370–372
    older adults, 336
    orgasmic disorder (OD), 323
    overweight and obesity, 157–158, 162

panic disorder, 122
peripartum depression, 354–355
personnel involved with, 19
physical inactivity, 169
planning for, 56
population health and, 19
prediabetes, 182
premature ejaculation (PE), 315
primary care provider (PCP) and, 65
problems and, 60
relationship, 319
self-management model of care and, 66
skill-based, 66
suicide, 430, 435
surgical for overweight and obesity, 167
tobacco use, 147, 148
unhealthy alcohol use, 273
unhealthy drug use, 288
Interviewing, motivational. *See* Motivational
    interviewing (MI)
Intimate partner distress. *See* Couple distress
Intimate partner violence (IPV), 395
    escape plans and, 412
    interventions for, 399, 412–413
    safety and, 412–413
    screening for, 399
Intravenous drug abuse, 228
IPV. *See* Intimate partner violence (IPV)
Irritable bowel syndrome (IBS), 268–269
    anxiety and, 269
    assertive communication and, 269
    chronic pain and, 268–269
    cognitive behavioral therapy (CBT) and,
        269
    depression and, 269
    interventions for, 269
    relaxation training and, 269
    stress and, 269
I statements, 404, 406

J

Jenny Craig, 160
Joiner's interpersonal theory of suicide, 422
Joint monitoring, 411
Juvenile-onset diabetes. *See* Type 1 diabetes

K

Kegel exercises, 325
    incontinence and, 338
Kidney disease and diabetes, 181

L

LABA (Long-acting β2-agonists), 201
Labeled praise, 380
LAMA (long-acting anticholinergics), 201

Latinxs con Diabetes en Acción (ALDEA),
    453
Leisure cognitive activity and cognitive
    functioning, 336
Lesbian, gay, bisexual, transgender, and
    queer or questioning (LGBTQ)
    older adults, 345
    suicide and, 424
    Trevor Project's 2022 National Survey,
        424
Levitra, 302
LGBTQ. *See* Lesbian, gay, bisexual,
    transgender, and queer or questioning
    (LGBTQ)
Lipoproteins, 229
Listening, 405–406
    effective communication and, 405
    pad-and-pencil technique for, 405
    speaker–listener technique for, 405
Long-acting anticholinergics (LAMA), 201
Long-acting β2-agonists (LABA), 201
Look AHEAD study, 182
Lung, 221, 229, 234

M

MacArthur Competence Assessment Tool,
    333
Macrovascular and microvascular diseases,
    179
Malingering, 267
Management, 52
Managing menopausal hot flashes with
    reassuring thinking form, 368, 369
Marijuana, 287
Marital distress. *See* Couple distress
Marketing
    daily check-ins, 37
    Problem of the Week flyer, 36–37
Marketing survey, 33
Marriage and health, 395
Masturbation training and orgasmic disorder
    (OD), 321, 323, 325
Maternal suicide, 350
MAT (Medication-assisted treatment), 266
Meals on Wheels, 334
Medication adherence
    asthma and, 214, 216, 221–222
    cardiovascular disease (CVD) and, 231,
        238, 246
    interventions for improving, 231
Medication-assisted treatment (MAT), 266
Medications
    asthma, 212–213, 222
    attention-deficit/hyperactivity disorder
        (ADHD), 390
    cardiovascular disease (CVD), 235
    chronic pain, 250, 263
    depression, 109

Medications (*continued*)
  diabetes, 180
  erectile disorder (ED), 302
  generalized anxiety disorder (GAD),
    117–118
  insomnia and, 139
  older adults, 336
  orgasmic disorder (OD), 320, 322
  overweight and obesity, 161
  pain and, 250
  peripartum depression, 353
  posttraumatic stress disorder (PTSD), 131
  tobacco use, 153
  weight loss, 161
Meditation, 74, 76
Mediterranean diet, 229
Meglitinides, 180
Memory
  cognitive exercises and, 336
  cues and devices, 336
  older adults, 334
  older adults and, 329–330
  physical activity and, 336–337
  relaxation techniques and, 336, 337
  significant decline of, 334
Menopause, 349, 361–372
  advise phase, 367–368
  agree phase, 369
  anxiety and, 364
  arrange phase, 370
  assess phase, 365–366
  assist phase, 370–372
  cognitive behavioral therapy (CBT) for,
    365
  cultural and diversity considerations,
    364–365
  definition of, 361
  depression and, 364
  environment and triggers and, 369
  flushes and, 363
  functional assessment questions, 366
  general education about, 367
  hormone replacement therapy for, 364
  hot flashes and, 363
  interventions for, 370–372
  monitoring symptoms, 367
  night sweats and, 363
  perimenopause, 361
  primary care adaptation, 365–370
  questioning thoughts, 367
  relaxation and, 367
  resources for, 371–372
  sleep behaviors and, 369
  sleep disturbances and, 364
  specialty mental health, 365
  symptoms of, 363
  vaginal dryness and, 364
  vasomotor symptom, 364

Mental health
  older adults and, 327
  suicide and, 435
Metformin, 180
  B12 deficiency and, 180
Methadone, 266
Methamphetamine, 287
Methylphenidate, 287, 390
Methylxanthines, 201
MI. *See* Motivational interviewing (MI)
Migraines, 267. *See also* Headaches
  biofeedback for, 267
  cognitive behavioral therapy and, 267
  relaxation training and, 267
Mindfulness-based stress reduction for
    chronic pain, 258
Mindfulness exercises, 65, 74–78
  advise phase, 75
  agree phase, 76
  arrange phase, 76
  assess phase, 75
  assist phase, 76
  behavioral interventions and, 65
  comfort zone and, 76
  opioid use and, 75
  overfocus and, 74
  pain management and, 75
  scripts, 75–76
  sensations and, 76
  suicide and, 436
Mini-Mental State Examination (MMSE),
    330
  measures of, 330
Mixed incontinence, 338
MMSE. *See* Mini-Mental State Examination
    (MMSE)
MoCA. *See* Montreal Cognitive Assessment
    (MoCA)
Modifying eating habits handout, 165
Monitoring behavioral triggers worksheet,
    96
Monitoring Pain handout, 266
Montreal Cognitive Assessment (MoCA),
    205, 330
  measures of, 330
Motivational enhancement, 90
  irritable bowel syndrome (IBS) and, 269
  questions, 161
  strategies, 408–410
  techniques, 89–90
Motivational interventions, 66. *See also*
    Behavioral interventions; Interventions
  behavioral self-analysis, 66
  motivational enhancement techniques, 66
  problem solving, 66
  self-monitoring, 66
Motivational interviewing (MI), 61, 89, 147, 408
  attention-deficit/hyperactivity disorder
    (ADHD) and, 393

couple distress and, 403
tobacco use and, 147
Multiple sclerosis
orgasmic disorder (OD) and, 320
premature ejaculation (PE) and, 313
Muscle tension, 260

N

Naltrexone, 266, 276
Narcolepsy, 139
National Academy of Medicine's Vital
Directions for Health and Health Care
series, 145
National Assembly for Wales, 442
National Committee for Quality Assurance
(NCQA), 20, 441
evaluation of patient-centered medical
home (PCMH) principles and, 22–23
National Domestic Violence Hotline, 413
National Heart, Lung, and Blood Institute,
158, 221, 229, 234
National Institute for Children's Health
Quality, 391
National Institute for Health and Care
Excellence (NICE), 11, 123, 337
National Institute of Diabetes and Digestive
and Kidney Diseases (NIDDK), 163,
196, 302
National Institute of Mental Health, 427
National Institute on Aging, 329
National Institute on Alcohol Abuse and
Alcoholism (NIAAA), 272
National Institute on Drug Abuse (NIDA),
287
National Suicide Hotline, 439
NCQA. *See* National Committee for Quality
Assurance (NCQA)
Negative affect, 155–156
Negative emotion and pain, 256
neonatal morbidity, 350
Neuromatrix, 250
NIAAA (National Institute on Alcohol Abuse
and Alcoholism), 272
NICE. *See* National Institute for Health and
Care Excellence (NICE)
Nicotine
chronic obstructive pulmonary disease
(COPD) and, 202
fading, 153
replacements for, 154
Nicotine cessation. *See* Tobacco cessation
Nicotine replacement therapy (NRT), 147
NIDA-Modified ASSIST V2.0, 291–295
NIDA (National Institute on Drug Abuse),
287
NIDA Quick Screen, 289
V1.01, 290

NIDDK. *See* National Institute of Diabetes
and Digestive and Kidney Diseases
(NIDDK)
Night sweats, 363
Nocturnal enuresis. *See* Bed-wetting
Noninsulin-dependent diabetes. *See* Type 2
diabetes
Nonnicotine medication, 147
Noom, 160
Nortriptyline, 147
No-suicide contracts, 433
NRT (nicotine replacement therapy), 147

O

Obesity. *See also* Overweight and obesity
guidelines for treating in children and
adolescents, 373
Obstetrics and gynecology (OB/GYN), 350
OD. *See* Orgasmic disorder (OD)
Older adults
abuse of, 329
Alzheimer's disease and, 329
anxiety and, 327, 342–343
behavioral health in primary care,
328–329
capacity evaluations of, 333
cerebrovascular diseases and, 329
cognitive exercises and, 336
cognitive impairment in, 329–337
cognitive interventions and, 335–336
cultural and diversity considerations, 328
decision making and, 333
dementia and, 329
depression and, 327, 342–343
erectile dysfunction (ED) and, 344
fall risk and, 344
finances and, 328
grief and, 345
interventions and, 336–337
lesbian, gay, bisexual, transgender, and
queer or questioning (LGBTQ), 345
medical care for, 327
medications and, 336
memory and, 329–330, 334
memory cues and devices for, 336
mental health and, 327
mild cognitive impairment and, 329
orgasmic disorder (OD) and, 344
pain and, 344
Parkinson's disease and, 329
physical activity and, 336–337
practical considerations for treating, 346
premature ejaculation (PE) and, 344
race and, 328
relaxation techniques and, 337
resources for, 335
retirement and, 345–346
screening for cognitive problems in, 331

Older adults (*continued*)
  screening for depression in, 342
  screening for memory problems in,
    331–332
  sexuality and, 344–345
  social roles and, 345–346
  social support structure and, 345–346
  specialty mental health, 328
  suicide and, 327, 342
  vaginal dryness and, 344
Onboarding activities, 31
Operation Enduring Freedom, 218
Operation Iraqi Freedom, 218
Opioids, 75, 250, 258, 287
Opioid use disorder (OUD), 266
  buprenorphine and, 266
  criteria for, 266
  methadone and, 266
  naltrexone and, 266
Oral candidiasis, 213
Oral Glucose Tolerance Test, 178
Orgasmic disorder (OD), 301, 319–325
  acquired vs. lifelong, 321
  advise phase, 323
  agree phase, 323–324
  anxiety and, 325
  arrange phase, 325
  assessment questions for, 322
  assess phase, 322–323
  assist phase, 324–325
  behavioral factors, 320
  behavioral health in primary care,
    321–324
  bupropion and, 320
  cultural and diversity factors, 321
  definition of, 319–320
  depression and, 323
  emotional and cognitive factors, 320
  environmental factors, 321
  heterosexual vs. lesbian women, 321
  interventions for, 323
  masturbation training and, 321, 323, 325
  medications and, 320, 322
  multiple sclerosis and, 320
  older adults and, 344
  pelvic nerve damage and, 320
  physical factors, 320, 322
  posttraumatic stress disorder (PTSD) and,
    323
  prevalence of, 320
  primary care adaptation, 322–325
  psychoeducation and, 324
  sample assessment questions handout,
    322
  selective serotonin reuptake inhibitors
    (SSRIs) and, 320
  sensate focus and, 321, 325
  sexual communication and, 325
  sildenafil citrate and, 320

specialty mental health, 321
  spinal cord injury and, 320
  systematic desensitization and, 321
  testosterone and, 320
  treatment for, 323
  vulvovaginal atrophy and, 320
Orlistat, 161
OUD. *See* Opioid use disorder (OUD)
Outcome Questionnaire Short Form, 41
Overactivity and underactivity cycle and
    chronic pain, 259
Overbreathing, 126, 213
Overflow incontinence, 338
Overfocus, 74
Overweight and obesity, 156–168. *See also*
    Weight loss
  advise phase, 160–161
  agree phase, 161
  arrange phase, 166–167
  assess phase, 158–160
  assist phase, 162–166
  behavioral health in primary care,
    157–158
  bingeing and, 160
  biopsychosocial factors, 157
  cultural and diversity considerations, 157
  diets for, 160
  eating disorders and, 159
  5As model of, 158–168
  intermittent fasting and, 160
  interventions for, 157–158, 162
  medications and, 161
  motivational enhancement questions and,
    161
  physical activity (exercise) and, 162, 166
  prevalence of, 156, 159
  primary care adaptation, 158–167
  purging and, 160
  specialty mental health, 157
  surgical interventions and, 167
  weight maintenance and, 166
Oxybutynin, 339, 340
Oxycodone, 287
OxyContin, 287
Oxygen therapy, 201

P

P4 screener, 427
Pacing activities for chronic pain, 259–261
Pacing Activities handout, 261
Pad-and-pencil technique, 405
Pain. *See also* Chronic pain; Pain disorders
  activation, 256
  acute, 251
  behavioral health consultants (BHCs)
    and, 250
  behavioral management of, 258
  biopsychosocial model of, 250

blocking, 255, 256–257
diagnoses of, 250–251
fibromyalgia and, 267–268
gate control theory of, 250
headaches and, 267
management and mindfulness exercises, 75
medications (misuse of), 250
monitoring form, 264, 266
negative emotion and, 256
neuromatrix theory of, 250
older adults and, 344
phantom, 256
recurrent, 251
signature, 256
suffering vs., 256
unhealthy beliefs about, 258–259
Pain catastrophizing, 258
cognitive behavioral therapy (CBT) and, 268
Pain disorders. *See also* Chronic pain; Pain
advise phase, 255–257
agree phase, 257–258
arrange phase, 264–266
assess phase, 254–255
assist phase, 258–264
behavioral health in primary care, 252–253
cultural and diversity considerations, 251
primary care adaptation, 253–266
specialty mental health, 251
Pain Self-Efficacy Questionnaire, 264
Panic disorder, 115, 122–129
advise phase, 123–124
agree phase, 124
arrange phase, 128–129
assess phase, 122–123
assist phase, 124–128
behavioral health in primary care, 122
changing thinking and, 126–128
definition of, 122
Diagnostic and Statistical Manual of Mental Disorders, Text Revision (*DSM-5-TR*), 122
education and, 124
5As model of, 122–129
functional assessment of, 123
interoceptive exposure and, 127
interventions for, 122
prevalence of, 116, 122
primary care adaptation, 122–129
relaxation training for, 127–128
resources for, 129
screening tools for, 123
selective serotonin reuptake inhibitors (SSRIs) and, 122
situational exposure and, 127
specialty mental health, 122
therapies for treatment of, 122
treatment options for, 123–124
ultrabrief interventions for, 122

Panic Disorder handout, 125–126
Parent–child interaction therapy (PCIT), 375
Parenting, 375
Parkinson's disease, 329
Paroxetine, 122, 130
Patient-centered care, 5
Patient-centered medical home (PCMH), 3, 17, 21–23
integrated behavioral health care and, 17
integrated behavioral health service in, 3
joint principles of and the Triple Aim approach, 21–22
National Committee for Quality Assurance (NCQA) evaluation and, 22–23
population health approach to, 17–20
primary care behavioral health (PCBH) model and, 17
primary care delivery and, 21
2014 expanded principles with behavior health integration, 22
2007 joint principles, 22
Patient Health Questionnaire-2 (PHQ-2), 108
Patient Health Questionnaire-9 (PHQ-9), 41, 107, 342, 427, 442
Patient self-management. *See* Self-management
PCBH model. *See* Primary care behavioral health (PCBH) model
PCIT (Parent–child interaction therapy), 375
PCMH. *See* Patient-centered medical home (PCMH)
PCMH Distinction in Behavioral Health Integration, 23
PCP. *See* Primary care provider (PCP)
PC-PTSD-5 (Primary Care PTSD Screen for the *DSM-5*), 131, 132–133
PE. *See* Premature ejaculation (PE)
Peak flow, 212
Pediatric Symptom Checklist (PSC), 378
PEG scale, 264
Pelvic floor muscle training (PFMT), 338
Pelvic nerve damage and orgasmic disorder (OD), 320
Penile hypersensitivity, 313
Percutaneous sacral nerve stimulation, 340
Performance anxiety and erectile disorder (ED), 312
Pericardial disease, 227
Perimenopause, 361
Periodic limb movements, 139
Peripartum depression, 349, 350–355. *See also* Depression
advise phase, 353–354
agree phase, 354
arrange phase, 355
assess phase, 351–352
assist phase, 354–355

Peripartum depression (*continued*)
  baby stroller walking group for, 354
  behavioral activation for, 354
  cognitive behavioral therapy (CBT) and, 351
  cognitive disputation for, 354
  communication training for, 354
  cultural and diversity considerations, 350–351
  Edinburgh Postnatal Depression Scale and, 352
  group treatments for, 353
  interventions for, 354–355
  maternal morbidity and, 350
  medications and, 353
  neonatal morbidity and, 350
  nonpharmacological treatments for, 353
  prevalence of, 350, 351
  primary care adaptation, 351–355
  psychotherapy for, 353
  resources for, 356
  screening for, 350, 351
  sleep strategies for, 355
  socioeconomic status and, 350
  specialty mental health, 351
  times for screening, 352–353
  treatments for, 353
Peripheral artery disease, 227
Personal Food Diary, 163
PFMT (pelvic floor muscle training), 338
Phantom pain, 256. *See also* Pain; Pain disorders
Phosphodiesterase-4 inhibitors, 201
Phosphodiesterase-5 inhibitors, 303
PHQ-2 (Patient Health Questionnaire-2), 108
PHQ-9. *See* Patient Health Questionnaire-9 (PHQ-9)
Physical activity, 65. *See also* Physical inactivity
  activity plan, 174
  arrange phase, 176
  assessing progress, 176
  asthma and, 223
  cardiovascular disease (CVD) and, 234, 244–246, 248
  cognitive functioning and, 336
  depression and, 113
  diabetes and, 195–196
  frequency and duration of, 173
  identify the activity, 173
  increasing handout, 174
  interventions and cardiovascular disease (CVD), 234
  measuring progress, 175
  memory and, 336–337
  moderate and vigorous, examples of, 172
  older adults and, 336–337

  overweight and obesity and, 162, 166
  prevent relapse and, 175
  setting specific goals for, 174
  standard assessment of, 171
  tracking devices, 175
  weight loss and, 162
Physical Activity Guidelines Advisory Committee, 113, 168
Physical Activity Vital Sign, 171
Physical inactivity, 168–176. *See also* Physical activity
  advise phase, 172–173
  agree phase, 173
  assess phase, 170–172
  assist phase, 173–175
  behavioral health concerns related to, 169
  behavioral health in primary care, 169
  cardiovascular disease (CVD) and, 169
  chronic obstructive pulmonary disease (COPD) and, 202
  cultural and diversity considerations, 168–169
  disease and, 168
  5As model and, 170–176
  interventions for, 169
  mental health and, 169
  primary care adaptation, 170–176
  resources for, 170
  specialty mental health, 169
Physical shared medical appointment (PSMA), 449–451. *See also* Shared medical appointments (SMAs)
  components of, 450
  duration of, 450
Pikes Peak Geropsychology Knowledge and Skill Assessment Tool, 328
Planning and Implementing Screening and Brief Intervention for Risky Alcohol Use: A Step-by-Step Guide for Primary Care Practices, 274
Play Nicely program, 382
PMR. *See* Progressive muscle relaxation (PMR)
Pneumonia, 199
Population health, 17–20
  integrated behavioral health care and, 17
  interventions and, 19
  management, 18, 20
  model, 19
  patient populations and, 19
  populations in, 17–18
  screening measure approach, 52
  Triple Aim and, 20
Positive attention, 380
Positive Parenting Program (Triple P), 375–376
Postpartum depression. *See* Peripartum depression

Posttraumatic stress disorder (PTSD), 105, 129–134
  advise phase, 131
  agree phase, 133–135
  arrange phase, 134
  assess phase, 131
  assist phase, 133
  behavioral health in primary care, 130–131
  cardiovascular disease (CVD) and, 231, 232–233, 247
  cultural and diversity considerations, 130
  diabetes and, 180
  Diagnostic and Statistical Manual of Mental Disorders, Text Revision (DSM-5-TR) definition of, 129–130
  5As model of, 131–134
  medications and, 131
  orgasmic disorder (OD) and, 323
  prevalence of, 130
  primary care adaptation, 131–134
  psychotherapy for, 131, 134
  resources for, 134
  screening for, 131, 132–133
  selective serotonin reuptake inhibitors (SSRIs) and, 130, 131
  serotonin and norepinephrine reuptake inhibitors (SNRIs) and, 131
  sexual and physical abuse and, 361
  specialty mental health, 130
  suicide and, 421
  therapies for, 130
  treatment for, 131, 133
PPAQ-2 (Primary Care Behavioral Health Provider Adherence Questionnaire), 46
Prediabetes, 177
  interventions for, 182
Predictions, 80
Pregabalin, 118
Premature Ejaculation Diagnostic Tool, 316
Premature ejaculation (PE), 301, 313–319
  advise phase, 316–317
  agree phase, 317
  anxiety and, 314
  arrange phase, 319
  assessment questions, 315–316
  assess phase, 315–316
  assist phase, 317
  behavioral factors, 314
  behavioral health in primary care, 315
  characterization of, 313
  child sexual abuse and, 314
  chronic prostatitis and, 313
  chronic renal insufficiency and, 313
  cultural and diversity considerations, 314
  education and, 317
  emotional and cognitive factors, 314
  environmental factors, 314
  epilepsy and, 313
  hyperthyroidism and, 313
  injections for, 314
  interventions for, 315
  lifelong vs. acquired, 313, 315
  medical conditions associated with, 313
  medications and, 313
  multiple sclerosis and, 313
  older adults and, 344
  pelvic or neurologic injury and, 313
  pharmacological approaches to, 314
  physical factors, 313–314
  prevalence of, 314
  primary care adaptation, 315–319
  relationship interventions and, 319
  social anxiety and, 314
  specialty mental health, 315
  squeeze technique and, 314
  stop–start technique and, 314
  surgical approaches to, 314
  treatment of, 315
Presbyterian Medical Group in New Mexico, 6
Presleep behaviors, 138
Primary care
  American Academy of Family Physicians definition of, 4
  behavioral health domains of, 46
  biopsychosocial factors in, 11
  clinical pathways to deliver, 441
  diabetes and, 183
  5As model and, 10
  integrating seamlessly into, 29
  learning the culture of, 38–40
  methods to deliver, 441
  pace of service, 38
  screening or assessment measures, 52
  time demands and practice expectations in, 7–8
  World Health Organization definition of, 4
Primary care behavioral health (PCBH) model, 5, 304
  collaboration and, 32
  definition of, 5
  depression and, 107
  ethical guidance for, 8
  GATHER acronym and, 5
  noteworthy system using, 6
  patient-centered medical home (PCMH) and, 17
  rationale behind, 6–7
  self-management and, 52
  transitioning to, 29–30
  Triple Aim and, 6
Primary Care Behavioral Health Provider Adherence Questionnaire (PPAQ-2), 46

Primary care provider (PCP), 5
  behavioral health consultants (BHCs)
    and, 5, 33–34
  behavioral health providers and, 5
  biopsychosocial management of health
    conditions and, 6
  depression and, 107
  interventions and, 65
  problem identification and, 55
  suicide and, 420
Primary Care PTSD Screen for the *DSM-5*
  (PC-PTSD-5), 131, 132–133, 359
Problem Areas in Diabetes Scale, 185
Problem of the Week flyers, 36–37
Problems
  change plan options and, 61
  conceptualization of, 60–61
  formulation of, 60
  interventions for, 60
  summary of, 60
Problem solving, 65, 90–92
  depression and, 114
  motivational interventions for, 66
  seven-step model for, 91
  therapy, 435
  training, 407–408
  treatment adherence and, 90–92
  worksheet for, 92
Pro forma, 30
Progressive muscle relaxation (PMR), 71–73,
  246
  for fibromyalgia, 268
Provider survey, 43–45
PSC (Pediatric Symptom Checklist), 378
Pseudoephedrine, 313
PSMA. *See* Physical shared medical
  appointment (PSMA)
Psychogenic pain, 249–250
Psychological jargon, 38
Psychotherapy
  peripartum depression and, 353
  posttraumatic stress disorder (PTSD) and,
    131, 134
PTSD. *See* Posttraumatic stress disorder (PTSD)
Purging, 160
Pursed-lip breathing, 208
Pursed-Lip Breathing for Asthma and COPD
  handout, 209

Q

Quadruple Aim, 3, 20–21
  behavioral health consultants (BHCs) and
    team-based primary care and, 21
  health care team well-being and, 21
Questionnaires. *See also* Forms; Handouts;
    Surveys; Worksheets
  Acceptance and Avoidance Questionnaire,
    version 2, 84

Diabetes Self-Management Questionnaire
    (DSMQ), 186
  Diabetes Self-Management
    Questionnaire, Revised (DSMQ-R), 186
  Outcome Questionnaire Short Form, 41
  Pain Self-Efficacy Questionnaire, 264
  Patient Health Questionnaire-2 (PHQ-2),
    108
  Patient Health Questionnaire-9 (PHQ-9),
    41, 107, 342, 427, 442
  Primary Care Behavioral Health Provider
    Adherence Questionnaire (PPAQ-2),
    46
  Strengths and Difficulties, 378–379
Questions
  focused vs. open-ended, 55–56
Quit plans, 151

R

Race
  asthma and, 210, 214
  cholesterol and, 233
  hypertension and, 233
  older adults and, 328
  suicide and, 423–424
Random blood glucose test, 178
Randomized controlled trials (RCTs), 199
Rapid Assessment of Physical Activity
    (RAPA), 171
RCTs (randomized controlled trials), 199
Readiness to change ruler, 86, 90, 91
Readiness to Quit Ladder, 148
Reasons for living list, 436
Recurrent pain, 251. *See also* Pain; Pain
    disorders
Reflective statements, 56
Rehabilitation Act, Section 504, and
    attention-deficit/hyperactivity disorder
    (ADHD), 393
Relapse prevention plan, 155
Relationship distress. *See* Couple distress
Relationship interventions, 319
Relaxation, 142
  blood pressure and, 246
  cardiovascular disease (CVD) and, 246
  chronic pain and, 262, 263
  cognitive functioning and, 336
  exercises and suicide, 436
  insomnia and, 142
  memory and, 336, 337
  menopause and, 367
  older adults and, 337
Relaxation training, 65, 66–74, 119, 208. *See
    also* Cue-controlled relaxation; Deep
    breathing; Guided imagery;
    Interventions; Progressive muscle
    relaxation
  advise phase, 67–68

agree phase, 68, 119
arrange phase, 74
assess phase, 67
assist phase, 68–74
behavioral interventions for, 65
chronic obstructive pulmonary disease
(COPD) and, 208
chronic pain and, 258, 262, 263
diabetes and, 196
erectile disorder (ED) and, 312
generalized anxiety disorder (GAD) and,
119
hypnosis vs., 74
irritable bowel syndrome (IBS) and, 269
meditation vs., 74
migraines and, 267
panic disorder and, 127–128
primary categories of, 68
scripts, 67
Resources
for anxiety, 129
for asthma, 225
for attention-deficit/hyperactivity disorder
(ADHD), 392
for bed-wetting, 388
for behavior management of children and
adolescents, 374
for cardiovascular disease (CVD), 230
for chronic obstructive pulmonary disease
(COPD), 211
for chronic pain, 265
for chronic pelvic pain (CPP), 362–363
for couple distress, 415–416
for depression, 115
for diabetes, 193–194
for erectile disorder (ED), 308–309
for insomnia, 144
for menopause, 371–372
for older adults, 335
for panic disorder, 129
for peripartum depression, 356
for physical inactivity, 170
for posttraumatic stress disorder (PTSD),
134
for shared medical appointments (SMAs),
454
for suicide, 438–440
for tobacco use, 156
for unhealthy alcohol use, 285–286
for weight loss, 167
Respiratory infections, 199
Responsiveness, 38
Restatements, 56
Restless leg syndrome, 139
Rethinking Drinking: Alcohol and Your Health,
278
Revised Dyadic Adjustment Scale, 401
Rheumatic heart disease, 228

Risperdal, 390
Risperidone, 390
Ritalin, 287, 390

S

SABA (short-acting β2-agonists), 201
Safety plans, 412–413
suicide and, 433
Saint Louis University Mental Status Exam,
331
SAMA (short-acting anticholinergics), 201
SAMHSA. *See* Substance Abuse and Mental
Health Services Administration
(SAMHSA)
Sample Assessment Questions for Female
Orgasmic Disorder handout, 322
SASQ (Single Alcohol Screening Question),
275
SBIRT (screening, brief intervention, and
referral to treatment), 273
Screening. *See also* Patient Health
Questionnaire-9 (PHQ-9)
Alcohol, Smoking and Substance
Involvement Screening Test, 289
AND I C REST mnemonic, 117, 118
Ask Suicide Screening Questions (ASQ),
427
Center for Epidemiologic Studies
Depression Scale-Revised and, 107
Child Behavior Checklist (CBCL), 392
clinical questions for suicide, 426
for cognitive problems, 331
Columbia-Suicide Severity Rating Scale,
427
for couple distress, 400
for depression, 107–109
for diabetes, 185
for intimate partner violence (IPV), 399
for memory problems, 331–332
NIDA Quick Screen, 289
older adults for depression, 342
P4 screener, 427
Patient Health Questionnaire-2 (PHQ-2),
108
Pediatric Symptom Checklist (PSC), 378
for peripartum depression, 350, 351
for posttraumatic stress disorder (PTSD),
131, 132–133
for primary care, 52
Strengths and Difficulties Questionnaire
and, 378–379
for suicide, 425–429
for tobacco use, 148
for unhealthy alcohol use, 273–275
for unhealthy drug use, 289–296
Zarit Burden Interview (ZBI) for caregiver
burden, 341

Screening, Brief Intervention, and Referral to Treatment for Substance Use: A Practitioners' Guide, 274
Screening, brief intervention, and referral to treatment (SBIRT), 273
Scripts
    acceptance and commitment therapy (ACT) introduction, 85
    assertive communication, 98
    behavioral self-analysis, 93–94
    cognitive disputation and unhelpful thinking, 81
    cue-controlled relaxation, 71
    deep breathing, 69–70
    follow-up appointment, 63
    guided imagery, 73
    initial consultation introduction to BHC services, 53
    mindfulness exercises, 75–76
    progressive muscle relaxation, 72
    provider survey introduction, 42
    relaxation training, 67
    stimulus control, 94–95
    summary statements and, 60
Sedatives, 287
Selective serotonin reuptake inhibitors (SSRIs), 107, 314
    generalized anxiety disorder (GAD) and, 117
    orgasmic disorder (OD) and, 320
    panic disorder and, 122
    posttraumatic stress disorder (PTSD) and, 130, 131
Self-management, 52
    definition of, 52
    efficacy of, 52
    model of care, 66
    primary care behavioral health (PCBH) model and, 52
    shared decision making and, 52
    strategies, 52
Self-monitoring, 92
    for motivational interventions, 66
Self-regulated behavior, 74
Semaglutide, 161
Sensate focus, 309–311
    orgasmic disorder (OD) and, 321, 325
Sensations and mindfulness exercises, 76
Serotonin and norepinephrine reuptake inhibitors (SNRIs), 107
    generalized anxiety disorder (GAD) and, 117
    posttraumatic stress disorder (PTSD) and, 131
Sertraline, 122, 130
Seven-step problem-solving model, 91
Sexual and physical abuse, 359
    chronic pelvic pain (CPP) and, 359
    posttraumatic stress disorder (PTSD) and, 361

Sexual dysfunctions
    chronic pelvic pain (CPP) and, 359–361
    description of, 301
Sexuality and older adults, 344–345
Sexual Problems and Self-Management Interventions handout, 310–311
SGLT2 inhibitors, 180
Shared decision making, 11, 63
    behavioral health consultants (BHCs) and, 11, 40
    follow-up appointments and, 63
    self-management and, 52
Shared medical appointments (SMAs), 441, 443–444. *See also* Cooperative health care clinic (CHCC); Drop-in group medical appointment (DIGMA); Physical shared medical appointment (PSMA)
    adaptations of, 452–454
    cultural considerations and, 453
    how they work, 443
    resources for, 454
    social considerations and, 453
Short-acting anticholinergics (SAMA), 201
Short-acting β2-agonists (SABA), 201
Short Blest Exam, 331
Short Portable Mental Status Exam, 331
Short Screening Instrument for Psychological Problems in Enuresis (SSIPPE), 385. *See also* Bed-wetting
Sibutramine, 161
SIGECAPS acronym (sleep, interest, guilt, energy, concentration, appetite, psychomotor agitation or retardation, suicidal ideation), 108
Sildenafil citrate, 302, 320
Single Alcohol Screening Question (SASQ), 275
Situational exposure, 127
Situational Exposure Hierarchy handout, 127–128
Sleep. *See also* Insomnia
    assessment of, 136–138
    diaries of, 136
    disturbances to, 364
    presleep behaviors, 138
    restrictions to, 142
    strategies for, 355
Sleep apnea, 139
Sleep hygiene, 65, 135, 136, 141, 142
Sleep, interest, guilt, energy, concentration, appetite, psychomotor agitation or retardation, suicidal ideation (SIGECAPS), 108
Sleep Restriction handout, 143
SMART (specific, measurable, achievable, relevant, and time-bound), 77–78
SMAs. *See* Shared medical appointments (SMAs)

Smoking. *See* Tobacco cessation; Tobacco use
  asthma and, 214
  chronic obstructive pulmonary disease
    (COPD) and, 201
Smoking and Substance Involvement
  Screening Test, 289
SNRIs. *See* Serotonin and norepinephrine
  reuptake inhibitors (SNRIs)
Social alienation and suicide, 422
Social anxiety and premature ejaculation
  (PE), 314
Social isolation and cardiovascular disease
  (CVD), 233
Social support and cardiovascular disease
  (CVD), 247–248
Socratic questioning for couple distress, 403
Somatic symptom disorder, 250
Sore throat, 213
Spanking, 381
Speaker–listener technique, 405
Specialty mental health care, 7
  asthma and, 215
  attention-deficit/hyperactivity disorder
    (ADHD) and, 390
  bed-wetting and, 383
  behavior management of children and
    adolescents and, 375–376
  cardiovascular disease (CVD), 234
  chronic obstructive pulmonary disease
    (COPD) and, 203–204
  chronic pelvic pain (CPP) and, 358
  couple distress and, 398–399
  definition of, 12
  depression and, 106–107
  diabetes and, 182–183
  erectile disorder (ED) and, 303–304
  generalized anxiety disorder (GAD) and,
    116
  insomnia and, 135–136
  menopause and, 365
  model, 7
  older adults and, 328
  orgasmic disorder (OD) and, 321
  overweight and obesity and, 157
  pain disorders and, 251
  panic disorder and, 122
  peripartum depression and, 351
  physical inactivity and, 169
  posttraumatic stress disorder (PTSD) and,
    130
  premature ejaculation (PE) and, 315
  suicide and, 424
  tobacco use and, 147–148
  unhealthy alcohol use and, 272
  unhealthy drug use and, 288
Specialty referrals, 40
Specific, measurable, achievable, relevant,
  and time-bound (SMART), 77–78

Spinal cord injury and orgasmic disorder
  (OD), 320
Sputum production, 200
Squeeze technique, 314
  goal of, 317
SSIPPE (Short Screening Instrument for
  Psychological Problems in Enuresis),
  385. *See also* Bed-wetting
SSRIs. *See* Selective serotonin reuptake
  inhibitors (SSRIs)
Statin therapy, 229
Staxyn, 302
Stendra, 302
Stepped-care approach, 109
Stimulants, 287
Stimulus control, 65, 94–95, 135, 141, 142
  advise phase, 95
  agree phase, 95
  arrange phase, 95
  assess phase, 94–95
  assist phase, 95
  holistic interventions and, 66
  insomnia and, 135, 142
  scripts and, 94–95
  worksheet, 97
Stop–start technique for premature
  ejaculation (PE), 314
  goal of, 317
Strategies to improve motivation to change
  form, 91
Strattera, 390
Strengths and Difficulties Questionnaire,
  378–379
Stress
  cardiovascular disease (CVD) and, 246
  diabetes and, 196
  incontinence and, 338
  irritable bowel syndrome (IBS) and, 269
Stress incontinence, 338
Stressors and hypertension, 232
Strokes, 227, 329
Study of Women's Health Across the Nation,
  364
Substance Abuse and Mental Health
  Services Administration-Health
  Resources and Services Administration,
  25
Substance Abuse and Mental Health Services
  Administration (SAMHSA), 271
  suicide rates, 419
Substance use disorder (SUD), 271
  diagnosis of, 289–290
  physician-prescribed opioids and, 266
  treatment for, 295–296
Sudden cardiac death, 227
Suffering vs. pain, 256
Suicide, 108
  adversarial confrontation and, 430
  advise phase, 430

Suicide (*continued*)
  age and, 423
  agree phase, 430
  anxiety and, 421
  apps, 438
  arrange phase, 437–439
  assess phase, 424–429
  assist phase, 430–437
  behavioral activation and, 436
  behavioral factors, 422–423
  behavioral health providers in primary
    care, 420
  brief contact interventions for, 435–436
  chronic illnesses associated with, 421
  chronic pain and, 421
  clinical question screening for, 426
  cognitive behavioral therapy (CBT) and,
    435
  cognitive factors, 421–422
  Columbia-Suicide Severity Rating Scale
    and, 427
  consultative model and, 420
  coping cards and, 436
  crisis response planning worksheet, 434
  cultural and diversity factors, 423–424
  dialectical behavior therapy and, 435
  emotional distress and, 421
  emotional factors, 421
  environmental factors, 423
  firearms and, 423
  four principles that guide care for suicidal
    patients in the primary care setting,
    420
  gender and, 423
  hotlines, 438
  inpatient treatment for, 437–438
  interventions for, 430, 435
  involuntarily hospitalization and, 437
  Joiner's interpersonal theory of, 422
  lesbian, gay, bisexual, transgender, and
    queer or questioning (LGBTQ) and,
    424
  low-risk monitoring and, 437
  maternal, 350
  mental disorder and, 435, 437
  mindfulness exercises and, 436
  multiple attempters, 422
  National Suicide Hotline, 439
  no-suicide contracts, 433
  older adults and, 327, 342
  P4 screener and, 427
  past attempts and, 422
  Patient Health Questionnaire-9 (PHQ-9)
    and, 427
  perceived burdensomeness and, 422
  physical factors, 421
  posttraumatic stress disorder (PTSD) and,
    421
  primary care adaptation, 424–439

  primary care provider (PCP) and, 420
  problem-solving therapy and, 435
  protective factors, 425
  race and, 423–424
  rates of, 419–420, 423–424
  reasons for living list and, 436
  recommended actions for levels of suicide
    risk, 431–432
  relaxation exercises and, 436
  resources for, 438–440
  risk assessment components, 429
  risk factors for, 422, 426
  risk levels, 431–432
  safety plan for, 433
  screening for, 425–429
  sense of low belongingness and, 422
  significant risk treatment and, 437–438
  social alienation and, 422
  specialty mental health, 424
  suicidal desire and ideation factors,
    421–422
  Suicide Crisis Hotline, 439
  survival kit/hope box and, 436
  trauma and, 421
  websites, 438
Suicide Crisis Hotline, 439
Sulfonylureas, 180
Summary statements, 56, 60–61
Support networks and chronic pain, 264
Surveys. *See also* Forms; Handouts;
    Questionnaires; Worksheets
  marketing survey, 33
  Provider Survey, 43
Survival kit/hope box, 436
Systematic desensitization and orgasmic
    disorder (OD), 321
Systolic blood pressure, 228

T

Tadalafil, 302
Tailoring, 8–9
Task Force on Clinical Practice Guidelines,
    228
Teamwork
  feedback and, 34
  informal leaders and, 36
Tegretol, 390
Telemedicine and diabetes, 183
Tenex, 390
Testosterone, 302, 320
  erectile disorder (ED) and, 302
  orgasmic disorder (OD) and, 320
Thiazolidinediones, 180
Threats, 381
Tic disorders, 392
Time-based pacing, 260
Time-outs, 380–381
Tirzepatide, 161

Tobacco cessation
  asthma and, 222
  chronic obstructive pulmonary disease
    (COPD) and, 199, 202, 204, 208
  counseling, 147
  handout, 151–152
Tobacco use, 19, 145–156
  advise phase, 150
  agree phase, 150–151
  arrange phase, 155–156
  assess phase, 148–150
  assist phase, 151–155
  aversive smoking, 153–154
  behavioral health in primary care, 148
  brand switching, 153, 154
  cardiovascular disease (CVD) and, 244
  Cochrane systematic review of, 147
  counseling and quit rates, 147
  cultural and diversity considerations, 146
  e-cigarette cessation interventions and,
    148
  5As model of, 148–156
  four As guide and, 154
  history of cessation attempts, 149
  interventions for, 147, 148
  maintaining cessation, 154–155
  motivational interviewing (MI) and, 147
  negative affect and, 155–156
  nicotine fading, 153
  nicotine replacements, 154
  nicotine replacement therapy (NRT) and,
    147
  nonnicotine medication and, 147
  pattern of use, 149
  pharmacological agents and, 147–148
  pharmacological therapies for, 148
  preparing to quit, 151–153
  prevalence of, 146
  primary care adaptation, 148–156
  quit plans and, 151
  quitting, 153–154
  readiness to change, 150
  relapse prevention plan, 155
  resources for, 156
  screening for, 148
  specialty mental health, 147–148
  tobacco cessation counseling and, 147
  tobacco cessation programs, 147
Tolterodine, 340
Tracking drinks, 281
Tranquilizers, 287
Trauma and suicide, 421
Treatment adherence
  behavioral self-analysis and, 92–94
  motivation enhancement techniques for,
    89–90
  problem solving and, 90–92
  self-monitoring and, 92

Treatment regimens
  communication and, 87
  complexity of, 86–87
  coordination and administration of, 87
  cultural and diversity considerations,
    87–88
  inaccurate beliefs and unrealistic
    expectations of, 87
  medication side effects of, 88
  motivational factors of, 88
  patient's understanding of, 87
Treatment regimens, enhancing motivation
    to change and adhere to, 86–94
  advise phase, 88–89
  agree phase, 89
  arrange phase, 94
  assess phase, 86–88
  assist phase, 89–94
  readiness to change ruler and, 86, 90
Trevor Project's 2022 National Survey on
    LGBTQ Youth's Mental Health, 424
Triple Aim, 3, 6, 20–21
  population health and, 20
  primary care behavioral health (PCBH)
    model and, 6
Triple P (Positive Parenting Program),
    375–376
2018 Physical Activity Guideline standards,
    168
Type 1 diabetes, 178. *See also* Diabetes
  causes of, 178
Type 2 diabetes, 178. *See also* Diabetes
  behavioral health consultants (BHCs)
    awareness of, 179
  depression and, 180
  emotional stress and elevated blood sugar,
    196

U

Understanding chronic pain handout, 257
Unhealthy alcohol use, 271–284, 289
  advise phase, 278, 279–281
  agree phase, 278–279
  alcohol use disorder diagnosis, 275–277
  arrange phase, 283
  assessment questions, 277
  assess phase, 274–277
  assist phase, 281–286
  awareness of consumption
    recommendations, 281
  behavioral health consultants (BHCs)
    and, 274
  brief interventions in the primary care
    setting for, 273
  cardiovascular disease (CVD) and,
    230–231, 246
  cultural and diversity considerations, 272
  drinking goals, 281

Unhealthy alcohol use (*continued*)
  harmful alcohol consumption, 272
  interventions for, 273
  pharmacotherapy for, 276–278
  prevalence of, 271
  primary care adaptation, 272–286
  primary care interventions and, 274
  reducing alcohol consumption, 282
  resources for, 285–286
  risky use, 272
  screening for, 273–275
  severity of, 277
  specialty mental health, 272
  specialty substance treatment and, 273
  stopping alcohol consumption, 283
  tracking drinks, 281
Unhealthy drug use, 287–299
  arrange phase, 296–298
  assess phase, 289–296
  assist phase, 298–299
  behavioral health consultants (BHCs)
    and, 297–299
  cultural and diversity considerations, 288
  definition of, 287
  factors associated with, 287
  interventions for, 288
  primary care adaptation, 288–299
  screening for, 289–296
  severity level, 289
  specialty mental health, 288
  substance use disorder diagnosis, 289–290
Unhealthy eating, 164
Unhealthy substance use. *See* Substance use
    disorder (SUD)
Unhealthy thinking
  common patterns of, 82
  how to question patients with, 79
University of Washington Health Promotion
    Research Center, 172
Urge incontinence, 338
U.S. Department of Defense (DoD), 252, 353
U.S. Department of Health and Human
    Services (DHHS), 145
U.S. Department of Veterans Affairs, 353
U.S. Department of Veterans Affairs and
    Department of Defense (VA/DoD), 130,
    199
U.S. Preventive Services Task Force
    (USPSTF), 106, 146, 235, 271, 330
  intimate partner violence (IPV) screening
    and, 400
  screening for depression
    recommendations, 342
  screening for peripartum depression
    recommendations, 351
  suicide screening and, 425
  unhealthy alcohol use screening, 274
  unhealthy drug use screening, 289

V

Vaginal dryness, 344, 364
Valium, 287
Valvular heart disease, 227–228
Vanderbilt Assessment Scale, 391
Vardenafil, 302
Varenicline tartrate, 147
Vasomotor symptoms, 363
  assessment and treatment of, 365–366
  hormonal changes and, 364
Vasopressin, 383
Venlafaxine, 117, 118, 122, 130
Veterans Health Administration, 6
Viagra, 302
Vicodin, 287
Violence
  couple distress and, 396
  safety plans and, 413
Vulvovaginal atrophy and orgasmic disorder
    (OD), 320
Vyvanse, 390

W

Warm handoff, 37
Weight
  cardiovascular disease (CVD) and, 244
  erectile disorder (ED) and, 312
Weight loss, 157. *See also* Overweight and
    obesity
  behavior change planning, 163–164
  Body Weight Planner and, 163
  calorie education and, 163
  C.A.M.E.S. approach, 164
  chronic obstructive pulmonary disease
    (COPD) and, 200
  counting calories and, 164
  diabetes and, 179
  distractions while eating and, 164
  eating rate and, 164
  goal setting and, 162–163
  heightened emotions and, 166
  medications for, 161
  motivational enhancement questions and,
    161
  personal food diary and, 163
  physical activity (exercise) and, 162, 166
  resources for, 167
  serving sizes and, 164
  strategies, 157, 160
  surgical interventions and, 167
  unhealthy eating and, 164
Weight maintenance, 166
  handout, 168
Weight Watchers, 160
Wellbutrin, 320, 390
What is a standard drink handout, 282
Woman Abuse Screening Tool, 401

Women's health clinics, 349
Worksheets. *See also* Forms; Handouts;
 Questionnaires; Surveys
 crisis response planning, 434
 monitoring behavioral triggers, 96
 problem solving, 92
 stimulus control plan, 97
World Health Organization (WHO),
 definition of primary care, 4
Worry log, 119
Worry Management handout, 121

X

Xanax, 287

XYZ* formula, 100

Z

Zarit Burden Interview (ZBI), 341

Zolpidem, 287

ABOUT THE AUTHORS

Christopher L. Hunter, PhD, ABPP, is board certified in clinical health psychology and codirects C & C Hunter Consulting. He has over 2 decades of experience developing and implementing integrated primary care behavioral health services in internal and family medicine clinics. He also has extensive experience training individuals to work in primary care and treat common mental health conditions, health behavior problems, and chronic medical conditions. He is a coauthor of the book *Integrating Behavioral Health Into the Medical Home: A Rapid Implementation Guide* (2016).

Jeffrey L. Goodie, PhD, ABPP, is a board-certified clinical health psychologist and a professor in the Department of Family Medicine, with a secondary appointment in the Department of Medical and Clinical Psychology, at the Uniformed Services University of the Health Sciences (USU) in Bethesda, Maryland. He currently serves as the deputy director of research in the family medicine department at USU. Dr. Goodie has extensive experience as a behavioral health consultant in family medicine, internal medicine, and obstetrics and gynecology clinics. His contributions extend to the training of psychology and social work residents and providers, focusing on delivering behavioral health interventions in integrated primary care settings. In addition to his work at USU, Dr. Goodie has held the position of president of the American Board of Clinical Health Psychology. He is a fellow of multiple organizations, including the American Psychological Association, the Society of Behavioral Medicine, and the Association of Behavioral and Cognitive Therapies.

Mark S. Oordt, PhD, ABPP, is a retired U.S. Air Force clinical health psychologist and a diplomate of the American Board of Professional Psychology in clinical health psychology. His specific professional interests include integrated behavioral health in primary care settings, assessment and treatment of suicidal risk, substance abuse prevention, and behavioral health care with military populations. He currently owns and operates a clinic providing rehabilitation services for individuals with neurological, vestibular, and orthopedic conditions.

Anne C. Dobmeyer, PhD, ABPP, is a clinical health psychologist who has been actively involved in implementation and training in integrated primary care for the past 2 decades. She has established fully integrated primary care behavioral health services in family medicine, internal medicine, and women's health clinics and provided training and consultation to clinics and medical centers across the country. Her publications and presentations primarily focus on training, implementation, and evaluation of integrated primary care programs. She has served as president of the American Board of Clinical Health Psychology and as a trustee of the American Board of Professional Psychology. She is the author of the book *Psychological Treatment of Medical Patients in Integrated Primary Care* (APA Books).